Novel Approaches for Drug Delivery

Raj K. Keservani
Rajiv Gandhi Proudyogiki Vishwavidyalaya, India

Anil K. Sharma
Delhi Institute of Pharmaceutical Sciences and Research, India

Rajesh Kumar Kesharwani
National Institute of Technology, Warangal, India

A volume in the Advances in Medical Technologies and Clinical Practice (AMTCP) Book Series

Medical Information Science Reference
An Imprint of IGI Global

Published in the United States of America by
Medical Information Science Reference (an imprint of IGI Global)
701 E. Chocolate Avenue
Hershey PA, USA 17033
Tel: 717-533-8845
Fax: 717-533-8661
E-mail: cust@igi-global.com
Web site: http://www.igi-global.com

Library of Congress Cataloging-in-Publication Data

Names: Keservani, Raj K., 1981- editor. | Sharma, Anil K., 1980- editor. | Kesharwani, Rajesh Kumar, 1978- editor.
Title: Novel approaches for drug delivery / Raj K. Keservani, Anil K. Sharma, and Rajesh Kumar Kesharwani, editors.
Description: Hershey, PA : Medical Information Science Reference, [2017] | Includes bibliographical references and index.
Identifiers: LCCN 2016017557| ISBN 9781522507512 (hardcover) | ISBN 9781522507529 (ebook)
Subjects: | MESH: Drug Delivery Systems
Classification: LCC RM301.25 | NLM QV 785 | DDC 615.1/9--dc23 LC record available at https://lccn.loc.gov/2016017557

This book is published in the IGI Global book series Advances in Medical Technologies and Clinical Practice (AMTCP) (ISSN: 2327-9354; eISSN: 2327-9370)

British Cataloguing in Publication Data
A Cataloguing in Publication record for this book is available from the British Library.

All work contributed to this book is new, previously-unpublished material. The views expressed in this book are those of the authors, but not necessarily of the publisher.

For electronic access to this publication, please contact: eresources@igi-global.com.

Advances in Medical Technologies and Clinical Practice (AMTCP) Book Series

Srikanta Patnaik
SOA University, India
Priti Das
S.C.B. Medical College, India

ISSN: 2327-9354
EISSN: 2327-9370

Mission

Medical technological innovation continues to provide avenues of research for faster and safer diagnosis and treatments for patients. Practitioners must stay up to date with these latest advancements to provide the best care for nursing and clinical practices.

The **Advances in Medical Technologies and Clinical Practice (AMTCP) Book Series** brings together the most recent research on the latest technology used in areas of nursing informatics, clinical technology, biomedicine, diagnostic technologies, and more. Researchers, students, and practitioners in this field will benefit from this fundamental coverage on the use of technology in clinical practices.

Coverage

- Nutrition
- Clinical Nutrition
- Telemedicine
- Patient-Centered Care
- Clinical High-Performance Computing
- Medical Imaging
- Biomedical Applications
- Diagnostic Technologies
- Clinical Data Mining
- Biomechanics

IGI Global is currently accepting manuscripts for publication within this series. To submit a proposal for a volume in this series, please contact our Acquisition Editors at Acquisitions@igi-global.com or visit: http://www.igi-global.com/publish/.

The Advances in Medical Technologies and Clinical Practice (AMTCP) Book Series (ISSN 2327-9354) is published by IGI Global, 701 E. Chocolate Avenue, Hershey, PA 17033-1240, USA, www.igi-global.com. This series is composed of titles available for purchase individually; each title is edited to be contextually exclusive from any other title within the series. For pricing and ordering information please visit http://www.igi-global.com/book-series/advances-medical-technologies-clinical-practice/73682. Postmaster: Send all address changes to above address.

Titles in this Series

For a list of additional titles in this series, please visit: www.igi-global.com

Emerging Research in the Analysis and Modeling of Gene Regulatory Networks
Ivan V. Ivanov (Texas A&M University, USA) Xiaoning Qian (Texas A&M University, USA) and Ranadip Pal (Texas Tech University, USA)
Medical Information Science Reference • copyright 2016 • 418pp • H/C (ISBN: 9781522503538) • US $195.00 (our price)

Applied Case Studies and Solutions in Molecular Docking-Based Drug Design
Siavoush Dastmalchi (Tabriz University of Medical Sciences, Iran) Maryam Hamzeh-Mivehroud (Tabriz University of Medical Sciences, Iran) and Babak Sokouti (Tabriz University of Medical Sciences, Iran)
Medical Information Science Reference • copyright 2016 • 367pp • H/C (ISBN: 9781522503620) • US $225.00 (our price)

Methods and Algorithms for Molecular Docking-Based Drug Design and Discovery
Siavoush Dastmalchi (Tabriz University of Medical Sciences, Iran) Maryam Hamzeh-Mivehroud (Tabriz University of Medical Sciences, Iran) and Babak Sokouti (Tabriz University of Medical Sciences, Iran)
Medical Information Science Reference • copyright 2016 • 456pp • H/C (ISBN: 9781522501152) • US $235.00 (our price)

Advancing Pharmaceutical Processes and Tools for Improved Health Outcomes
Tagelsir Mohamed Gasmelseid (International University of Africa, Sudan)
Medical Information Science Reference • copyright 2016 • 388pp • H/C (ISBN: 9781522502487) • US $185.00 (our price)

Classification and Clustering in Biomedical Signal Processing
Nilanjan Dey (Techno India College of Technology, India) and Amira Ashour (Tanta University, Egypt)
Medical Information Science Reference • copyright 2016 • 463pp • H/C (ISBN: 9781522501404) • US $225.00 (our price)

Virtual Reality Enhanced Robotic Systems for Disability Rehabilitation
Fei Hu (University of Alabama, USA) Jiang Lu (University of Houston -Clear Lake, USA) and Ting Zhang (University of Alabama, USA)
Medical Information Science Reference • copyright 2016 • 383pp • H/C (ISBN: 9781466697409) • US $210.00 (our price)

Editorial Advisory Board

Table of Contents

Detailed Table of Contents

Section 7
Liquid Crystals

Liquid crystalline system is a thermodynamically stable phase which is characterized by anisotropy. Liquid Crystals (LCs) are also termed as mesophase as they exhibit isotropic properties and liquid like behavior under some conditions (alter in temperature and concentration). Liquid crystals are influenced by number of parameters includes concentration, temperature, pH, and presence of salt. Liquid crystals are divided on the basis of shape of the molecules into two groups one is calmitic and other is discotic. A range of liquid crystalline phase (called mesophases) can be categorized by their sort of arrangement. The alignment of fragments in liquid crystalline phases is extensive on the molecular scale. Liquid crystal technology has a most important influence on several areas of pharmacy science and engineering, as well as device technology. As a novel type of drug delivery system, liquid crystals are explored and examined, definitely achieve mounting significance in industrial and scientific purposes.

Liquid crystals have been recently studied as novel drug delivery system. The reason behind this is their similarity to colloidal systems in living organisms. They have proven to be advantageous over Traditional, Dermal, Parentral and Oral Dosage forms. Liquid crystals are thermodynamically stable and possess long shelf life. Liquid crystals show bio adhesive properties and sustained release effects. Objective of this book chapter is to provide in-depth information of Pharmaceutical crystal technology. It shall deal with cubic and hexagonal liquid crystal and their applications in Drug delivery system.

Section 8
Dendrimers

Dendrimers are nanosized, monodisperse, highly branched polymers with well-defined topological structure which have attracted much attention for drug delivery recently. To further improve the performance of

Section 10
Nanotechnology

Nanofibers as a main group of nanoparticles have a vast range of applicability for therapeutic purposes, duo to their outstanding attributes such as very large surface to volume ratio and high porosity. These types of nanoparticles are more known as tissue scaffolds and drug delivery carriers. Nanofiber-based carriers are able to control the release pattern of drugs. In addition, they can act as multidrug-loaded materials with programed dual release profile. Electrospinning is a simple method, which is recognized as the most efficient approach for the fabrication of nanofibers. Production of ultrafine fibers based on various natural or synthetic polymers is possible by means of electrospinning. In this chapter, a comprehensive review is presented on various medical applications of electrospun nanofibers in the case of tissue engineering and drug delivery. Several investigations on therapeutic nanofibers and their processing methods are also summarized in this chapter.

Small colloidal particles having their diameter in the range of 50 to 500nm are defined as Nanoparticles. These are usually prepared either by using biodegradable or non-biodegradable polymers and are usually classified in two broad categories: (1) Nanocapsules: a type of reservoir system in which an oil or aqueous core is surrounded by a polymeric membrane. (2) Nanospheres: a type of matrix system. Preparation of nanoparticle as a drug delivery system is one of the most widely accepted approach since the prepration of nanoparticle were easy and convenient to scale up. Their high stability and conveniently easy to freeze-dried their preparations provide some additional advantages to choose Nanoparticles as a good drug delivery system. Inspite of them Nanoparticles were were able to achieve with success tissue targeting of many drugs (antibiotics, cytostatics, peptides and proteins, nucleic acids, etc.).

The most exciting advancement in the fields of biomaterial science is its ability to engineer new materials at the nanoscale level for various biological applications particularly drug and gene delivery for therapeutic applications. The main focus of this chapter is to review the therapeutic applications of different nanobiomaterials. Thus, it is proposed to discuss type of nanobiomaterials, general biological barriers for therapeutics, surface functionalization of nanobiomaterials and their therapeutics application in the present chapter. The therapeutic applications are explained on the basis of type of nanobiomaterials. The biocompatibility and toxicological response towards nanobiomaterials is an important issue that requires investigation for clinical development and their commercialization. The commercial prospects and future challenges in development of nanobiomaterials particularly for drug delivery are also discussed in the present chapter.

Foreword

The targeted drug delivery concept which has been predicted by Paul Ehrlich in 1891 has been not only successfully realized, but also achieved a tremendous advance in the research, development and implementation during the last decade, and is one of the frontiers based on the integrated multidisciplinary approach. The Drug Delivery Systems (DDS) which use variety of carriers, such as soluble polymers, nanoparticles, nanocapsules, lipoproteins, liposomes, micelles, cells ghosts, phytosomes, transfersomes, ethosomes, microspheres, emulsions, were timely developed in order to minimize drug degradation, to prevent side-effects, to increase drug bioavailability and drug targeting systems are currently under the development. The DDS, from drugs to therapeutic peptides, viral vectors, vaccines, gene therapy which were created for traditional oral and intravenous administration, have been expanded to transdermal, nasal, ocular, buccal, intramuscular, rectal, intrauterine, vaginal and pulmonary administration, ceramic implants, etc. The main factors in selection of the drug delivery route such as solubility, pH, ionization, concentration, particle size, temperature, crystallinity, molecular affinity, degree of absorption, state of hydration, resistance to an enzymatic and bacterial degradation, as well as drug biological interactions, distribution and ways of elimination, play crucial role in formulation, development and effective implementation of every type of the DDS.

Drugs delivery efficiency, targeting and safety concerns, solubility and cells microenvironment problems have created a huge demand for development of a new highly effective DDS. In order to be effective, the basic requirements for the DDS are: easy crossing biological barriers, maintaining concentrations of a drug in plasma over extended period of time, low cytotoxicity and ability to overcome host defence mechanism, reduction of the side-effects and dependency, bio-degradability, high absorption rate, physical and chemical stability, biocompatibility, guaranteed targeted and controlled drugs release in vivo based on molecular imprinting technology, reduced time of exposure at non-targeting tissues, ability to be mass-produced at the possibly low costs, reduced frequency of drug administrations per day which will improve patient compliance and overall wellbeing.

The amount of the Novel Drug Delivery Systems (NDDS) based on the achievements in pharmacodynamics, pharmacokinetics, bio-recognition, immunogenicity and nonspecific toxicity, as well as using modern advanced materials and progressive technologies has significantly increased during the past few years and will exponentially increase in the near future. The global market for drug delivery systems is expected to reach about \$175.6 billion by 2016, \$212.8 billion in 2018 and will continue to grow impressively. Novel carriers need to be designed out of a unique advanced material to enable the controlled release of active molecules, and new concepts of the NDDS formulation, development and applications need to be submitted for future publications.

The "Handbook of Research on Novel Approaches for Drug Delivery" which is an essential resource for anyone venturing into the area of drug development, is well written book based on the connection between pharmaceutical, biomedical and medical science. It is not only a comprehensive overview of various established and novel approaches to drug delivery systems and targeting, but it is also in depth discussion of a modern research and a critical analysis of the available information on NDDS and their numerous modern therapeutic and commercial applications. The handbook is not only containing available results and description for the NDDS, but also provide their comprehensive analysis and evaluation, integrate a variety of case studies, research results, existing and modern theories, but also summarize the diversity, method of preparation, efficiency, route of administration, biological activity and a variety of theoretical approaches. All the contributing authors demonstrate an exceptional expertise in the field of NDDS research and development, and provide a global perspective on current and future advances and discovery of new market opportunities.

Mila Emerald
Phytoceuticals International, Canada & Novotek Global Solutions, Canada

Preface

What really knocks me out is a book that, when you're all done reading it, you wish the author that wrote it was a terrific friend of yours and you could call him up on the phone whenever you felt like it. That doesn't happen much, though. – J.D. Salinger

This book i.e., Novel approaches for drug delivery systems was motivated by the desire we and others have had to further the evolution of the core course in Pharmaceutical Science. This book has novel aim for novel drug delivery system and covers maximum part of novel drug delivery systems to provide scattered information in gathered form under one roof. This book offers an overview of the therapeutic application of drug delivery strategies, liposomes, niosomes, pharmacosomes, transfersomes and pro-transfersomes, red blood cells (resealed erythrocytes), liquid crystals, dendrimers, polymeric system, nanotechnology, nanomedicine, biosimilars with special emphasis on their pharmaceutical applications in different disease which really helps authors and readers.

The content of these chapters is written by highly skilled, experienced and renowned scientists, researchers across all over the world with updated knowledge to provide drug delivery information to readers, researchers, academician, scientists and industrialists around the globe.

CHAPTER COMPOSITION

This book has 15 chapters and divided into 10 sections. Section 1 comprises of Chapter 1, "An Overview of Therapeutic Applications," structured by Sandeep Waghulde and Pravin Naik from India, provides an overview of therapeutic applications with great emphasis on drug delivery. The authors have also revealed that the drugs can improve the strength of pharmacological action and reduce the ill effect all over the body, for they release in the target organs. There has been an attempt to compile information concerned to variety of drug carriers encompassing target specific drug delivery systems. The adequate drug carriers are described in detail availing their pros and cons. The chapter also entails regarding safety profile of different polymers/ materials used. The chapter has provided a general description of several drug carriers with their possible applications in therapeutics.

Section 2 has two chapters, Chapter 2, "Liposomes: Properties and Therapeutic Applications," written by Ljiljana Djekic from Serbia, describes formulation methodologies, lipids employed in preparation and evaluation of liposomal vesicular drug delivery system. Further, the authors have strived to put together facts pertaining to progress in optimizing physicochemical features with emphasis on safety of this drug carrier. The vesicular carrier might be a viable substitute for traditional drug delivery system which sometimes lacks the specificity to deliver the drug at target site. Moreover, the lipids employed in preparations also enhance their acceptability by biological system as these are physiological lipids in chemical composition which is akin to natural ones. Chapter 3, "Liposomes: Concept and Therapeutic Applications," written by Mangal Shailesh Nagarsenker and Megha Sunil Marwah from India provides historical developments of liposomes concept and its therapeutic applications in drug delivery and have offered an overview of primary therapeutic and diagnostic applications and a brief insight into the in vivo behavior of liposomes. The authors have taken the scale up potential of liposomes during manufacturing into consideration. The feasibility assessment of scale may help in commercialization in effective fashion. Moreover, it may lower the cost of such products.

Section 3 contains Chapter 4, "Non-Ionic Surfactant Vesicles (Niosomes) as New Drug Delivery Systems," well written by Abbas Pardakhty from Iran about the non-ionic surfactant vesicles (niosomes) as new drug delivery systems with its various method of preparation and its application in the field of pharmaceutical science. This chapter presents a detailed discussion about niosomes forming components, methods of preparation and routes of administration. Many examples for drug delivery potential of niosomes are also available in this review. This drug carrier system could administer via injection, oral, pulmonary, vaginal, rectal, ophthalmic, nasal or transdermal routes with penetration enhancing potential. The topical drug delivery mediated by niosomes could bypass the side/adverse effects linked with oral drug application in case of several drugs.

Section 4 has Chapter 5, "Vesicular Drug Delivery Systems: A Special Emphasis on Pharmacosomes," structured by Preeti Khulbe from India gives significance of pharmacosomes in the field of drug delivery. This special carrier covalently binds with drug molecules thus, ensuring maximum drug encapsulation. This chapter includes the basic introduction, applications, methods of preparation, characterization, advantages, some research experiences and future prospects of pharmacosomes. These vesicular carriers are similar to others except for covalent binding with the drug molecules. The pharmacosomes are promising candidates for organ specific drug targeting.

Section 5 has only one chapter on transfersomes and protransfersome, Chapter 6, "Transfersomes and Protransfersomes: Ultradeformable Vesicular System," written by Bhusan Rajendra Rane and Nayan Ashok Gujarathi from India shared that vesicular system brings several possible advantages over conventional route of drug delivery system via this chapter. The deformability possessed by these vesicles is the highlight of this chapter which has conferred them the ability to traverse through gaps/pores present on bio-membranes. By virtue of this these vesicles can act as a carrier for wide variety of drugs.

In Section 6, Chapter 7, "Biosimilars: Concept and Regulation," written by Anil K. Sharma, Raj K. Keservani, and Rajesh K. Kesharwani, from India, describes biosimilar overview and introduces the fundamentals of biologics and to explain how they are different and what these differences mean for pharmacists. This chapter is an attempt to make its readers familiar about alternatives of synthetic drugs prevalent in the market in the form of biologicals as future drugs. The chapter has given a list of such products which are marketed recently. The global perspectives of such products are discussed with appropriate examples. Further, the regulations prevailing for these products in different countries have been described.

Section 7 has two chapters. Chapter 8, "Liquid Crystalline System: A Novel Approach in Drug Delivery," by Nayan Ashok Gujarathi, Bhushan Rajendra Rane, and Raj K. Keservani from India, has described applications of liquid crystal technology in several areas of pharmacy, science and engineering, as well as device technology. The chapter dealt with detailed discussion about liquid crystals, their morphology, preparation and evaluation of formulations in particular drug delivery science. Besides these other applications are also covered in present chapter. As a novel type of drug delivery system, liquid crystals are explored and examined, definitely achieve mounting significance in industrial and scientific purposes. The advent of liquid crystals has opened many avenues for variety of applications. These structures are able to carry both hydrophilic and hydrophobic molecules for therapeutic purposes. This feature has made them carriers of choice for topical drug delivery. Chapter 9, "Liquid Crystal Systems in Drug Delivery," written by Kamal Kumar Chaudhary, Pooja Kannojia and Nidhi Mishra from India provides in-depth information of pharmaceutical crystal technology. It deals with cubic and hexagonal liquid crystal and their applications in drug delivery system exclusively. The formulation and evaluation relevant to pharmacy has been covered exhaustively in present chapter. The applied aspect has been reinforced by adequate examples wherever necessary.

Section 8 dealt with Chapter 10, "Multifunctional Dendrimers for Drug Nanocarriers," by Tingbin Zhang, Chunqiu Zhang, Jinfeng Xing, Jing Xu, Chan Li, Paul C Wang, Ling Peng and Xing-jie Liang from China, describing dendrimers as drug nanocarriers and provide the ideas for designing the dendrimers based nanocarriers for controllable drug delivery and let more people know the development of dendrimers for drug delivery in recent years. The chapter has discussed genesis of dendrimers, synthesis schemes for different generations along with their testing for drug delivery ability. The enhanced permeation effect (EPR) exhibited by these nanocarriers in cancers is one of the most significant utility in the pharmaceutical field. The inherent structure of dendrimers provides space for hydrophobic as well as hydrophilic molecules thereby facilitating their delivery in single carrier. The sizes of magnitudes of nanometric range have enabled the entry of such carriers to interiors of the body artifacts. The surface of dendrimers may be designed to impart them acceptable biopharmaceutical characteristics.

Section 9 has two chapters. Chapter 11, "Smart Hydrogels for Pharmaceutical Applications," is by Snezana S Ilic-Stojanovic, Ljubisa B Nikolic, Vesna D Nikolic and Slobodan D. Petrovic from Serbia, well written and describes smart hydrogels with different physical and chemical properties, chemical structure and technology of obtaining, show great potential for application in the pharmaceutical industry. The application of smart hydrogels is very promising and at the beginning of the development and exploitation. The hydrogels being hydrophilic can absorb up to 50% of their original weight. Further, stimulus responsive hydrogels have added new dimensions to the attributes of hydrogels conferring them nomenclature of smart hydrogels. The stimulus may be pH, temperature etc. The drug effect is a function of behavior exhibited by hydrogels under the influence of certain stimuli. Based on this the drug delivery may be optimized. Chapter 12, "Rational Design of Polymeric Micelles for Cancer Therapy," is written by Yixian Huang, Jingjing Sun, Song Li from USA states that clinical application of anticancer drugs is limited by problems such as low water solubility, lack of tissue-specificity and toxicity. Formulation development represents an important approach to these problems. This book chapter provides a brief review of recent advancements in developing environmentally responsive micellar systems for controlled delivery of chemotherapeutic agents to tumor tissues. The emphasis is placed on the discussion of several dual functional nanomicellar systems that were recently developed in our laboratory as well as a new strategy of improving micellar formulations via incorporation of an interfacial drug-interactive motif(s). This is a known fact that micelles are responsible for improvement in solubility of drug molecules over their critical content. The retention of actives in tumor cells is of prime concern while developing a robust drug delivery strategy. The micelles because of the zwitterion nature may act to facilitate increased residence in tumor cells.

Section 10 has three chapters. Chapter 13, "Pharmaceutical and Medical Applications of Nanofibers," by Khosro Adibkia, Shadi Yaqoubi and Solmaz Maleki Dizaj from Iran deals with several investigations on therapeutic nanofibers and their processing methods are also summarized. Nanofibers as a main group of nanoparticles have a vast range of applicability for therapeutic purposes, duo to their outstanding attributes such as very large surface to volume ratio and high porosity. These types of nanoparticles are more known as tissue scaffolds and drug delivery carriers. Nanofiber-based carriers are able to control the release pattern of drugs. The utility of such fibers is discussed with suitable instances relevant to drug delivery. Chapter 14, "Application of Nanoparticles as a Drug Delivery System," by Vijay Kumar Singh and Raj K. Keservani from India demonstrates nanoparticles and its different approaches for the treatment of diseases. Preparation of nanoparticle as a drug delivery system is one of the most widely accepted approach since the preparation of nanoparticle were easy and convenient to scale up. Their high stability and conveniently easy to freeze-dried preparations provide some additional advantages to choose nanoparticles as a good drug delivery system. These nanostructures are capable of targeting to variety of tissues or organs. Chapter 15, "Therapeutic Applications of Nanobiomaterials," is written by Anuj Garg from India and summarized commercial prospects and future challenges in development of nanobiomaterials particularly for drug delivery. The chapter has discussed type of nanobiomaterials, general biological barriers for therapeutics, surface functionalization of nanobiomaterials and their therapeutic application. The nanobiomaterial encompasses natural ones as well as derived from synthesis. These are mostly able to control drug release and are devoid of toxicity.

This book presents recent technology and future prospective and different drug delivery in addition highlighted its pharmaceutical and medical application. The present endeavor does not boast that this has been one of its kinds but it enriches the pool of scientific information already present. We are quite hopeful that this particular compilation would receive the interest of its target audience. The editors are an email away to accept any suggestion, comment or critics. In last section book contains compilation of references, list of contributors and subject index.

Raj K. Keservani
Rajiv Gandhi Proudyogiki Vishwavidyalaya, India

Anil K. Sharma
Delhi Institute of Pharmaceutical Sciences and Research, India

Rajesh K. Kesharwani
National Institute of Technology, Warangal, India

Acknowledgment

We would like to acknowledge the people who were associated in long due project. Without their hearty support this book would not be completed.

We would like to thanks all the authors who spent their time, expertise, and sincere efforts to accomplish this book. We acknowledge our respected reviewers for their valuable contribution in improving the quality and presentation of the content. The authors also serve as referees; we greatly appreciated their dual role. Last but not the least we are also thankful to members of Editorial Advisory Board. We also express our Special thanks to Dr. Mila Emerald for writing the foreword.

It would be appropriate to mention that the IGI Global publishers have availed the scientific platform to us by exhibiting confidence and motivation to take this liaison in future too. Their publishing assistants deserve our thanks for extending support as and when desired.

During the Preparation of this book projects something happened very good and we started a new journey of life, Saritha a wife of Rajesh K. Kesharwani and Nidhi a wife of Raj K. Keservani received the gift of seeing the birth of sons Vihaan and Atharva respectively. Anil enjoyed life with his wife Ritu and girl Aashna. This book is dedicated to them.

Section 1
Introduction

Chapter 1
An Overview of Therapeutic Applications

Sandeep Waghulde
University of Mumbai, India

Pravin Naik
University of Mumbai, India

ABSTRACT

Over the last few years' great advances have been made on the development drug delivery systems for different purposes for targeting the diseased conditions. Novel drug delivery originates from polymers or associated with some devices is generally related with the emergence of novel characteristics. These changes are what eventually comprise the value of drug delivery system and Novel drug delivery system. Novel properties become existed without making new materials. Novel drug delivery system comparable to traditional system, following Targeted Drug Delivery System (TDDS) is also called targeting drug system. A new drug delivery system makes the drugs densely gather pathological-change structures, and has an improved healing effect and less toxic side effects. The drugs can improve the strength of pharmacological action and reduce the bad effect all over the body, for they release in the target organs.

INTRODUCTION

The method of treating infection and illness as we enter in next era twenty first century includes the subsequent forms of treatment a. surgery, b. psychotherapy, c. physical therapy, d. radiation and e. chemo or pharmacotherapy. The most commonly used is treatment method (Banker, Siepmann; Rhodes, 2002).

Novel drug delivery system whether it originates from polymers or associated with some devices is generally related with the emergence of novel characteristics. The most extensive results of their minute size, dosage form or targets are without distrust the change in their final properties. Next in significance are changes in other properties, both physical and chemical. These changes are what eventually comprise the value of drug delivery system and Novel drug delivery system. Novel properties become existed without making new materials.

DOI: 10.4018/978-1-5225-0751-2.ch001

Role of Targeted Drug Delivery System (TDDS)

Novel drug delivery system comparable to traditional system, following Targeted drug delivery system (TDDS) is also called targeting drug system'. A new drug delivery system makes the drugs densely gather pathological-change structures, and has an improved healing effect and less toxic side effects. The drugs can improve the strength of pharmacological action and reduce the bad effect all over the body, for they release in the target organs (Chaturvedi et al., 2011).

Carrier-mediated drug delivery has emerged as a powerful line of attack for the action of various pathologies. The therapeutic index of conventional and novel drugs is enhanced via the increase of specificity due to target of drugs to a particular tissue, cell or intracellular segment, the control over release kinetics, the protection of the active agent or a combination of the above. Nanoparticles (NPs) were proposed as drug carriers over 30 years ago and have received increasing attention since, mainly due to their stability, improved loading capabilities and control over physicochemical properties. The unique pathophysiology of solid tumors allows passive accrual of NPs at these sites upon intravenous injection. Furthermore, stealth NPs with long circulation times is better organized in reaching tumor tissue.

Drug activity is a result of molecular interaction(s) in certain cells; it is therefore easily deduced that it is essential for the drug to reach one way or another site of action following administration (oral, intravenous, local, transdermal, etc.) at sufficient concentrations. The systematic field dealing with this issue is known as drug delivery and has fundamentally the following aim: to deliver the drug at the exact place, at the right concentration for the right period. This is not possible by simply selecting a suitable administration route, or if such administration causes patient uneasiness, strategies based on the involvement of the drug with a carrier. Additional motivations for such approaches include the reduction of required resources for therapy, accomplished by an increase of the drug's therapeutic index and the prevention of frequent, unpleasant or expensive treatments.

Role of Drug Delivery System Other than TDDS

Drug delivery systems, ranging from implantable electronic devices to single polymer chains, are required to be well suited with processes in the body (biocompatibility) as well as with the drug to be delivered. DDS alter the biodistribution and pharmacokinetics of the associated drug: that is the time-dependent proportion of the administered dose in the different organs of the body. Furthermore, obstacles arising from little drug solubility, degradation (environmental or enzymatic), fast clearance rates, non-specific toxicity, in ability to cross biological barriers, just to mention a few, may be dealing by drug delivery system. Overall, the challenge of increasing the therapeutic outcome of drugs, with a simultaneous minimization of side effects, can be tackled from side to side-appropriate design and engineering of the DDS, in a case-to-case manner (Kelner, 2005; Mann et al, 2001; Pathak et al, 1992).

Even the most difficult part in all Drug delivery systems development actions, the accomplishment of release of the drugs, can be controlled suitably. This is true of both Drug delivery systems and novel drug delivery systems. Because of the extensive history of development, there has been profusion of time to develop perfect Drug delivery systems to novel one. One decisive finding opened up completely novel strategies for both traditional systems and Drug delivery systems the make use of polymers, frequently consisting of organic molecules. Such interesting molecules not only support the delivery systems by their kinetic and size-limiting function; they also make the drugs soluble in solvents, depending on the chemical character of the delivery systems.

Role of Novel Drug Delivery Systems (NDDS)

However, novel drug delivery systems have also had a notable revival after a hundred years' sleep. This is in particular true of delivery systems. Apart from leading to an increase in our information of delivery systems, these offer unimagined application possibilities. Although novel delivery systems are currently, being used in numerous industrial and medical applications, organized research into the novel delivery systems of drugs needs some attention.

It is apparent, for any variety of chemical approach, that dependence on the present-day pattern of information exchange in logic fundamentals or memory devices will entail defect-tolerant computer architectures with suitable, intellectual software. On the other hand, it may be promising to develop other routes which require more complex architectures and unlike principles of information exchange where the problems associated with idleness, current density, recital speed, and especially contact confrontation and charge redistribution at the lead-to-molecule interface are less relevant (Schmid, 2011).

Role of Novel Drug Delivery Systems with Its Different Application

Most of the anti hyperlipidimic drugs have reduced water solubility hence poor dissolution, which lead to reduced bioavailability. Therefore, when these drugs are given in predictable dosage forms they do not meet the therapeutic requirements therefore are given in large doses, which show the various side effects. Therefore, it is the essential to formulate that type of dosage form in which the drug shows better bioavailability and not as much of side effects (Farooq et al, 2013). Researchers are going on in this field and a variety of novel drug delivery systems are formulated and evaluated which have exposed the intensify the bioavailability of these drugs. Some of the novel drug delivery systems for antihyperlipimic drugs are:

1. **Self-Micro Emulsifying Drug Delivery System:** Self-emulsifying formulations enhance readily in the GI tract, and the digestive motility of the stomach and the intestine make available the agitation essential for self-emulsification. Lovastatin is inadequately soluble in gastric fluid when administered throughout predictable dosage forms like tablet, so SMEDDS are formulated to enhance the solubility of drug in gastric fluid and therefore improving the bioavailability by rising gastrointestinal absorption through passive diffusion. Fenofibrate is a (BCS) Class II drug with a high dose number. Thus, has little oral bioavailability due to its solubility and dissolution limits. An optimized SMEDDS formulation consisting of Labrafac CM10 (31.5% wt/wt), Tween 80 (47.3% wt/wt), PEG 400(12.7% wt/wt), and fenofibrate (8.5% wt/wt) has been developed with an improved dissolution rate, increased solubility therefore, improved bioavailability of a poorly water-soluble drug. Supersaturated drug delivery systems include the drug in a high-energy or rapidly dissolving form, which allows the solution to have drug concentrations higher than the solubility limit. (Cowan-Lincoln)
2. **Ternary Solid Dispersions:** Solid dispersions have been generally used to enhance the solubility, dissolution rate, and bioavailability of poorly soluble drugs. There are different types of solid dispersion systems categorized according to the physical states of the drug and the mover in the systems. It may be a molecular solid solution, a dispersion of amorphous or crystalline drug particles in an amorphous carrier matrix or an arrangement of a solution and distribution of solids. Fenofibrate compound is almost insoluble in water and has high lipophilicity. Therefore, the dissolution rate

of fenofibrate is likely to limit its absorption from the gastrointestinal tract. The solid dispersion of the fenofibrate was prepared by spray drying method using Poloxamer 188 as carrier and TPGS as surfactant shows highest solubility improvement of fenofibrate. Solid dispersion along with an adsorption method that employs a water-soluble adsorbent can be used to improve the dissolution of Ezetimibe, which may effect from the combined effect of hydrophilic carriers and improved surface area. Many drugs can be given in such form which will improve the efficiency of the drug. (Bhise, 2011; Parmar et al, 2011)

3. **Nano Suspension:** Nano suspensions not only increase the surface area but also at the same time enhance the saturation solubility and the solution velocity by raising the vapor pressure of the particles. Here the dissolution velocity slowly is improved due to decrease in the diffusional distance on the surface of drug nanoparticles. The saturation solubility gets affected through in situ generation of energies throughout alter of drug microcrystals to nanoparticles. Fenofibrate is a Nano suspension currently marketed in the name of Tricor. Nanosuspensionsmake use of some technique to decrease the particle size to the nano level which help to enhance the solubility of the drug suitable to small particle size. (Selvamuthukumar et al, 2012)
4. **Ion Exchange Resins:** Cholestyramine resin USP, when used as an active ingredient, binds bile acids; this leads to replacement of bile acids; through improved metabolism of serum cholesterol resultant in lowered serum cholesterol levels. Ion exchange resins no uncertainty are very effective in improving the bioavailability of the drugs but due to the use of some polymers it also enhances the charge of the delivery system. (Pande et al, 2011; Srikanth et al, 2010)
5. **Nanosponge Drug Delivery:** Nanosponges are a new class of materials and prepared of microscopic particles with few nanometers wide cavities, in which a huge variety of substances can be encapsulated. These particles are capable of carrying equally lipophilic and hydrophilic substances and of enhancing the solubility of poorly water-soluble molecules. This technology offers entrapment of ingredients and is supposed to decrease side effects by controlling the release, develop stability, enhance elegance and enhance formulation flexibility. These complexes can be also used to enhance the dissolution rate and solubility, to cover unpleasant flavors and to convert liquid substances to solids. By calculating the ratio of polymer to the cross-linker the particle size and release rate can be modulated. Nanosponges facilitate the insoluble drugs, protect the active moieties from physico-chemical degradation, and controlled release. Atorvastatin, Fenofibrate, Glibenclamide, Glipizide, Lovastatin can be formulated into nanosponges. Nanospongesdevelop the solubility of the drugs efficiently but the technology employed in this process is not cost effective as this technique utilizes some polymers which are costly in nature. (Sharma & Pathak, 2010)
6. **Nanoparticle Formulation:** Nanoparticulate drug delivery as the biological dimension of nano-technology has been developed, which may help generate useful formulations of OA for clinical applications. Nanoparticulate drug delivery system increases the dissolution rate and bioavailability of OA, providing a practical formulation method for clinical applications. (Chen et al, 2011)
7. **Mucoadhesive Microcapsules:** Simvastatin (SV) is a cholesterol-lowering agent that is resulting synthetically from a fermentation product of *Aspergillus terreus* and is widely used to treat hy-percholesterolemia. Microcapsules of Simvastatin were prepared by complexation with HPBCD and by this means including this complex in the polymeric matrix by make use of orifice gelation method resulted in more improved drug delivery. (Bal et al, 2012)
8. **Pulsatile Drug Delivery System:** Pulsatile Drug Delivery System is helpful in the diseases in which the drug release is timed to counterpart rhythms of the disease to optimize the beneficial

effect and reduce the side effects. Circadian rhythm occurs during hepatic cholesterol synthesis, which is higher during the night than daylight and diurnal synthesis represent upto 30-40% of daily cholesterol synthesis. The maximal production occurs in the morning. So there is a regular require for new delivery systems that can offer improved therapeutic benefits to the patients by delivering drug at the right time, right place & in right amounts to correspond with circadian rhythm of body. These dosage forms offer several advantages, such as almost stable plasma drug level without any fluctuations, decrease in dose of drug, decreased dosage frequency, least side effects, and enhanced patient compliance. Various systems like capsular system, osmotic system, and single multiple unit system based on the use of soluble or erodible polymer coating and use of repturable membrane. (Rajput et al., 2012; Rasve et al, 2011)

Ternary solid dispersion and ion exchange resins are the systems which improve the solubility of drugs largely and hence the bioavailability but it utilizes the variety of polymers which are costly in nature hence they may enhance the cost of the medication. Gastric floating drug delivery system is helpful in improving the solubility of those drugs, which are less soluble in acidic pH, and the drug waste is much more. This system is helpful in prolongs the gastric retention of the drugs and therefore increases the solubility of the drugs. While as pulsatile drug, delivery system is the system, which responds to the circadian rhythms of the body, and as a result, this system is very useful because cholesterol synthesis depends on circadian rhythms. SMEDD Scan is used to improve the solubility of the drugs by lessening the particle size in the emulsion base, which will efficiently enhance the bioavailability of the drug. Among all the systems above SMEDDS seems to be the most successful delivery system for antihyperlipidemic drugs because it is very easy to formulate and does not require any costly polymers, which make it effective in therapy as well as in cost. Many other novel drug delivery systems can be used to enhance the efficiency of these drugs.

Role of Novel Drug Delivery Systems in Cancer

Over the past several years, great advances have been made on expansion of novel drug delivery systems of anticancer drug (NDDS). The selection of novel formulations like polymeric nanoparticles, nanocapsules, liposomes, phytosomes, nanoemulsions, microsphere, hydrogels has been reported using bioactive and plant extracts. The novel formulations are reported to have extraordinary advantages over conventional formulations of anticancer, which include improvement of solubility, bioavailability, and protection from toxicity, improvement of pharmacological activity, improvement of stability, better tissue macrophages distribution, sustained delivery, and protection from physical and chemical degradation. (Kushwaha et al, 2012).

Role of Polymers in Drug Delivery Systems

Multiple synthetic and natural biodegradable polymers have been investigated for these purposes, with polyesters, polyether's, poly amino-acids, polysaccharides, and proteins (Medina et al, 2004). These polymers are employed as injectable drug delivery system, and especially as injectable drug delivery system for cancer chemotherapy, and have been investigate dynamically so as to reduce the toxic side effects and increase the carcinostatic pharmaceutical effects (Heller & Hoffman, 1996).

Methods of local administration of drug delivery system, nanoparticles (Barraud et al., 2005; Brannon-Peppas & Blanchette, 2012; Panyam & Labhasetwar, 2003), microspheres(Freiberg & Zhu, 2004; Kakinoki et al., 2003), polymeric micelles (Hrubý et al., 2005; Nishiyama et al, 2005; Rapoport et al, 2003), liposomes (Abraham et al., 2005; Goyal et al., 2005; Kaneda, 2000; Saul, et al., 2003), and hydrogel systems (H. He et al, 2004; Ruel-Gariepy & Leroux, 2004)for targeting and controlled release have been investigated with non-biodegradable polymers. However, the targeting drug delivery system has not been acceptably achieved. Accordingly, the injectable in situ formulating a drug delivery system with hydrogel system, that demonstrates a sol–gel transition in a physiological environment, has many uses (Packhaeuser et al, 2004). For example, water-soluble polymers with stimuli responsiveness have been widely used as injectable drug delivery system.

For the last few years, novel drug delivery systems have been investigated to conquer the control of the conventional systems. Cancer chemotherapy and DNA-based vaccines have been well known as special areas of need for improved drug delivery. Lipoproteins as drug delivery systems have turn out to be an attractive area of research and they are considered admirable candidates as novel drug delivery systems. Herbal drugs have massive therapeutic impending, which should be explored through some significance additional drug delivery systems. Lipid solubility and molecular size are the major restraining factors for drug molecules to pass the biological membrane to be absorbed systematically follows oral or topical administration. Several plant extracts and phytomolecules, despite having exceptional bioactivity in vitro show fewer or no in vivo actions due to their poor lipid solubility absorption and reduced bioavailability. Standardized plant extracts or mainly polar phytoconstituents like flavonoids, terpenoids, tannins, xanthones when administered through novel drug delivery system show much improved absorption profile, which enables them to cross the biological membrane, resulting enhanced bioavailability. Hence, extra amount of active constituent becomes present at the site of action (liver, brain, heart, kidney, etc.) at similar or less dose as compared to the conventional plant extract or phytomolecule. Therefore, the therapeutic action becomes improved, more detectable and prolonged. Several excellent phytoconstituents have been successfully delivered using NDDS. Hence, there is a great potential in the development of novel drug delivery systems for the plant actives and extracts.

Previously used for simple encapsulation of cells or drugs, in homogenous materials, today's hydrogels are new complex smart polymers with different types of ligands and cross-links allowing for highly regulated structures and different bio responsive functionalities. Hydrogels that undergo swelling changes in response to specific biomolecules have become ever more important because of their potential applications in the development of biomaterials and drug delivery systems and the biomedical applications of the hydrogels. We concentrate on the bio responsive hydrogels and sensors, also introduces the physical background of the special properties of stimuli-responsive hydrogels; use of the variety of transducers describing changes in physical properties of the hydrogels. It considers the opportunity of using artificial neural network models to identify model for swelling behavior as new techniques.

Molecular imprinting involves forming a pre-polymerization complex between the template molecule and functional monomers or functional oligomers (or polymers) (Lim & Sun, 1980) with detailed chemical structures interrelate with the template either by covalent (Wulff, 1995), non-covalent chemistry (Kirsch, et al, 2000). Formerly the pre-polymerization complex was formed, the polymerization reaction occurs in the presence of a cross linking monomer and an appropriate solvent which controls the overall polymer morphology and macro porous structure. Once the template is removed, the product is a hetero polymer matrix with specific known elements for the template molecule. It is explaining the upcoming field of molecular imprinting and designed molecular recognition (Takeuchi & Haginaka, 1999). The macromolecular architecture must be planned in a different way than more traditional dense network and must contain a spatially varying cross-linking density (micro and macro-porous regions). A density fluctuation in the polymer network generates regions or microgels of localized higher cross-linking, which contain an effective imprinting structure and suitable rigidity to produce enough specificity (areas or patches of recognition).

Hydrogel Applications (Kalshetti, et al, 2012)

1. Biological molecules can be covalently built-in into hydrogel structures.
2. Hydrogels has mechanical properties, which are highly elastic, and elasticity can be tailored by modifying cross-link densities.
3. Hydrogels provide appropriate semi wet and three-dimensional environments for molecular-level biological interactions.
4. Many hydrogels shows inert surfaces that prevent nonspecific adsorption of proteins, known as antifouling.
5. Hydrogels can be designed to alter properties due to externally useful factors, such as temperature, ionic strength, solvent polarity, electric /magnetic field, light, or small biomolecules.

The objective of every drug delivery system is to give a therapeutic amount of drug to the proper target site in the body and then maintain the desired drug concentration. A well-designed controlled drug delivery system can overcome some of harms of conservative therapy and improve therapeutic efficacy of the given drug. There are various approaches in delivering therapeutic substance to the target site in sustained and controlled release fashion. One such approach is using microspheres as carriers for drug. Microspheres are characteristically free flowing powders consisting of proteins or synthetic polymers, which are biodegradable in nature ideally, have particle size less than 200μm.Various synthetic and natural materials are used for the preparation of microspheres. These are prepared by techniques like Single emulsion, Double emulsion, Polymerization, Phase separation co acervation, Emulsion solvent evaporation and solvent diffusion. Microspheres are having wide range of applications because of controlled and sustained release. Most important use is that it is used for targeting tumours usinganti cancer drugs. It is important carrier for safe and effective in vivo drug delivery (see Table 1). (Kotta et al., 2012; J. Silva et al., 2014; Thiagarajan, 2011)

Role of Microencapsulation in NDDS

Microencapsulation is used to alter and delayed drug release of pharmaceutical dosage forms. A well-planned controlled drug delivery system can overcome the problems of traditional therapy and improves the therapeutic efficacy of a drug. It is the dependable way to deliver the drug to the target site with specificity, if modified, and to retain the desired concentration at the site of interest without untoward effects. Microspheres received much attention not only for extended release, but also for targeting of anticancer drugs to the tumor. The objective is to draw attention to the potential of microencapsulation technique as a vital method in novel drug delivery. Polymerization is a relatively new microencapsulation technique utilizes polymerization technique to from protective microcapsule coatings in situ. The methods involve the reaction of monomeric units located at the interface existing between a core material substance and a continuous phase in which the core material is dispersed. The continuous or core

Table 1. Microsphere applications

Type of Microspheres	Applications
Bio-adhesive microspheres	Buccal, oral, ocular, nasal, colonic drug delivery Nasal - Gentamicin, Insulin (Farraj et al.,1990), GI –Glipizide (Kyyrönen et al., 1992) Colonic – Insulin (Geary & Schlameus, 1993), Ocular - Methyl prednisolone (J. Patel et al., 2004)
Magnetic microspheres	Used in DNA analysis, cell isolation, protein purification and targeting drugs to tumour sites(Doxorubicin) (Pawan& Hemchand, 2009)
Floating microspheres	Carriers for drugs like antiviral, antifungal and antibiotic agents (so called absorption windows), non-steroidal anti-inflammatory drugs, Prednisolone, Lansoprazole (Garima Chawla et al., 2013; Shirwaikar et al., 2006)
Radioactive microspheres	For diagnostic purpose - Diagnostic radio embolization: 99mTc-macroaggregated human serum albumin (MAA) (Ercan, 1992), Thrombus imaging in deep vein thrombosis: 99mTc-sulfur colloid (Knight, 1986) For therapeutic purpose – Radio embolization of liver and spleen tumours: 90Ymicrospheres, Local radiotherapy: 212Pb-sulfur colloid (Russell et al., 1988).
Polymeric microspheres Vaccine delivery:	Hepatitis, Influenza, Pertussis, Diphtheria toxoid (Haefeli et al., 1992), Oral drug delivery of easily degraded drugs: Gene therapy with DNA plasmids; delivery of insulin, LHRH Controlled drug delivery after local application: Release of proteins, hormones and peptides over extended times

Prasanth, et al., 2011; Ramteke et al., 2012.

material supporting phase is usually a liquid or gas, and therefore the polymerization reaction occurs at a liquid-liquid, liquid-gas, solid-liquid, or solid-gas interface (Venkatesan et al., 2009). Microspheres are typically free flowing powders consisting of synthetic polymers which are biodegradable in nature and ideally having particle size less than 200 μM (N. Jain, 2002). There are many reasons why drugs and related chemicals have been microencapsulated (N. K. Jain, 1997; Lachman et al., 1986).

The technology has been used widely in design and proposes of controlled release and sustained release dosage forms.

1. To mask the bitter taste of drugs like Paracetamol, Nitrofurantoin, etc.
2. Many drugs have been microencapsulated to reduce gastric and other G.I. tract irritations. Sustained release Aspirin preparations have been reported to cause significantly less G.I. bleeding than conventional preparations.
3. A liquid can be converted to a pseudo-solid for easy handling and storage. e.g. Eprazinone.
4. Hygroscopic properties of core materials may be reduced by microencapsulation e.g. Sodium chloride.
5. Carbon tetra chlorides and a number of other substances have been microencapsulated to reduce their odor and volatility.
6. Microencapsulation has been employed to provide protection to the core materials against atmospheric effects, e.g. Vit. A. Palmitate.
7. Separation of irreconcilable substance has been achieved by encapsulation.

Role of Nanoemulsions in NDDS

Nanoemulsions are novel drug delivery systems containing emulsified oil and water systems with mean droplet diameters ranging from 50 to 1000 nm. Usually, droplet size is between 100 and 500 nm and can exist as oil-in-water (o/w) or water-in-oil (w/o) form, where the core of the particle is either oil or water, respectively. Nanoemulsions are made from pharmaceutical surfactants that are generally regarded as safe (GRAS) (Chime et al., 2014).

The major advantages of nanoemulsions as drug delivery carriers comprises of increased drug loading, improved drug solubility and bioavailability, reduced patient variability, controlled drug release, and protection from enzymatic degradation (Kotta et al., 2012). A range of novel strategies are currently being developed for capable delivery of poorly water-soluble drugs, such as the formulation of amorphous solid form, nanoparticles, microemulsions, solid dispersions, melt extrusion, salt formation and formation of water-soluble complexes. Among all, the most accepted approach is the lipid-based formulation approach (Dixit & Nagarsenker, 2008; Shafiq et al., 2007).

Recently importance of nanoemulsions have become increasing as good vehicles for the controlled delivery of cosmetics and for the optimized dispersion of active ingredients in particular skin layers. Nanoemulsions are suitable in cosmetics because there is no chance of creaming, sedimentation, flocculation or coalescence, which is observed within microemulsions. The incorporation of potentially nauseating surfactants can be avoided by using high-energy equipment during manufacturing process. PEG free nanoemulsions for cosmetics have also been developed and formulations shown good stability (Chime et al., 2014; Lovelyn & Attama, 2011; Thiagarajan, 2011).

A characteristic of the nanoemulsions is their highly selective toxicity to microbes at concentration range that are non-irritating to skin or mucous membrane. The safety range of nanoemulsions is because of the minute amount of detergent in each droplet, so far when acting in concert; these droplets have enough energy and surfactant to destabilize targeted microbes without affect healthy cells. Nanoemulsions can get a level of current antimicrobial activity, which can only be formerly achieved by systemic antibiotics.

The US Army (RestOps) checked the broad-spectrum nanoemulsions on surfaces in Dec 1999 for decontamination of Anthrax spore. It was checked again by RestOps in March 2001 as a chemical decontamination agent. This tool has been tested on gangrene and clostridium botulism spores, and can even be used on infected wounds to salvage limbs. The first applications as vaccine, an influenza vaccine and an HIV vaccine, can proceed to clinical trials. The nanoemulsion causes proteins useful to the mucosal surface to be adjuvant and it help uptake by antigen presenting cells. This results in the significant systemic and mucosal immune response due to that the production of specific IgG and IgA antibody as well as cellular immunity. Research has been ongoing to complete the evidence of concept in animal trials for other vaccines including Anthrax and Hepatitis B. The University of Michigan has licensed this technology to NanoBio (Chime et al., 2014).

Another interesting application, which is experiencing an active development, is the use of nanoemulsion formulations, for controlled drug delivery and targeting (Wang et al., 2007). The development of magnetic nanoemulsions is an innovative approach for cancer therapy. These can transport photosensitizers as ifFoscan® to deep tissue layers crossways the skin thereby inducing hyperthermia for subsequent free radical generation. This method can be used for the treatment of cancer in the type of photodynamic therapy (Primo et al., 2007).

Among the possible delivery systems, the use of nano based carriers hold a great promise to protect the biomolecules, promote nanocarrier interface with mucosa and to direct antigen to the lymphoid tissues. As a result, the use of nanoemulsions in intranasal drug delivery system is set to transport about important results in targeting drugs to the brain in treatment of diseases correlated to the central nervous system (Clark et al., 2001). Major clinical and pre-clinical trials have therefore been carried out with parenteral nanoemulsion based carriers. The advances in these novel drug delivery systems have been reviewed by Patel and Patel (R. Patel & Patel, 2010). Nanoemulsions overloaded with thalidomide have been synthesized where a dose as low as 25mg leads to plasma concentrations which can be therapeutic (Araújo et al., 2011). However, a significant reduce in the drug substance of the nanoemulsion was observed at 0.01% drug formulation after two months' storage which could be overcome by the addition of polysorbate 80. Chlorambucil, a lipophilic anticancer agent has been used against breast and ovarian cancer. Lipid formulations are used to treat cardiovascular diseases since they accrue in the walls of injured vessels, transporting the drug to the place of vascular injury and to protect it from rapid inactivation by the lungs (Hoshi, 1996; Igarashi et al., 2001; Momma, 1996; Scheffler et al., 1996). Nanoemulsions are proposed for numerous applications in pharmaceuticals as drug delivery systems because of their ability to solubilize non-polar active compounds. Future perspectives of nanoemulsion are very hopeful in diverse fields of therapeutics or application in development of cosmetics for hair or skin. One of the versatile applications of nanoemulsions is in the part of drug delivery where they act as efficient carriers for bioactive, facilitating administration by various routes.

Role of Microbubbles in NDDS

Ultrasound-mediated microbubbles destruction has been planned as a novel method for noninvasive delivering of drugs and genes to different tissues. Microbubbles are used to carry a drug or gene until a specific area of importance is reached, and then ultrasound is used to burst the microbubbles, causing site-specific delivery of the bioactive materials. In addition, the capacity of albumin-coated microbubbles to adhere to vascular regions with glycocalix damage or endothelial dysfunction is another probable mechanism to deliver drugs even in the absence of ultrasound. Microbubbles that give those therapeutic properties and some important aspects of ultrasound parameters that are known to control microbubble-mediated drug delivery (Majumdar & Chowdhury, 2010).

In addition, current studies relating this novel therapeutic use of microbubbles (Majumdar & Chowdhury, 2010; Tsutsui, Xie, & Porter, 2004) have shown that microbubbles targeted to AlphaV, BetaIII can be used to measure the temporal expression of this integrin in association with angiogenesis. A contrast agent targeted to endothelial- based markers of angiogenesis might be used to develop diagnosis and treatment of disorders affected by angiogenesis. Other endothelialbased targets such as P-selectin might be shown to develop targeted imaging agents for detecting inflammation. Vulnerable plaques are those that have been infiltrated by macrophages, and are undergoing inflammation (Majumdar & Chowdhury, 2010). Inflammation can show the way to rupture of vulnerable plaque and formation of thrombus, as in stroke and myocardial infarct. Vulnerable plaques may lie unknown as unseen threats, liable to cause morbidity and sudden death.

Microbubbles accelerate the rate of SonoLysis. Improvement is greater for the targeted molecular ultrasound contrast agent, MRX-408, than for the non-targeted agent. Hynynen has shown (O'Reilly & Hynynen, 2012) that intravenous doses of microbubbles and transcranial function of ultrasound can be used to reversibly open the blood brain barrier. Laser-induced bubble formation around nanoparticles may play a crucial role in selective laser nanophoto thermolysis of cancer cells targeted with nanoparticles. Progress in cardiovascular gene therapy has been vulnerable by concerns over the safety and practicality of viral vectors and the ineffectiveness of current nonviral transfection techniques. Ultrasound exposure (USE) enhances transgene expression in vascular cells by up to 10-fold after naked DNA transfection, and enhances lipofection by up to three-fold. The presence of gas in the gene-filled microbubble allows ultrasound energy to "pop" the bubble. An energetic wave is then created which allows the genetic material to enter surrounding cells (Lawrie et al., 2000).

Microbubbles are presently used clinically as contrast agents in ultrasound (US) diagnostics and experimentally as drug or nucleic acid carriers. The protective blood-brain barrier blocks many drugs from acting on brain cells. Now, a new technique for delivering drugs directly to the affected area may enhance the effectiveness of chemotherapy in brain tumors and reduce its toxic effect on healthy cells. Researchers at the University of California are developing a novel technique that uses ultrasound and drug-laden "microbubbles" to deliver concentrated chemotherapy drugs to the inner lining of blood vessels. Doctors already use ultrasound to recognize tumors and leads to biopsy procedures. Ultrasound pulse sequences can also guide micro-packaged medications to specific parts of the body (Shortencarier et al., 2004).

The purpose of nanotechnology in the field of health care has come under great attention in recent times. There are many treatments today that take a lot of time and are also very costly. Using nanotechnology, quicker and much cheaper treatments can be developed. By performing further research on this technology, cures can be found for diseases that have no cure today. We could make surgical instruments of such accuracy and precision that they could operate on the cells and even molecules from which we are made - something well beyond today's medical technology. (Bhowmik et al., 2009)

Role of Vesicular Systems in NDDS

Novel drug delivery attempts to either sustain drug action at a fixed rate, or by maintaining a relatively constant, effective drug level in the body with related minimization of undesirable side effects. The vesicular systems are highly ordered assemblies of one or several concentric lipid bilayers formed, when certain amphiphillic building blocks are confronted with water. The vesicular system such as liposomes, niosomes, sphingosomes, ethosomes, transferosomes and pharmacosomesare used to develop the therapeutic index of both existing and new drug molecules by encapsulating an active medicament inside vesicular structure in one such system. It prolongs the existence of the drug in systemic circulation and finally reduces the toxicity. Such different systems are widely used in gene delivery, tumor targeting, oral formulations, in stability and permeability problems of drugs. Now a day's vesicle as a carrier system have become the vehicle of choice in drug delivery and lipid vesicles were found to be of value in immunology, membrane biology and diagnostic technique and most recently in genetic engineering (Jadhav, et al., 2012).

Different types of pharmaceutical carriers such as particulate, polymeric, macromolecular and cellular are present. Particulate type carrier also known as colloidal carrier system, includes lipid particles (low and high density lipoprotein-LDL and HDL, respectively), microspheres, nanoparticles, polymeric micelles and vesicular like liposomes, sphingosome, niosomes, transferosomes, pharmacosomes, virosomes (Sezaki & Hashida, 1985).

The cells of RES preferentially take up the vesicles. The uptake of niosomes by the cells is also by circulating serum factors known as opsonins, which mark them for approval. Such limited to a small area drug accumulation has, however, been exploited in treatment of animal tumors known to metastasize to the liver and spleen and in parasitic infestation of liver (Malhotra & Jain, 1994).

Niosomeshave been used for studying the nature of the immune response provoked by antigens. Brewer and Alexanderhave reported niosomes as potent adjuvant in terms of immunological selectivity, small toxicity and stability (Brewer & Alexander, 1992).

Transferosomes improve the site specificity, overall drug safety and lesser the doses quite a lot of times than the currently available formulations for the treatment of skin diseases. Because of their excellent penetration power and flexibility, transferosomes formulations are used for useful delivery of non-steroidal anti-inflammatory agents like ibuprofen and diclofenac. Transferosomes not only enhance the penetration of diclofenac through intact skin, but also transfer these agents directly into the depth of the soft tissues under the application site (Cevc, 1996).

Ethosomes have high penetration rate through the skin as compared to liposomes therefore these can be used commonly in place of liposomes. Although, the exact mechanism for better penetration into deeper skin layers from ethosomes is still not clear. The synergistic effects of combination of phospholipids and high concentration of ethanol in vesicular formulations have been recommended to be responsible for deeper distribution and penetration in the skin lipid bilayers. The size range of ethosomes may differ from tens of nanometers to microns (Dayan & Touitou, 2000; S. Patel, 2007). Ethosomesare mainly used as replacement of liposomes mainly for the transdermal route of drug delivery.

Sphingosomes solve the major disadvantage of vesicle system (liposomes) like less stability, less in vivo circulation time, low tumor loading efficiency in case of cancer therapy. Sphingosomes are clinically used delivery system for chemotherapeutic agent, biological macromolecule and diagnostics. Due to flexibility in size and composition, different types of sphingosomes have been developed (Saraf, Gupta, Kaur, & Saraf, 2011). Sphingosomal products such as Marqibo(TM) (sphingosomal vincristine) are loaded with active, cell cycle-specific anticancer agents that may help from increased targeting and longtime drug exposure at the tumor site. Vincristine, vinorelbine and topotecan are approved cancer therapies which have been chosen for sphingosomal formulation specifically for their ability to help from this novel encapsulation.

Pharmacosomes are the colloidal dispersions of drugs covalently bound to lipids and may be present as ultrafine vesicular, micellar or hexagonal aggregates, depending on the chemical structure of the drug–lipid complex (Semalty, Semalty, Rawat, Singh, & Rawat, 2009). Because the system is formed by involving a drug (pharmakon) to a carrier (soma), they are called pharmacosomes. Any drug possessing a free carboxyl group or an active hydrogen atom (–OH, NH2) can be esterified (with or without a spacer group) to the hydroxyl group of a lipid molecule, thus generating an amphiphilic prodrug, which will facilitate membrane, tissue, or cell wall transport, in the organism. Any drug with a definite cut-off molecular weight may be formulated as pharmacosomes provided it has active functional groups to integrate with the vesicle-forming amphiphilic molecule.

Various amphipathic liponucleotideprodrugs, 1-β-D-arabinofuranosylcytosine 5'-Diacylglycerols (Ryu et al., 1982) (containing either dimyristoyl, dipalmitoyldistearoyl free fatty acid side chains) and determined the aggregational and morphological character of their sonicated dispersions in relation to alter in temperature. The sonication at low temperature gave turbid solutions containing big bilayer sheets. On increasing the temperature, a transition temperature (tg) was reached at which a stable three dimensional cross-linked network of small interlocking bilayer stacks was formed. Sonication at the temperature close up to tg produced small disc-shaped micellar structures. These micelles were shown to be present in another aggregational equilibrium consisting of stacking-destacking process. In contrast, the prodrug containing unsaturated fatty acid chain gave multilamellar liposomes. Improved biological activity after incorporation of drug into pharmacosomes was found in case of Taxol and Cytarabin.

Role of Nanocarriers in NDDS

Nanocarriers with optimized physicochemical and biological properties are in use up by cells more easily than larger molecules, so they can be effectively used as delivery tools for currently existing bioactive compounds (Suri, Fenniri, & Singh, 2007). It is usually accepted that nanoparticles with a hydrodynamic diameter of 10–100 nm have best possible pharmacokinetic properties for *in vivo* applications. Smaller nanoparticlesare subjects to tissue extravasations and renalclearance whereas larger are rapidly opsonized and removed from the bloodstream *via* the macrophages of the reticuloendothelial system (Cole et al., 2011).

Once the drug-nanocarrier conjugates reach the diseased tissues, the therapeutic agents are released. A controlled release of drugs from nanocarriers can be achieved during changes in physiological environment such as temperature, pH, osmolality, or *via* an enzymatic activity. Nanocarriers used for medical applications have to be biocompatible (able to integrate with a biological system without eliciting immune response or any negative effects) and nontoxic (harmless to a given biological system) (Wilczewska et al., 2012).

SLN (solid lipid nanoparticles), NLC (nanostructured lipid carriers) and LDC (lipid drug conjugates) are types of carrier systems based on solid lipid matrix, i.e., lipids solid at the body temperature (Wissing et al., 2004). They have been exploited for the dermal (Abdel-Mottaleb et al., 2011), peroral (Muchow et al., 2008), parenteral (Nayak et al., 2010), ocular (Attama et al., 2007), pulmonary (Liu et al., 2008), and rectal (Sznitowska et al., 2001) delivery.

The application of biodegradable nanosystems for the development of nanomedicines is one of the most successful ideas. Nanocarriers composed of biodegradable polymers undergoes hydrolysis in the body, produces biodegradable metabolite monomers, such as lactic acid and glycolic acid. Kumari et al. (Kumari et al., 2010) reported a minimal systemic toxicity related with using of PLGA for drug delivery or biomaterial applications. Such nanoparticles are biocompatible with tissue and cells (Panyam & Labhasetwar, 2003). Drug-biodegradable polymeric nanocarrier conjugates used for drug delivery are stable in blood, non-toxic, and non-thrombogenic. They are also non-immunogenic as well as non-pro inflammatory, and they neither activate neutrophils nor affect reticuloendothelial system (des Rieux et al. 2006).

Silica materials used in controlled drug delivery systems are classified as xerogels (Czarnobaj, 2008) and mesoporous silica nanoparticles (MSNs), e.g., MCM-41 (Mobil Composition of Matter) and SBA-15 (Santa Barbara University mesoporous silica material) (Wei, Hu, & Zhang, 2010). They exhibit several advantages as carrier systems, including biocompatibility, highly porous framework and an ease in terms of functionalization (Amato, 2010). Among inorganic nanoparticles, silica materials are the carriers which most often are chosen for biological purposes (Slowing, Trewyn, Giri, & Lin, 2007). Xerogels used in controlled drug release (Quintanar-Guerrero et al., 2009). Phenytoin (Fidalgo et al., 2009), doxorubicin (Prokopowicz et al., 2010), cisplatin (Katarzyna et al., 2007), metronidazole (Katarzyna et al., 2012), nifedipine (Maver et al., 2007), diclofenac (Katarzyna Czarnobaj & Czarnobaj, 2008), and heparin (Ahola et al., 2001) are examples of drugs which have been loaded into xerogels using this technique.

The best known types of mesoporous silica nanomaterials are MCM-41 with a hexagonal arrangement of the mesopores and SBA-15 with a well-ordered hexagonal connected system of pores. The MSNs, in comparison with xerogels, possess more homogenous structure, lower polydispersity and higher surface area for adsorption of therapeutic or diagnostic agents (Di Pasqua et al., 2009). The mechanism of drug loading into mesoporous silica material is a chemical or physical adsorption. By these processes, diverse types of drugs, including anticancer drugs (Q. He et al., 2011), antibiotics (Li et al., 2010), and heart disease drugs (Popovici et al., 2011) have been embedded into MNSs.

Carbon nanocarriers used in DDS are differentiated into nanotubes (CNTs) and nanohorns (CNH). CNTs are characterized by unique architecture formed by rolling of single (SWNCTs – single walled carbon nanotubes) or multi (MWCNTs – multi walled carbon nanotubes) layers of graphite with an enormous surface area and an excellent electronic and thermal conductivity (Beg et al., 2011). Drug release from carbon nanotubes can be electrically or chemically controlled. To prevent the unwanted release of the drug, the open ends of CNTs were sealed with polypyrrole (PPy) films [129]. Homing devices, i.e., folic acid [130] and epidermal growth factor (Bhirde et al., 2009), were attached to improve selectivity of such drug delivery systems. Newer studies have pointed out the similarity in carcinogenic potential between CNT and asbestos. (Poland et al., 2008). Carbon nanotubes have been shown to cause necrosis or apoptosis of macrophage cell lines and changes in cell morphology (Jia et al., 2005). Radomski et al. (Radomski et al., 2005) studied the effects of engineered carbon nanoparticles (MWCNT and SWCNT) on human platelet aggregation *in vitro* and rat vascular thrombosis *in vivo*. Incubation of platelets with carbon nanomaterials caused platelet aggregation with little or no granular release.

Therapeutic activity of diverse drugs incorporated into iron oxide nanocarriers have been tested and reported. Magneic Nano Particals have been examined for multitasking treatment as biosensors (diagnosis) and drug carriers (therapy) simultaneously. Concomitant use of magnetic resonance or magnetofluorescent imaging and targeted therapy (*via* conjugation of targeting moieties) can enhance effectiveness of cancer therapy (Chomoucka et al., 2010). Magnetic nanoparticles promote activation of phagocytotic and cytokine-release functions of macrophages (Dobrovolskaia& McNeil, 2007). Gas vesicles were observed in MNPs treated cells with increased granularity of the cells (Mahmoudi et al., 2010). Magnetite nanoparticles have the potency of causing oxidative DNA lesions in cultured A549 cells (the human lung epithelial cell line) (Karlsson, Cronholm, Gustafsson, & Moller, 2008). They also cause transient increase of ALT (serum alanine aminotransferase), AST (aspartate aminotransferase), and ALP (alkaline phosphatase) levels. (Jain TK et al., 2007)

Most of the applications of nanotechnology in medicine are still under development nanocrystalline silver is used already as an antimicrobial agent in the treatment of wounds. Qdots will be useful to identify the location of cancer cells in the body. Use of nanoparticles that can deliver chemotherapeutic drugs directly to cancer cells which minimizes damage to the healthy cells. Nanoshells concentrate the heat from infrared light to destroy cancer cells with minimal damage to surrounding healthy cells. Nanotubes used in the broken bones to provide a structure for newbone material to grow. Nanoparticles that can attach to cells infected with various diseases and permit a doctor to identify, in a blood sample, the particular disease (Bhowmik et al., 2009).

Nanomedicine refers to future developments in medicine that will be based on the ability to build nanorobots. In the future, these nanorobots could actually be programmed to repair specific diseased cells, functioning in a similar way to antibodies in our natural healing processes. Nanomedicines would be able to eliminate of bacterial infections in a patient within minutes as an alternative of using treatment with antibiotics over a period of weeks, also able to perform surgery at the cellular level, removing individual diseased cells and even repairing defective portions of individual cells. Significant lengthening of the human lifespan by repairing cellular level conditions that cause the body to age.

Nanoparticles can be planned with a structure very similar to the bone structure. An ultrasound is performed on existing bone structures and then bone like nanoparticles are created using the results of the ultrasound (G. A. Silva et al., 2004). The bone-like nanoparticles are inserted into the body in a paste form (Adhikari, Kundu, & Rao, 2013). When they arrive at the fractured bone, they accumulate themselves to form an ordered structure which later becomes part of the bone.

Another key use for nanoparticles is the treatment of injured nerves. Samuel Stupp and John Kessler at Northwestern University in Chicago have made tiny rod like nano-fibers called *amphiphiles*. They have kept capped with amino acids and are known to spur the growth of neurons and prevent scar tissue formation. Experiments have shown that rat and mice with spinal injuries recovered when treated with these nano-fibers.

The use of RNA interference (RNAi) to down regulate several targets has emerged as a treatment modality of exceptional promise for cancer treatment (Fire et al., 1998). The RNAi approach uses small RNA molecules which bind to messenger RNAs (mRNA) by complementary base pairing, to induce degradation of the mRNA and/or block protein synthesis. The small RNA molecules are included and processed into cellular RNA processing machinery to induce their inhibitory effects in one RNAi-based therapy modality, a 21-27 base pair double stranded RNA (siRNAs) is introduced into the cells, where it binds to its specific complementary mRNA sequence and inhibits protein synthesis (this effect is commonly called RNA silencing) (Elbashir et al., 2001). SiRNAs are designed to target only one gene which is normally over expressed in cancer cells compared with normal cells. As a result, it is highly desirable to use siRNAs targeting key genes involved in cancer cell migration, invasion, and metastasis. Before RNAi discovery, sequence-specific inhibition of gene expression was possible using nucleic acid-based antisense technology. One of the major advantages of RNAi over antisense based approaches is that the RNAi depends on the cellular machinery to target complementary transcripts resulting in efficient and potent down-regulation of gene expression (Aagaard & Rossi, 2007). Furthermore, the use of the RNAi strategy is highly specific when modulation of a particular target is desired. In this scenario, lower side effects are expected compared to conventional chemotherapy.

CONCLUSION

In this chapter we explore different therapeutics applications of different Novel Drug Delivery System which will be providing complete set of information about drug delivery systems are being of great concern due to their sole purposes. The significance of different drug delivery and targeted drug therapy is to carry a drug directly to the centre of the disease under physiological condition and thereby treat it purposely, with neither effect on the body. This is particularly significant in cancer chemotherapy and enzyme substitute treatment. Drug targeting is the delivery of drugs to receptors or organs of the body to which one hopes to deliver the drug entirely. The targeted delivery of drugs is truly a very inviting aim because these supply one of the most potential ways to develop therapeutic index of the drugs. Previous work done between late 1960s and the mid-1980s stressed the need for drugs carrier system originally to alter the pharmacokinetics of the before proven drugs whose efficacy might be improved by changing the rates of metabolism in liver or clearance by the kidneys. These approaches commonly were not focused to achieve site specific or targeted delivery such as getting a cytotoxic drug to cancerous tissue while sparing other normal, though equally sensitive tissue with the progress in the carrier technology the issue of delivering either single or the entire carrier to the specific site has been addressed during the last few years. The effective use of applications in targeted drug delivery relies on a number of different factors all play a key role in determining the effectiveness of magnetic drug delivery.

REFERENCES

Aagaard, L., & Rossi, J. J. (2007). RNAi therapeutics: Principles, prospects and challenges. *Advanced Drug Delivery Reviews*, *59*(2), 75–86. doi:10.1016/j.addr.2007.03.005 PMID:17449137

Abdel-Mottaleb, M. M., Neumann, D., & Lamprecht, A. (2011). Lipid nanocapsules for dermal application: A comparative study of lipid-based versus polymer-based nanocarriers. *European Journal of Pharmaceutics and Biopharmaceutics*, *79*(1), 36–42. doi:10.1016/j.ejpb.2011.04.009 PMID:21558002

Abraham, S. A., Waterhouse, D. N., Mayer, L. D., Cullis, P. R., Madden, T. D., & Bally, M. B. (2005). The liposomal formulation of doxorubicin. *Methods in Enzymology*, *391*, 71–97. doi:10.1016/S0076-6879(05)91004-5 PMID:15721375

Adhikari, T., Kundu, S., & Rao, A. S. (2013). Impact of SiO2 and Mo Nano Particles on Seed Germination of Rice (Oryza Sativa L.). *Int J Agric Food Sci Tec*, *4*, 809–816.

Ahola, M. S., Säilynoja, E. S., Raitavuo, M. H., Vaahtio, M. M., Salonen, J. I., & Yli-Urpo, A. U. (2001). In vitro release of heparin from silica xerogels. *Biomaterials*, *22*(15), 2163–2170. doi:10.1016/S0142-9612(00)00407-5 PMID:11432596

Amato, G. (2010). Silica-encapsulated efficient and stable Si quantum dots with high biocompatibility. *Nanoscale Research Letters*, *5*(7), 1156–1160. doi:10.1007/s11671-010-9619-9 PMID:20596494

Araújo, F., Kelmann, R., Araujo, B., Finatto, R., Teixeira, H., & Koester, L. (2011). Development and characterization of parenteral nanoemulsions containing thalidomide. *European Journal of Pharmaceutical Sciences*, *42*(3), 238–245. doi:10.1016/j.ejps.2010.11.014 PMID:21130164

Attama, A., Schicke, B., Paepenmüller, T., & Müller-Goymann, C. (2007). Solid lipid nanodispersions containing mixed lipid core and a polar heterolipid: Characterization. *European Journal of Pharmaceutics and Biopharmaceutics*, *67*(1), 48–57. doi:10.1016/j.ejpb.2006.12.004 PMID:17276663

Bal, T., Murthy, P. N., & Sengupta, S. (2012). Preparation and evaluation of mucoadhesive simvastatin microcapsules using orifice gelation technique. *Asian Journal of Pharmaceutics*, *6*(1), 74. doi:10.4103/0973-8398.100152

Banker, G. S., Siepmann, J., & Rhodes, C. (2002). *Modern pharmaceutics*. CRC Press. doi:10.1201/9780824744694

Barraud, L., Merle, P., Soma, E., Lefrançois, L., Guerret, S., Chevallier, M., & Vitvitski, L. et al. (2005). Increase of doxorubicin sensitivity by doxorubicin-loading into nanoparticles for hepatocellular carcinoma cells in vitro and in vivo. *Journal of Hepatology*, *42*(5), 736–743. doi:10.1016/j.jhep.2004.12.035 PMID:15826724

Beg, S., Rizwan, M., Sheikh, A. M., Hasnain, M. S., Anwer, K., & Kohli, K. (2011). Advancement in carbon nanotubes: Basics, biomedical applications and toxicity. *The Journal of Pharmacy and Pharmacology*, *63*(2), 141–163. doi:10.1111/j.2042-7158.2010.01167.x PMID:21235578

Bhirde, A. A., Patel, V., Gavard, J., Zhang, G., Sousa, A. A., Masedunskas, A., & Rusling, J. F. et al. (2009). Targeted killing of cancer cells in vivo and in vitro with EGF-directed carbon nanotube-based drug delivery. *ACS Nano*, *3*(2), 307–316. doi:10.1021/nn800551s PMID:19236065

Bhise, S. D. (2011). Ternary solid dispersions of fenofibrate with Poloxamer 188 and TPGS for enhancement of solubility and bioavailability. *Int J Res Pharm Biomed Sci*, *2*(2), 583–595.

Bhowmik, D., Chiranjib, C. R., & Jayakar, B. (2009). Role of nanotechnology in novel drug delivery system. *Journal of Pharmaceutical Science and Technology*, *1*(1), 20–35.

Brannon-Peppas, L., & Blanchette, J. O. (2012). Nanoparticle and targeted systems for cancer therapy. *Advanced Drug Delivery Reviews*, *64*, 206–212. doi:10.1016/j.addr.2012.09.033 PMID:15350294

Brewer, J., & Alexander, J. (1992). The adjuvant activity of non-ionic surfactant vesicles (niosomes) on the BALB/c humoral response to bovine serum albumin. *Immunology*, *75*(4), 570. PMID:1592432

Cevc, G. (1996). Transfersomes, liposomes and other lipid suspensions on the skin: permeation enhancement, vesicle penetration, and transdermal drug delivery. *Critical Reviews™ in Therapeutic Drug Carrier Systems, 13*(3-4).

Chaturvedi, M., Kumar, M., Sinhal, A., & Saifi, A. (2011). Recent development in novel drug delivery systems of herbal drugs. *International Journal of Green Pharmacy*, *5*(2), 87. doi:10.4103/0973-8258.85155

Chen, M., Zhong, Z., Tan, W., Wang, S., & Wang, Y. (2011). Recent advances in nanoparticle formulation of oleanolic acid. *Chinese Medicine*, *6*(1), 20. doi:10.1186/1749-8546-6-20 PMID:21619582

Chime, S., Kenechukwu, F., & Attama, A. (2014). Nanoemulsions—Advances in Formulation, Characterization and applications in drug delivery. In Application of nanotechnology in drug delivery. Croatia: In Tech.

Chomoucka, J., Drbohlavova, J., Huska, D., Adam, V., Kizek, R., & Hubalek, J. (2010). Magnetic nanoparticles and targeted drug delivering. *Pharmacological Research*, *62*(2), 144–149. doi:10.1016/j.phrs.2010.01.014 PMID:20149874

Clark, M. A., Jepson, M. A., & Hirst, B. H. (2001). Exploiting M cells for drug and vaccine delivery. *Advanced Drug Delivery Reviews*, *50*(1), 81–106. doi:10.1016/S0169-409X(01)00149-1 PMID:11489335

Cole, A. J., Yang, V. C., & David, A. E. (2011). Cancer theranostics: The rise of targeted magnetic nanoparticles. *Trends in Biotechnology*, *29*(7), 323–332. doi:10.1016/j.tibtech.2011.03.001 PMID:21489647

Cowan-Lincoln, M. (n.d.). *FORMULATION-Solubility| Improve the Bioavailability of Poorly Soluble Drugs*. Academic Press.

Czarnobaj, K. (2008). Preparation and characterization of silica xerogels as carriers for drugs. *Drug Delivery*, *15*(8), 485–492. doi:10.1080/10717540802321495 PMID:18798086

Czarnobaj, K., & Czarnobaj, J. (2008). Sol–gel processed porous silica carriers for the controlled release of diclofenac diethylamine. *Journal of Biomedical Materials Research. Part B, Applied Biomaterials*, *87*(1), 114–120. doi:10.1002/jbm.b.31076 PMID:18437709

Czarnobaj, K., & Łukasiak, J. (2007). In vitro release of cisplatin from sol–gel processed organically modified silica xerogels. *Journal of Materials Science. Materials in Medicine*, *18*(10), 2041–2044. doi:10.1007/s10856-007-3139-x PMID:17558477

Czarnobaj, K., & Sawicki, W. (2012). The sol-gel prepared SiO2-CaO-P2O5 composites doped with Metronidazole for application in local delivery systems. *Pharmaceutical Development and Technology*, *17*(6), 697–704. doi:10.3109/10837450.2011.572894 PMID:21480825

Dayan, N., & Touitou, E. (2000). Carriers for skin delivery of trihexyphenidyl HCl: Ethosomes vs. liposomes. *Biomaterials*, *21*(18), 1879–1885. doi:10.1016/S0142-9612(00)00063-6 PMID:10919691

des Rieux, A., Fievez, V., Garinot, M., Schneider, Y.-J., & Préat, V. (2006). Nanoparticles as potential oral delivery systems of proteins and vaccines: A mechanistic approach. *Journal of Controlled Release*, *116*(1), 1–27. doi:10.1016/j.jconrel.2006.08.013 PMID:17050027

Di Pasqua, A. J., Wallner, S., Kerwood, D. J., & Dabrowiak, J. C. (2009). Adsorption of the PtII anticancer drug carboplatin by mesoporous silica. *Chemistry & Biodiversity*, *6*(9), 1343–1349. doi:10.1002/cbdv.200900021 PMID:19774597

Dixit, R., & Nagarsenker, M. (2008). Self-nanoemulsifying granules of ezetimibe: Design, optimization and evaluation. *European Journal of Pharmaceutical Sciences*, *35*(3), 183–192. doi:10.1016/j.ejps.2008.06.013 PMID:18652892

Dobrovolskaia, M. A., & McNeil, S. E. (2007). Immunological properties of engineered nanomaterials. *Nature Nanotechnology*, *2*(8), 469–478. doi:10.1038/nnano.2007.223 PMID:18654343

Elbashir, S. M., Lendeckel, W., & Tuschl, T. (2001). RNA interference is mediated by 21-and 22-nucleotide RNAs. *Genes & Development*, *15*(2), 188–200. doi:10.1101/gad.862301 PMID:11157775

Ercan, M. T. (1992). Rapid determination of hydrolyzed-reduced technetium-99m in particulate radiopharmaceuticals. *International Journal of Radiation Applications and Instrumentation. Part A, Applied Radiation and Isotopes*, *43*(9), 1175–1177. doi:10.1016/0883-2889(92)90065-M

Farooq, S. A., Saini, V., Singh, R., & Kaur, K. (2013). Application of novel drug delivery system in the pharmacotherapy of Hyperlipidemia. *Journal Of Chemical and Pharmaceutical Sciences*, *6*(3), 138–144.

Farraj, N., Johansen, B., Davis, S., & Illum, L. (1990). Nasal administration of insulin using bioadhesive microspheres as a delivery system. *Journal of Controlled Release*, *13*(2), 253–261. doi:10.1016/0168-3659(90)90016-M

Fidalgo, A., Lopez, T. M., & Ilharco, L. M. (2009). Wet sol–gel silica matrices as delivery devices for phenytoin. *Journal of Sol-Gel Science and Technology*, *49*(3), 320–328. doi:10.1007/s10971-008-1880-3

Fire, A., Xu, S., Montgomery, M. K., Kostas, S. A., Driver, S. E., & Mello, C. C. (1998). Potent and specific genetic interference by double-stranded RNA in Caenorhabditis elegans. *Nature, 391*(6669), 806-811.

Freiberg, S., & Zhu, X. (2004). Polymer microspheres for controlled drug release. *International Journal of Pharmaceutics*, *282*(1), 1–18. doi:10.1016/j.ijpharm.2004.04.013 PMID:15336378

GarimaChawla, P. G., Koradia, V., & Bansal, A. K. (2013). *Gastroretention, a means to address regional variability in intestinal drug absorption*. Academic Press.

Geary, R. S., & Schlameus, H. W. (1993). Vancomycin and insulin used as models for oral delivery of peptides. *Journal of Controlled Release*, *23*(1), 65–74. doi:10.1016/0168-3659(93)90071-C

Goyal, P., & Goyal, K., Kumar, S. G. V., Singh, A., Katare, O. P., & Mishra, D. N. (2005). Liposomal drug delivery systems-clinical applications. *Acta Pharmaceutica (Zagreb, Croatia)*, *55*(1), 1–25. PMID:15907221

Haefeli, U., Atcher, R., Morris, C., & Beresford, B. (1992). Polymeric radiopharmaceutical delivery systems. *Radioactivity and Radiochemistry*, *3*, 11–11.

He, H., Cao, X., & Lee, L. J. (2004). Design of a novel hydrogel-based intelligent system for controlled drug release. *Journal of Controlled Release*, *95*(3), 391–402. doi:10.1016/j.jconrel.2003.12.004 PMID:15023451

He, Q., Gao, Y., Zhang, L., Zhang, Z., Gao, F., Ji, X., & Shi, J. et al. (2011). A pH-responsive mesoporous silica nanoparticles-based multi-drug delivery system for overcoming multi-drug resistance. *Biomaterials*, *32*(30), 7711–7720. doi:10.1016/j.biomaterials.2011.06.066 PMID:21816467

Heller, J., & Hoffman, A. (1996). Drug delivery systems. *Biomaterials science: An introduction to materials in medicine*, 346-356.

Hoshi, K. (1996). Approved indications of lipo-PGE 1 in Japan. *Advanced Drug Delivery Reviews*, *20*(2), 171–176. doi:10.1016/0169-409X(95)00120-V

Hrubý, M., Koňák, Č., & Ulbrich, K. (2005). Polymeric micellar pH-sensitive drug delivery system for doxorubicin. *Journal of Controlled Release*, *103*(1), 137–148. doi:10.1016/j.jconrel.2004.11.017 PMID:15710507

Igarashi, R., Takenaga, M., Takeuchi, J., Kitagawa, A., Matsumoto, K., & Mizushima, Y. (2001). Marked hypotensive and blood flow-increasing effects of a new lipo-PGE 1 (lipo-AS013) due to vascular wall targeting. *Journal of Controlled Release*, *71*(2), 157–164. doi:10.1016/S0168-3659(00)00373-4 PMID:11274747

Jadhav, S. M., Morey, P., Karpe, M., & Kadam, V. (2012). *Novel vesicular system: An overview*. Academic Press.

Jain, N. (2002). *Targeted and Controlled Drug Delivery*. New Delhi: CBS Publishers and Distributors.

Jain, N. K. (1997). *Controlled and novel drug delivery*. CBS Publishers & Distributors.

Jia, G., Wang, H., Yan, L., Wang, X., Pei, R., Yan, T., & Guo, X. et al. (2005). Cytotoxicity of carbon nanomaterials: Single-wall nanotube, multi-wall nanotube, and fullerene. *Environmental Science & Technology*, *39*(5), 1378–1383. doi:10.1021/es0487291 PMID:15787380

Kakinoki, S., Yasuda, C., Kaetsu, I., Uchida, K., Yukutake, K., Nakayama, M., & Ohyanagi, H. et al. (2003). Preparation of poly-lactic acid microspheres containing the angiogenesis inhibitor TNP-470 with medium-chain triglyceride and the in vitro evaluation of release profiles. *European Journal of Pharmaceutics and Biopharmaceutics*, *55*(2), 155–160. doi:10.1016/S0939-6411(02)00156-X PMID:12637091

Kalshetti, P. P., Rajendra, V. B., Dixit, D. N., & Parekh, P. P. (2012). Hydrogels as a drug delivery system and applications: A review. *International Journal of Pharmacy and Pharmaceutical Sciences*, *4*(1), 1–7.

Kaneda, Y. (2000). Virosomes: Evolution of the liposome as a targeted drug delivery system. *Advanced Drug Delivery Reviews*, *43*(2), 197–205. doi:10.1016/S0169-409X(00)00069-7 PMID:10967226

Karlsson, H. L., Cronholm, P., Gustafsson, J., & Moller, L. (2008). Copper oxide nanoparticles are highly toxic: A comparison between metal oxide nanoparticles and carbon nanotubes. *Chemical Research in Toxicology*, *21*(9), 1726–1732. doi:10.1021/tx800064j PMID:18710264

Kelner, A., & Schacht, E. H. (2005). Tailor-made polymers for local drug delivery: Release of macromolecular model drugs from biodegradable hydrogels based on poly (ethylene oxide). *Journal of Controlled Release*, *101*(1), 13–20. doi:10.1016/j.jconrel.2004.09.010 PMID:15588890

Kirsch, N., Alexander, C., Lübke, M., Whitcombe, M., & Vulfson, E. (2000). Enhancement of selectivity of imprinted polymers via post-imprinting modification of recognition sites. *Polymer*, *41*(15), 5583–5590. doi:10.1016/S0032-3861(99)00782-X

Knight, L. (1986). *Thrombus-localizing radiopharmaceuticals. In Radiopharmaceuticals: Progress and clinical perspectives* (pp. 23–40). Boca Raton, FL: CRC Press.

Kotta, S., Khan, A. W., Pramod, K., Ansari, S. H., Sharma, R. K., & Ali, J. (2012). Exploring oral nanoemulsions for bioavailability enhancement of poorly water-soluble drugs. *Expert Opinion on Drug Delivery*, *9*(5), 585–598. doi:10.1517/17425247.2012.668523 PMID:22512597

Kumari, A., Yadav, S. K., & Yadav, S. C. (2010). Biodegradable polymeric nanoparticles based drug delivery systems. *Colloids and Surfaces. B, Biointerfaces*, *75*(1), 1–18. doi:10.1016/j.colsurfb.2009.09.001 PMID:19782542

Kushwaha, S. K., Rastogl, A., Rai, A., & Singh, S. (2012). Novel drug delivery system for anticancer drug: A review. *International Journal of Pharm Tech Research*, *4*(2), 542–553.

Kyyrönen, K., Hume, L., Benedetti, L., Urtti, A., Topp, E., & Stella, V. (1992). Methylprednisolone esters of hyaluronic acid in ophthalmic drug delivery: In vitro and in vivo release studies. *International Journal of Pharmaceutics*, *80*(1), 161–169. doi:10.1016/0378-5173(92)90274-6

Lachman, L., Lieberman, H. A., & Kanig, J. L. (1986). *The theory and practice of industrial pharmacy*. Academic Press.

Lawrie, A., Brisken, A., Francis, S., Cumberland, D., Crossman, D., & Newman, C. (2000). Microbubble-enhanced ultrasound for vascular gene delivery. *Gene Therapy*, *7*(23), 2023–2027. doi:10.1038/sj.gt.3301339 PMID:11175314

Li, Z., Su, K., Cheng, B., & Deng, Y. (2010). Organically modified MCM-type material preparation and its usage in controlled amoxicillin delivery. *Journal of Colloid and Interface Science*, *342*(2), 607–613. doi:10.1016/j.jcis.2009.10.073 PMID:19948346

Lim, F., & Sun, A. M. (1980). Microencapsulated islets as bioartificial endocrine pancreas. *Science*, *210*(4472), 908–910. doi:10.1126/science.6776628 PMID:6776628

Liu, J., Gong, T., Fu, H., Wang, C., Wang, X., Chen, Q., & Zhang, Z. et al. (2008). Solid lipid nanoparticles for pulmonary delivery of insulin. *International Journal of Pharmaceutics*, *356*(1), 333–344. doi:10.1016/j.ijpharm.2008.01.008 PMID:18281169

Lovelyn, C., & Attama, A. A. (2011). Current state of nanoemulsions in drug delivery. *Journal of Biomaterials and Nanobiotechnology*, *2*(05), 626–639. doi:10.4236/jbnb.2011.225075

Mahmoudi, M., Simchi, A., Imani, M., Shokrgozar, M. A., Milani, A. S., Häfeli, U. O., & Stroeve, P. (2010). A new approach for the in vitro identification of the cytotoxicity of superparamagnetic iron oxide nanoparticles. *Colloids and Surfaces. B, Biointerfaces*, *75*(1), 300–309. doi:10.1016/j.colsurfb.2009.08.044 PMID:19781921

Majumdar, S., & Chowdhury, S. (2010). Novel therapeutic application of microbubbles for targeted drug delivery. *International Journal of Pharma and Bio Sciences, 1*(3).

Malhotra, M., & Jain, N. (1994). Niosomes as drug carriers. *Indian Drugs-Bombay*, *31*, 81–81.

Mann, B. K., Gobin, A. S., Tsai, A. T., Schmedlen, R. H., & West, J. L. (2001). Smooth muscle cell growth in photopolymerized hydrogels with cell adhesive and proteolytically degradable domains: Synthetic ECM analogs for tissue engineering. *Biomaterials*, *22*(22), 3045–3051. doi:10.1016/S0142-9612(01)00051-5 PMID:11575479

Maver, U., Godec, A., Bele, M., Planinšek, O., Gaberšček, M., Srčič, S., & Jamnik, J. (2007). Novel hybrid silica xerogels for stabilization and controlled release of drug. *International Journal of Pharmaceutics*, *330*(1), 164–174. doi:10.1016/j.ijpharm.2006.09.024 PMID:17055199

Medina, O. P., Zhu, Y., & Kairemo, K. (2004). Targeted liposomal drug delivery in cancer. *Current Pharmaceutical Design*, *10*(24), 2981–2989. doi:10.2174/1381612043383467 PMID:15379663

Momma, K. (1996). Lipo-PGE 1 treatment of the neonate with critical congenital heart disease and ductus-arteriosus dependent circulation. *Advanced Drug Delivery Reviews*, *20*(2), 177–180. doi:10.1016/0169-409X(95)00121-M

Muchow, M., Maincent, P., & Müller, R. H. (2008). Lipid nanoparticles with a solid matrix (SLN®, NLC®, LDC®) for oral drug delivery. *Drug Development and Industrial Pharmacy*, *34*(12), 1394–1405. doi:10.1080/03639040802130061 PMID:18665980

Nayak, A. P., Tiyaboonchai, W., Patankar, S., Madhusudhan, B., & Souto, E. B. (2010). Curcuminoids-loaded lipid nanoparticles: Novel approach towards malaria treatment. *Colloids and Surfaces. B, Biointerfaces*, *81*(1), 263–273. doi:10.1016/j.colsurfb.2010.07.020 PMID:20688493

Nishiyama, N., Bae, Y., Miyata, K., Fukushima, S., & Kataoka, K. (2005). Smart polymeric micelles for gene and drug delivery. *Drug Discovery Today. Technologies*, *2*(1), 21–26. doi:10.1016/j.ddtec.2005.05.007 PMID:24981751

O'Reilly, M. A., & Hynynen, K. (2012). Ultrasound enhanced drug delivery to the brain and central nervous system. *International Journal of Hyperthermia*, *28*(4), 386–396. doi:10.3109/02656736.2012.666709 PMID:22621739

Packhaeuser, C., Schnieders, J., Oster, C., & Kissel, T. (2004). In situ forming parenteral drug delivery systems: An overview. *European Journal of Pharmaceutics and Biopharmaceutics*, *58*(2), 445–455. doi:10.1016/j.ejpb.2004.03.003 PMID:15296966

Pande, S., Kshirsagar, M., & Chandewar, A. (2011). Ion exchange resins pharmaceutical applications and recent advancement. *International Journal of Advances in Pharmaceutical Sciences, 2*(1).

Panyam, J., & Labhasetwar, V. (2003). Biodegradable nanoparticles for drug and gene delivery to cells and tissue. *Advanced Drug Delivery Reviews*, *55*(3), 329–347. doi:10.1016/S0169-409X(02)00228-4 PMID:12628320

Parmar, K. R., Shah, S. R., & Sheth, N. R. (2011). Studies in dissolution enhancement of ezetimibe by solid dispersions in combination with a surface adsorbent. *Dissolut Technol*, *8*(3), 55–61. doi:10.14227/DT180311P55

Patel, J., Bharadia, P., Amin, A., & Patel, M. (2004). Formulation optimisation and evaluation of controlled release mucoadhesive microspheres of glipizide for oral delivery using factorial design. *Drug Delivery*, *4*, 48–53.

Patel, R., & Patel, K. P. (2010). Advances in novel parentral drug delivery systems. *Asian Journal of Pharmaceutics*, *4*(3), 193. doi:10.4103/0973-8398.72117

Patel, S. (2007). Ethosomes: A promising tool for transdermal delivery of drug. *Pharmainfo. Net, 5*(3), 345-350.

Pathak, C. P., Sawhney, A. S., & Hubbell, J. A. (1992). Rapid photopolymerization of immunoprotective gels in contact with cells and tissue. *Journal of the American Chemical Society*, *114*(21), 8311–8312. doi:10.1021/ja00047a065

Pawan, C., & Hemchand, P. (2009). Magnetic microsphere: as targeted drug delivery. *Journal of Pharmacy Research, 2*(5).

Poland, C. A., Duffin, R., Kinloch, I., Maynard, A., Wallace, W. A., Seaton, A., & Donaldson, K. et al. (2008). Carbon nanotubes introduced into the abdominal cavity of mice show asbestos-like pathogenicity in a pilot study. *Nature Nanotechnology*, *3*(7), 423–428. doi:10.1038/nnano.2008.111 PMID:18654567

Popovici, R., Seftel, E., Mihai, G., Popovici, E., & Voicu, V. (2011). Controlled drug delivery system based on ordered mesoporous silica matrices of captopril as angiotensin-converting enzyme inhibitor drug. *Journal of Pharmaceutical Sciences*, *100*(2), 704–714. doi:10.1002/jps.22308 PMID:20740675

Prasanth, V., Moy, A. C., Mathew, S. T., & Mathapan, R. (2011). Microspheres-An Overview. *International Journal of Research in Pharmaceutical and Biomedical Sciences*, *2*(2), 332–338.

Primo, F. L., Michieleto, L., Rodrigues, M. A., Macaroff, P. P., Morais, P. C., Lacava, Z. G., & Tedesco, A. C. et al. (2007). Magnetic nanoemulsions as drug delivery system for Foscan®: Skin permeation and retention in vitro assays for topical application in photodynamic therapy (PDT) of skin cancer. *Journal of Magnetism and Magnetic Materials*, *311*(1), 354–357. doi:10.1016/j.jmmm.2006.10.1183

Prokopowicz, M. (2010). Synthesis and in vitro characterization of freeze-dried doxorubicin-loaded silica xerogels. *Journal of Sol-Gel Science and Technology*, *53*(3), 525–533. doi:10.1007/s10971-009-2126-8

Quintanar-Guerrero, D., Ganem-Quintanar, A., Nava-Arzaluz, M. G., & Piñón-Segundo, E. (2009). *Silica xerogels as pharmaceutical drug carriers*. Academic Press.

Radomski, A., Jurasz, P., Alonso-Escolano, D., Drews, M., Morandi, M., Malinski, T., & Radomski, M. W. (2005). Nanoparticle-induced platelet aggregation and vascular thrombosis. *British Journal of Pharmacology*, *146*(6), 882–893. doi:10.1038/sj.bjp.0706386 PMID:16158070

Rajput, M., Sharma, R., Kumar, S., Jamil, F., Sissodia, N., & Sharma, S. (2012). Pulsatile drug delivery system: A review. *International Journal of Research in Pharmaceutical and Biomedical Sciences*, *3*(1), 118–124.

Ramteke, K., Jadhav, V., & Dhole, S. (2012). Microspheres: As carriers used for novel drug delivery system. *IOSR Journal of Pharmacy*, *2*(4), 44–48. doi:10.9790/3013-24204448

Rapoport, N., Pitt, W. G., Sun, H., & Nelson, J. L. (2003). Drug delivery in polymeric micelles: From in vitro to in vivo. *Journal of Controlled Release*, *91*(1), 85–95. doi:10.1016/S0168-3659(03)00218-9 PMID:12932640

Rasve, G., Borade, G., Deshmukh, S., & Tagalpallewar, A. (2011). Pulsatile drug delivery system: current scenario. *International Journal of Pharma and Bio Science, 2*(3).

Ruel-Gariepy, E., & Leroux, J.-C. (2004). In situ-forming hydrogels—review of temperature-sensitive systems. *European Journal of Pharmaceutics and Biopharmaceutics*, *58*(2), 409–426. doi:10.1016/j.ejpb.2004.03.019 PMID:15296964

Russell, J., Carden, J., & Herron, H. (1988). Dosimetry calculations for yttrium-90 used in the treatment of liver cancer. *Endocurietherapy/Hyperthermia Oncology, 4*(171-1), 86.

Ryu, E. K., Ross, R. J., Matsushita, T., MacCoss, M., Hong, C. I., & West, C. R. (1982). Phospholipid-nucleoside conjugates. 3. Syntheses and preliminary biological evaluation of 1-. beta.-D-arabinofuranosylcytosine 5'-monophosphate-L-1, 2-dipalmitin and selected 1-. beta.-D-arabinofuranosylcytosine 5'-diphosphate-L-1, 2-diacylglycerols. *Journal of Medicinal Chemistry*, *25*(11), 1322–1329. doi:10.1021/jm00353a010 PMID:7143370

Saraf, S., Gupta, D., Kaur, C. D., & Saraf, S. (2011). Sphingosomes a novel approach to vesicular drug delivery. *Int J Cur Sci Res.*, *1*(2), 63–68.

Saul, J. M., Annapragada, A., Natarajan, J. V., & Bellamkonda, R. V. (2003). Controlled targeting of liposomal doxorubicin via the folate receptor in vitro. *Journal of Controlled Release*, *92*(1), 49–67. doi:10.1016/S0168-3659(03)00295-5 PMID:14499185

Scheffler, P., Gross, J., Markwirth, T., Maier, J., & Schieffer, H. (1996). Progress in the prostaglandin E1-therapy of the intermittent claudication by means of bolus injections of LIPO-prostaglandin E1 (LIPO-PGE1). *European Journal of Clinical Pharmacology*, *51*(3-4), 235–239. doi:10.1007/s002280050190 PMID:9010691

Schmid, G. (2011). *Nanoparticles: from theory to application*. John Wiley & Sons.

Selvamuthukumar, S., Anandam, S., Krishnamoorthy, K., & Rajappan, M. (2012). Nanosponges: A novel class of drug delivery system-Review. *Journal of Pharmacy & Pharmaceutical Sciences*, *15*(1), 103–111. doi:10.18433/J3K308 PMID:22365092

Semalty, A., Semalty, M., Rawat, B. S., Singh, D., & Rawat, M. (2009). *Pharmacosomes: the lipid-based new drug delivery system*. Academic Press.

Sezaki, H., & Hashida, M. (1985). Macromolecules as drug delivery systems *Directed*[Springer.]. *Drug Delivery*, 189–208.

Shafiq, S., Shakeel, F., Talegaonkar, S., Ahmad, F. J., Khar, R. K., & Ali, M. (2007). Development and bioavailability assessment of ramipril nanoemulsion formulation. *European Journal of Pharmaceutics and Biopharmaceutics*, *66*(2), 227–243. doi:10.1016/j.ejpb.2006.10.014 PMID:17127045

Sharma, R., & Pathak, K. (2010). Nanosponges: emerging drug delivery system. *Pharma Stud*, 33-35.

Shirwaikar, A., Kumar, S., Jacob, S., Rashi, W., & Ravi, K. (2006). Recent developments in floating drug delivery systems for gastric retention of drugs, an overview. *INDIAN DRUGS-BOMBAY*, *43*(9), 697.

Shortencarier, M. J., Dayton, P., Bloch, S. H., Schumann, P., Matsunaga, T. O., & Ferrara, K. W. (2004). A method for radiation-force localized drug delivery using gas-filled lipospheres. *Ultrasonics, Ferro-electrics, and Frequency Control. IEEE Transactions on*, *51*(7), 822–831.

Silva, G. A., Czeisler, C., Niece, K. L., Beniash, E., Harrington, D. A., Kessler, J. A., & Stupp, S. I. (2004). Selective differentiation of neural progenitor cells by high-epitope density nanofibers. *Science*, *303*(5662), 1352–1355. doi:10.1126/science.1093783 PMID:14739465

Silva, J., Fernandes, A. R., & Baptista, P. V. (2014). Application of nanotechnology in drug delivery. *Application of Nanotechnology in Drug Delivery*.

Slowing, I. I., Trewyn, B. G., Giri, S., & Lin, V. Y. (2007). Mesoporous silica nanoparticles for drug delivery and biosensing applications. *Advanced Functional Materials*, *17*(8), 1225–1236. doi:10.1002/adfm.200601191

Srikanth, M., Sunil, S., Rao, N., Uhumwangho, M., & Murthy, K. R. (2010). Ion-exchange resins as controlled drug delivery carriers. *Journal of Scientific Research*, *2*(3), 597. doi:10.3329/jsr.v2i3.4991

Suri, S. S., Fenniri, H., & Singh, B. (2007). Nanotechnology-based drug delivery systems. *Journal of Occupational Medicine and Toxicology (London, England)*, *2*(1), 16. doi:10.1186/1745-6673-2-16 PMID:18053152

Sznitowska, M., Gajewska, M., Janicki, S., Radwanska, A., & Lukowski, G. (2001). Bioavailability of diazepam from aqueous-organic solution, submicron emulsion and solid lipid nanoparticles after rectal administration in rabbits. *European Journal of Pharmaceutics and Biopharmaceutics*, *52*(2), 159–163. doi:10.1016/S0939-6411(01)00157-6 PMID:11522481

Takeuchi, T., & Haginaka, J. (1999). Separation and sensing based on molecular recognition using molecularly imprinted polymers. *Journal of Chromatography. B, Biomedical Sciences and Applications*, *728*(1), 1–20. doi:10.1016/S0378-4347(99)00057-2 PMID:10379652

Thiagarajan, P. (2011). Nanoemulsions for drug delivery through different routes. *Research in Biotechnology*, *2*(3).

Tsutsui, J. M., Xie, F., & Porter, R. T. (2004). The use of microbubbles to target drug delivery. *Cardiovascular Ultrasound*, *2*(1), 23. doi:10.1186/1476-7120-2-23 PMID:15546496

Venkatesan, P., Manavalan, R., & Valliappan, K. (2009). Microencapsulation: A vital technique in novel drug delivery system. *J Pharm Sci Res*, *1*(4), 26–35.

Wang, L., Li, X., Zhang, G., Dong, J., & Eastoe, J. (2007). Oil-in-water nanoemulsions for pesticide formulations. *Journal of Colloid and Interface Science*, *314*(1), 230–235. doi:10.1016/j.jcis.2007.04.079 PMID:17612555

Wei, L., Hu, N., & Zhang, Y. (2010). Synthesis of polymer—mesoporous silica nanocomposites. *Materials (Basel)*, *3*(7), 4066–4079. doi:10.3390/ma3074066

Wilczewska, A. Z., Niemirowicz, K., Markiewicz, K. H., & Car, H. (2012). Nanoparticles as drug delivery systems. *Pharmacological Reports*, *64*(5), 1020–1037. doi:10.1016/S1734-1140(12)70901-5 PMID:23238461

Wissing, S., Kayser, O., & Müller, R. (2004). Solid lipid nanoparticles for parenteral drug delivery. *Advanced Drug Delivery Reviews*, *56*(9), 1257–1272. doi:10.1016/j.addr.2003.12.002 PMID:15109768

Wulff, G. (1995). Molecular imprinting in cross-linked materials with the aid of molecular templates—a way towards artificial antibodies. *Angewandte Chemie International Edition in English*, *34*(17), 1812–1832. doi:10.1002/anie.199518121

Section 2
Liposomes

Chapter 2
Liposomes:
Properties and Therapeutic Applications

Ljiljana Djekic
University of Belgrade, Serbia

ABSTRACT

This chapter reviews the current progress in liposome based pharmaceuticals with particular emphasis on the carrier design, size, surface properties, drug delivery performances and therapeutic applications for different routes of administration. There were described selected examples of encapsulation of drug substances by liposomes which allowed improvement of therapeutic index of cytotoxic drugs (such as antineoplastics, antibiotics) or sustained drug release and reduction of the frequency of administration of analgesics and local anesthetics, and potentiate the immunogenicity of vaccines against hepatitis A and influenza. Furthermore, the performances of the marketed pharmaceuticals which represent pulmonary surfactant substituents (in the form of liposome vesicles) in premature infants and topical preparations with high molecular weight actives (e.g., heparin sodium) encapsulated in liposomes, were highlighted. The most important factors that affect the development of new drugs with this type of nanomaterials and their safety were commented.

INTRODUCTION

Liposomes were first investigated in 1976 as colloidal carriers for insulin in order to protect the drug against potential proteolysis in gastrointestinal tract (GIT) (Dapergolas & Gregoriadis, 1976). Until now, this field of investigations is at the preclinical level, primarily due to limited stability of liposomal carriers in the GIT. On the other hand, encapsulation of drug substances in this type of carriers becomes important strategy in development of pharmaceutical preparations for different routes of administration (De Villiers et al., 2009; Farokhzad & Langer, 2009; Park, 2007). Curently available pharmaceutical products based on liposomes are predominantly parenteral preparations for intravenous (*i.v.*), intramuscular (*i.m.*), subcutaneous (*s.c.*), and intrathecal (*i.t.*) administration. Liposomal based products for cutaneous and intratracheal administration are also on the market (Table 1).

DOI: 10.4018/978-1-5225-0751-2.ch002

Table 1. Marketed pharmaceutical products comprising drug substances encapsulated in liposome-type carriers

Name of the Medicinal Product	Pharmaceutical Form	Qualitative and Quantitative Composition	Carrier	List of Excipients	Manufacturer	Indications
Caelyx®/ Doxil®	Concentrate for solution for infusion	Doxorubicin hydrochloride 20 mg/10 ml 50 mg/25 ml	PEGylated liposomes (80 – 100 nm)	α- (2- [1,2-distearoyl-sn-glycero (3) fosfooksi] ethylcarbamoyl) -ω-methoxypoly (oxyethylene) -40 sodium salt (MPEG-DSPE), hydrogenated soy phosphatidylcholine (HSPC), cholesterol, ammonium sulfate, sucrose, histidine, Water for injections hydrochloric acid, sodium hydroxide	Janssen-Cilag, UK / Ortho Biotech, Johnson & Johnson, USA	Metastatic breast cancer, ovarian cancer, multiple myeloma, Kaposi's sarcoma in patients with AIDS
Myocet®	A powder, a dispersion and a solvent for dispersing the concentrate for infusion	Doxorubicin hydrochloride 50 mg	Small unilamellar liposomes	**Powder:** Lactose **Dispersion:** Phosphatidylcholine, Cholesterol, Citric acid, Sodium hydroxide, Water for injections **Solvent:** Sodium carbonate, Water for injections	Cephalon, USA	Metastatic breast cancer
DaunoXome®	Concentrate for solution for infusion	Daunorubicin hydrochloride 50 mg/25 ml	Small unilamellar liposomes (35 – 65 nm)	**Liposomes:** Distearoilfosfatidilholin (28.16 mg/ml), Cholesterol (6.72 mg/ml), citric acid **Vehicle:** Sucrose (2,125 mg), Glycine (94 mg), Calcium chloride, dihydrate (7 mg), Water for Injection (q.s. ad 25 ml) pH 4.9 - 6.0	Nextar Pharmaceuticals/ Gilead Sciences, USA	Kaposi's sarcoma in patients with AIDS
Marqibo®	A solution for injection (vincristine sulfate 5 mg/5 ml). Dispersion of liposomes. Buffer solution.	Vincristine sulfate 5 mg/31 ml	Liposomes (~100 nm)	**A solution for injection of vincristine sulfate of mannitol.** **Dispersion of liposomes:** sphingomyelin, cholesterol, sodium citrate, citric acid. **Buffer:** Sodium phosphate, sodium chloride.	Talon Therapeutics, USA	Acute lymphoblastic leukemia
AmBisome®	Powder for solution for infusion	Amphotericin B 50 mg	Conventional bilamellar liposomes (<100 nm)	Hydrogenated soy phosphatidylcholine (213 mg), cholesterol (52 mg), distearoylphosphatidylglycerol (84 mg), alpha-tocopherol (0.64 mg), sucrose (900 mg), disodium succinate hexahydrate (27 mg), sodium hydroxide, hydrochloric acid. pH 5-6 (after reconstitution of the powder with water for injection)	NeXstar Pharmaceuticals/ Gilead, USA	Severe systemic fungal infections (disseminated candidiasis, aspergillosis, mycetoma, cryptococcal meningitis, visceral leishmaniasis)

continued on following page

Table 1. Continued

Name of the Medicinal Product	Pharmaceutical Form	Qualitative and Quantitative Composition	Carrier	List of Excipients	Manufacturer	Indications
Nyotran®	Powder for solution for infusion	Nystatin 50 mg 100 mg	Multilamellar liposomes	Dimyristoyl, dimyristoyl phosphatidylglycerol	Aronex-Roche, USA	Severe systemic fungal infections (disseminated candidiasis, aspergillosis)
Visudyne®	Powder for solution for infusion	Verteporfin 15 mg	Liposomes	Lactose monohydrate, eggs phosphatidylglycerol, dimyristoyl phosphatidylcholine, ascorbyl palmitate, butylated hydroxytoluene (BHT) (E321)	Novartis, Switzerland	Photodynamic therapy of age-related macula degeneration
DepoCyt®	Suspension for injection	Cytarabine 50 mg/5 ml	DepoFoam® multivesicular liposomes	Cholesterol (4.4 mg/ml), triolein (1.2 mg/ml), dioleoylphosphatidylcholine (DOPC) (5.7 mg/ml), dipalmitoylphosphatidylglycerol (DPPG) (1.0 mg/ml), sodium chloride 0.9% w/v, water for injections. (pH 5.5 - 8.5)	Pacira, USA	Lymphomatous meningitis
DepoDur®	Suspension for injection	Morphine sulfate pentahydrate 10 mg/1 ml 15 mg/1,5 ml 20 mg/2 ml	DepoFoam® multivesicular liposomes	Dioleoylphosphatidylcholine (DOPC), dipalmitoilfosfatidildiglicerol (DPPG), cholesterol, triolein, tricaprylin, sodium chloride, hydrochloric acid, diluted (10%), water for injections.	Flynn Pharma, Ireland	Postoperative treatment of pain
Exparel®	Suspension for injection	Bupivacaine hydrochloride 300 mg/20 ml	DepoFoam® multivesicular liposomes	Cholesterol (4.7 mg/ml), 1,2-dipalmitoyl-sn-glycero-3-phospho-rac- (1-glycerol) (DPPG) (0.9 mg/ml), tricaprylin (2.0 mg/ml), 1,2- dierucoyl phosphatidylcholine (DEPC) (8.2 mg/ml). pH 5.8 - 7.4	Pacira, SAD	Postoperative treatment of pain (local and regional infiltrative anesthesia)
Epaxal®	Suspension for injection in a pre-filled syringe	Inactivated hepatitis A virus (strain RG-SB), grown in human diploid (MRC-5) cells. ≥24 IU/0,5 ml	Immunopotentiating reconstituted influenza virosomes (IRIV)	**Virosomes:** Highly purified influenza virus surface antigens (hemagglutinin 10 mg) A/Singapore/6/86 (H1N1) strain, phospholipids lecithin (80 mg), kefalin (20 mg) **Vehicle:** Sodium chloride, Water for injections	Crucell, Switzerland	Hepatitis A vaccine
Inflexal® V	Suspension for injection in a pre-filled syringe	Inactivated Influenza virus surface antigens (haemagglutinin and neuraminidase) strains: • A/California/7/2009 (H1N1), A/Perth/16/2009 (H3N2) -A/Victoria/210/2009 • B/Brisbane/60/2008 • 15 µg haemagglutinin/ 0,5 ml	Immunopotentiating reconstituted influenza virosomes (IRIV)	Sodium chloride, disodium phosphate dihydrate, potassium dihydrogen phosphate, lecithin, water for injections.	Crucell, Switzerland	Influenza vaccine

continued on following page

Table 1. Continued

Name of the Medicinal Product	Pharmaceutical Form	Qualitative and Quantitative Composition	Carrier	List of Excipients	Manufacturer	Indications
Survanta®	Suspension for endotracheopulmonary instillation	Beractant (25 mg/ml) (The extract of bovine lungs, comprising: phospholipids (25 mg/ml) (including saturated phosphatidylcholines) (11.0 to 15.5 mg/ml), triglycerides (from 0.5 to 1.75 mg/ml), free fatty acids (1.4 to 3.5 mg/ml) protein (0.1 – 1.0 mg/ml).	Liposomes	Sodium chloride, palmitic acid, dipalmitoylphosphatidylcholine, tripalmitin, sodium hydroxide, hydrochloric acid, water for injection	AbbVie, USA	Prevention and therapy of respiratory distress syndrome (RDS) in premature infants
Alveofact®	Suspension for endotracheopulmonary instillation	Bovactant (120 mg/1.5 ml and 240 mg/3 ml) (The extract of bovine lungs, comprising: phospholipids (92%), cholesterol (3.2%), a surfactant complex/hydrophobic protein (0.6%), free fatty acids (0.4%).	Liposomes	Sodium chloride, sodium hydrogen carbonate, water for injection	Boehringer Ingelheim GmbH, Germany	Prevention and therapy of respiratory distress syndrome (RDS) in premature infants
Curosurf®	Suspension for endotracheopulmonary instillation	Poractant alpha (80 mg/ml) (Phospholipids (74 mg/ml), low molecular weight hydrophobic proteins (0.9 mg/ml).	Liposomes	Sodium chloride, sodium hydrogen carbonate, water for injection	Chiesi Farmaceutici SpA, Italy	Prevention and therapy of respiratory distress syndrome (RDS) in premature infants
ViaTromb®	Spray gel	Heparin sodium (2400 i.j./g)	Liposomes	Soybean lecithin, ethanol (96%), potassium dihydrogen phosphate, sodium hydroxide, water, purified	Pharbil Waltrop, Germany	Relieve symptoms of varicose veins and superficial thrombophlebitis

Liposomal encapsulation of drug substances allowed increase in therapeutic index of cytotoxic drugs, prolonged release and reduced frequency of administration of analgesics and local anesthetics, and potentiated the immunogenicity of vaccines against hepatitis A and influenza. Furthermore, pharmaceutical products for substitution of pulmonary surfactant in premature infants comprise active substances in the form of liposomal vesicles. On the European market there are spray gel products for dermal application of heparin sodium encapsulated in liposomal carriers (ViaTromb®, Lipohep®). Delivery of the encapsulated drug substances mainly depends on the physicochemical properties of the ingredients of the carrier, its size, structure, and surface properties, the administered dose and route of administration. This chapter aims to describe the main aspects of pharmaceuticals and vaccines with active substances encapsulated in liposomes.

BACKGROUND

Phospholipide drug delivery carriers have significant potential to meet current requirements regarding biocompatibility and nanoencapsulation or microencapsulation of active substances of different physicochemical properties (Djekic et al., 2015; Elnaggar et al., 2014; Li et al., 2015). Phospholipids are compatible with biological membranes. They are also suitable for covalent attachment of active substances (e.g., polyphenols) (Djekic et al., 2015) and specific ligands (e.g., monoclonal antibodies, mannose, folic acid, peptides) in order to increase selectivity and specificity of drug delivery in the target tissue (Torchilin, 2005). Liposomes are spherical vesicles with an aqueous core surrounded by a lipid bilayer (*unilamellar liposomes*) or a larger number of lipid bilayers between which is a water phase, resembling onion layers (i.e., *multilamellar liposomes*). Typical ingredients of the lipid bilayers are phospholipids and cholesterol. Phospholipids in the liposomal vesicles may be of natural origin (i.e., egg and soy lecithin), semi-synthetic or synthetic origin (e.g., phosphatidylcholine, phosphatidylethanolamine, phosphatidylglycerol, dioleoyltrimethylammoniumpropane, dilaurylphosphatidylcholine, dimiristoylphosphatidylethanolamine, dilaurylphosphatidylglycerol, dilaurylphosphatidylglycerol). In conventional liposomes, for the purpose of stabilizing the lipid bilayers, phospholipids are usually combined with cholesterol at a molar ratio of 1:1 or 2:1. Lipid bilayers may also contain sphingolipids, glycolipids, long chain fatty acids, and proteins. The polar moieties of the amphiphilic molecules are oriented towards the aqueous phase, while their nonpolar parts are in the interior of the bilayer. Size of liposomes is typically in the range of 20 nm - 20 µm. Clasification of liposomal vesicles in accordance with their size and structure is presented in Table 2. The relevant literature describes unilamellar liposomes smaller than 100 nm as *nanosomes* (Castor, 2005; Gopalakrishnan et al., 2013). A larger number of liposomal vesicles fused within a single vesicle are referred as *multivesicular vesicles*.

Drawbacks in development of the liposomal carriers, such as high cost of ingredients and unsatisfactory physicochemical stability, encourage design of different types of the related elastic vesicular carriers with the increased flexibility and deformability of the membrane, such as Rovisome®, flexosomes, and ethosomes. This is achieved by increasing the amount of lipids with unsaturated fatty acids or by introduction of surface active agents (e.g., polysorbate 20, polysorbate 80, sodium cholate) and/or ethanol in the membrane. Rovisome® liposomes, patented by ROVI Cosmetics, Germany, contain a high proportion of phospholipids with linoleic acid and other unsaturated fatty acids, which make the bilayer more flexible, but also more susceptible to oxidation (van den Bergh et al., 2001). Ethosomes are vesicles consisting of phospholipids (0.5 - 10%), alcohol (ethanol, isopropanol) (20 - 50%), ethylene

Table 2. Classification of liposomal vesicles according to their size and structure

Type of Liposome Vesicles	Size
Small unilamellar vesicles (SUV)	20 - 100 nm
Medium unilamellar vesicles (MUV)	>100 nm
Large unilamellar vesicles (LUV)	>100 nm
Giant unilamellar vesicles (GUV)	>1 μm
Oligolamellar vesicle (OLV)	0.1 - 1 μm
Multilamellar vesicles (MLV)	>0.5 μm
Multivesicular vesicles	>1 μm

glycol, propylene glycol, or diethylene glycol monoethyl ether (2 - 20%), cholesterol (0.1 - 1%), and water (Torchilin, 2005). Ethosomes may also contain nonionic surfactants from the group of macrogol ethers of fatty alcohols and cationic lipids (e. g., cocamides, polyethoxylated alkyl amines, dodecylamines, and cetrimide) (Mbah et al., 2014; Touitou et al., 2000; Tyagi et al., 2013). Flexosomes are ultradeformable vesicles whose main ingredient is soybean phosphatidylcholine (> 80%) with a high content of linoleic acid, sodium and calcium cholate, sodium deoxycholate, potassium glycyrrhizinate and nonionic surfactants (10 - 25%), such as polysorbate 80 and polysorbate 20. Also, flexosomes usually contain 3 - 10% of ethanol. The average size of flexosomes obtained by patented technology Transfersome® (IDEA, Germany) is 200 - 300 nm (Kumar et al., 2012).

Phospholipide drug delivery carriers have significant potential to meet current requirements regarding biocompatibility and nanoencapsulation or microencapsulation of active substances of different physicochemical properties (Djekic et al., 2015; Elnaggar et al., 2014; Li et al., 2015). Phospholipids, as the main structural components, are compatible with biological membranes. They are also suitable for covalent attachment of active substances (e.g., polyphenols) (Djekic et al., 2015) and specific ligands (e.g., monoclonal antibodies, mannose, folic acid, peptides) in order to increase selectivity and specificity of drug delivery in the target tissue (Torchilin, 2005). In the liposomal vesicles may be introduced ingredients which enable sensitivity of the carrier to variations in the pH, temperature or concentration of particular metabolites in the pathological tissue, and thus control release of the encapsulated active substance.

PROPERTIES AND THERAPEUTIC APPLICATIONS OF LIPOSOMES

Methods of Preparation of Liposomes

Technological expansion over the last 20 years, including rapid progress of nanotechnology, has enabled the design of various types of liposomes and the development and implementation of procedures for their preparation. Liposomes preparation procedures are based on the association of molecules of starting materials and formation of supramolecular associates of bilayer types that form vesicles. The major prerequisite is appropriate selection of the building blocks molecules and their quantitative relationship to form vesicles that have acceptable physical stability. The most important factors that influence the thermodynamic of the self-association process and physicochemical characteristics of the vesicles are: type and concentration of monomers, HLB value and geometry of amphiphilic molecules, and geometry and symmetry of the bilayer membrane. The geometry of the amphiphilic molecule usually is described by the critical packing parameter (cpp), which is determined by the volume of the lipophilic chain, the size of the oil/water interface, and the maximum length of the molecule. Bilayers form tensides in which is $1/2 \leq cpp \leq 1$ (Marianeci et al., 2014). The association of amphiphilic molecules in the bilayer membrane and formation of vesicles is not a spontaneous process, but requires input of energy to the system in the form of agitation (shaking, stirring), warming or ultrasound. The type and size of the liposomal vesicles may be influenced by adjusting the concentration of the starting ingredients, agitation speed, temperature and pressure. A number of methods for the preparation of liposomes are already developed. They can be classified into conventional methods (e.g., lipid hydration based methods, lipid solution injection based methods, and lipid emulsification solution based methods), and novel methods, including microfluidic methods, supercritical fluids based methods, freeze drying of double emulsions, membrane contactor method, hydration of phospholipids deposited on nanostructured materials, and curvature-tuning (spontaneous vesiculation) method. This section commented the most important aspects of the main methods of liposome preparation.

Lipid Hydration Based Methods

The oldest method for preparation of liposomes is lipid hydration method (hydration of dried lipid films, Bangham method, film method) (Bangham et al., 1965). The lipids are dissolved in a suitable organic solvent (e.g., chloroform, methylene chloride, methanol, *tert*-butanol), and then the solvent is removed under reduced pressure (vacuum) or heating, to yield a dry film, paste or a compact pellet. The residue after removal of organic solvent is added to the aqueous phase, wherein the lipids hydrate and form liposomes. Hydration of a phospholipid film may perform as gentle hydration (natural swelling methods), under strong hydrodynamic flows, or the phospholipid film is deposited on electrodes and subsequently hydrated for a couple of hours in the presence of an electric field (*electro-formation*). Substances for encapsulation are dissolved in the organic solvent or the aqueous phase, according to their solubility. The film method is simple and can be applied for a great number of active substances, however, encapsulation efficiency is generally low. In this way are obtained dispersions of large multilamellar vesicles of various sizes, which are further processed by high pressure homogenization (HPH), ultrasound or extrusion, in order to reduce the size and number of lipid bilayers, and to increase uniformity in size of the liposomes. HPH is carried out in microfluidizers or piston homogenizers at a pressure of 0 - 200 bar, for a few thousand cycles. In this way may be obtained the liposomes with the size of 50 - 200 nm. The process is suitable for industrial production of liposomes, including the preparation of sterile liposomal dispersions. Reduction of the size of liposomes by extrusion is performed by using extruders, such as Lipex™ extruder system (Northern Lipids Inc., Canada) and Maximator® HPE (Chemisch-pharmazeutisches Labor, Germany), equipped with filters of defined pore size and under pressure from 5 - 120 bar. The pressure applied in the processing of liposomes by extrusion, as compared to HPH, is lower, thus the possibility of physical destabilization of the vesicles is reduced. Although the extrusion process has better reproducibility than HPH, a major drawback of this process is the risk of clogging of the filter of extruder (Gregoriadis, 2007; Mozafari, 2005; Patil & Jadhav, 2014; Riaz, 1996; Wagner & Vorauer-Uhl, 2011).

Lipid Solution Injection/Emulsification Based Methods

Preparation of liposomes by applying methods based on injection or emulsification of the solution of lipids (solvent injection technique and emulsion technique, respectively) starts with dissolution of lipids in a suitable solvent which is miscible with water (ethanol or propylene glycol) or immiscible with water, respectively. The lipid solution in ethanol or propylene glycol is then injected into the aqueous phase, under vigorous stirring (injection of organic solvent with dissolved phospholipids into an aqueous phase method). Thereafter the solvent was removed by evaporation under reduced pressure, by heating in a water bath, in the chromatography column, by filtration or dialysis. In the modified procedure, the lipids are dissolved in an organic solvent which is immiscible with water, and then the solution was gradually added to the water phase and emulsifies under vigorous stirring (solvent spherule method, reverse phase evaporation method). After that, the organic phase removes with subsequent formation of large unilamellar, oligolamellar, or multilamellar vesicles with high capacity for the encapsulation of active substances, including macromolecules. Liposomes obtained by this procedure do not have a uniform size. Large unilamellar liposomes can be prepared from the dispersion of mixed micelles, which are formed from a suitable lipid and a surfactant (such as cholate, alkyl polyglucosides, octylphenol ethoxylates), with subsequent removal of the surfactant by suitable method (dialysis, gel chromatography, membrane filtration, adsorption on hydrophobic resins or cyclodextrins) (methods based on the removal of a surfactant, detergent dialysis method). The advantages of these methods are high reproducibility and uniformity in the size of liposomes (Gregoriadis, 2007; Mbah et al., 2014; Mozafari 2005; Patil & Jadhav, 2014; Riaz, 1996; Touitou et al., 2000; Tyagi et al., 2013; Wagner & Vorauer-Uhl, 2011).

Novel Methods for Liposome Preparation

Generally, the implementation of liposome preparation procedures in the pharmaceutical industry is related to a number of problems. The development of the liposome manufacturing process and quality control are extremely complicated, thus increase the price of the final product. The presence of organic solvents may damage the encapsulated active ingredient of protein nature. Residues of organic solvents and surfactants in the final pharmaceutical formulation are not desirable because they are potentially toxic and can contribute to physical destabilization and release ("leakage") of encapsulated active ingredient during storage. It is therefore necessary that the method for producing liposomes include time-consuming and expensive purification techniques such as gel filtration and dialysis, as well as to determine the residue content in the final product (Gregoriadis, 2007; Mozafari 2005Riaz, 1996; Wagner & Vorauer-Uhl, 2011). Novel preparation methods, such as microfluidic methods, supercritical reverse phase evaporation method, supercritical anti-solvent (SAS) method, freeze drying of double emulsions, membrane contactor method, hydration of phospholipids deposited on nanostructured materials, and curvature-tuning (spontaneous vesiculation) method, were recently developed in order to overcome the problems that occur with conventional methods (Laouini et al., 2012; Patil & Jadhav, 2014).

Microfluidic methods for liposome formation involves fluid flow in channels having crosssectional dimensions, typically in the range of 5–500 μm. In the last decade, several novel microfluidics-based techniques have been developed to produce liposomes, including micro hydrodynamic focusing (MHF), microfluidic droplets for formation of giant vesicles, pulsed jet flow microfluidics for giant vesicles, thin film hydration in microtubes. In MHF, an aqueous buffer flows along two opposite walls of a specific rectangular or circular micro-channels, while a phospholipid solution in isopropyl alcohol or ethanol flows between the aqueous layers along the axis of the channel. Counter diffusion of water and isopropyl alcohol leads to regions with low alcohol fraction where phospholipids are forced to self-assemble into bilayers which eventually close into liposomes. Liposome formation by MHF method in presence of sonication resulted in smaller liposomes. The features of microfluidic systems that can be used to advantage in liposome production include ability to accurately dispense nanoliter volumes, precise control over the position of the interface, diffusion-dominated axial mixing and continuous mode of operation at low volumes. Formation of giant vesicles in microfluidic droplets can be achieved when two immiscible phases such as oil and water are allowed to flow in a microchannel, under certain conditions. Recently, a novel microfluidic device was developed in which the generation water in oil-emulsion, subsequent removal of the oil phase and transfer of giant vesicles into an aqueous phase takes place on the same device. Water-in-oil-in-water double emulsions prepared by microfluidic method with the phospholipid dissolved in the middle oil phase which was a volatile mixture of toluene and chloroform are used to obtaned giant vesicles when the organic layer removed by evaporations. This method is suitable for incorporation of both hydrophilic and hydrophobic drugs into the vesicles, as well as proteins, cells and microparticles. Pulsed jet flow microfluidics for giant vesicles involves a pulsed jet flow of an aqueous solution from a micro-capillary at a phospholipid bilayer generated by bringing two macro-sized aqueous drops together in a phospholipid containing oil phase. As the oil film between the drops drains, a planar bilayer is formed into which a pulsed jet of aqueous solution is injected using a microdispensor. In thin film hydration in microtubes method, phospholipids dissolved in chloroform were dried inside microtubes of diameters ranging from 200 to 530 µm, and the resulting thin film was hydrated by perfusing an aqueous buffer through the tube. The main features of microfluidic systems that can be used to advantage in liposome production include ability to accurately dispense nanoliter volumes, precise control over the position of the interface, diffusion-dominated axial mixing and continuous mode of operation at low volumes. A possible drawback is the presence of residual organic solvent in the final liposome product (Laouini et al., 2012; Patil & Jadhav, 2014).

Supercritical fluids (SCFs), predominantly carbon dioxide, are increasingly replacing organic solvents in liposome preparation as they enable more efficient separation and purification and the drug encapsulation efficiency. In the first method, the compressed mixture of the phospholipid, SCF and organic cosolvent is injected into the aqueous phase through a nozzle. In the second method, the aqueous phase is first mixed with the phospholipid, SCF and co-solvent mixture and later decompressed rapidly by spraying through a nozzle. In a supercritical reverse phase evaporation method the system pressure reduces gradually by using a variable volume chamber. A supercritical anti-solvent (SAS) method use spraying of the organic co-solvent containing the phospholipid into the supercritical fluid, which acts as the antisolvent, leading to precipitation of micronized particles of the lipids. The particles are hydrated in an aqueous buffer to obtain liposomes. The size of liposomes formed by the SAS method is a functon of the pressure of the system as well as the SCF/co-solvent ratio. The important advantage of the SCF methods is their suitability for scale-up (Laouini et al., 2012; Patil & Jadhav, 2014).

Other novel methods for preparing liposomes such as freeze drying of double emulsions, membrane contactor, hydration of phospholipids deposited on nanostructured materials, and curvature-tuning method, are also reported. Freeze drying of liposome forming lipids and water-soluble carrier materials dissolved in tert-butyl alcohol/water co-solvent systems results in cakes of an isotropic monophasic solution. On addition of water, the freezedried product spontaneously forms a homogenous dispersion of multilamellar vesicles which may then be downsized by extrusion. The important limitation of freeze drying was the relatively low encapsulation efficiency of liposomes, and it may enhance by drying of a water/oil/

water emulsion, where oil phase is the organic solution of phospholipid. Freeze drying technique is also used to solve the long term liposome stability. A modified ethanol injection method where phospholipid solution in ethanol was extruded into an aqueous phase using a membrane contactor enable a high drug encapsulation efficiency (over 90%), enhanced control on liposome size, and continuous operation and scale-up of the process. Hydration of phospholipids deposited on electrospun amphiphilic nanofibres, composed of the hydrophilic polymer polyvinyl pyrrolidone and soybean lecithin was used to prepared monodisperse liposomes which size was modulated by varying the phospholipid/polymer ratio. The spontaneous vesiculation in mixtures of different lipids, sterols, and proteins, induced by rapid change of pH after adding to an aqueous buffer, is introduced as a solvent-free method for the preparation of monodisperse small unilamellar liposomes which size, shape and polydispersity depend mainly on the time interval of pH jump, equilibration time, temperature, and lipid type (Laouini et al., 2012; Patil & Jadhav, 2014).

Encapsulation of Active Substances

The active substances may be encapsulated: passively (on the surface or into the interior of the carrier, by adding the drug during formation of the vesicle); actively (in the prepared vesicle by using mechanisms based on ionic gradient). The efficiency of encapsulation is in the range of 1 - 90%, depending on the structure and the size of liposome and the properties of the active substance. The choice of encapsulation method is also directly reflected on the entrapment efficiency (Marianeci et al., 2014). Passive encapsulation can be carried out physically, by the establishment of hydrogen bonds or hydrophobic interactions between the active substance and the carrier, by dissolving in the aqueous core of the vesicle or by incorporation into the phospholipid bilayer. In passive encapsulation, water-soluble drug substance is dissolved in the aqueous phase used for hydration of lipides. In this case, the amount of encapsulated substance increases with the increase of its solubility in the aqueous phase and the volume of the water phase that fills the core of the liposome. The liposoluble active ingredients are dissolved in an organic solvent, together with a mixture of lipids incorporated into the lipid bilayer of the liposomes. The efficiency of encapsulation depends on the lipophilic drug solubility, molecular size, chemical structure, oil/water partition coefficient, and geometry of the lipid bilayer. Additional approach of passive encapsulation uses the covalent coupling of an active substance to a suitable starting material (e.g., a phospholipid, a polymer, or a protein). The selection of the molecule via which they associate (linker) is essential, since it has to ensure that the conjugate is stable in the biological environment, as well as that the active substance can be released from the carrier at the site of action, under the influence of enzymes or by hydrolysis. The covalent binding of active substances to bilayer constituents has a significant potential in achieving of controlled release (Djekic et al., 2015; Mishra et al., 2010). The passive encapsulation methods which has been proposed for the encapsulation of proteins is based on a cyclic procedure including lyophilisation, rehydration and extrusion of a dispersion of small unilamellar liposomes, which were prepared by the film method and using the solution of the drug substance (i.e., *f*reeze-thaw extrusion, extrusion dehydration-rehydration methods). These methods enable formation of large multilamellar or oligolamelar liposomes (Samad et al., 2007). Part of the drug substance that is not encapsulated usually removes by dialysis, chromatographic techniques, filtration, centrifugation or by using ion-exchange resins (Gregoriadis, 2007; Kumar et al., 2012; Lasic, 1998; Malam et al., 2009; Mozafari, 2005; Riaz, 1996; Storm & Crommelin, 1998).

The active encapsulation is efficient mechanism for the drug molecules which are weak bases or acids. The drug is encapsulated into previously prepared liposomes by adjusting the concentration of hydrogen, manganese, sulfate, acetate or citrate ions (method of pH gradient; gradient method of manganese, sulfate, acetate or citrate ions). Drug substance in the aqueous phase is in the non-ionised form and then diffuses into or through the lipid bilayer (into the liposome). Then, the pH or the concentration of the respective ions is adjusted to a value at which the drug substance is again in an ionized form so as to establish ionic interactions with the lipid bilayer or form poorly soluble salt into the aqueous core, thereby preventing its diffusion out of the liposomes. In the biological environment protons can pass through the lipid bilayer, suppress the ionization of the drug substance, and subsequently, the drug molecules release from the liposomes by diffusion. This encapsulation mechanism is suitable for unstable drugs, so their encapsulation is integrated with drug reconstitution prior administration (Gubernator et al., 2014; Wang et al., 2013).

Characteristics of Liposome Based Pharmaceuticals

Dosage forms of currently marketed liposome based pharmaceutical products are:

- Solutions and suspensions for injection/infusion,
- Powders (lyophilisates) for solutions/suspensions for injection/infusion,
- Suspensions for endotracheopulmonary instillation,
- Liquid spray preparations for cutaneous application (Table 1).

Production of sterile pharmaceutics performs under aseptic conditions and by using sterile starting materials of high purity. The main steps in production process are: preparation of liposomes, reduction of the vesicles size by extrusion, sonication, or HPH, and encapsulation of the drug substance. The excess of the drug removes by dialysis, chromatography, filtration or centrifugation. Membrane filtration is a suitable sterilization method for aqueous dispersions of liposomes smaller than 150 nm. Dispersions of larger liposomes can be sterilized by γ-irradiation. Steam sterilization is not a recommended method because in most cases liposomes destabilize (Lasic, 1998).

Liposomes are susceptible to chemical degradation (by hydrolysis or oxidation of the phospholipids), and physical destabilization in the presence of oils, emulsifying agents, and preservatives, that are common ingredients of pharmaceutical preparations, as well as at high and low temperatures, which leads to aggregation and fusion of the vesicles, and premature release of the encapsulated active substance. Nanosomes are characterized by high surface energy and they are particularly prone to spontaneous agglomeration and aggregation, especially when dispersed in the aqueous vehicles. Disturbation of the physical stability of the carrier may compromise the expected therapeutical and safety profile of the drug. Physical and chemical destabilization of liposomes is particularly pronounced in aqueous vehicles. With the increase in the content of unsaturated fatty acids in the lipid bilayer, increases flexibility of the vesicles as well as their susceptibility to oxidation. Oxidation of double bonds in unsaturated fatty acids of phospholipids results in formation of peroxides, which destabilizes the vesicles and irritate at the site of application. The dispersions of liposomes in the aqueous vehicles are prone to the growth of microorganisms. However, addition of preservatives may also destabilize the liposomal membrane (Gregoriadis, 2007; New, 1990; Sirisha et al., 2012). Acceptable stability during 1 - 3 years of liquid pharmaceutical formulations comprising liposomes can be accomplished by:

- Storing in a refrigerator (2 - 8 °C),
- Adjusting the pH (generally in the range of 5.5 - 8.5),
- Packaging in the presence of liquid nitrogen,
- Addition of antioxidants (tocopherols, butylhydroxyanisole (BHA), butylhydroxytoluene (BHT)), and chelating agents (disodium edetate),
- Using the containers that protects the product from light and oxygen.

Liposomes may irreversibly destabilize at low temperatures, thus the liquid pharmaceutical formulations should not freeze (Lasic, 1998; Wagner & Vorauer-Uhl, 2011). Sterile preparations of liposomes are usually packed in a single dose bottles or the pre-filled syringe of neutral glass Type I. Lyophilization of liposomal dispersions significantly reduce the risk of chemical destabilization, agglomeration, aggregation, and subsequent "leakage" of the drug substance, as well as the growth of microorganisms. Shelf-life of liposomal drugs in the form of powders for injection/infusion is 2 - 4 years at room temperature. Freeze-drying also may cause physical destabilization of the liposomes and the "leakage" of encapsulated active substance. Typically, trehalose is used as a cryoprotectant. Powders for injection/infusion require reconstitution prior to use, by addition of a suitable vehicle (e.g., water for injection, glucose 5% solution for infusion, sodium chloride 0.9% solution for infusion). Rehydration of small unilamellar liposomes is associated with the risk for the conversion into the multilamellar vesicles and the release of the drug substance. Trehalose also effectively prevents fusion of liposomes during reconstitution (Gregoriadis, 2007; Sirisha et al., 2012; Wagner & Vorauer-Uhl, 2011). Drug loaded liposomes for cutaneous administration are suitable for incorporation in vehicles such as aqueous solutions, hydrogels of carbomers or cellulose ethers (e.g., hypromellose, methylcellulose), and hydrophilic creams with a low content of the oil phase and emulsifiers. Avoidance of high temperatures and stirring speeds during the production process is often recommended (Gregoriadis, 2007; Sirisha et al., 2012). In general, the lipid bilayer is permeable for water and sensitive to changes in osmotic parameters in the biological environment after application, which may be related with the risk for physical destabilization. Furthermore, dilution of the drug in the bloodstream (particularly in cases where a volume of distribution is large) can reduce the concentration of carrier ingredients below the critical association concentration, and destabilize the carrier with premature and/or sudden release of encapsulated active substance. When applying cutaneously, conventional liposomes are also prone to physical destabilization mainly on the skin surface (Gregoriadis, 2007; Samad et al., 2007; Sirisha et al., 2012; Wagner & Vorauer-Uhl, 2011).

Parenteral Drug Delivery

Encapsulation of drug substances into the liposomes is important strategy in development of parenteral preparations, which may enable significant improvements of their biopharmaceutical profile and delivery to the site of action, and thus increase therapeutic efficacy and/or reduce side effects, compared with the conventional pharmaceutical preparations (De Villiers et al., 2009; Farokhzad & Langer, 2009; Park, 2007). Currently available pharmaceuticals are designed for intravenous (*i.v.*), intramuscular (*i.m.*), subcutaneous (*s.c.*), and intrathecal (*i.t.*) administration, and for local tissue infiltration (Table 1). Parenteral preparations that have been developed on the principles of microencapsulation/nanoencapsulation of the drug substances into the liposomal carriers enable:

- Increased therapeutic index of cytotoxic drug substances;
- Sustained release of analgesics, anesthetics and antineoplastic agents;
- Enhanced antigenicity of vaccines.

Active substance from the group of antineoplastic agents and antibiotics which are applied intravenously as solutions for injection/infusion, frequently exhibit myelotoxicity, nephrotoxicity, and cardiotoxicity, due to large volume of distribution. In clinical studies it was shown that after *i.v.* application of liposomal dispersions, such drugs in the bloodstream remain encapsulated in the carrier, eliminated much more slowly and passively directed towards tissues affected by a pathological process (the passive targeted drug delivery). In this way their toxicity drastically reduces, and there is possibility to decrease the therapeutic dose of the drug (Mishra et al., 2010; Samad et al., 2007; Sirisha et al., 2012). In biological environment, the biomolecules such as plasma proteins, adsorbe on the carrier in order to reduce the surface energy (opsonization), which is crucial for their biodistribution and recognition by the cells of the reticuloendothelial system (RES) such as liver, spleen and bone marrow. Conventional liposomes larger than 150 nm, particularly with larger zeta-potential, are quickly removed from the circulation by phagocytosis in the RES. This may be employed for passive targeting of malignant and infectious diseases of the RES tissues and organs, particularly with the negatively-charged liposomes having a size in the range of 100-1000 nm. Modification of surface of the liposomes by coating hydrophilic polymers such as polyethylene glycols, linear dextrans, polyvinylpyrrolidone, and polyvinyl alcohol, create steric hindrance for opsonization. This makes them "invisible" for RES and ensures their retention in the systemic circulation (PEGylated, Stealth, long-circulating, sterically stabilized liposomes). Coating of liposomes with PEGs of molecular weight of 1000 - 5000 g/mol extends retention time in the systemic circulation to 45 h and more, while it is up to several hours in conventional liposomes. Small unilamellar liposomes ($\leq$ 100 nm), with rigid bilayer, or PEGylated liposomes with size from 50 - 150 nm and minimal electrical charge, are developed as carriers for antibiotics, antineoplastic drugs, and corticosteroids, for passive targeting of infections, malignant diseases, and inflammatory processes in the not-RES tissues and organs, respectively. PEGylated liposomes pass from the systemic circulation and retain to a greater extent in tissues where the permeability of the vascular endothelium is increased and lymphatic drainage decreased, such as tumor tissues and tissues with inflammation (Enhanced Permeability and Retention (EPR) effect), which is not the case in healthy tissues. PEGylation and the EPR effect are the main mechanisms for passive targeted drug delivery in the treatment of malignancies and other disorders in non-RES tissues and organs in which traditional formulating strategies generally do not provide a satisfactory therapeutic index (Frank et al., 2014; Lammers et al., 2012).

Passive drug targeting restricts the distribution of the drug substance in healthy tissues and organs and reduces elimination through the kidneys. Thus, encapsulation of the drug substance in the liposome-type carriers aims to increase drug bioavailability over corresponding conventional pharmaceutical preparations. Furthermore, nephrotoxicity and other adverse effects that occur after the use of conventional pharmaceutics, are reduced (Qian et al., 2012; Samad et al., 2007; Sirisha et al., 2012; Storm & Crommelin, 1998; Torchilin, 2005; Ye et al., 2000). For example, amphotericin B-loaded liposome (AmBisome® powder for infusion (Table 1) has from 50 to 70 times lower toxicity, while therapeutic doses may be 5 times higher, than those of conventional formulations. The drugs encapsulated in such carriers are also effective against intracellular infections (Schiffelers et al., 2001). Nyotran® powder for solution for infusion (Table 1) comprises nystatin loaded multilamellar liposomes with the drug concentration of 10% w/w. It was categorized by FDA and EMA in 2000, as an orphan drug for the treatment of invasive systemic fungal infections in patients infected with HIV. Therapeutic efficiency of Nyotran® liposomal nystatin in the treatment of systemic mycoses is comparable with *i.v.* applied Fungizone® (Farmar L'Aigle, France) amphotericin B solution for infusion, while nephrotoxicity was observed in 14% and 37% of patients, respectively. Although this study included a relatively small number of patients, the obtained results indicate the possibility of applying Nyotran® liposomal nystatin in the treatment of severe systemic aspergillosis and candidiasis, especially in cases where conventional preparations with other antifungal agents (e.g., itraconazole, posakonazole, amphotericin B) are not effective. There are other examples which demonstrate the improvement of safety profile of pharmaceutical preparations, which has been achieved by encapsulation of the active substance into the liposomes. For instance, Visudyne® powder for solution for infusion (Novartis Europharm, United Kingdom) (Table 1) contains a photosensitive active substance verteporfin in conventional liposomal vesicles. The drug was approved by the EMA for the photodynamic treatment of exudative age-related macular degeneration and secondary subfoveal choroidal neovascularization. After 15 minutes from the application of the infusion, the drug substance is activated under the influence of laser light ($\lambda = 689$ nm; the recommended light intensity of 600 mW/cm^2). Encapsulation reduces distribution of the drug substance and the risk of side effects. Nevertheless, the drug distributed to other parts of the body is not activated, so the patients should not be exposed to direct sunlight or the light of medical devices (lamps in operating rooms, dental offices) for 48 hours after application.

The extravasation of liposomes into interstitial fluid of the tumor likely leads to their physical and chemical destabilization at low pH and under the influence of tissue lipase. Doxil® concentrate for solution for infusion is the first drug with liposomes that has been approved for human use in 1995 in the United States and after that in Europe under the name Caelyx®. It is applied in the form of slow *i.v.* infusion as monotherapy of metastatic breast cancer in patients with high risk for heart disease, in the treatment of multiple myeloma and Kaposi's sarcoma in patients with AIDS and in the treatment of advanced ovarian cancer when they are not achieved improvement after application of platinum derivatives, which are the first line chemotherapeutic. Doxil®/Caelyx® contains doxorubicin sulfate, which is encapsulated in the core of the long-circulated liposomes with the average size from 80 - 100 nm. On the surface of liposomes are hydrophilic linear segments of methoxypolyethylene which diminish the opsonization. In clinical studies it has been shown that doxorubicin remains in circulation for several days ($t_{1/2} \sim 55$h), wherein at least 90% of the drug substance remains encapsulated in the carrier. Cardiotoxicity is 4.5 times lower, and myelosuppression milder. Nausea, vomiting and alopecia are less severe or do not occur. DaunoXome® concentrate for solution for infusion contains daunorubicin citrate encapsulated in the aqueous core of the small unilamellar liposomes (35 - 65 nm) with a lipid bilayer of distearoylphosphatidylcholine and cholesterol (in a ratio of 2:1). In clinical trials conducted in 13 medical centers in the US, it was found that the therapeutic efficacy of this drug is similar to the conventional solution for injection (Adriamycin®, Pharmacia & Upjohn, USA), while the toxicity is reduced. Bioavailability has increased 36 times. Sterically-stabilized liposomes comprising soy phosphatidylcholine, cholesterol, and dipalmitoylphosphatidyl MPEG-DSPE, are under clinical evaluation as carriers for cisplatin (Lipoplatin™, Regulon, USA) and oxaliplatin (Lipoxal™, Regulon, USA) for the treatment of various types of cancer (adenocarcinoma of the pancreas, cancer of the head, neck, breast). According to the obtained results, the therapeutic efficacy of the encapsulated drug is better or similar to conventional formulations of cisplatin. Elimination half-life is 5 days. The concentration of cisplatin in organized tumors is 10 - 200 times higher compared to other tissues. Renal toxicity, peripheral neuropathy, ototoxicity, myelotoxicity, nausea, vomiting and asthenia associated with using conventional preparation of cisplatin, were reduced after applying Lipoplatin™ (Boulikas, 2009). FDA in 2012 gave an initial approval for commercial use of the drug Marqibo® solution for infusion of vincristine sulfate (Table 1). It is categorized as a drug for rare diseases and is indicated in progressive stages of acute lymphoblastic leukemia. The active substance is encapsulated in the liposome vesicles of sphingomyelin and cholesterol, with the average size of 100 nm. The encapsulation of the drug substance increases the retention time of the drug in the bloodstream (plasma clearance of 345 ml/h) almost 30 times as compared with a solution of unencapsulated substance (plasma clearance of 11.34 ml/h), and the bioavailability of vincristine sulfate is significantly higher.

The development of the third generation of liposomes aims to increase the specificity of delivery of the drug substance in the target tissue and to achieve the active targeted drug delivery. The introduction of lipids and polymers in the phospholipid bilayer of sterically stabilized liposomes, that are sensitive to variation of factors in the biological environment (pH, temperature, specific enzymes), is potentially useful for controlled (triggered) activation of the drug release in the diseased tissue or organ (Lammers et al., 2012; Liu et al., 2010). Thermosensitive liposomes comprise phospholipids which are transformed from the crystalline state to the gel at temperatures slightly higher than physiological (39 - 42 °C). The described transformation enables formation of channels through which the encapsulated drug substance releases. Moreover, the increased temperature of the tissue enhances vascular permeability and extravasation of the drug (Couvreur & Vauthier, 2006; Koo et al., 2005; Torchilin, 2005). Patented technology platform Lysolipid Thermally Sensitive Liposomes (LTSL) (Celsion Corporation, USA) was employed for development of ThermoDox® solution for infusion of thermosensitive liposomes with doxorubicin. After *i.v.* administration a target area is exposed to radio waves, microwaves or ultrasound, to cause mild local hyperthermia (39 - 42 ° C) which triggers the release of doxorubicin from the carrier. In vivo animal studies showed that the concentration of doxorubicin in tumor tissue after application of ThermoDox® infusion was 25 times higher compared to conventional solution for infusion and 5 times higher compared to the reference liposome based preparation. The clinical trials for primary and metastatic tumors of the liver, for ThermoDox® in combination with radiofrequency ablation, are completed. The liposomes with a pH-sensitive polymer in the lipid bilayer (pH-sensitive liposomes) are physically unstable in the acidic environment of the tumor tissue, where the drug substances release. The development of this strategy requires to design liposomes that are sensitive to changes in pH from 7.4 (systemic circulation) to 6.5 (tumor tissue) or 5.0 (cell organelles such as lysozyme, endosomes). Phospholipid degradation under the influence of enzymes whose level is elevated in tumor tissue, such as phospholipases and alkaline phosphatase, also may enable release of the encapsulated drug. The recent research studies also demonstrated examples of the use of ultrasoud, light or magnetic field to trigger drug release from the echogenic ("bubble") liposomes, photo-sensitive liposomes, and magnetically responsive liposomes, respectively (Allen & Cullis, 2013). The surface of the long-circulating liposomes may be modified by the covalent attachment of ligands for molecular recognition of the receptor on the surface of tumor cells, such as monoclonal antibodies specific for the tumor cells membrane antigen, transferrin, folic acid, and mannose. The presence of the antibody and the proteins on the surface of the liposomes increases their immunogenicity and risk of uptake in the RES. Therefore, preference is given to the small molecules such as folic acid and mannose (Lammers et al., 2012; Mishra et al., 2010).

The subcutaneous (*s.c.*) and intramuscular (*i.m.*) administration of parenteral preparations containing liposomes is suitable to achieve sustained release of encapsulated drug substances in order to reduce toxicity and/or frequency of application (Glantz et al., 1999). For this purpose, large multilamellar liposomes and multivesicular vesicles are preferred due to longer retention on the application site, in comparison with small unilamellar vesicles. Pacira Pharmaceuticals (USA) patented technology DepoFoam® multivesicular vesicles provide sustained release of encapsulated active substances up to 30 days. So far, this technology has been used in development of: suspension for intrathecal injection of cytarabine (DepoCyt®), suspension for epidural injection of morphine chloride (DepoDur®), and suspension for injection for local and regional infiltration of bupivacaine hydrochloride (Exparel®) (Table 1). The DepoFoam® carrier consists of numerous water compartments separated with phospholipid bilayers composed of cholesterol, dioleoylphosphatidylcholine, dipalmitoylphosphatidylcholine, and triglycerides. Size of DepoFoam® multivesicular liposomes is approximately several tens of micrometers, and they have high capacity for the drug encapsulation. Thus, the relatively large amount of active substance may be administered in a small volume of the pharmaceutical formulation (Mantripragada, 2002). The main mechanism of drug release is gradual erosion and reorganization of the lipid membranes. The release rate depends on quantitative and qualitative composition of lipids in the bilayers (100 - 230 h, 48 h, or 72 h, from DepoCyt®, DepoDur®, and Exparel®, respectively) (Bramlett et al., 2012; Chahar & Cummings, 2012; Gambling et al., 2005; Glantz et al., 1999; Nagle & Gerancher, 2007; Richard et al., 2011; White et al., 2009; Ye et al., 2000).

Vaccine Adjuvants

Specific unilamellar vesicles may be used as carriers of antigens in vaccines (adjuvants) to raise their immunogenicity and accelerate, enhance and/or prolong the protective effect (immunopotentiating reconstituted influenza virosomes, IRIV) (Gregoriadis, 2007). Size of virosomes (~ 150 nm) and their structure is very similar to the capsid of influenza virus. In the phospholipid bilayer of virosomes are embedded influenza hemagglutinin and neuraminidase. These are functional glycoproteins that play a key role for adjuvant properties of virosomes. Virosomes allow delivery of the encapsulated antigen into the cytoplasm of antigen-presenting cells (macrophages and dendritic cells). After *i.m.* administration of IRIV based vaccines, the presence of specific antigens initiates a cascade of processes that activate cellular and humoral immune response. Virosomes as adjuvants in vaccines represent an alternative to standard adjuvants such as aluminum hydroxide and aluminum phosphate, which cause a variety of local adverse reactions upon vaccine administration. Vaccines developed on virosomes have no adverse effects after parenteral (*i.m.*) administration (Glück, 1999; Herzog et al., 2009; Holzer et al., 1996), although, the use of virosomes in vaccines for mucosal immunization is associated with a certain risk. For example, the virosome based vaccine for nasal immunization against influenza virus (NasalFlu®) was withdrawn from the market after several months, because of increased risk to cause facial paralysis (Couvreur & Vauthier, 2006; Lewis et al., 2009).

Dermal and Transdermal Drug Delivery

The research on potential application of vesicular nanocarriers for dermal and transdermal drug delivery has been intensified over the past decade. Encapsulation of active substances in liposomes increases their stability, prolongs their retention on skin and improves their percutaneous penetration and permeation. Numerous investigations at the pre-clinical and clinical level, on a large number of formulations comprising encapsulated active substances, showed improvement in percutaneous delivery of nonsteroidal antiinflammatory drugs, hormones, antiviral and antifungal drugs, cytostatics and antiparkinsonians (Marianeci et al., 2014; Neubert, 2011). Transdermal drug delivery is considered a significant alternative route of administration that enables to avoid irritation and bypass degradation of the drug in the GIT as well as to achieve a therapeutic effect with significantly less systemic side effects. However, the structure and function of the skin as the outer barrier restrict the ability of the large number of substances to penetrate the skin in appropriate extent and rate. Results of pre-clinical studies indicate that conventional liposomes can improve penetration and permeation of drug substances in deeper layers of skin or to provide transdermal delivery of poorly soluble drug substances by:

- Increasing their solubility,
- Fusion of the lipid bilayer with the cell membrane,
- Release of the encapsulated drug and distribution into the skin,
- Influence of phospholipides from the liposomal bilayers as penetration/permeation enhancers.

Although liposomes are generally suitable for the encapsulation of various active substances, this type of carriers is scarcely used in development of pharmaceutical preparations for cutaneous application. For instance, unilamellar liposomes are used as carriers for transdermal delivery of water-soluble polysaccharide heparin sodium which is dissolved in aqueous core of the carrier. The drug loaded vesicles are dispersed in a mixture of water and ethanol. Such products (Heparin PUR/-Forte Ratiopharm®, Lipohep®, ViaTromb®) (Table 1) are used to relieve the symptoms of varicose veins. Rades et al. (1997) found that heparin sodium loaded liposomes do not penetrate into the skin, but after evaporation of the liquid phase, they transform into multilamellar vesicles and lamellar liquid crystal mesophase ("gel"), so that penetration enhancing effect of heparin can be attributed to phospholipids from the liposomes. Clinical trials that have been conducted in patients with superficial thrombophlebitis (Górski et al., 2005; Katzenschlager et al., 2003; Katzenschlager et al., 2007) demonstrated similar efficacy for relieving pain, redness, and limiting the size of thrombus was observed in the liposome based product applied on the skin at a dose of 1832 IU once daily during 1 to 2 weeks, in comparison with a subcutaneously administered dose of 40 mg of enoxaparin-sodium solution (Clexane®). It is well established that the deeper layers of the skin can reach only nanosomes with a diameter of <50 nm, and vesicles similar to liposomes with the high degree of flexibility and deformability of the membrane such as Rovisome®, flexosomes and ethosomes, which comprise an increased fraction of single-chain lipids, surfactants (polysorbate 20, polysorbate 80, sodium cholate) and ethanol, respectively. Nonionic surfactants provide elasticity and deformability of the membrane. As the contents of sodium cholate and sodium deoxycholate increase, diameter of the flexosomes decreases. For example, the average size of flexosomes produced by patented technology Transfersome® (IDEA, Germany) is 200-300 nm (Kumar et al., 2012). It is assumed that the shape of these vesicles adjusted so that they can penetrate through intact skin in the direction of osmotic gradient, carrying the active substance to the deeper layers of the skin, however, the detailed mechanism is not elucidate (Cevc, 2004; Honeywell-Nguyen & Bouwstra, 2005). As established, these mechanisms are likely similar to those proposed for vesicular carriers based on nonionic surfactants (niosomes), which have a structure similar to liposomes. Furthermore, ethosomes have a high ethanol content, which affects the polar groups of lipid molecules of stratum corneum increasing his fluidity. In addition, ethanol may partially extract lipids from the surface layer of the skin and increase the intercellular permeability.

By using this type of carrier and adjusting the contents of ethanol, water and/or a polyol, transdermal drug delivery may significantly enhance (Dubey et al., 2007; Elsayed et al., 2007). Diractin® gel (IDEA, Germany) containing ketoprofen 22.9 mg/g in Transfersome® flexosomes is under current clinical trials and it is intended for alleviating inflammation and pain in superficial joints affected by osteoarthritis. The aim of ketoprofen encapsulation is to provide its permeation together with the carrier to the deep layers of the skin, where it is gradually released from the carrier and delivered into the subcutaneous tissue. Clinical evaluation of the preparation TDT® 067 have shown that the encapsulation of terbinafine (1.5%) in the Transfersome® carrier allows penetration into the nail plate and surrounding tissue, as well as in the hyphae of dermatophytes, and thus provides more efficient suppression of onychomycosis, as compared to conventional preparations (Ghannoum et al., 2012). Of particular importance is the possibility of transdermal application of insulin encapsulated in flexosomes. The company IDEA (Germany) patented Transfersulin® flexosomes with human recombinant insulin, 40 IU/ml. Several clinical studies have shown a significant reduction in therapeutic application of blood glucose after percutaneous administration of Transfersulin®. The encapsulation of insulin into flexosomes allows drug substance to reach the systemic circulation and maintaining normoglycemia over several hours, similar to subcutaneously injected insulin preparations.

Pulmonary Surfactant Substitutes

Pharmaceutical preparations for prevention and therapy of the respiratory distress syndrome (RDS), hyaline membrane disease (HMD), or surfactant deficiency in newborn babies, include ingredients that are similar to the pulmonary surfactant (phospholipids and specific proteins). RDS is a major cause of acute mortality and acute morbidity in the preterm baby and may also be related for long term respiratory and neurologic sequelae. Lung surfactant is a mixture of substances, mainly phospholipids and specific proteins, lining the internal surface of alveoli and stabilising alveoli from collapse at end-expiration. Pulmonary surfactant substitutes for intratracheal administration were developed to replace this deficiency of endogenous pulmonary surfactant. Marketed sterile suspensions for intratracheal administration for surfactant replacement contain constituents of pulmonary surfactant of synthetic or animal origin and associated into liposomal vesicles (Couvreur & Vauthier, 2006; Fox & Sothinathan, 2005). The pionir products of this type are Alveofact® (Dr Karl Thomae GmbH, Germany) and Surfacten® (Surfactant TA, Tokyo Tanabe, Japan), and they were placed on the market in the late 1980s. After that, several similar drugs (Curosurf®; Survanta®) (Table 1) have been approved for human use. These pharmaceutical products contain pulmonary surfactants of natural origin: beractant (bovine lung extract) and poractant alpha (extract of porcine lungs) isolated by extraction with organic solvents (e.g., chloroform, methanol). Inactive ingredients are suitable phospholipids, fatty acids, triglycerides, and hydrophobic proteins, which are added to standardize the formulation regarding the capability of lowering the surface tension as in human pulmonary surfactant. Excipients and pulmonary surfactant components form liposomal vesicles. For instance, Survanta® consists of about 45% of lamellar-vesicular forms and 55% of crystals, as demonstrated by electron microscopy. Such products are available as unit dosage forms in ready to use clear colourless Type I glass vials that should be stored in a refrigerator at +2°C to +8°C. The vial should be warmed to room temperature before administration, for example by holding it in the hand or by standing at room temperature for 20 minutes, and gently turned upside down a few times, without shaking, in order to obtain a uniform suspension. After intratracheal instillation, the product quickly spreads across the air-liquid interfaces of the alveoli, prevents their collapse during respiration and provide an increase in alveolar ventilation. In most cases, the effect lasts for at least 72 h after administration of a single dose of a suspension for endotracheopulmonary instillation.

FUTURE RESEARCH DIRECTIONS

The use of liposomes as carriers for encapsulation of the drug substances is an important tool for therapeutic improvements that cannot be achieved by conventional technological processing. It is of particular importance for cytotoxic agents whose administration is associated with severe side effects and low therapeutic efficiency. The majority of marketed liposome based pharmaceuticals employ the first or the second generation of liposomes. The current development is focused on design of a more complex third generation of liposomes by using principles of the active targeted drug delivery. An increased number of new pharmaceutical preparations employing the third generation liposomes is in the stage of clinical trials. In addition, development of multifunctional liposomal carriers that could be used for simultaneous active targeted delivery of imaging diagnostic agents and active substances (theranostics) is a growing research field. There is a significant effort for further development of different liposome related carriers, by modifying their nature and/or structure, in order to manipulate membrane flexibility, physicochemical stability, surface properties in biological environment, and drug delivery potential. The main challenges in the future may appear during the development and approval process for liposome based pharmaceutical products that cannot be clearly classified as pharmaceutics, biopharmaceutics, diagnostic agents, or medical devices, and which may require additional evaluation of the quality, safety and efficiency.

CONCLUSION

Liposomes is the overall term for a group of vesicular carriers which may consist of one or more bilayers formed by association of suitable amphiphilic molecules (phospholipids, cholesterol, ethanol, and/or surfactants), in such a way that the polar end oriented towards the aqueous phase, the non-polar portion of the molecule is in the interior of the bilayer, and the aqueous phase is located in the core, and possibly between bilayers. They are suitable for encapsulation of hydrophilic, lipophilic and amphiphilic active substances. Depending on the composition, physical and chemical stability, suitability to modify the surface properties and flexibility of the membrane vesicles, they are designated as conventional liposomes, liposomes of the second and the third generation designed for targeted drug delivery, and related vesicular carriers such as ethosomes, flexosomes, virosomes, and multivesicular vesicles. Furthermore, they differ from each other in terms of the capacity for encapsulation of the active substances and potential for their delivery in biological systems. Liposomes are generally considered as biocompatible vesicular carriers suitable for microencapsulation and nanoencapsulation of drug substances with various physicochemical characteristics. A numerous pharmaceutical products with drug loaded liposomes are already developed for different routes of application (parenteral, oral, cutaneous, pulmonal), with significant improvements of their biopharmaceutical profile and potential for delivery of active agents to site of action, thus increased therapeutic efficacy and/or reduced side effects, in comparison with their conventional equivalents. The current number of the marketed liposome based pharmaceutics is much lower compared to the vast research in this area in numerous academic and clinical centers worldwide. The main reasons for this are: low reproducibility of the results obtained from investigations on *in vitro* and *in vivo* models, due to the high complexity of the mechanisms of active targeted delivery and variability in physicochemical properties of drug loaded carriers and biological systems; complex process control and quality control of the manufacturing process; high risk for physicochemical destabilization, including aggregation/agglomeration; high production costs; poorly developed regulatory framework on pharmaceuticals based on drug nanoencapsulation strategies.

REFERENCES

Allen, T. M., & Cullis, P. R. (2013). Liposomal drug delivery systems: From concept to clinical applications. *Advanced Drug Delivery Reviews*, *65*(1), 36–48. doi:10.1016/j.addr.2012.09.037 PMID:23036225

Bangham, A. D., Standish, M. M., & Watkins, J. C. (1965). Diffusion of univalent ions across the lamellae of swollen phospholipids. *Journal of Molecular Biology*, *13*(1), 238–252. doi:10.1016/S0022-2836(65)80093-6 PMID:5859039

Boulikas, T. (2009). Clinical overview on Lipoplatin™: A successful liposomal formulation of cisplatin. *Expert Opinion on Investigational Drugs*, *18*(8), 1–22. doi:10.1517/13543780903114168 PMID:19053877

Bramlett, K., Onel, E., Viscusi, E. R., & Jones, K. (2012). A randomized, double-blind, dose-ranging study comparing wound infiltration of DepoFoam bupivacaine, an extended-release liposomal bupivacaine, to bupivacaine HCl for postsurgical analgesia in total knee arthroplasty. *The Knee*, *19*(5), 530–536. doi:10.1016/j.knee.2011.12.004 PMID:22285545

Castor, T. P. (2005). Phospholipid nanosomes. *Current Drug Delivery*, *2*(4), 329–340. doi:10.2174/156720105774370195 PMID:16305436

Cevc, G. (2004). Lipid vesicles and other colloids as drug carriers on the skin. *Advanced Drug Delivery Reviews*, *56*(5), 675–711. doi:10.1016/j.addr.2003.10.028 PMID:15019752

Chahar, P., & Cummings, K. C. III. (2012). Liposomal bupivacaine: A review of a new bupivacaine formulation. *Journal of Plant Research*, *5*, 257–264. PMID:23049275

Couvreur, P., & Vauthier, C. (2006). Nanotechnology: Intelligent Design to Treat Complex Disease. *Pharmaceutical Research*, *23*(7), 1417–1450. doi:10.1007/s11095-006-0284-8 PMID:16779701

Dapergolas, G., & Gregoriadis, G. (1976). Hypoglycaemic effect of liposome-entrapped insulin administered intragastrically into rats. *Lancet, 2*(7990), 824-827.

De Villiers, M. M., Aramwit, P., & Kwon, G. S. (Eds.). (2009). *Nanotechnology in drug delivery*. New York, NY: Springer. doi:10.1007/978-0-387-77667-5

Djekic, L., Krajisnik, D., Martinovic, M., Djordjevic, D., Primorac, M. (2015). Characterization of gelation process and drug release profile of thermosensitive liquid lecithin/poloxamer 407 based gels as carriers for percutaneous delivery of ibuprofen. *International Journal of Pharmaceutics, 490*(1-2), 180-189.

Djekic, L., Krajisnik, D., & Micic, Y. (2015). Polyphenolics-Phospholipid Complexes as Natural Cosmetic Ingredients: Properties and Application. Tenside, Surfactants. *Detergents*, *52*(3), 186–192.

Dubey, V., Mishra, D., Nahar, M., & Jain, N. K. (2007). Vesicles as tools for the modulation of skin permeability. *Expert Opinion on Drug Delivery*, *4*(6), 579–593. doi:10.1517/17425247.4.6.579 PMID:17970662

Elnaggar, Y. S., El-Refaie, W. M., El-Massik, M. A., & Abdallah, O. Y. (2014). Lecithin based nanostructured gels for skin delivery: An update on state of art and recent applications. *Journal of Controlled Release*, *180*, 10–24. doi:10.1016/j.jconrel.2014.02.004 PMID:24531009

Elsayed, M. M. A., Abdallah, O. Y., Naggar, V. F., & Khalafallah, N. M. (2007). Lipid vesicles for skin delivery of drugs: Reviewing three decades of research. *International Journal of Pharmaceutics*, *332*(1-2), 1–16. doi:10.1016/j.ijpharm.2006.12.005 PMID:17222523

Farokhzad, O. C., & Langer, R. (2009). Impact of nanotechnology on drug delivery. *ACS Nano*, *3*(1), 16–20. doi:10.1021/nn900002m PMID:19206243

Fox, G. F., & Sothinathan, U. (2005). The choice of surfactant for treatment of respiratory distress syndrome in preterm infants: A review of the evidence. *Infant*, *1*, 8–12.

Frank, D., Tyagi, C., Tomar, L., Echoonara, Y., du Toit, L. C., Kumar, P., & Pillay, V. et al. (2014). Overview of the role of nanotechnological innovations in the detection and treatment of solid tumors. *International Journal of Nanomedicine*, *9*, 589–613. PMID:24489467

Gambling, D., Hughes, T., Martin, G., Horton, W., & Manvelian, G. (2005). A comparison of Depodur, a novel, single-dose extended-release epidural morphine, with standard epidural morphine for pain relief after lower abdominal surgery. *Anesthesia and Analgesia*, *100*(4), 1065–1074. doi:10.1213/01.ANE.0000145009.03574.78 PMID:15781524

Ghannoum, M., Isham, N., Henry, W., Kroon, H.-A., & Yurdakul, S. (2012). Evaluation of the Morphological Effects of TDT 067 (Terbinafi ne in Transfersome) and Conventional Terbinafi ne on Dermatophyte Hyphae In Vitro and In Vivo. *Antimicrobial Agents and Chemotherapy*, *56*(5), 2530–2534. doi:10.1128/AAC.05998-11 PMID:22354309

Glantz, M. J., LaFollette, S., Jaeckle, K. A., Shapiro, W., Swinnen, L., Royental, J. R., & Howell, S. B. et al. (1999). Randomized trial of a slow-release versus a standard formulation of cytarabine for the intrathecal treatment of lymphomatous meningitis. *Journal of Clinical Oncology*, *17*, 3110–3116. PMID:10506606

Glück, R. (1999). Adjuvant activity of immunopotentiating reconstituted influenza virosomes (IRIVs). *Vaccine*, *17*(13-14), 1782–1787. doi:10.1016/S0264-410X(98)00440-X PMID:10194840

Gopalakrishnan, A. M., Kundu, A. K., Mandal, T. K., & Kumar, N. (2013). Novel nanosomes for gene delivery to Plasmodium falciparum-infected red blood cells. *Scientific Reports*, *3*, 1534. doi:10.1038/srep01534 PMID:23525038

Górski, G., Szopiński, P., Michalak, J., Marianowska, A., Borkowski, M., Geremek, M., & Noszczyk, W. et al. (2005). Liposomal heparin spray: A new formula in adjunctive treatment of superficial venous thrombosis. *Angiology*, *56*(1), 9–17. doi:10.1177/000331970505600102 PMID:15678251

Gregoriadis, G. (Ed.). (2007). Liposome Technology. New York, NY: Informa Healthcare.

Gubernator, J., Lipka, D., Korycińska, M., Kempińska, K., Milczarek, M., Wietrzyk, J., & Kozubek, A. et al. (2014). Efficient Human Breast Cancer Xenograft Regression after a Single Treatment with a Novel Liposomal Formulation of Epirubicin Prepared Using the EDTA Ion Gradient Method. *PLoS ONE*, *9*(3), e91487. doi:10.1371/journal.pone.0091487 PMID:24621591

Herzog, C., Hartmann, K., Künzi, V., Kürsteiner, O., Mischler, R., Lazar, H., & Glück, R. (2009). Eleven years of Inflexal® V-a virosomal adjuvanted influenza vaccine. *Vaccine*, *27*(33), 4381–4387. doi:10.1016/j.vaccine.2009.05.029 PMID:19450630

Holzer, B. R., Hatz, C., Schmid-Sissolak, D., Glück, R., Althaus, B., & Egger, M. (1996). Immunogenicity and adverse effects of inactivated virosome versus alum-adsorbed hepatitis A vaccine: A randomized controlled trial. *Vaccine*, *14*(10), 982–986. doi:10.1016/0264-410X(96)00042-4 PMID:8873392

Honeywell-Nguyen, P. L., & Bouwstra, J. A. (2005). Vesicles as a tool for transdermal and dermal delivery. *Drug Discovery Today. Technologies*, *2*(1), 67–74. doi:10.1016/j.ddtec.2005.05.003 PMID:24981757

Katzenschlager, R., Ugurluoglu, A., Minar, E., & Hirschl, M. (2003). Liposomal heparin-spraygel in comparison with subcutaneous low molecular weight heparin in patients with superficial venous thrombosis. A randomized, controlled, open multicentre study. *Journal für Kardiologie*, *10*, 375–378.

Katzenschlager, R., Ugurluoglu, A., Sipos, G., Bihari, I., Anyova, E. B., Hirschl, M., & Cencora, A. et al. (2007). Efficacy and tolerability of liposomal heparin spraygel as an add-on treatment in the management of superficial venous thrombosis. *Angiology*, *58*(1SSuppl 1), S27–S35. doi:10.1177/0003319706297741 PMID:17478880

Koo, O. M., Rubinstein, I., & Onyuksel, H. (2005). Role of nanotechnology in targeted drug delivery and imaging: A concise review. *Nanomedicine; Nanotechnology, Biology, and Medicine*, *1*(3), 193–212. doi:10.1016/j.nano.2005.06.004 PMID:17292079

Kumar, A., Pathak, K., & Bali, V. (2012). Ultra-adaptable nanovesicular systems: A carrier for systemic delivery of therapeutic agents. *Drug Discovery Today*, *17*(21/22), 1233–1241. doi:10.1016/j.drudis.2012.06.013 PMID:22766375

Kumar, K. P. S., Bhowmik, D., & Deb, L. (2012). Recent Trends in Liposomes Used As Novel Drug Delivery System. *The Pharma Innovation Journal, 1*, 29-38. Available from The Pharma Innovation Journal Web site: http://www.thepharmajournal.com

Lammers, T., Kiessling, F., Hennink, W. E., & Storm, G. (2012). Drug targeting to tumors: Principles, pitfalls and (pre-) clinical progress. *Journal of Controlled Release*, *161*(2), 175–187. doi:10.1016/j.jconrel.2011.09.063 PMID:21945285

Laouini, A., Jaafar-Maalej, C., Limayem-Blouza, I., Sfar, S., Charcosset, C., & Fessi, H. (2012). Preparation, Characterization and Applications of Liposomes: State of the Art. *Journal of Colloid Science and Biotechnology*, *1*(2), 147–168. doi:10.1166/jcsb.2012.1020

Lasic, D. D. (1998). Novel applications of liposomes. *Trends in Biotechnology*, *16*(7), 307–321. doi:10.1016/S0167-7799(98)01220-7 PMID:9675915

Lewis, D. J. M., Huo, Z., Barnett, S., Kromann, I., Giemza, R., Galiza, E., Woodrow, M., Thierry-Carstensen, B., Andersen, P., Novicki, D., Del Giudice, G., Rappuoli, R. (2009). Transient Facial Nerve Paralysis (Bell's Palsy) following Intranasal Delivery of a Genetically Detoxified Mutant of Escherichia coli Heat Labile Toxin. *PLoS One, 4*(9), e6999. doi:10.1371/journal.pone.0006999

Li, J., Wang, X., Zhang, T., Wang, C., Huang, Y., Luo, X., & Deng, Y. (2015). A review on phospholipids and their main applications in drug delivery systems. *Asian Journal of Pharmaceutical Sciences*, *10*(2), 81–98. doi:10.1016/j.ajps.2014.09.004

Liu, Y., Niu, T., Zhang, L., & Yang, J. (2010). Review on nano-drugs. *Natural Science*, *2*(01), 41–48. doi:10.4236/ns.2010.21006

Malam, Y., Loizidou, M., & Seifalian, A. M. (2009). Liposomes and nanoparticles: Nanosized vehicles for drug delivery in cancer. *Trends in Pharmacological Sciences*, *30*(11), 592–599. doi:10.1016/j.tips.2009.08.004 PMID:19837467

Mantripragada, S. (2002). A lipid based depot (DepoFoam® technology) for sustained release drug delivery. *Progress in Lipid Research*, *41*(5), 392–406. doi:10.1016/S0163-7827(02)00004-8 PMID:12121719

Marianeci, C., Marzio, L., Rinaldi, F., Celia, F., Paolino, D., Alhaique, F., & Carafa, M. et al. (2014). Niosomes from 80s to present: The state of the art. *Advances in Colloid and Interface Science*, *205*, 187–206. doi:10.1016/j.cis.2013.11.018 PMID:24369107

Mbah, C. C., Builders, P. F., & Attama, A. A. (2014). Nanovesicular carriers as alternative drug delivery systems: Ethosomes in focus. *Expert Opinion on Drug Delivery*, *11*(1), 45–59. doi:10.1517/17425247.2013.860130 PMID:24294974

Mishra, B., Patel, B. B., & Tiwari, S. (2010). Colloidal nanocarriers: A review on formulation technology, types and applications toward targeted drug delivery. *Nanomedicine; Nanotechnology, Biology, and Medicine*, *6*(1), 9–24. doi:10.1016/j.nano.2009.04.008 PMID:19447208

Mozafari, M. R. (2005). Liposomes: An overview of manufacturing techniques. *Cellular & Molecular Biology Letters*, *10*, 711–719. PMID:16341279

Nagle, P., & Gerancher, J. C. (2011). DepoDur® (extended-release epidural morphine): A review of an old drug in a new vehicle. *Techniques in Regional Anesthesia & Pain Management*, *11*(1), 9–18. doi:10.1053/j.trap.2007.02.011

Neubert, R. H. H. (2011). Potentials of new nanocarriers for dermal and transdermal drug delivery. *European Journal of Pharmaceutics and Biopharmaceutics*, *77*(1), 1–2. doi:10.1016/j.ejpb.2010.11.003 PMID:21111043

New, R. R. C. (Ed.). (1990). *Liposomes a pratical approach.* Oxford, UK: Oxford University Press.

Park, K. (2007). Nanotechnology: What it can do for drug delivery. *Journal of Controlled Release*, *120*(1-2), 1–3. doi:10.1016/j.jconrel.2007.05.003 PMID:17532520

Patil, Y. P., & Jadhav, S. (2014). Novel methoda for liposome preparation. *Chemistry and Physics of Lipids*, *177*, 8–18. doi:10.1016/j.chemphyslip.2013.10.011 PMID:24220497

Qian, S., Li, C., & Zuo, Z. (2012). Pharmacokinetics and disposition of various drug loaded liposomes. *Current Drug Metabolism*, *13*(4), 372–395. doi:10.2174/138920012800166562 PMID:22443534

Rades, T., Gerke, A., Schutze, W., & Muller-Goymann, C. C. (1997). Characterization of a commercial liposome spray. *Die Pharmazie*, *52*(1), 44–50. PMID:9035234

Riaz, M. (1996). Liposomes preparation methods. *Pakistan Journal of Pharmaceutical Sciences*, *19*, 65–77. PMID:16414777

Richard, B., Merryman, T., Newton, P., Ott, L., Haan, D., Brubaker, A., . . . One, E. (2011). *Safety Evaluation of a Novel Pharmaceutical Excipient (DEPC) in EXPAREL™, an Extended-Release Liposomal Formulation of Bupivacaine*. The 38th Annual Meeting & Exposition of the Controlled Release Society, National Harbor, MD. Retrieved from Pacira Pharmaceuticals Inc. Web site: http://investor.pacira.com/phoenix.zhtml?c=220759&p=irol-newsArticle&ID=1591609

Samad, A., Sultana, Y., & Aqil, M. (2007). Liposomal Drug Delivery Systems: An Update Review. *Current Drug Delivery*, *4*(4), 297–305. doi:10.2174/156720107782151269 PMID:17979650

Schiffelers, R., Storm, G., & Bakker-Woudenberg, I. (2001). Liposome-encapsulated aminoglycosides in pre-clinical and clinical studies. *The Journal of Antimicrobial Chemotherapy*, *48*(3), 333–344. doi:10.1093/jac/48.3.333 PMID:11532996

Sirisha, V. N. L., BhavaniHarika, I., Sruthi, B., Namrata, M., Kirankumar, P., Kiran Kumar Rao, Y., … UmaMaheshwaraRao, O. (2012). Liposomes – the potential drug carriers. *IOSR Journal of Pharmacy*, *2*, 26-38.

Storm, G., & Crommelin, D. (1998). Liposomes: Quo vadis? *Pharmaceutical Science & Technology Today*, *1*(1), 19–31. doi:10.1016/S1461-5347(98)00007-8

Torchilin, V. (2005). Recent advances with liposomes as pharmaceutical carriers. *Nature Reviews. Drug Discovery*, *4*(2), 145–160. doi:10.1038/nrd1632 PMID:15688077

Touitou, E., Dayan, N., Bergelson, L., Godin, B., & Eliaz, M. (2000). Ethosomes – novel vesicular carriers for enhanced delivery: Characterization and skin penetration properties. *Journal of Controlled Release*, *65*(3), 403–418. doi:10.1016/S0168-3659(99)00222-9 PMID:10699298

Tyagi, L. K., Kumar, S., Maurya, S. S., & Kori, M. L. (2013). Ethosomes: Novel Vesicular Carrier for enhanced transdermaldrug delivery system. *Bulletin of Pharmaceutical Research*, *3*(1), 6–13.

van den Bergh, B. A., Wertz, P. W., Junginger, H. E., & Bouwstra, J. A. (2001). Elasticity of vesicles assessed by electron spin resonance, electron microscopy and extrusion measurements. *International Journal of Pharmaceutics*, *217*(1-2), 13–24. doi:10.1016/S0378-5173(01)00576-2 PMID:11292538

Wagner, A., & Vorauer-Uhl, K. (2011). Liposome Technology for Industrial Purposes. *Journal of Drug Delivery*. 10.1155/2011/591325

Wang, Y., Tu, S., Pinchuk, A. N., & Xiong, M. P. (2013). Active drug encapsulation and release kinetics from hydrogel-in-liposome nanoparticles. *Journal of Colloid and Interface Science*, *406*, 247–255. doi:10.1016/j.jcis.2013.05.081 PMID:23809875

White, P. F., Ardeleanu, M., Schooley, G., & Burch, R. M. (2009). *Pharmacokinetics of DepoBupivacaine Following Infiltration in Patients Undergoing Two Types of Surgery and in Normal Volunteers.* The International Anesthesia Research Society Annual Meeting, San Diego, CA. Retrieved from: http://www.google.rs/url?sa=t&rct=j&q=&esrc=s&frm=1&source=web&cd=1&ved=0CBwQFjAA&url=http%3A%2F%2Fphx.corporate-ir.net%2FExternal.File%3Fitem%3DUGFyZW50SUQ9NDI4NTE2fENoaWxkSUQ9NDQ1NDk1fFR5cGU9MQ%3D%3D%26t%3D1&ei=DDOHVfTGBoSrUePzmbAN&usg=AFQjCNH6FX5VmgkfXPINYvRCdmKCUx0B-g&sig2=QB1d8uciRRRy5RpYJLHqEQ

Ye, Q., Asherman, J., Stevenson, M., Brownson, E., & Katre, N. V. (2000). DepoFoam® technology: A vehicle for controlled delivery of protein and peptide drugs. *Journal of Controlled Release*, *64*(1-3), 155–166. doi:10.1016/S0168-3659(99)00146-7 PMID:10640654

KEY TERMS AND DEFINITIONS

Flexosomes: Liposomes with increased bilayer membrane elasticity.

Immunopotentiating Reconstituted Influenza Virus Virosomes: Specific unilamellar vesicles with encapsulated influenza hemagglutinin and neuraminidase which enhance and/or prolong the protective effect of vaccines and may be used as carriers for antigens of other viruses.

Liposomes: Spherical microvesicles or nanovesicles with an aqueous core surrounded by one or more phospholipid bilayers between which is a water phase; the polar moieties of the amphiphilic molecules are oriented towards the aqueous phase, while their nonpolar parts are in the interior of the bilayer.

Long-Circulating Liposomes: Liposomes with increased hydrophilicity of surface by attachment of polymers such as polyethylene glycols, which makes them unrecognizable in reticuloendothelial system (RES).

Microencapslation/Nanoncapsulation: Encapsulation of the active substances into the carrier with diameter at microscale /nanoscale, respectively.

Multilamellar Vesicles: Liposomes with larger number of concentrically arranged phospholipid bilayers.

Multivesicular Vesicles: Vesicles comprising larger number of fused liposomal phospholipid bilayers.

Nanosomes: Liposomes with diameter up to 100 nm.

Sustained Release Drug Delivery: A drug delivery prolonged over an extended period of time on single dose.

Targeted Drug Delivery: Delivery of drug in a manner that increases its concentration in organs and tissues affected by pathological process, relative to others.

Chapter 3
Liposomes:
Concept and Therapeutic Applications

Mangal Shailesh Nagarsenker
Bombay College of Pharmacy, India

Megha Sunil Marwah
Bombay College of Pharmacy, India

ABSTRACT

The science of liposomes has expanded in ambit from bench to clinic through industrial production in thirty years since the naissance of the concept. This chapter makes an attempt to bring to light the impregnable contributions of great researchers in the field of liposomology that has witnessed clinical success in the recent times. The journey which began in 1965 with the observations of Bangham and further advances made en route (targeting/stealthing of liposomes) along with alternative and potential liposome forming amphiphiles has been highlighted in this chapter. The authors have also summarised the conventional and novel industrially feasible methods used to formulate liposomes in addition to characterisation techniques which have been used to set up quality control standards for large scale production. Besides, the authors have provided with an overview of primary therapeutic and diagnostic applications and a brief insight into the in vivo behaviour of liposomes.

INTRODUCTION AND BACKGROUND

A Historical Perspective

The advent of liposomology in the domain of nanoscience has revolutionised clinical therapy in the recent times (Lian & Ho, 2001). 'Liposomes', now a benchmark in drug delivery science, was conceptualized by Alec Bangham as 'multilamellar smectic mesophases' in the year 1964(Deamer, 2010). These bilayer structures were serendipitously observed by Bangham in the process of artificially emulating cell membranes while investigating properties of cellular constituents of blood. They were formerly referred to as 'Banghasomes'. Gerald Weissmann suggested the term 'liposomes' to describe microscopic vesicles composed of one or more lipids (Sessa & Weissmann, 1968).

DOI: 10.4018/978-1-5225-0751-2.ch003

Jointly with Horne, Bangham demonstrated the existence of multilamellar phospholipid vesicles through electron micrographs (A. D. Bangham & Horne, 1964). His pioneering work ascertained that lipids were the primary permeability barrier to ions and large molecules (A. BanghamStandish & Weissmann, 1965; A. BanghamStandish & Watkins, 1965) following which scientists like Gregory Gregoriad is extrapolated the concept of liposomes to drug delivery in the 1970s (Gregoriadis, 1976a, 1976b). This led to a dissemination of liposomal systems into cell biology, medicine, chemistry and biophysics.

Twenty years after the introduction of liposomes to drug delivery, the pharmaceutical industry witnessed a paradigm shift with USFDA approval of Doxil™ (Alza Corporation) in the year 1995 (Weissig, 2010). It was the first marketed injectable liposomal formulation that corroborated the prescience of Bangham and associated scientists. This journey of liposomes from bench to clinic cannot disparage the efforts of Gregoriadis, Ryman, Weissmann and Papahadjopoulos who embarked upon the application of liposomes in drug delivery and formulation sciences. Following this, the subsequent years saw a precipitous rise in the number of patents and research articles emerging in the arena of liposomology and its applications in drug delivery.

Further investigations carried out to establish liposomes in the clinic emphasized on problems like inadequate comprehension of liposomal stability, circulation time *in vivo*, lipid-drug interactions and lipid-cell interactions (Lian & Ho, 2001). A consequent milestone in this field was laid by the work of Crowes who highlighted the potential of liposomes to be freeze dried and reconstituted. The invincible efforts of researchers like Gregoriadis, Papahadjopoulos, Lasic and their team led to the landmark discovery of long circulating liposomes, wherein, they tested the antitumour efficacy of polymer bearing lipids *in vivo* (Lasic & Martin, 1995).

Given the background of the discovery of liposomes and the work carried out towards the growth of this discipline in delivery science, we would like to draw the reader's attention to how liposomes came into being much before they were discovered (Lasic & Barenholz, 1996). The use of liposomes dates back to the prehistoric man when eggs, which contain lecithin and cholesterol, were beaten in water. Virchow, in 1854, first described the swelling of lipids that he observed after transferring nerve cores in water. Later, many others like Lehmann (1911) and Reinitzer, who discovered liquid crystals, made similar observations, but failed to realize the presence of liposomes. In the course of analysing the cell structure and its constituents, Gortel and Wendelin 1926, introduced the concept of bilayered structure of cell membranes. This was followed by Danielli and Davson, who familiarised the world with the existence of a sandwich of proteins between the bilayers in 1935. Singer and Nicholson subsequently instituted the theory of the fluid-mosaic model. However, it was Bangham who comprehended the presence of an enclosed aqueous phase within the liposomes and thus laid the foundation for innovation in various disciplines.

Liposomes: Concept and Practice

In accordance with the observation of Bangham, liposomes are defined as microscopic spheres consisting of lipid bilayers encompassing an aqueous core. These vesicular structures are colloidal in nature and form when natural or synthetic phospholipids are dispersed in water. Phospholipids are amphiphilic in nature and consist of a hydrophilic head group and a hydrophobic hydrocarbon chain. When dispersed in water, the phospholipid molecules assume different morphologies depending on the phospholipid: water ratio and a few physicochemical properties of the lipid molecules (this part is dealt with later in the chapter) (Bordi et al., 2006; Vemuri & Rhodes, 1995). Among the different forms adopted by lipid molecules, liposomes are those capable of spontaneous assembly to bilayers as a means to overcome the entropically unfavourable interaction of hydrophobic chains with water. The resulting structures are a consortium of lipid molecules with the head groups oriented towards the aqueous phase and the hydrocarbon chains facing each other as shown in Figure 1 (Vemuri & Rhodes, 1995). The thermodynamic instability in the form of entropic gain and self- association characteristics of bilayers aid assembly of the latter into a closed sphere with an aqueous core within (Akbarzadeh et al., 2013). One or more bilayers comprising a liposome are referred to as lamella (e). The number of bilayers in a liposome defines multiple properties like size and the capacity to carry hydrophilic/hydrophobic solutes and can be controlled by the method employed to formulate liposomal systems.

The amphiphilic nature of phospholipids and their ability to form bilayers makes them suitable for drug delivery (Laouini et al., 2012). Liposomes serve as carriers of hydrophilic molecules in the aqueous core and hydrophobic ones in the lipid bilayer. Thus, liposomal drug delivery approach offers the advantage of formulating an array of chemically different molecules which is a formidable challenge for researchers globally. A few examples of molecules belonging to different chemical and therapeutic categories that have been incorporated into liposomal vesicles and have witnessed market success are enlisted in Table 1.

Biodegradability, biocompatibility and non-immunogenicity are biologically desirable properties possessed by phospholipids that make them amenable to the intravenous route of drug administration. Besides, *in vivo* protection against enzymatic degradation offers a platform for protein and gene delivery. Also, vesicular entrapment of drugs having poor solubility facilitates improved bioavailability of the latter.

A major achievement with liposomal systems was the ability to passively and/or actively navigate them to a specific organ or tissue. The small size of liposomes enables passive targeting by evading opsonisation by the reticulo-endothelial system (RES). Moreover, they are amenable to physical and chemical surface modification which aids active targeting to specific receptors thereby reducing off-target toxicity(dealt with in detail later in the chapter). Modification of liposomal composition by the addition of long chain hydrophilic polymers like polyethylene glycol (PEG) also abets prolonged residence time in the circulation.

A plethora of advantages offered by liposomes in drug delivery has made them the system of choice in the recent times. The following sections will delve into a few details with a view to give an insight into liposomes.

Figure 1. Entropy driven self-assembly process of amphiphilic molecules

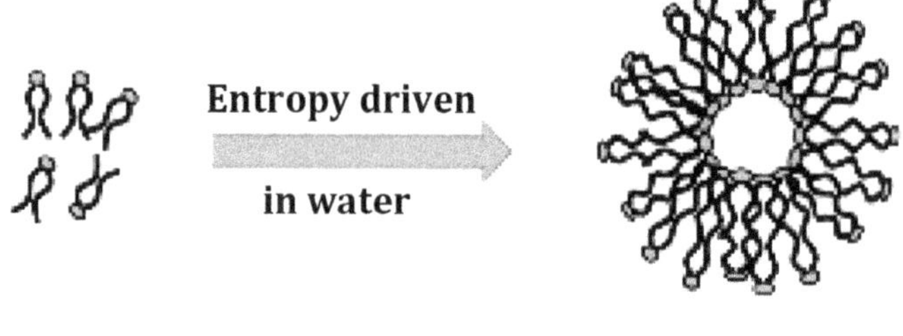

Table 1. Liposomal products: marketed and pipeline products

Liposomal Product	Drug	Lipid Composition	Pharmacological Category/Applications of Drug	Year of Approval	Reference(s)
			Approved Products		
Ambisome (Gilead)	Amphotericin B	HSPC, DSPG and cholesterol	Antileishmanial, Antifungal	1990 (Europe), 1997 (USA)	(Hann & Prentice, 2001)
Doxil/Caelyx (Johnson and Johnson)	Doxorubicin	HSPC, cholesterol and DSPE-PEG$_{2000}$	• Anticancer • Kaposi's sarcoma • Ovarian cancer • Breast cancer • Multiple myeloma+Velcade	• 1995 • 1999 • 2003 • 2007 (Europe, Canada)	(Y. C. Barenholz, 2012; Bladé et al., 2011; James et al., 1994; Muggia et al., 1996)
DaunoXome (Galen)	Daunorubicin	DSPC and cholesterol	• Anticancer • Kaposi's sarcoma	1996 (Europe, USA)	(Petre & Dittmer, 2007)
DepoDur (Pacira)	Morphine sulphate	DOPC, DPPG cholesterol and triolein	• Analgesic • Pain following surgery	2004	(Gambling et al., 2005)
Visudyne (QLT Phototherapeutics, Inc)	Verteporfin	EPG and DMPC	Age-related macular degeneration	2000	(Bressler & Bressler, 2000)
			Pipeline Products		
ThermoDox	Doxorubicin	DPPC, MSPC, DSPE-PEG$_{2000}$	• Anticancer • Nonresectable hepatocellular carcinoma	III	(Yarmolenko et al., 2010)
Endo-Tag-1 (Medigene)	Cationic liposomal paclitaxel	DOTAP, DOPC	• Pancreatic cancer • Triple negative breast cancer(Semple et al., 2010)	II II	(Fasol et al., 2012)
ALN-VSP (Alnylam)	• siRNA targeting PCSK9 • RNAi targeting • liver cancer	DLinDMA, DSPC, mPEG$_{2000}$-cDMA, cholesterol	• Hypercholesterolemia • Liver cancer and liver metastasis	I I	(Semple et al., 2010; Zimmermann et al., 2006)

Abbreviations: HSPC-Hydrogenated soyabean phosphatidyl choline, DSPG- Distearoyl phosphatidyl glycerol, DSPE-PEG$_{2000}$ – Distearoyl phosphatidyl ethanolamine-polyethylene glycol 2000, DPPG- Dipalmitoyl phosphatidyl glycerol, DSPC- Distearoyl phosphatidyl choline, DMPC- Dimyristoyl phosphatidyl choline, EPG-Egg phosphatidyl glycerol, DLinDMA- 1,2-dilinoleyloxy-3-dimethylaminopropane, mPEG$_{2000}$- cDMA-(3-*N*-[(methoxy poly(ethylene glycol)2000)carbamoyl]-1,2-dimyrestyloxypropylamine), siRNA- small interfering RNA, RNAi- RNA interference.

Classification of Liposomes

Liposomes, being multifaceted systems, can be classified in many ways, few of which have been described below (Figure 2):

1. Based on structural parameters (Laouini et al., 2012; Sharma & Sharma, 1997):
   a. Unilamellar Vesicles (UV):
      i. **Small Unilamellar Vesicles (SUV):** Less than 100nm.
      ii. **Large Unilamellar Vesicles (LUV):** More than 100nm but less than 1000nm (Bordi et al., 2006).
      iii. **Giant Unilamellar Vesicles (GUV):** More than 1000nm.

Figure 2. Classification of liposomes based on structural parameters

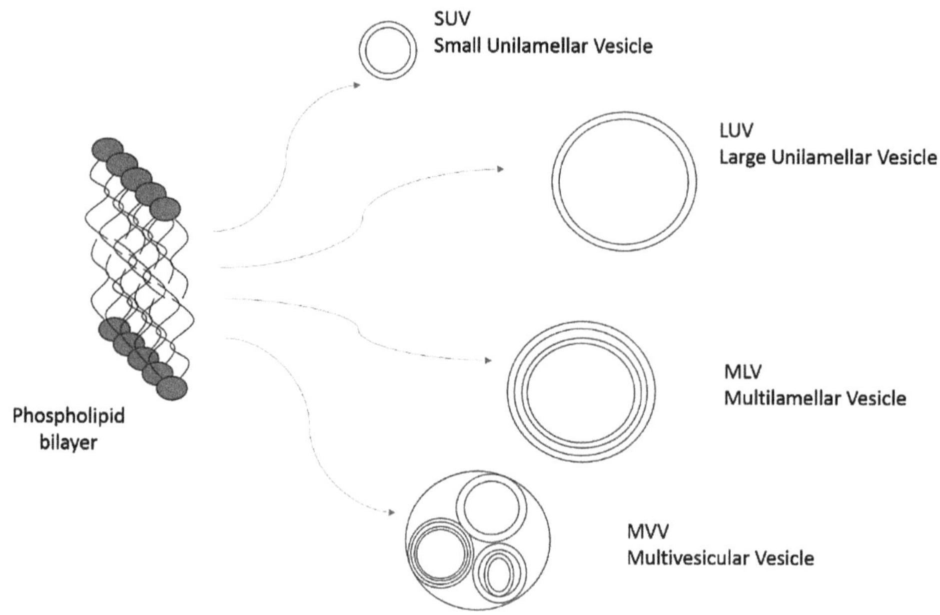

b. **Oligolamellar Vesicles (OLV):** 100 nm to 500nm.
c. **Multilamellar Vesicles (MLV):** More than 500nm.
d. Double liposomes (DL) (Ebato et al., 2003).
e. Multivesicular vesicles (MVV).

2. Based on method of preparation (Kreuter, 1994; Vemuri & Rhodes, 1995):
   a. Reverse-phase evaporation vesicles (REV) (SUV/OLV/MLV).
   b. French press vesicles (FPV).
   c. Ether injection vesicles (EIV).
   d. Stable Plurilamellar vesicles (SPLV).
   e. Frozen and thawed MLV (FAT-MLV).
   f. Vesicles prepared by extrusion method (VET).
   g. Vesicles prepared by fusion (FUV).
   h. Dehydration-rehydration vesicles (DRV).
   i. Bubblesomes (BSV).
3. Based on composition and mechanism of intracellular delivery (Sharma & Sharma, 1997):
   a. Conventional liposomes.
   b. Cationic liposomes.
   c. Surface modified liposomes (Immunoliposomes/Ligand decorated liposomes).
   d. Triggerable liposomes.
   e. Long circulating liposomes.

The varied classification approaches delineated above are independent of each other. For example, SUV, MLV or OLV may be produced by employing reverse phase evaporation method. Therefore, a completely defined liposomal system entails size, lamellarity as well as method of preparation of the said vesicles (Swarbrick & Boylan, 1993).

The size and lamellarity govern the *in vivo* circulation time and encapsulation of solutes in liposomes. Smaller the size (less than 200nm) (Guo & Huang, 2011), longer is the residence time of the liposomal system in blood circulation. This is because the RES is unable to recognize particles less than 200nm in size. (Size of particulate delivery systems is one of many critical factors that dictate opsonisation by the RES). Besides, vesicles with larger size and more number of bilayers warrant greater capture of hydrophilic/hydrophobic drugs/macromolecules and are more stable than the ones with a smaller size and fewer lamellae (Sharma & Sharma, 1997).

Vesicle size and number of bilayers are also significantly influenced by the method of preparation of liposomes. Literature reports identify vesicular systems as thermodynamically unstable or metastable assemblies. Thus, energy supplied by the formulation approach employed helps surmount the kinetic barrier for vesicle formation or traps them in the metastable thermodynamic state and liposomes of different sizes are formed. A size distribution is obtained in the resultant vesicles since the liposomes occupy different local free energy minima depending on the method of preparation (Lasic & Barenholz, 1996; Swarbrick & Boylan, 1993). However, few amphiphiles are capable of spontaneous assembly and form thermodynamically equilibrated systems when mixed; for example, oppositely charged amphiphiles can spontaneously assemble into vesicles.

Liposomal architecture and composition are imperative to its interaction with blood components and cells *in vivo*. The composition with respect to charge density, bilayer fluidity, surface modification and addition of polymers, influences the communication of the vesicular system with cells and receptors, thereby affecting cellular uptake of the latter. Thus, the composition of liposomal systems is a prerequisite to the determination of mechanism of its intracellular delivery. This is very well exemplified by Magee and Miller who demonstrated the necessity to include a cationic lipid into liposomes with a view to improve their adsorption to cells in tissue culture (Magee et al., 1974). Surface modification of liposomes may serve dual purpose depending on the surface modifying agent employed. Incorporation of a few hydrophilic molecules like carbohydrates, polymers or glycolipids may not only increase the circulation time of the system, but also aid interaction with a particular receptor on a specific organ or tissue (targeting) (Allen et al., 1995).

Liposomes can be exploited to deliver the drugs effectively to the target site by using a number of triggering modalities. The latter can be categorized into internal and external triggers (Ganta et al., 2008; Puri, 2013), depending on the location of the stimulus responsible for causing release of the drug from liposomes. Internal triggers typically involve utilization of:

1. Acidic pH of endosomes/lysosomes (Puri, 2013),
2. Enzymes overexpressed in certain pathological conditions,
3. Tunable redox potential of liposomes.

External triggers, on the other hand, entail the use of:

1. Heat (Thermosentive liposomes),
2. Light (Photosensitive liposomes),
3. Magnetic field,
4. Ultrasound (Ganta et al., 2008).

These strategies have gained clinical importance with Thermodox® (thermosensitive liposomes) and Visudyne® (photosensitive liposomes) having witnessed *in vivo* success for the treatment of cancer and age related macular degeneration respectively. Besides, the temporal and spatial dissemination of magnetically triggered liposomal systems can be controlled and used for image-guided drug delivery with the aid of contrast agents like superparamagnetic iron oxide particles (SPION) which also possess magnetic properties (Puri, 2013).

In addition, intracellular triggers like differential pH across the cell, overexpression of enzymes such as Phospholipase A2 and disparate expression of redox enzymes in pathological conditions like cancer have been utilized in the arena of drug delivery by liposomes.

Site specificity coupled with stimuli sensitivity exploited in the fabrication of liposomal drug delivery systems bear potential to benefit a number of formidable therapies including cancer.

Liposome Forming Amphiphiles: Types and Role

Before taking a look at the components of a liposome, it is important to answer a few questions like 'What type of materials can form vesicles? What are the essential requirements in an amphiphile for bilayer and vesicle formation? How does vesicle formation take place? Can vesicle forming materials also form other supramolecular assemblies like micelles and associated structures?'

Let us try and answer these questions one by one.

Molecules with amphiphilicity are a prerequisite to self- assembly, that is, the molecule, must necessarily possess a hydrophilic component (head group) and a lipophilic component (the hydrophobic tail) within the same structure. When such molecules are dispersed in water, an interplay of a number of diverse forces give rise to self-assembled supramolecular aggregates.

This can be explained as follows: The hydrocarbon-water interface is confronted with opposing forces exerted by the hydrophobic tail group in the form of 'hydrophobic attractive forces' and the hydrophilic head group in the form of 'steric or ionic repulsive forces' (Figure 3). The attractive forces tend to decrease the interfacial area, 'a', by exerting a pull on the molecules away from the outer aqueous medium, while the repulsive forces coerce the entire molecule towards the outer aqueous phase, with a concomitant effort to increase 'a'. The result is an increased interfacial free energy owing to simultaneous action of opposite forces at the interface.

The system holistically tries to minimise the total interfacial free energy by decreasing the exposure of its hydrophobic chains to water, thereby giving rise to the concept of an optimal area per head group, 'a_0'. It is a compromise made by the system to balance the two disparate forces acting at the interface. In the process, the system concludes into a supramolecular aggregate in coherence with entropic requisites.

The interdependence of interfacial free energy and surface area per head group can be mathematically expressed as follows (Israelachvili, 2011):

$$\mu_N^{\circ} = 2\gamma a_0 + \frac{\gamma}{a}\left(a - a_0\right)^2 \quad (1)$$

where,

μ°_N: Interfacial free energy per molecule.

Figure 3. Forces acting at the interface of a self-aggregating molecule

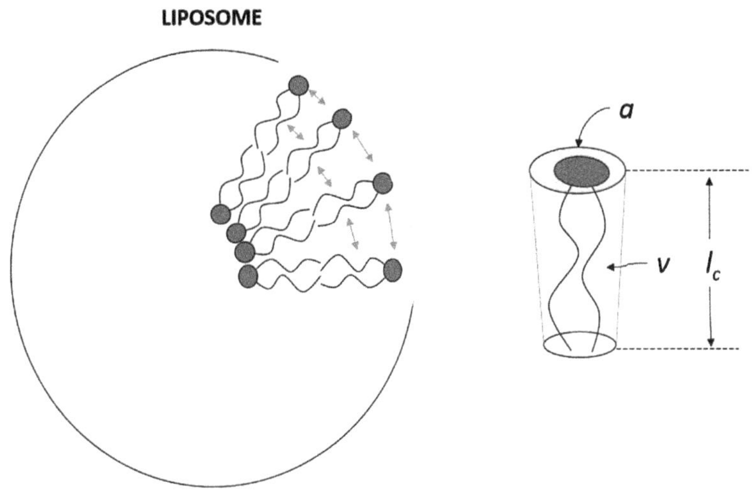

γ: Interfacial free energy per unit area.

a_0: Optimal surface area per molecule $a_0 = \sqrt{\frac{K}{\gamma}}$

K: Constant.
a: Surface area occupied per head group.

The total interfacial free energy of the system varies parabolically with the surface area per head group and is found to be minimum at a certain optimum surface area per head group.

With the aid of 'optimum surface area per head group, a_0' of an amphiphile in conjunction with two other parameters, viz., 'volume of the hydrocarbon chain, v' and 'critical chain length, l_c', Israelachvili and co-workers predicted the various molecular shapes that any amphiphile could assume (Kreuter, 1994) in an aqueous dispersion. They introduced the concept of 'critical packing parameter, p', a dimensionless number, mathematically expressed in Equation 2, which can be used to ascertain the packing properties of an amphiphile (Israelachvili, 2011).

$$p = \frac{v}{a_0 l_c} \tag{2}$$

In Equation 2, critical chain length, l_c, is the maximum effective length that the chains can assume when fluid. It represents the limiting value for the distance to which the chains can extend when deformed and is less than the fully extended molecular length, l_{max}, of the chains which is in congruence with energetic and entropic requirements.

Numerical description of the packing parameter allows the revelation of the shape associated with it. As the value of 'p' increases from 0 to 1 and above, the shape and packing properties of an aggregate change from spherical micelles ($0<p<1/3$) to nonspherical micelles ($1/3 <p< 1/2$) to cylindrical micelles

(p ~ ½) to interconnected structures (1/2 $<p<$ 1) to vesicles and planar bilayers (p ~ 1) and ultimately to inverted structures like inverted cone, inverted hexagonal and inverted cubic structures ($p>$ 1). The different types of amphiphiles along with their examples that lead to different aggregate structures are summarised in Table 2 (Israelachvili, 2011; Kreuter, 1994).

Table 2. Amphiphiles and their aggregate geometries

Lipid/Amphiphile	Examples	Critical Packing Parameter	Critical Packing Shape	Geometry of Aggregate
Single-chained lipids with large head group areas	SLS, Tweens, Spans	< 1/3	Cone 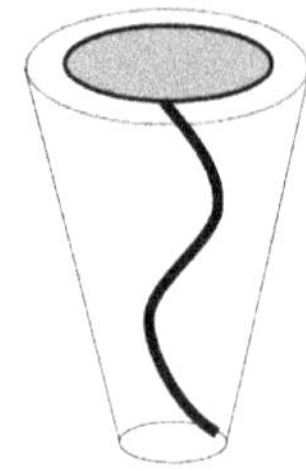	Spherical micelles
Single-chained lipids with small head group areas	SLS, CTAB in high salt, lipids with uncharged, non-ionic, zwitterionic head groups insensitive to salt content like lysolecithin	1/3-1/2	Truncated cone 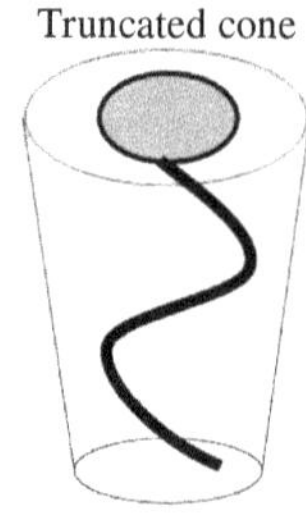	Cylindrical micelles
Double-chained lipids with large headgroup areas (fluid chains), Single chained lipids with sterols	PC, PS, PI, PG, sphingomyelin, dialkyl dimethyl ammonium salts, Lysolecithins with cholesterol	½-1	Truncated wedge 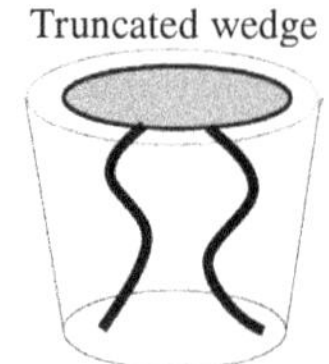	Flexible bilayers, vesicles
Double-chained lipids with small head group areas (frozen chains)	PE, PS + Ca^{+2}	~ 1	Cylinder 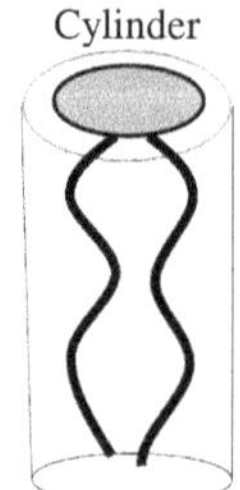	Planar bilayers
Double-chained lipids with smaller headgroup areas	PE, Cardiolipin + Ca+2	>1	Inverted truncated cone or wedge 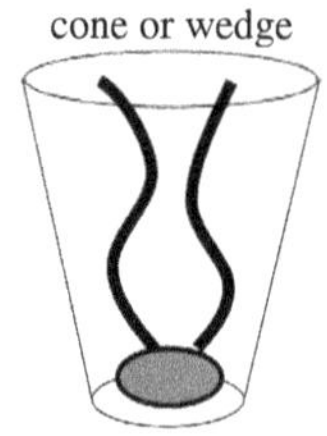	Inverted micelles

Kreuter, 1994.

Bilayer Formation and Vesiculation: An Insight into Amphiphile Geometry

Antonietti et al have suggested a two-staged process for vesicle formation for an amphiphile, the first step being bilayer formation followed by closure into a vesicle (Antonietti & Förster, 2003). It is, therefore, noteworthy to consider factors affecting both bilayer and vesicle formation.

From the above discussion, it is evident that for an amphiphile to form bilayers, the packing parameter should approach unity. The amphiphiles belonging to this category have the following peculiarities:

1. They generally have two tails, since, in order to meet the requirement of $p = 1$, the amphiphile must preferably possess two times the hydrocarbon volume 'v' vis-à-vis the same required to form a micelle, keeping a_0 and l_c constant. For example, double chain amphiphiles like dipalmitoylphosphatidyl choline (DPPC) and dimyristoylphosphatidyl choline (DMPC) easily form bilayers, whereas single chain amphiphiles like lysophosphatidylcholine preferably form micelles. Besides, owing to the larger volumes of their hydrocarbon chains and relatively small surface areas for their head groups, such amphiphiles find it difficult to pack into micellar structures ($0 < p < 1/2$).

However, some single chained amphiphilic molecules like lysophosphatidyl choline in the presence of fatty acids are capable of assuming a bilayer morphology (Israelachvili, 2011; Kreuter, 1994).

2. The higher hydrophobicity of these amphiphiles contributes to a lower critical micelle concentration (CMC), hydrophilic-lipophilic balance (HLB) and higher residence time within the aggregate as compared to micelles.

Under certain conditions, these bilayer forming amphiphiles close into a vesicle in order to minimise exposure of their edges and the resulting increased interfacial tension. At the same time, a low bending elasticity and a higher curvature due to uneven distribution in the number of amphiphiles constituting the inner and outer leaves of the bilayer contribute to closure of the hull. A depth into the mathematics of the mean curvature 'H' and Gaussian curvature 'K' can be found in literature (Antonietti & Förster, 2003; Israelachvili, 2011; Kreuter, 1994).

The packing parameter of amphiphiles can be adjusted to unity by the following methods (Antonietti & Förster, 2003; Israelachvili, 2011; Mark, 2013):

1. For a fixed length 'l_c', increasing volume 'v' by swelling with organic solvents or altering the same by means of modification of solute concentrations shifts the value of 'p' towards unity.
2. Decreasing head group repulsive forces by decreasing 'a' or hydrophilic fraction at constant 'l_c' contribute to a higher value of 'p'. This may be realized by a change in pH/temperature or electrolyte /polymer addition which bring about shielding of electrostatic repulsion.
3. Amphiphile concentration also plays an important role in maintaining the aggregate structureof a particular type. A higher concentration may result in increased repulsion and lower hydration resulting in inverted structures (Israelachvili, 2011). This corroborates the idea of a single amphiphile forming varied structures under different conditions.

The proposition of the packing parameter and vesiculation mechanisms throws light on the most suitable types of amphiphiles for formulating bilayers and vesicular structures. Phospholipids, which are a vital component of biological cells, were deemed to possess the characteristics of a bilayer forming amphiphile and were explored in liposomological research areas key components. The following gives a brief account of the various amphiphiles that have been employed in the formulation of liposomes.

The chief constituents of liposomes are phospholipids which are amphiphilic in nature. Chemically, phospholipids bear a glycerol backbone and are esters of phosphatidic acid. They are generally represented by the structure shown in Figure 4. The hydroxyl groups at positions 1 and 2 of the glycerol backbone are conjugated with fatty acids, while the one at position 3 is chemically tethered to an oxygen of the phosphate group of phosphatidic acid by ester bonds. The remaining oxygen of the phosphate group is chemically appended to a small organic molecule like choline/ethanolamine/glycerol/inositol or serine. Thus, the amphiphilic phospholipid molecule comprises of a fatty acid tail coexistent with a head group which entails a small organic molecule esterified to the phosphate group of phosphatidic acid (Lian & Ho, 2001). Examples of phospholipids include phosphatidyl choline (PC), phosphatidyl ethanolamine (PE), phosphatidyl glycerol (PG), phosphatidyl inositol (PI) and phosphatidyl serine (PS).

Phospholipids used in the formulation of lipid bilayers are primarily obtained from egg yolks or soyabeans. The two sources differ in the nature and content of their fatty acids. The phospholipids obtained from egg yolks essentially contain a saturated fatty acyl chain at position 1 and an unsaturated one at position 2, while the ones isolated from soyabeans have unsaturated fatty acyl chains at both, positions 1 and 2 (linoleic acid is one of the chief components of phospholipids obtained from soyabeans). This is an important aspect to be considered while selecting lipids for formulating liposomes since the degree of branching, degree of saturation, fatty acyl chain length, location of double bond and such other facets of fatty acid composition affect the bilayer permeability, hydrophobicity, lipid bilayer-drug interaction and thus *in vitro* and *in vivo* performance of these lipid vesicles (Cevc, 1987, 1991; Swarbrick & Boylan, 1993). Five categories of phospholipids along with their sources, chemistry and applications are summarised in Table 4. Phospholipids employed in the preparation of liposomes can also be classified into

Figure 4. Chemical structures of phospholipids and sphingolipids

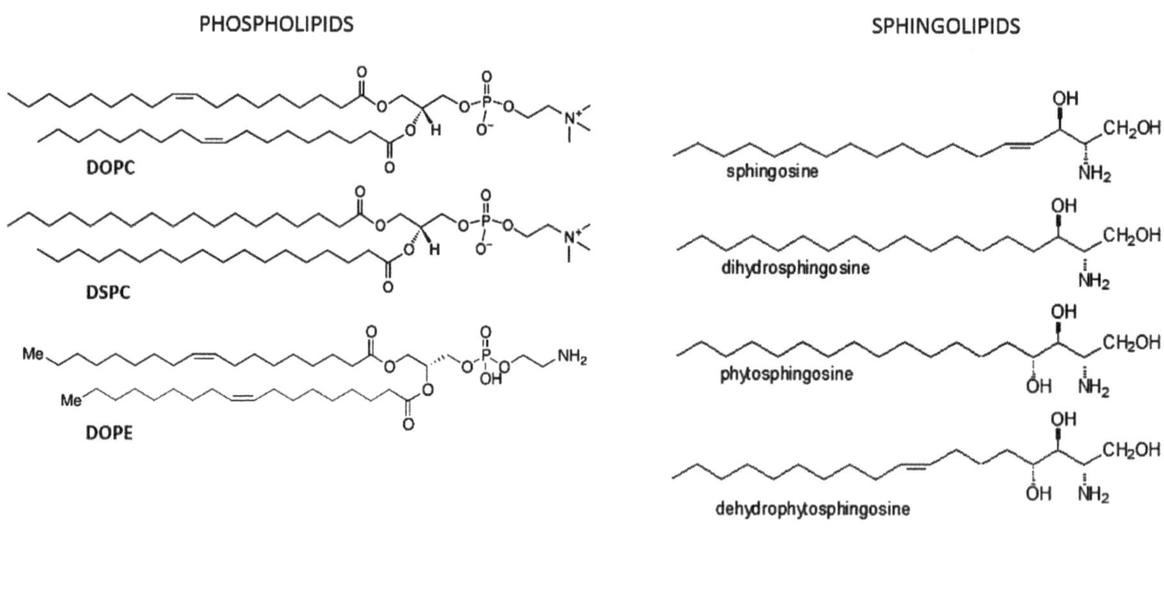

Table 3. Classification of phospholipids/their derivatives on the basis of overall charge on molecule

Phospholipid Type	Charge on Molecule	Examples
Cationic	Positive	DOTAP, DOGS, DOTMA
Anionic	Negative	DPPA, DPPG and other PG, PS, PI, PA.
Nonionic	Neutral	DOPC, DPPC

anionic, cationic and neutral on the basis of the overall charge on the lipid. A brief insight into this classification system is provided with in Table 3.

Besides phospholipids, sphingolipids like sphingomyelin, cardiolipin and ceramides are also ubiquitously employed in liposomal formulations. Sphingosine, an aliphatic amino alcohol sphingoid base, forms the backbone of these lipids. The general structure of sphingolipids is as shown in Figure 4. In case of a sphingolipid, the fatty acyl chain is chemically linked to the amino group of sphingoid base by an amide bond vis-à-vis ester bond in phospholipids. This difference in chemical structure influences bilayer properties, a gist of which is given in Table 4.

Phospholipids in bilayers exhibit a unique phenomenon of structural phase transition, wherein they transit from the gel state to the more fluid liquid crystalline state. The temperature associated with this transition is called as chain – melting/main transition temperature or the phase transition temperature (T_m) (Sackmann, 1995). The bilayer lipids are relatively more ordered and rigid in the gel state. When the temperature is increased to T_m and higher, the lipids lose their order and rigidity, thereby engender-

Table 4. Phospholipids/Sphingolipids classification based on their source, chemistry, and applications

Phopholipid	Source	Chemistry	General Applications/ Remarks
Natural Phospholipids (PC, PE, PG, PI, PS, PA, SPM)	Natural: • Egg (one saturated and one unsaturated acyl chain) • Soy (two unsaturated acyl chains)	Mixed acyl ester phospholipids	May be used for any route including parenteral
Modified natural phospholipid (HSPC)	Partially/fully hydrogenated using enzymes like phospholipase D	Saturated/partially saturated acyl chains	Improving oxidative stability, purity.
Semisynthetic phospholipids	Semisynthetic: PLA2 used to cleave acyl chains on Carbon position '2'	Unsaturated acyl chains replaced.	Improved reproducibility in different batches.
Fully synthetic (e.g. cationic phospholipids like DOPC)	Synthetic: Enzymes used to sterespecifically produce phospholipids	Mixed acyl ester phospholipids	Specifically used for parenteral administration. Improving intracellular delivery.
Phospholipids with non-natural head groups (PEGylated phospholipids, Monoclonal antibody linked phospholipids, protein conjugated phospholipids)	Synthetic	PEG- conjugated mixed acyl ester phospholipids/Functional groups like –COOH, -NH2, vicinal –OH, -SH may be employed for head groups.	Parenteral administration. Improving residence time in circulation, targetability
Sphingolipids (ceramides, sphingomyelin)	Natural/synthetic	Mixed acyl chain amides containing sphingoid base	Parenteral route and other routes.

Kreuter, 1994; Swarbrick & Boylan, 1993; van Hoogevest & Wendel, 2014.

ing the fluid liquid crystalline state. They are more permeable and leakier in this disordered state. For this reason, drug encapsulation in liposomes is carried out above the transition temperature of the lipids comprising it.

The transition temperature is influenced by a number of factors and one of them is the presence of additives. Liposomes often contain cholesterol in addition to the lipids that are commonly used. Cholesterol, being a sterol with amphipathic nature, positions itself within the bilayer with the sterol rings wrung between the fatty acyl chains and the hydroxyl group facing the aqueous phase (Vemuri & Rhodes, 1995) (Figure 5). By its presence, cholesterol abolishes structural phase transition of bilayer lipids and improves rigidity by reducing permeability of the liposomes. It also decreases interactions of the vesicles with blood proteins like albumin, thereby enhancing the *in vivo* stability of the system on the whole.

Recent progress in liposomology has recognised non-phospholipid molecules capable of forming lamellar self-assemblies. These include sterols in conjunction with single-chain amphiphiles, which, under certain conditions, can self-assemble into stable fluid bilayer structures (Cui & Lafleur, 2014). The geometry of the resultant structure is determined by the packing parameter of the mixture. As mentioned previously, an amphiphile with an overall packing parameter of 1 assumes bilayer geometry. Therefore, the putative consequence of mixing a cone-shaped sterol like cholesterol (packingparameter: 1.08) (Chen & Rand, 1997; Ipsen et al., 1987; Thewalt & Bloom, 1992) with an inverted cone-shaped single chain amphiphile (packing parameter < 0.5) is a bilayerstructure. As an example of this phenomenon, 1-palmitoyl-sn-glycerol-3-phosphocholine (lysoPPC), a single chain amphiphile that forms micelles readily in water, was shown to form MLVs and SUVs when mixed with an equimolar ratio of cholesterol (Ramsammy & Brockerhoff, 1982). Vesicles of single-chain amphiphiles in combination with cholesterol exhibit limited

Figure 5. Interaction of cholesterol with bilayer lipids

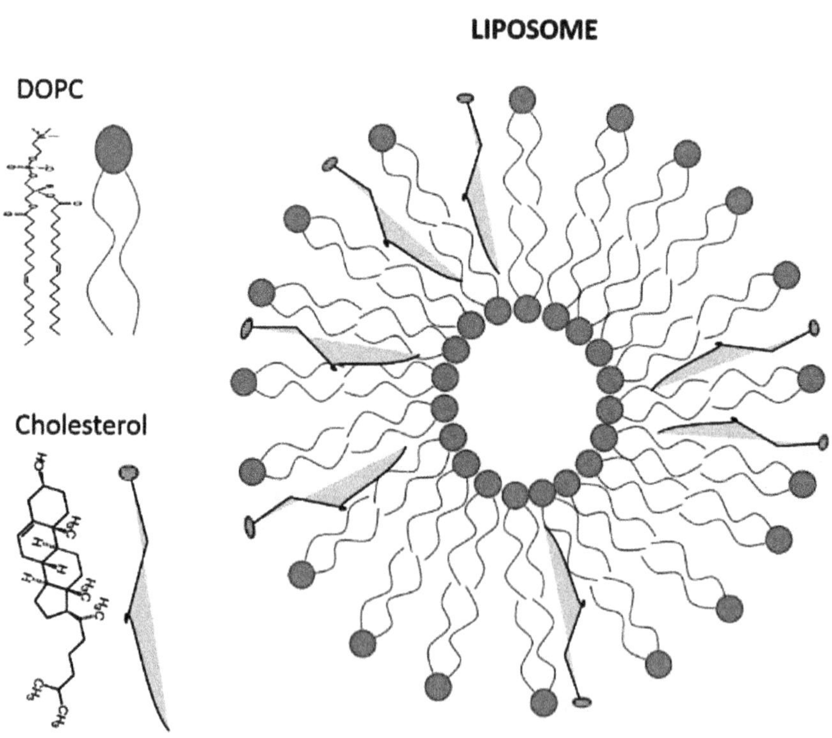

permeability, good stability and are amenable to functionalization and surface modification. Besides, the former are easy to obtain, handle, transport and store and would therefore serve as prospective alternatives to phospholipids. Interested readers are recommended to read the review on self-assembly of single chain amphiphiles by Z.K Cui and M. Lafleur to get a detailed comprehension of the topic.

The discovery of archaeol lipids (also known as bolaamphiphiles) has opened new avenues in the realm of liposomes for drug and vaccine delivery. This new generation of structural analogues of phospholipids consist of branched and saturated phytanyl chains (20-40 carbons long) appended via ether bonds to the 2nd and 3rd carbons of sn-glycerol which forms the backbone. Archaeol lipids are capable of self-assembly into monolayers/bilayers/a blend of the two called archaeosomes, a novel class of liposomes. The bilayers are composed of monopolararchaeol (diether) lipids, while bipolar caldarchaeol (tetraether) lipids comprise the monolayers. The archaeol lipids used for formulation development may be obtained naturally (from archaea organism) or may be partially or fully synthetic in origin.

Archaeosomes have been reported to be extremely stable to severe temperatures, high pressures, acidic and alkaline pH, oxidation, action of enzymes like phospholipases, bile salts and serum proteins. In addition, owing to the presence of ether linkages and ring structures, the permeability and crystallinity at ambient conditions are abated, thereby increasing packing rigidity and decreasing bilayer fluidity (Benvegnu et al., 2009). Moreover, archaeosomal vesicles can be formulated by conventional liposome formulation techniques like thin film hydration, extrusion and detergent removal (discussed in detail later in the chapter). This new addition to the family of liposomes has been identified as a potential delivery system for incorporation of thermally labile drugs and adjuvants for vaccines and gene delivery. Readers are recommended to read patents and reviews on bolaamphiphiles and archaeosomes by (Chong et al., 2012; Fariya et al., 2014) for further details on the topic.

Selection of Appropriate Amphiphilic Lipids for Bilayer Formation: Polymorphism and Formulation Aspects

The discussion in the above section suggests that amphiphiles with a '*p*' value in the range of 0.5 to 1 have a very high proclivity towards bilayer formation and vascularisation. However, while designing a liposomal system for drug delivery, many other factors contribute to and affect the *in vivo* behaviour of the system and must be taken into consideration while selecting lipids for the preparation of such systems.

In addition to theoretical property predictors like critical packing parameter and HLB, the choice of the lipid(s) to be employed for bilayer/vesicle formation for the purpose of drug delivery are more concretely governed by the following as depicted in Figure 6 (Li et al., 2015; New et al., 1995).

1. Lipid properties,
2. Availability and cost of the end product,
3. Therapeutic applications,
4. Drug Properties/BCS class of drug,

Methods of Preparation of Liposomes: From Lab Scale to Large Scale

Liposomes are generally regarded as thermodynamically unstable or metastable systems and the methods employed to prepare them are energy-intensive leading to differently sized vesicles, each bearing a distinct

Figure 6. Factors governing the choice of lipid for formulation into vesicles/bilayers

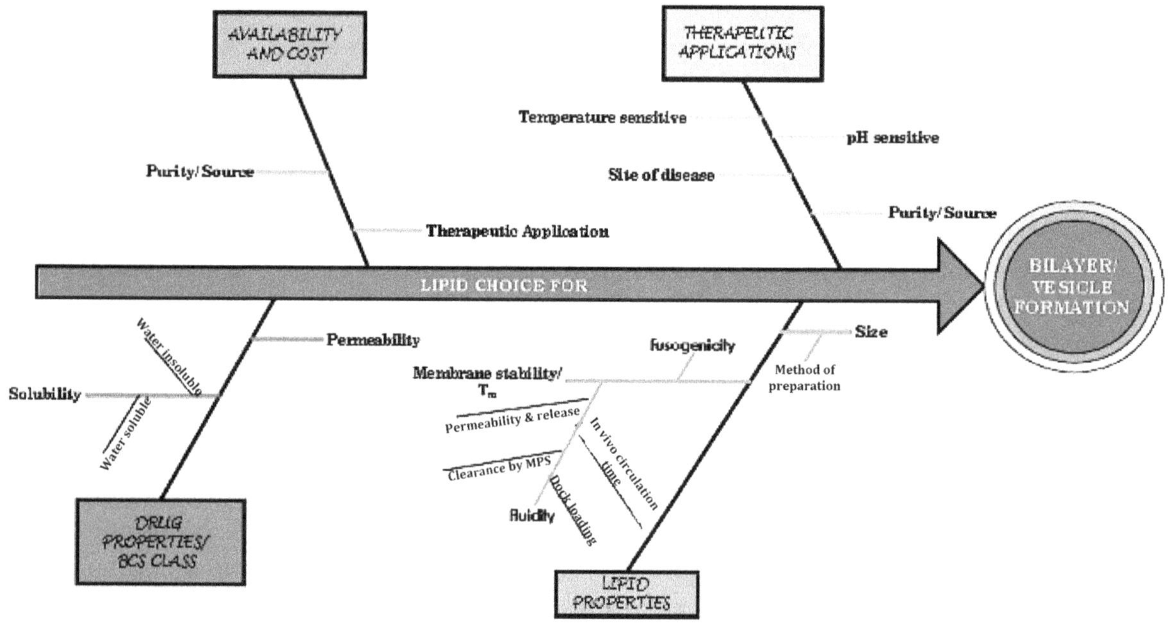

energy minimum. The formulation approach, therefore, critically determines the size and lamellarity of the resulting liposomes and is broadly composed of two steps:

1. Hydration of lipids,
2. Downsizing/Size reduction,

The most suitable method for the preparation of liposomes as a drug delivery system would therefore involve an appropriate execution of the above mentioned steps using the most congruent technique for a particular drug and a specific application. This has been exemplified in reports by the reverse phase evaporation technique for encapsulation of water soluble drugs wherein the lipids are hydrated in the presence of an organic solvent and particle size control is achieved by means of sonication (Kreuter, 1994). Besides, for drugs which do not exhibit a very high affinity to the bilayer and significantly remain unentrapped are required to be eliminated. This can be achieved by employing techniques like dialysis, ultracentrifugation, gel permeation chromatography and ion-exchange resins (Kreuter, 1994).

A number of theories in literature have attempted to explain the underlying mechanisms of liposome formation by the various methods that have been utilised till date. Of these, the 'budding off model' and the 'bilayer phospholipid fragment' theory unambiguously vindicate the vesiculation process. The former discusses the involvement of a combination of forces confronted by hydrated lipids causing them to 'bud-off' and reduce in size. The latter, on the other hand, elucidates vesicle formation through an intermediate stage structure called the bilayer phospholipid fragment (BPF), which is a planar bilayer composed of hydrated lipid. The BPF, undergoes folding of its lamellae owing to the thermodynamic instability associated with the exposure of its hydrophobic surface to water (Lasic, 1988; Lichtenberg & Barenholz, 1988).

The methods used to formulate liposomes can be largely categorized under the following heads (Table 5) (Amselem et al., 1993; A. Bangham, 1982; Lasic, 1988; Lichtenberg & Barenholz, 1988; Nässander et al., 1990; New, 1990; Szoka Jr & Papahadjopoulos, 1980):

1. Mechanical dispersion methods,
2. Solvent dispersion methods,
3. Detergent Removal methods,
4. Size transformation and fusion methods,
5. Methods based on pH adjustment.

Each of the methods mentioned in Table 5 will be dealt with shortly in the following section.

1. **Mechanical Dispersion Methods:**
    a. **Thin Film Hydration Method:** The thin film hydration approach also known as the classical Bangham method involves dispersing the lipids in an organic solvent and depositing a lipid film along a glass wall. The lipid film so formed is then hydrated with an aqueous buffer above the T_m. The resulting vesicles are heterogeneously sized and shaped MLVs which can be reduced to a uniformly sized population (SUVs) by employing ultrasonication or low pressure extrusion through polycarbonate filters (Kreuter, 1994; Laouini et al., 2012).
    b. **Ultrasonication/High Pressure Extrusion/Microfluidization/Low Pressure Extrusion:** Techniques like ultrasonication, high pressure extrusion, microfluidization and low pressure extrusion have been employed in literature to obtain a narrow vesicle size distribution after liposome preparation (Kreuter, 1994; Laouini et al., 2012). Notwithstanding that the approaches differ in the mechanisms by which size reduction is achieved resulting in differences in the final size attained at the end of each process, they provide with a uniform size distribution which is reproducible. Lapinski et al provided direct comparison of liposomes formed by extrusion and sonication employed for size reduction and found that the two techniques yield a difference in mean diameter and size distribution of the vesicles. However, they also concluded that the molecular organization of liposomes is governed by the nature of their constituents and the interactions between them, rather than the modus operandi employed for formulation (Lapinski et al., 2007). In addition to using them as post preparation size reduction tools, the above mentioned techniques have also been utilized to directly obtain vesicles of the desired size distribution. Brandl et al developed a single-step method of preparation of lecithin SUVs with size ranging between 25-50nm using a Gaulin Micron Lab 40 high pressure homogenizer (Brandl et al., 1990).
    c. **Bubbling of an Inert Gas:** With a view to eliminate the use of organic solvents and detergents, Talsma et al developed a low shear technique which entailed the introduction of nitrogen gas into a dispersion of solid powdered lipids to form liposomes with a mean particle size in the range of 0.2 to 0.5μ (Talsma et al., 1994). The resulting vesicles possessed a higher aqueous captured volume as compared to those prepared by conventional methods like thin film hydration.

Table 5. Methods of preparation and their advantages and disadvantages

Method of Preparation	Type of Liposome Formed	Advantages	Disadvantages	References
Mechanical Dispersion Methods				
Thin film hydration (Vortex/hand shaking)	MLV	• Easy to handle • Very good upscaling feasibility	• Not suitable for entrapment of water soluble drugs • Traces of organic solvent-critical for parenteral delivery.	(Laouini et al., 2012), (Kreuter, 1994)
Ultrasonication/ High Pressure Extrusion/ Microfluidization/ French pressure cell extrusion	Mainly SUV	• Avoids use of organic solvents/ detergents. • High pressure homogenizers can handle high concentration of lipids and are amenable to scale-up. • Both hydration and downsizing are achieved in a single step. • Uniform particle size distribution is obtained with good reproducibility.	• Surface erosion from high pressure homogenizers/probe sonicators may result in contamination of product. • Low aqueous capture volumes, hence unsuitable for entrapment of water soluble drugs.	(Laouini et al., 2012), (Kreuter, 1994; Lapinski et al., 2007).
Bubbling of inert gas	BSV	• Eliminates use of organic solvents and detergents, utilizes low shear. • High aqueous captured volume-suitable for loading of proteins.	• Very large sized vesicles obtained. • Mild phospholipid degradation (hydrolysis) could take place.	(Kreuter, 1994), (Talsma et al., 1994).
Solvent Dispersion Methods				
Ether injection method/Ethanol injection method	MLV, OLV, SUV, LUV	• Methods involving use of water-miscible solvents are amenable to scale-up. • Small liposomes with a narrow size distribution can be prepared without the need for sonication or extrusion.	• Many lipids are insoluble in ethanol. • Traces of organic solvent may restrict parenteral use of the preparation. • Not suitable for encapsulation of biological molecules like proteins, enzymes, DNA, RNA.	(Laouini et al., 2012), (Jaafar-Maalej et al., 2010), (Akbarzadeh et al., 2013).
Reverse phase evaporation method	LUV, OLV, MLV, MLV-REV, SPLV	• High aqueous space-to-lipid ratio. • High encapsulation efficiencies for water-soluble molecules.	• Exposure of molecules to be entrapped to organic solvents limiting their use for parenteral administration • Not suitable for encapsulation of biological molecules that degrade in presence of organic solvents.	(Akbarzadeh et al., 2013), (Vemuri & Rhodes, 1995), (Lu et al., 2014).
Detergent Removal Methods				
Dialysis/Gel permeation chromatography/ Dilution/ Adsorption onto polymeric beads.	SUV, OLV, MLV, LUV	• This method precludes the use of organic solvents. • Adsorption onto polymeric beads ensures removal of detergents with very low CMCs. • The method is amenable to scale-up for preparation of OLV.	• Not suitable for entrapment of molecules with low affinity for lipid bilayers. • Safety concerns about residual detergents limits parenteral use.	(Akbarzadeh et al., 2013), (Vemuri & Rhodes, 1995), (Lu et al., 2014).
Size Transformation and Fusion Methods				
Freeze drying/ Freeze thawing/ Dehydration-rehydration of SUV	LUV, OLV, MLV	• Enables loading of labile molecules without exposure to organic solvents or detergents. • Freeze thawing improves encapsulation efficiency of bilayer by eliminating bilayer stacks and improved swelling.	• High concentrations of cryoprotectant may interfere with the entrapment of molecules. • Freezing may be destructive to labile molecules, limiting this method for their use. • These methods may not be suitable for drugs which do not exhibit 100% entrapment of require removal of the unentrapped portion.	(Kreuter, 1994)
pH adjustment methods	SUV, LUV		• Heterogeneity in size distribution of formed vesicles. • Low encapsulation efficiency. • High cost of ionic lipids.	

2. **Solvent Dispersion Methods:**
    a. **Ether Injection Method/Ethanol Injection Method:** Ether injection and ethanol injection methods enable the preparation of liposomes of small size (100nm) without the aid of sonication and extrusion techniques (Kreuter, 1994; Laouini et al., 2012). The methods consist of injecting an ethanolic or etheric dispersion of lipids into aqueous media followed by removal of the organic solvents at elevated temperatures and/or under reduced pressures to obtain liposomes. Other water miscible solvents like methanol, isopropyl alcohol and water immiscible solvents like chloroform, freonscan also be employed. An aerosolised spray form of a liposomal dispersion prepared using water, ethanol and chlorofluorocarbons as vehicle has been suggested in literature (McGurk et al., 1986). ChirazJaafar-Maalej et al employed the ethanol injection method to produce multilamellar vesicles with sizes ranging from 80 to 170nm. These liposomes were successfully used to encapsulate a hydrophobic drug, beclomethasonedipropionate (100%) and a hydrophilic drug, cytarabine (16%) for pulmonary delivery (Jaafar-Maalej et al., 2010).
    b. **Reverse Phase Evaporation:** The reverse phase evaporation technique of preparing liposomes comprises of preparation of water-in-oil emulsion of lipids and buffer/aqueous phase in excess of organic solvent by sonication. The organic solvent is then eliminated gradually under reduced pressure resulting in the formation of a gel-like viscous intermediate. At a critical point in the procedure, the gel collapses and gives rise to liposomes (Lu et al., 2014; Vemuri & Rhodes, 1995). Organic solvents like isopropyl ether, diethyl ether, chloroform and mixtures thereof are employed in this method.

Szoka et al demonstrated the application of REV method in encapsulating water soluble molecules like drugs, proteins and nucleic acids with an appreciable retention of activity (for example, 41% for alkaline phosphatase) despite the use of organic solvents (Szoka & Papahadjopoulos, 1978).

3. **Detergent Removal Methods:**
    a. **Dialysis/Gel Permeation Chromatography/Dilution/Adsorption onto Polymeric Beads:** Detergents like glycocholate and deoxycholate are often used to solubilise lipids by formation of mixed micelles. The removal of detergent precedes the formation of a lipid rich phase which later culminates into liposomes. Dialysis, gel permeation chromatography, dilution with buffer and adsorption onto beaded organic polystyrene adsorbers facilitate formation of liposomes by elimination of detergent. Milsmann et al substantiated dialysis as a method for obtaining homogeneous liposomes from phosphatidylcholine/cholate mixed micelles (Milsmann et al., 1978).

Techniques like dialysis have also been used to obtain liposomes of a predetermined size and size distribution. Bosworth et al corroborated the utility of dialysis in succession with extrusion for controlling the lower end of the size frequency distribution of liposomes (Bosworth et al., 1982).

4. **Size Transformation and Fusion Methods:**
    a. **Freeze Drying/Freeze Thawing/Dehydration-Rehydration of SUV:** These processes essentially involve the use of 'freezing' for the formation of multilamellar or large unilamellar liposomes. Process variables like freezing time, freezing rate and freezing temperature can

be controlled to obtain desired liposomes. Besides, cryoprotectant concentration and type plays an important role in determining the encapsulation efficiency of the molecule(s) to be entrapped. Evans et al patented the process for preparing liposomes by freeze drying and evinced the benefits of the latter (Evans et al., 1983).

5. **pH Adjustment Methods:** This method utilizes surface charge density of the lipid molecule to promote vesiculation and thus liposome formation. pH of the dispersion medium, thus, critically governs the process of liposome formation by this method. Formation of phosphatidic acid SUV at higher pH values (~7 to 8) was shown by Hauser and Gains (Hauser & Gains, 1982).

Loading of Liposomes with Molecules of Biological Interest

Liposomes have been exploited for pharmaceutical applications as carriers of drugs and other molecules of biological interest like deoxyribonucleic acid (DNA), ribonucleic acid (RNA), and genetic material of therapeutic value. These molecules either occupy the bilayer space or the aqueous lacuna offered by the liposomes. Bilayer properties (fluidity of the bilayer, aqueous volume, charge, size and lamellarity) in addition to the physicochemical properties (bilayer/water partition coefficient) of the cargo to be encapsulated determine the type of interaction between them and the stability of such cargo loaded liposomal systems. Loading of the agent of interest may be carried out by one of the following methods:

1. **Passive Loading:** Wherein the molecule of interest is loaded within the liposome during their preparation. The extent of loading achieved with this method is governed by the type of interaction between the cargo and the liposome. Bilayer composition, aqueous volume available and drug bilayer/water partition coefficient are predisposing factors to hydrophobic or electrostatic interaction which facilitate the loading of the cargo into the liposomal system (Kreuter, 1994). Besides, the osmotic gradient established after hydration of lipids in the process of liposome formation also influences the encapsulation of a cargo within the vesicles.

Cullis et al have reviewed the requirements of a system to achieve high trapping efficiencies for various cargos by means of passive loading techniques (Cullis et al., 1989).

2. **Active Loading/Remote Loading:** wherein a 'driving force' is employed to load the molecule of interest within the vesicles after their preparation, without perturbing the integrity of the vesicle membrane. A pH gradient, a membrane potential or an ammonium sulphate gradient could be utilised to attain a driving force sufficient to aid encapsulation of drugs into liposomal systems. Many amine drugs belonging to different therapeutic categories have been loaded into liposomes using active loading technique. Examples include doxorubicin, daunorubicin, serotonin, imipramine, lidocaine, quinidine and a few others (Bally et al., 1988; Vemuri & Rhodes, 1995).

Novel Industrial Methods

Methods based on the use of supercritical fluid technology, dual asymmetric centrifugation, membrane contractor method, cross flow filtration detergent depletion method, freeze drying double emulsion method have been shown to possess large scale feasibility.

Table 6 provides a summary of these novel techniques that have been developed for the preparation of liposomes in the recent times and can be utilised at the industrial scale.

Characterisation

Characterization of liposomal systems is critical for defining quality standards and obtaining reproducibility for bench work and manufacturing process. Some of the characterization tools employed for liposomal systems are as stated in Table 7.

Applications of Liposomes

The myriad properties and advantages of liposomes make them amenable to a number of applications. However, due to space restrictions, we shall focus on the therapeutic and diagnostic applications in this section of the chapter.

Table 6. Novel methods for industrial scale production of liposomes

Method	Description	Comments
Supercritical fluid technology: Suprcriticalantisolvent/ reverse phase evaporation method (100-10,000nm)	• Organic solvent used to dissolve lipids is evaporated in a supercritical fluid CO_2 environment, thereby precipitating lipids in the form of extremely small particles. Liposomes are obtained by hydrating this deposited film of ultrafine lipid particles. • Supercritical reverse phase evaporation method entails the use of supercritical fluid CO_2 for dissolution of lipids.	• Ensures complete removal of organic solvent. • Particle size, entrapment efficiency comparable with that of Bangham method obtained.
Dual Asymmetric centrifugation (DAC) (70-120nm)	Two overlaying movements of sample material (vials turn around the main axis-rotation at fixed speed and distance, as well as around their own centres) in a centrifugation vial bring about liposome formation and size reduction comparable to homogenization technique.	• Good reproducibility in size is obtained. • DAC is a small and easy to operate equipment. • Water-soluble drugs have high entrapment efficiency in liposomes prepared by this method. • Organic solvent free method. • Used for prepation of vesicular phospholipid gels.
Membrane contractor technology (~100nm)	Similar to ethanol injection method, wherein liposomes are formed by mixing of lipid and aqueous phases under pressure in a membrane contractor module, accompanied by removal of organic solvent like ethanol.	• Homogeneous and small particle size obtained with multilamellar vesicle formation. • Useful for entrapment of lipophilic drugs. • Scale-up is easy.
Cross-flow filtration detergent depletion method (~50nm)	Based on detergent depletion method of liposome formation with feasibility for continuous, sterile operation using a cross-flow filtration assembly to facilitate complete detergent removal.	• Sterile liposomes with small particle size and homogeneity prepared quickly. • Recycling of waste filtrate enables reduction of cost.
Freeze drying double emulsion method	A double emulsion of the form W/O/W of lipids and aqueous phase is subjected to freeze drying in the presence of cryoprotectants.	• Sterile liposomes with good shelf life can be obtained. • Cryoprotectants limit the use of such preparation in diabetic patients.

Huang et al., 2014.

Table 7. Characterization techniques for liposomes

Characterization Parameter	Characterization Method
Physical Characterization	
Particle size and size distribution analysis	Static or Dynamic light scattering, coulter counter, HPLC-SEC, Field flow fractionation, Polarization intensity differential scattering
Lamellarity determination	SAXS, NMR, Electron microscopy, Use of fluorescent probes.
Determination of entrapped volume	Coloured or fluorescent probes
Zeta potential determination	Light scattering techniques, microelectrophoresis, zeta potential probes.
Structural and motional characterization	NMR, ESR, DSC
Encapsulation efficiency	Ultracentrifugation, Size Exclusion Chromatography(SEC), Dialysis
In vitro drug release	Dialysis
Chemical Characterization	
Lipid analysis	Bartlett assay, complexation techniques, Fluorescence assay, Enzymatic assays, Chromatographic techniques like HPLC, GC, TLC
Biological Characterization	
Sterility	Aerobic and anaerobic bottle cultures
Pyrogenicity	Rabbit or LAL tests
Animal Toxicity	Histology, pathology, survival

Laouini et al., 2012; Swarbrick & Boylan, 1993.

Therapeutic and Diagnostic Applications

Targeting: Exploitation of Liposomes for Site Specific Drug Delivery

Drug delivery science witnessed a paradigm shift with the introduction of the concept of 'targeting' laid down by Paul Ehrlich, who described it as a 'magic bullet' remedy. Targeting essentially involves interaction between a targeting moiety (as a part of the delivery system) and a target (as a receptor or enzyme in a specific location of the body) resulting in accrual of an API at the target site vis-à-vis other locations *in vivo* (V. P. Torchilin, 2010). Nanosystems utilise 'the targeting approach' to deliver drugs to specific locations thereby minimising off-target toxicity.

Drug delivery can be effected by 'passive' or 'active' targeting. Passive targeting utilizes physical properties of the delivery system like particle size and accumulation at the target site is achieved by means of the enhanced permeation and retention (EPR) effect. The latter entails extravasation (particles sized between 10 to 500nm) through leaky vasculature observed in tumours, infarcts and inflammations (V. P. Torchilin, 2010). Therefore, it is important to note that the pathophysiology of a particular tissue or organ enables passive targeting of a drug loaded delivery system. However, vascular permeability is not affected in many diseases and that may forbid the entry of a delivery system via EPR effect. In such situations, active targeting can be employed to achieve high concentrations of the API at the target site. A target receptor specific ligand or antibody can be appended to the delivery system housing the API thereby facilitating recognition and interaction with the target organ and intracellular drug delivery.

Liposomes have been widely exploited for targeted drug delivery in clinical conditions like cancer. Properties like biocompatibility, biodegradability, ability to modify pharmacokinetics of the encapsulated drug, amenability to surface modification by ligands and antibodies make liposomes suitable for passive and active targeted drug delivery (Sawant & Torchilin, 2012).

In addition to properties like optimum particle size, prolonged residence time in circulation is a prerequisite to passive targeting of liposomes. The increase in the circulation time of liposomes can be achieved by utilizing a hydrophilic polymer like PEG on the liposomal surface (Sawant & Torchilin, 2012; V. P. Torchilin, 2010). Such 'stealthing' in the form of a well solvated and flexible hydrophilic coating not only prolongs the in vivo circulation time, but also prevents opsonisation and impedes RES uptake of the delivery system. Steric stabilisation of liposomes can be employed for both passive and active targeting of the delivery system.

Surface modification of liposomes by PEG can be accomplished by physical adsorption, incorporation during liposome preparation as PEG-lipid conjugate or by tethering reactive chemical groups on liposomal surface (Immordino et al., 2006). Sant et al corroborated the concept of stealthing with a novel PEG-Lipid conjugate, viz, PEG-Cholesterol (V. P. Sant & Nagarsenker, 2011) and demonstrated a two-fold increase in the antimetastatic activity of pentoxifylline when incorporated in sterically stabilised liposomes (V. Sant et al., 2000). Sant et al have also evaluated the effect of steric stabilisation on the cytotoxic activity of a combination of etoposide and pentoxifylline incorporated in stealth liposomes and envisaged clinical potential for the same independent of sequence of administration (V. P. Sant et al., 2003).

Stealthing of liposomes has also been exploited for drug delivery to organs of infection, in addition to its use in cancer treatment. Studies on stealthing of amphotericin B liposomes by Jadhav et al provide proof of concept for increased residence time of the liposomes in circulation which further opens avenues to improvement in the therapeutic efficacy of such drugs indicated in fungal infections (Jadhav et al., 2011).

Recent developments in the realm of sterically stabilised liposomes suggest alteration in their pharmacokinetic behaviour on multiple dosing of PEG-grafted liposomes. Rapid elimination of a second dose of PEGylated liposomes followed by their accumulation in liver and spleen was observed when the former was administered after an interval of several days from the first dose. This phenomenon is called accelerated blood clearance (ABC) (Ishida et al., 2005; Ishida & Kiwada, 2008; Laverman, Boerman et al., 2001; Laverman, Carstens et al., 2001).

Immordino et al have reviewed stealthing of liposomes and further details on this topic can be found in the same (Immordino et al., 2006).

Active targeting has largely been utilized with a view to overcome the limitations of passive targeting which is accompanied by an increased interstitial fluid pressure when targeting tumours. Active targeting of drugs using delivery systems like liposomes to sites of biological interest is realized with the aid of homing molecules like ligands and antibodies (immunoliposomes). Ligands may be carbohydrates/lipids/proteins in nature and are employed for surface modification of liposomes. The recognition of target receptors by such targeting molecules facilitates site specific intracellular drug delivery, in addition to surmounting the barrier of drug resistance (Sawant & Torchilin, 2012). Site specificity can thus be achieved in various clinical conditions with improved therapeutic efficacy and abated off target toxicities. The following reports provide a deeper insight into active targeting:

Shah et al have provided preclinical evidence for the targetability of palmitoylated arabinogalactan (Shah et al., 2013), a carbohydrate based ligand specific to ASGPR receptors expressed on hepatocytes in HCC. Besides, they have also demonstrated significantly higher tumour suppression in immunocompromised mice facilitated by active targeting with the arabinogalactan based ligand modified liposomes as compared to conventional liposomes (Shah et al., 2014). Also, Pathak et al have synthesized cholesteryl derivative of arabinogalactan and utilized it for surface modification of liposomes. They have substantiated increased uptake of such ligand modified liposomes vis-à-vis conventional liposomes in ASGPR positive HepG2 cell line and presaged such actively targeted systems as potential alternatives to existing treatment of HCC (Pathak et al., 2015).

Jain et al have reported active targeting with the aid of an antineoplastic drug molecule like tamoxifen. They are the first ones to utilize an anticancer molecule like tamoxifen as a ligand for active targeting of doxorubicin loaded liposomes. They have successfully proved its utility in providing significantly greater inhibition of estrogen receptor positive MCF-7 cell based tumour growth in nude mice, when compared with doxorubicin solution and doxorubicin liposomes. The study has positively brought to light the dual role of targetability and therapeutic efficacy attainable with an anticancer molecule like tamoxifen (Jain et al., 2014).

Targeting approaches also make use of stimuli-sensitivity such as slightly raised temperature or low pH observed in certain pathological conditions like tumours and inflammations in addition to the active and passive processes mentioned above. Shah et al and Jain et al have demonstrated higher release of doxorubicin from surface modified liposomes at tumour pH(5.5) compared to blood pH (7.4) thus corroborating stimuli-sensitive delivery of the drug(Jain et al., 2014; Shah et al., 2014).

Biological Molecules: Utilising Liposomes for Gene Delivery

Genetic dysfunction is responsible for a number of pathological conditions including cancer. Identification of the non-functional gene or its respective translated protein has intuitively shown the path towards treatment of such clinical conditions. Until the revelation of the role of liposomes in the delivery of such materials to specific cellular targets, viral vectors were being used to achieve gene delivery owing to their high transgene expression and transduction efficiency (Monteiro et al., 2014). However, they possessed multiple drawbacks like mutagenesis, lack of target specificity, immunogenicity of the viral components and recombination engendering infectious virions (Barua et al., 2011; Kawakami et al., 2008; Vo et al., 2012). Felgner et al introduced cationic lipids like N-[1-(2,3-dioleyloxy)propyl]-N,N,N-trimethylammonium chloride(DOTMA) capable of spontaneous assembly and association with DNA. They further vindicated efficient uptake of the lipid-DNA complex leading to expression of complexed DNA, thus providing utility of cationic liposomes for gene delivery (Felgner et al., 1987). Many transfection kits are commercially available since then and various cationic lipids are being explored for their role in transfection (Y. Barenholz, 2001).

Liposomes used for gene delivery are essentially composed of cationic lipids (e.g. 1,2-bis(oleoyloxy)-3-(trimethylammonio)propane (DOTAP), dioctadecylamidoglycylspermine (DOGS), DOTMA,3β[N-(N,N-dimethylaminoethane)-carbamoyl] cholesterol DC-chol) and neutral lipids (eg.Dioleoylphosphatidylethanolamine (DOPE), Dioleoylphosphatidylcholine(DOPC)), the latter also commonly known as helper lipids. The advantage of non-viral vectors over their viral counterparts is the lack of untoward effects and immunogenicity and their ability to transfect large-sized genetic materials (Lian & Ho, 2001; Sharma & Sharma, 1997).

Current research on gene delivery of liposomes entails exploration of novel cationic lipids and augmenting their transfection efficiency with improved cellular targeting. On these lines, Dhawan et al have demonstrated utility of novel cationic lecithin nanoparticles in inducing apoptosis leading to their use in oral anticancer delivery (Dhawan et al., 2014).

Liposomes as Immunological Adjuvants for Vaccine Delivery

The physicochemical properties of liposomes enable targeting of the immune system including the RES. The potential of large sized liposomes has been explored for delivering antigens to the cells of immune system. Liposomes are capable of inducing both humoral and cellular immunity by presenting the antigen to dendritic cells, endothelial cells and Langerhans cells in addition to macrophages by engaging both MHC-I and MHC –II presentation mechanisms. This facilitates the induction of a stronger immune response as compared to conventional adjuvants like Freund's adjuvant (Lian et al., 1999; V. Torchilin, 2012). Mucosal immunity can also be accessed with the aid of liposomal antigen delivery via the oral route.

The use of immune stimulators like amphiphilic muramyl peptides, lipid A and lipopolysaccharides in conjunction with liposomes fosters immunological adjuvanticity of the latter. Besides physicochemical properties of liposomes like bilayer fluidity charge density and epitope density modulate the immune response to the antigen incorporated in the liposomes (Kersten & Crommelin, 1995).

Liposomal vaccine containing Hepatitis A virions is the first such vaccine to be approved for human use in Switzerland. A number of clinical trials are being conducted to develop liposomal vaccines for cancer, infectious diseases like influenza and other pathological conditions (Gregoriadis, 1995).

Miscellaneous Applications: Unmitigated Scope of Liposomes

Commencement of commercialization of liposomal drug delivery systems in the mid 90's persuaded researchers to exploit their utility for various drug/gene delivery applications. Notwithstanding their valuable contribution to site specific drug delivery, gene delivery and vaccine delivery, liposomes have also been employed for topical, ocular and pulmonary delivery owing to their ability to hold an array of different molecules and sustain their release over time. Nagarsenker et al. demonstrated the superiority of sodium chromoglycate loaded REV liposomes in comparison with drug solution when evaluated in sensitized guinea pig model for treatment of asthma (Nagarsenker & Londhe, 2003). The formulated liposomes have been shown to inhibit neutrophil influx even at 24h from administration thereby proving advantage of liposomal treatment employed for pulmonary disorders.

In addition, liposomes also find wide application for drug delivery through skin. Nagarsenker et al have explored the role of liposomes containing cyclodextrin complex of Ketorolac acid for transdermal delivery and found that the liposomes slowed the permeation of drug through skin when compared with drug solution and cyclodextrin complex of drug (Nagarsenker et al., 2008). Besides, Shah et al have conducted a detailed study comparing three vesicular systems (liposomes, invasomes and leciplex) employed for treatment of acne, while Date et al have reviewed liposomes as one of the novel systems employed in topical treatment of acne (Naik & Nagarsenker, 2006; Shah et al., 2015).

The benefits of liposomes also extend to diagnostic purposes, wherein, imaging and contrasting agents can be incorporated into liposomal bilayers/aqueous core/adsorbed onto the surface. As a development on this front, amphiphilic polymers have been introduced into liposomes with a view to augment the load of contrasting agents and reporter metals facilitating improved visualization in various diagnostic techniques.

Al-Jamal et al have additionally reported theranostic application of liposomes when fabricated as hybrids with nanoparticles. They have shown improved dispersibility of quantum dots in liposomal bilayers thereby providing dual advantage of imaging and cytotoxicity when loaded with doxorubicin (Al-Jamal & Kostarelos, 2011).

The unassailable contribution to applications of liposomes on targeting by Torchilin et al (V. P. Torchilin, 2010), sterically stabilised liposomes by Lasic et al (Papahadjopoulos et al., 1991),preparation of liposomes mimicking erythrocyte membrane using gangliosides and sialic acid derivatives by Allen et al, Gabizon et al (Allen et al., 1989; Gabizon & Papahadjopoulos, 1988)and demonstration of decreased MPS uptake by surface modification using gangliosides by Yamauchi et al(Yamauchi et al., 1995) facilitated intense research and growth in liposomology.

In Vivo Behaviour/Fate of Liposomes

The ultimate aim of a formulation scientist is to reach the delivery system to its target site of action *in vivo*. In case of liposomes, the *in vivo* behaviour is critically dictated by the route of administration. Intravenous administration of liposomes results in concentration of the vesicles in the RES, particularly, macrophages of the liver, spleen, bone marrow and circulation. The presence of a tumorous or infectious site predisposes the distribution of liposomes *in vivo* owing to a compromised vasculature and increased permeability. Subcutaneous or intramuscular injection of liposomes leads to the formation of a sustained release depot at the site of administration, with maximum retention occurring in the lymph nodes.

Once in circulation, the liposomes encounter a number of different cells in the body resulting in different types of interactions. Lipid-cell communication *in vivo*, is affected by various factors like bilayer fluidity, surface hydration and charge, particle size and excipients like polymers, ligands and antibodies. The various pathways by which liposome-cell interaction occurs is shown in Figure 7. These pathways are described in brief below (Allen et al., 1995; Marcolis, 1984; Pagano & Weinstein, 1978):

Figure 7. Liposome-cell interaction and mechanisms of cell uptake

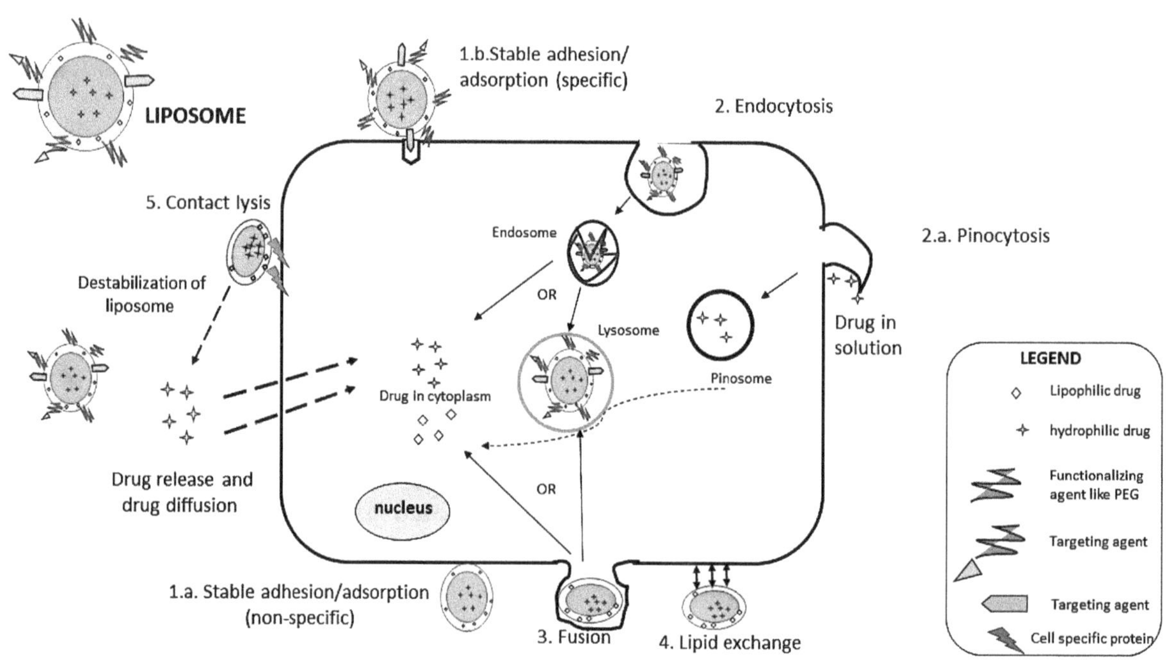

1. **Stable Adhesion/Adsorption:** Stable adhesion or adsorption refers to nonspecific interaction through hydrophobic bonds/Van der Waals forces or specific interaction through antibodies or surface proteins, of liposomes with cells without undergoing further modification.
2. **Endocytosis:** Endocytosis may be receptor mediated through presence of specific ligands or antibodies on the surface of liposomes or via clathrin coated pits which result in the formation of endosomes or lysosomes containing the endocytosed liposomes. In some cases, however, it may be possible to escape the endosomal capture of liposomes. Endocytosis may also be mediated via pinosomes, in the event of the drug/payload being released in the outer medium. Macrophage mediated endocytosis of liposomes is usually observed *in vivo* and is more commonly referred to as phagocytosis.
3. **Fusion:** Fusion implies the amalgamation of the liposomal membrane with the plasma membrane resulting in concurrent release of the liposomal contents into the cytoplasm.
4. **Lipid Exchange between Liposomal and Plasma Membrane:** This process refers to the exchange of plasma membrane lipids with those of liposomes resulting in a leaky liposomal membrane. The process culminates into the release of liposomal contents into the cytoplasm of the cell. Lipid transfer process has been reported to find application in the modulation of cholesterol content of liposomes and cells.
5. **Contact Lysis of Liposomes:** This process suggests the destabilization of liposomes and simultaneous release of their contents upon contacting the cells. This process is mediated by certain proteins present on the surface of particular cells.

One or more of the aforementioned processes may be involved in liposome-cell interactions. Besides, these liposome-cell interactions can be tuned to favour a particular process based on the need and application to be catered to. For example, gene delivery into the cell can be accomplished by employing a fusion peptide like 'Tat-peptide', the latter being capable of favouring the destabilization of the gene loaded liposomes following the fusion process.

The liposomes are cleared from the circulation by destabilization into their individual components. Phospholipids and cholesterol, like the endogenous lipids, are finally taken up by the liver and acted upon by enzymes therein (Cevc, 1993; Williams et al., 1984).

CONCLUSION

The plethora of opportunities and advantages offered by liposomes makes them one of the most successful clinical translations in the realm of nanotechnology. The market capture attained with the sales of Doxil® and Ambisome® validates the industrial scalability of these nanosystems. The structural features of liposomal constructs allow loading of a variety of molecules along with surface functionalization. This renders them amenable to passive and active targeting permitting accumulation of incorporated molecules directly into the cell. A blend of physicochemical properties of liposomes and the pathological features of target site enable designing of 'smart vesicular fabricates'. These specially fabricated liposomes possess PEG chain tethered to the liposomal surface via a biologically cleavable bond like pH sensitive hydrazone bond. This confers long *in vivo* circulation time and deshielding of the surface of liposomes containing an active targeting ligand/antibody on reaching the target cell by cleavage of the labile bond. Smart liposomes thus provide an insight into versatility of these nanosystems.

A lot of efforts are being directed towards meeting the regulatory and quality requirements for industrially feasible production methods. Further, there is a need to achieve sterile, stable and standard liposomal systems for making scalability a success for the numerous methods employed to prepare liposomes on lab scale. An important area of liposomology that deserves consideration is the intracellular delivery of liposomes and elucidation of mechanisms for antigen delivery by liposomes. Products in pipeline like transferrin surface modified liposomes (MBP-426 Phase I/II trial) (Etheridge et al., 2013) are representative of attempts made to improve intracellular delivery of liposomes.

Extensive and encouraging research on liposomes envisages them as promising systems with potential clinical success for a number of applications in the subsequent decades.

REFERENCES

Akbarzadeh, A., Rezaei-Sadabady, R., Davaran, S., Joo, S. W., Zarghami, N., Hanifehpour, Y., & Nejati-Koshki, K. (2013). Liposome: Classification, preparation, and applications. *Nanoscale Research Letters*, *8*(1), 102. PMID:23432972

Al-Jamal, W. T., & Kostarelos, K. (2011). Liposomes: From a clinically established drug delivery system to a nanoparticle platform for theranostic nanomedicine. *Accounts of Chemical Research*, *44*(10), 1094–1104. doi:10.1021/ar200105p PMID:21812415

Allen, T. M., Hansen, C., & Rutledge, J. (1989). Liposomes with prolonged circulation times: Factors affecting uptake by reticuloendothelial and other tissues. *Biochimica et Biophysica Acta (BBA)-. Biomembranes*, *981*(1), 27–35. doi:10.1016/0005-2736(89)90078-3

Allen, T. M., Hansen, C. B., & de Menezes, D. E. L. (1995). Pharmacokinetics of long-circulating liposomes. *Advanced Drug Delivery Reviews*, *16*(2), 267–284. doi:10.1016/0169-409X(95)00029-7

Amselem, S., Gabizon, A., & Barenholz, Y. (1993). A large-scale method for the preparation of sterile and non-pyrogenic liposomal formulations of defined size distributions for clinical use. *Liposome Technology, 1*, 501-525.

Antonietti, M., & Förster, S. (2003). Vesicles and liposomes: A self-assembly principle beyond lipids. *Advanced Materials*, *15*(16), 1323–1333. doi:10.1002/adma.200300010

Bally, M. B., Mayer, L. D., Loughrey, H., Redelmeier, T., Madden, T. D., Wong, K., & Cullis, P. R. et al. (1988). Dopamine accumulation in large unilamellar vesicle systems induced by transmembrane ion gradients. *Chemistry and Physics of Lipids*, *47*(2), 97–107. doi:10.1016/0009-3084(88)90078-3 PMID:2457454

Bangham, A. (1982). Techniques in the Life Science, B4/11. *Lipid and Membrane Biochemistry B*, *420*, 1–25.

Bangham, A., Standish, M., & Weissmann, G. (1965). The action of steroids and streptolysin S on the permeability of phospholipid structures to cations. *Journal of Molecular Biology*, *13*(1), 253–IN228. doi:10.1016/S0022-2836(65)80094-8 PMID:5859040

Bangham, A., Standish, M. M., & Watkins, J. (1965). Diffusion of univalent ions across the lamellae of swollen phospholipids. *Journal of Molecular Biology*, *13*(1), 238–IN227. doi:10.1016/S0022-2836(65)80093-6 PMID:5859039

Bangham, A. D., & Horne, R. (1964). Negative staining of phospholipids and their structural modification by surface-active agents as observed in the electron microscope. *Journal of Molecular Biology*, *8*(5), 660–IN610. doi:10.1016/S0022-2836(64)80115-7 PMID:14187392

Barenholz, Y. (2001). Liposome application: Problems and prospects. *Current Opinion in Colloid & Interface Science*, *6*(1), 66–77. doi:10.1016/S1359-0294(00)00090-X

Barenholz, Y. C. (2012). Doxil®—the first FDA-approved nano-drug: Lessons learned. *Journal of Controlled Release*, *160*(2), 117–134. doi:10.1016/j.jconrel.2012.03.020 PMID:22484195

Barua, S., Ramos, J., Potta, T., Taylor, D., Huang, H.-C., Montanez, G., & Rege, K. (2011). Discovery of cationic polymers for non-viral gene delivery using combinatorial approaches. *Combinatorial Chemistry & High Throughput Screening*, *14*(10), 908–924. doi:10.2174/138620711797537076 PMID:21843141

Benvegnu, T., Lemiègre, L., & Cammas-Marion, S. (2009). New generation of liposomes called archaeosomes based on natural or synthetic archaeal lipids as innovative formulations for drug delivery. *Recent Patents on Drug Delivery & Formulation*, *3*(3), 206–220. doi:10.2174/187221109789105630 PMID:19534669

Bladé, J., Sonneveld, P., San Miguel, J. F., Sutherland, H. J., Hajek, R., Nagler, A., & Zhuang, S. H. et al. (2011). Efficacy and safety of pegylated liposomal doxorubicin in combination with bortezomib for multiple myeloma: Effects of adverse prognostic factors on outcome. *Clinical Lymphoma Myeloma and Leukemia*, *11*(1), 44–49. doi:10.3816/CLML.2011.n.005 PMID:21454189

Bordi, F., Cametti, C., & Sennato, S. (2006). Electrical properties of aqueous liposome suspensions. *Advances in Planar Lipid Bilayers and Liposomes*, *4*, 281–320. doi:10.1016/S1554-4516(06)04009-9

Bosworth, M. E., Hunt, C. A., & Pratt, D. (1982). Liposome dialysis for improved size distributions. *Journal of Pharmaceutical Sciences*, *71*(7), 806–812. doi:10.1002/jps.2600710722 PMID:7120068

Brandl, M., Bachmann, D., Drechsler, M., & Bauer, K. (1990). Liposome preparation by a new high pressure homogenizer Gaulin Micron Lab 40. *Drug Development and Industrial Pharmacy*, *16*(14), 2167–2191. doi:10.3109/03639049009023648

Bressler, N. M., & Bressler, S. B. (2000). Photodynamic therapy with verteporfin (Visudyne): Impact on ophthalmology and visual sciences. *Investigative Ophthalmology & Visual Science*, *41*(3), 624–628. PMID:10711673

Cevc, G. (1987). How membrane chain melting properties are regulated by the polar surface of the lipid bilayer. *Biochemistry*, *26*(20), 6305–6310. doi:10.1021/bi00394a002 PMID:3427005

Cevc, G. (1991). How membrane chain-melting phase-transition temperature is affected by the lipid chain asymmetry and degree of unsaturation: An effective chain-length model. *Biochemistry*, *30*(29), 7186–7193. doi:10.1021/bi00243a021 PMID:1854729

Cevc, G. (1993). *Phospholipids handbook*. CRC Press.

Chen, Z., & Rand, R. (1997). The influence of cholesterol on phospholipid membrane curvature and bending elasticity. *Biophysical Journal*, *73*(1), 267–276. doi:10.1016/S0006-3495(97)78067-6 PMID:9199791

Chong, P. L.-G., Ayesa, U., Prakash Daswani, V., & Hur, E. C. (2012). On physical properties of tetraether lipid membranes: Effects of cyclopentane rings. *Archaea (Vancouver, B.C.)*, 2012. PMID:23028246

Cui, Z.-K., & Lafleur, M. (2014). Lamellar self-assemblies of single-chain amphiphiles and sterols and their derived liposomes: Distinct compositions and distinct properties. *Colloids and Surfaces. B, Biointerfaces*, *114*, 177–185. doi:10.1016/j.colsurfb.2013.09.042 PMID:24184913

Cullis, P., Mayer, L., Bally, M., Madden, T., & Hope, M. (1989). Generating and loading of liposomal systems for drug-delivery applications. *Advanced Drug Delivery Reviews*, *3*(3), 267–282. doi:10.1016/0169-409X(89)90024-0

Deamer, D. W. (2010). From "Banghasomes" to liposomes: A memoir of Alec Bangham, 1921–2010. *The FASEB Journal*, *24*(5), 1308–1310. doi:10.1096/fj.10-0503 PMID:20430797

Dhawan, V. V., Joshi, G. V., Jain, A. S., Nikam, Y. P., Gude, R. P., Mulherkar, R., & Nagarsenker, M. S. (2014). Apoptosis induction and anti-cancer activity of LeciPlex formulations. *Cellular Oncology*, *37*(5), 339–351. doi:10.1007/s13402-014-0183-7 PMID:25204961

Ebato, Y., Kato, Y., Onishi, H., Nagai, T., & Machida, Y. (2003). In vivo efficacy of a novel double liposome as an oral dosage form of salmon calcitonin. *Drug Development Research*, *58*(3), 253–257. doi:10.1002/ddr.10162

Etheridge, M. L., Campbell, S. A., Erdman, A. G., Haynes, C. L., Wolf, S. M., & McCullough, J. (2013). The big picture on nanomedicine: The state of investigational and approved nanomedicine products. *Nanomedicine; Nanotechnology, Biology, and Medicine*, *9*(1), 1–14. doi:10.1016/j.nano.2012.05.013 PMID:22684017

Evans, J. R., Fildes, F. J., & Oliver, J. E. (1983). *U.S. Patent No. 4,370,349*. Washington, DC: U.S. Patent and Trademark Office.

Fariya, M., Jain, A., Dhawan, V., Shah, S., & Nagarsenker, M. S. (2014). Bolaamphiphiles: A Pharmaceutical Review. *Advanced Pharmaceutical Bulletin, 4*(Suppl 2), 483.

Fasol, U., Frost, A., Büchert, M., Arends, J., Fiedler, U., Scharr, D., & Mross, K. et al. (2012). Vascular and pharmacokinetic effects of EndoTAG-1 in patients with advanced cancer and liver metastasis. *Annals of Oncology*, *23*(4), 1030–1036. doi:10.1093/annonc/mdr300 PMID:21693769

Felgner, P. L., Gadek, T. R., Holm, M., Roman, R., Chan, H. W., Wenz, M., & Danielsen, M. et al. (1987). Lipofection: A highly efficient, lipid-mediated DNA-transfection procedure. *Proceedings of the National Academy of Sciences of the United States of America*, *84*(21), 7413–7417. doi:10.1073/pnas.84.21.7413 PMID:2823261

Gabizon, A., & Papahadjopoulos, D. (1988). Liposome formulations with prolonged circulation time in blood and enhanced uptake by tumors. *Proceedings of the National Academy of Sciences of the United States of America*, *85*(18), 6949–6953. doi:10.1073/pnas.85.18.6949 PMID:3413128

Gambling, D., Hughes, T., Martin, G., Horton, W., & Manvelian, G. (2005). A comparison of Depodur™, a novel, single-dose extended-release epidural morphine, with standard epidural morphine for pain relief after lower abdominal surgery. *Anesthesia and Analgesia*, *100*(4), 1065–1074. doi:10.1213/01.ANE.0000145009.03574.78 PMID:15781524

Ganta, S., Devalapally, H., Shahiwala, A., & Amiji, M. (2008). A review of stimuli-responsive nanocarriers for drug and gene delivery. *Journal of Controlled Release*, *126*(3), 187–204. doi:10.1016/j.jconrel.2007.12.017 PMID:18261822

Gregoriadis, G. (1976a). The carrier potential of liposomes in biology and medicine. *The New England Journal of Medicine*, *295*(13), 704–710. doi:10.1056/NEJM197609232951305 PMID:958245

Gregoriadis, G. (1976b). The carrier potential of liposomes in biology and medicine (second of two parts). *The New England Journal of Medicine*, *295*(14), 765–770. doi:10.1056/NEJM197609302951406 PMID:785256

Gregoriadis, G. (1995). Engineering liposomes for drug delivery: Progress and problems. *Trends in Biotechnology*, *13*(12), 527–537. doi:10.1016/S0167-7799(00)89017-4 PMID:8595139

Guo, S., & Huang, L. (2011). Nanoparticles escaping RES and endosome: Challenges for siRNA delivery for cancer therapy. *Journal of Nanomaterials*, *2011*, 11. doi:10.1155/2011/742895

Hann, I. M., & Prentice, H. G. (2001). Lipid-based amphotericin B: A review of the last 10 years of use. *International Journal of Antimicrobial Agents*, *17*(3), 161–169. doi:10.1016/S0924-8579(00)00341-1 PMID:11282260

Hauser, H., & Gains, N. (1982). Spontaneous vesiculation of phospholipids: A simple and quick method of forming unilamellar vesicles. *Proceedings of the National Academy of Sciences of the United States of America*, *79*(6), 1683–1687. doi:10.1073/pnas.79.6.1683 PMID:6952221

Huang, Z., Li, X., Zhang, T., Song, Y., She, Z., Li, J., & Deng, Y. (2014). Progress involving new techniques for liposome preparation. *Asian Journal of Pharmaceutical Sciences*, *9*(4), 176–182. doi:10.1016/j.ajps.2014.06.001

Immordino, M. L., Dosio, F., & Cattel, L. (2006). Stealth liposomes: Review of the basic science, rationale, and clinical applications, existing and potential. *International Journal of Nanomedicine*, *1*(3), 297. PMID:17717971

Ipsen, J. H., Karlström, G., Mourtisen, O., Wennerström, H., & Zuckermann, M. (1987). Phase equilibria in the phosphatidylcholine-cholesterol system. *Biochimica et Biophysica Acta (BBA)-. Biomembranes*, *905*(1), 162–172. doi:10.1016/0005-2736(87)90020-4

Ishida, T., Harada, M., Wang, X. Y., Ichihara, M., Irimura, K., & Kiwada, H. (2005). Accelerated blood clearance of PEGylated liposomes following preceding liposome injection: Effects of lipid dose and PEG surface-density and chain length of the first-dose liposomes. *Journal of Controlled Release*, *105*(3), 305–317. doi:10.1016/j.jconrel.2005.04.003 PMID:15908032

Ishida, T., & Kiwada, H. (2008). Accelerated blood clearance (ABC) phenomenon upon repeated injection of PEGylated liposomes. *International Journal of Pharmaceutics*, *354*(1), 56–62. doi:10.1016/j.ijpharm.2007.11.005 PMID:18083313

Israelachvili, J. N. (2011). *Intermolecular and surface forces* (3rd ed.). Academic Press.

Jaafar-Maalej, C., Diab, R., Andrieu, V., Elaissari, A., & Fessi, H. (2010). Ethanol injection method for hydrophilic and lipophilic drug-loaded liposome preparation. *Journal of Liposome Research*, *20*(3), 228–243. doi:10.3109/08982100903347923 PMID:19899957

Jadhav, M., Nagarsenker, M. S., Gaikwad, R., Samad, A., & Kshirsagar, N. A. (2011). Formulation and evaluation of long circulating liposomal amphotericin B: A scinti-kinetic study using 99mTc in BALB/C mice. *Indian Journal of Pharmaceutical Sciences*, *73*(1), 57. doi:10.4103/0250-474X.89757 PMID:22131622

Jain, A. S., Goel, P. N., Shah, S. M., Dhawan, V. V., Nikam, Y., Gude, R. P., & Nagarsenker, M. S. (2014). Tamoxifen guided liposomes for targeting encapsulated anticancer agent to estrogen receptor positive breast cancer cells: In vitro and in vivo evaluation. *Biomedicine and Pharmacotherapy*, *68*(4), 429–438. doi:10.1016/j.biopha.2014.03.004 PMID:24721327

James, N., Coker, R., Tomlinson, D., Harris, J., Gompels, M., Pinching, A., & Stewart, J. (1994). Liposomal doxorubicin (Doxil): An effective new treatment for Kaposi's sarcoma in AIDS. *Clinical Oncology*, *6*(5), 294–296. doi:10.1016/S0936-6555(05)80269-9 PMID:7530036

Kawakami, S., Higuchi, Y., & Hashida, M. (2008). Nonviral approaches for targeted delivery of plasmid DNA and oligonucleotide. *Journal of Pharmaceutical Sciences*, *97*(2), 726–745. doi:10.1002/jps.21024 PMID:17823947

Kersten, G. F., & Crommelin, D. J. (1995). Liposomes and ISCOMS as vaccine formulations. *Biochimica et Biophysica Acta (BBA)-. Reviews on Biomembranes*, *1241*(2), 117–138.

Kreuter, J. (1994). *Colloidal drug delivery systems* (Vol. 66). CRC Press.

Laouini, A., Jaafar-Maalej, C., Limayem-Blouza, I., Sfar, S., Charcosset, C., & Fessi, H. (2012). Preparation, characterization and applications of liposomes: state of the art. *Journal of Colloid Science and Biotechnology, 1*(2), 147-168.

Lapinski, M. M., Castro-Forero, A., Greiner, A. J., Ofoli, R. Y., & Blanchard, G. J. (2007). Comparison of liposomes formed by sonication and extrusion: Rotational and translational diffusion of an embedded chromophore. *Langmuir*, *23*(23), 11677–11683. doi:10.1021/la7020963 PMID:17939695

Lasic, D. D. (1988). The mechanism of vesicle formation. *The Biochemical Journal*, *256*(1), 1–11. doi:10.1042/bj2560001 PMID:3066342

Lasic, D. D., & Barenholz, Y. (1996). *Handbook of nonmedical applications of liposomes: Theory and basic sciences* (Vol. 1). CRC Press.

Lasic, D. D., & Martin, F. J. (1995). *Stealth liposomes* (Vol. 20). CRC press.

Laverman, P., Boerman, O. C., Oyen, W. J., Corstens, F. H., & Storm, G. (2001). In vivo applications of PEG liposomes: unexpected observations. *Critical Reviews™ in Therapeutic Drug Carrier Systems, 18*(6).

Laverman, P., Carstens, M. G., Boerman, O. C., Dams, E. T. M., Oyen, W. J., van Rooijen, N., & Storm, G. et al. (2001). Factors affecting the accelerated blood clearance of polyethylene glycol-liposomes upon repeated injection. *The Journal of Pharmacology and Experimental Therapeutics*, *298*(2), 607–612. PMID:11454922

Li, J., Wang, X., Zhang, T., Wang, C., Huang, Z., Luo, X., & Deng, Y. (2015). A review on phospholipids and their main applications in drug delivery systems. *Asian Journal of Pharmaceutical Sciences*, *10*(2), 81–98. doi:10.1016/j.ajps.2014.09.004

Lian, T., Bui, T., & Ho, R. J. (1999). Formulation of HIV-envelope protein with lipid vesicles expressing ganglioside GM1 associated to cholera toxin B enhances mucosal immune responses. *Vaccine*, *18*(7), 604–611. doi:10.1016/S0264-410X(99)00315-1 PMID:10547418

Lian, T., & Ho, R. J. (2001). Trends and developments in liposome drug delivery systems. *Journal of Pharmaceutical Sciences*, *90*(6), 667–680. doi:10.1002/jps.1023 PMID:11357170

Lichtenberg, D., & Barenholz, Y. (1988). Liposomes: Preparation, characterization, and preservation. *Methods of Biochemical Analysis*, *33*, 337–462. doi:10.1002/9780470110546.ch7 PMID:3282152

Lu, W., Zhan, C., & Hou, H. (2014). *Targeted Liposomes and Micelles as Carriers for Cancer Therapy. In Nano-Oncologicals* (pp. 95–122). Springer.

Magee, W. E., Goff, C. W., Schoknecht, J., Smith, M. D., & Cherian, K. (1974). The interaction of cationic liposomes containing entrapped horseradish peroxidase with cells in culture. *The Journal of Cell Biology*, *63*(2), 492–504. doi:10.1083/jcb.63.2.492 PMID:4138544

Marcolis, L. B. (1984). Cell interaction with model membranes probing, modification and simulation of cell surface functions. *Biochimica et Biophysica Acta (BBA)-. Reviews on Biomembranes*, *779*(2), 161–189.

Mark, H. F. (2013). *Encyclopedia of polymer science and technology, concise.* John Wiley & Sons.

McGurk, J., Ross, A., & Gilroy, G. (1986). A Novel Method for the In-Situ Preparation of Liposomes Using an Aerosol Delivery System. *The Journal of Pharmacy and Pharmacology*, *38*(S12), 20P–20P. doi:10.1111/j.2042-7158.1986.tb14249.x

Milsmann, M. H., Schwendener, R. A., & Weder, H.-G. (1978). The preparation of large single bilayer liposomes by a fast and controlled dialysis. *Biochimica et Biophysica Acta (BBA)-. Biomembranes*, *512*(1), 147–155. doi:10.1016/0005-2736(78)90225-0

Monteiro, N., Martins, A., Reis, R. L., & Neves, N. M. (2014). Liposomes in tissue engineering and regenerative medicine. *Journal of the Royal Society, Interface*, *11*(101), 1–24. doi:10.1098/rsif.2014.0459 PMID:25401172

Muggia, F., Hainsworth, J., Jeffers, S., Groshen, S., Tan, M., & Greco, F. (1996). *Liposomal doxorubicin (Doxil) is active against refractory ovarian cancer.* Paper presented at the Proc Am Soc Clin Oncol.

Nagarsenker, M., Amin, L., & Date, A. A. (2008). Potential of cyclodextrin complexation and liposomes in topical delivery of ketorolac: In vitro and in vivo evaluation. *AAPS PharmSciTech*, *9*(4), 1165–1170. doi:10.1208/s12249-008-9157-2 PMID:19016331

Nagarsenker, M., & Londhe, V. (2003). Preparation and evaluation of a liposomal formulation of sodium cromoglicate. *International Journal of Pharmaceutics*, *251*(1), 49–56. doi:10.1016/S0378-5173(02)00583-5 PMID:12527174

Naik, B., & Nagarsenker, M. (2006). Novel drug delivery systems: Potential in improving topical delivery of antiacne agents. *Skin Pharmacology and Physiology*, *19*(1), 2–16. doi:10.1159/000089138 PMID:16247244

Nässander, U., Storm, G., Peeters, P., & Crommelin, D. (1990). Liposomes. *Drugs and the Pharmaceutical Sciences, 45*, 261-338.

New, R. R. (1990). *Liposomes: a practical approach*. IRL Press.

New, R. R., Philippot, J., & Schuber, F. (1995). *Influence of liposome characteristics on their properties and fate*. New York, NY: CRC Press.

Pagano, R. E., & Weinstein, J. N. (1978). Interactions of liposomes with mammalian cells. *Annual Review of Biophysics and Bioengineering*, *7*(1), 435–468. doi:10.1146/annurev.bb.07.060178.002251 PMID:352245

Papahadjopoulos, D., Allen, T., Gabizon, A., Mayhew, E., Matthay, K., Huang, S., & Redemann, C. et al. (1991). Sterically stabilized liposomes: Improvements in pharmacokinetics and antitumor therapeutic efficacy. *Proceedings of the National Academy of Sciences of the United States of America*, *88*(24), 11460–11464. doi:10.1073/pnas.88.24.11460 PMID:1763060

Pathak, P. O., Nagarsenker, M. S., Barhate, C. R., Padhye, S. G., Dhawan, V. V., Bhattacharyya, D., & Fahr, A. et al. (2015). Cholesterol anchored arabinogalactan for asialoglycoprotein receptor targeting: Synthesis, characterization, and proof of concept of hepatospecific delivery. *Carbohydrate Research*, *408*, 33–43. doi:10.1016/j.carres.2015.03.003 PMID:25841057

Petre, C. E., & Dittmer, D. P. (2007). Liposomal daunorubicin as treatment for Kaposi's sarcoma. *International Journal of Nanomedicine*, *2*(3), 277. PMID:18019828

Puri, A. (2013). Phototriggerable liposomes: Current research and future perspectives. *Pharmaceutics*, *6*(1), 1–25. doi:10.3390/pharmaceutics6010001 PMID:24662363

Ramsammy, L. S., & Brockerhoff, H. (1982). Lysophosphatidylcholine-cholesterol complex. *The Journal of Biological Chemistry*, *257*(7), 3570–3574. PMID:7061497

Sackmann, E. (1995). Physical basis of self-organization and function of membranes: physics of vesicles. Handbook of Biological Physics, 1, 213-304.

Sant, V., Nagarsenker, M., Rao, S., & Gude, R. (2000). Enhancement of Anti-metastatic Activity of Pentoxifylline by Encapsulation in Conventional Liposomes and Sterically Stabilized Liposomes in Murine Experimental B16F10 Melanoma Model. *The Journal of Pharmacy and Pharmacology*, *52*(12), 1461–1466. doi:10.1211/0022357001777667 PMID:11197073

Sant, V. P., & Nagarsenker, M. S. (2011). Synthesis of Monomethoxypolyethyleneglycol—Cholesteryl Ester and Effect of its Incorporation in Liposomes. *AAPS PharmSciTech*, *12*(4), 1056–1063. doi:10.1208/s12249-011-9674-2 PMID:21853369

Sant, V. P., Nagarsenker, M. S., Rao, S. A., & Gude, R. P. (2003). Sterically stabilized etoposide liposomes: Evaluation of antimetastatic activity and its potentiation by combination with sterically stabilized pentoxifylline liposomes in mice. *Cancer Biotherapy & Radiopharmaceuticals*, *18*(5), 811–817. doi:10.1089/108497803770418355 PMID:14629829

Sawant, R. R., & Torchilin, V. P. (2012). Challenges in development of targeted liposomal therapeutics. *The AAPS Journal*, *14*(2), 303–315. doi:10.1208/s12248-012-9330-0 PMID:22415612

Semple, S. C., Akinc, A., Chen, J., Sandhu, A. P., Mui, B. L., Cho, C. K., & Yaworski, E. et al. (2010). Rational design of cationic lipids for siRNA delivery. *Nature Biotechnology*, *28*(2), 172–176. doi:10.1038/nbt.1602 PMID:20081866

Sessa, G., & Weissmann, G. (1968). Phospholipid spherules (liposomes) as a model for biological membranes. *Journal of Lipid Research*, *9*(3), 310–318. PMID:5646182

Shah, S. M., Ashtikar, M., Jain, A. S., Makhija, D. T., Nikam, Y., Gude, R. P., & Fahr, A. et al. (2015). LeciPlex, invasomes, and liposomes: A skin penetration study. *International Journal of Pharmaceutics*, *490*(1-2), 391–403. doi:10.1016/j.ijpharm.2015.05.042 PMID:26002568

Shah, S. M., Goel, P. N., Jain, A. S., Pathak, P. O., Padhye, S. G., Govindarajan, S., & Gopal, V. et al. (2014). Liposomes for targeting hepatocellular carcinoma: Use of conjugated arabinogalactan as targeting ligand. *International Journal of Pharmaceutics*, *477*(1), 128–139. doi:10.1016/j.ijpharm.2014.10.014 PMID:25311181

Shah, S. M., Pathak, P. O., Jain, A. S., Barhate, C. R., & Nagarsenker, M. S. (2013). Synthesis, characterization, and in vitro evaluation of palmitoylated arabinogalactan with potential for liver targeting. *Carbohydrate Research*, *367*, 41–47. doi:10.1016/j.carres.2012.11.025 PMID:23298829

Sharma, A., & Sharma, U. S. (1997). Liposomes in drug delivery: Progress and limitations. *International Journal of Pharmaceutics*, *154*(2), 123–140. doi:10.1016/S0378-5173(97)00135-X

Swarbrick, J., & Boylan, J. C. (1993). *Encyclopedia of Pharmaceutical Technology: Volume 9-Liposomes as Pharmaceutical Dosage Forms to Microencapsulation*. CRC Press.

Szoka, F., & Papahadjopoulos, D. (1978). Procedure for preparation of liposomes with large internal aqueous space and high capture by reverse-phase evaporation. *Proceedings of the National Academy of Sciences of the United States of America*, *75*(9), 4194–4198. doi:10.1073/pnas.75.9.4194 PMID:279908

Szoka, F. Jr, & Papahadjopoulos, D. (1980). Comparative properties and methods of preparation of lipid vesicles (liposomes). *Annual Review of Biophysics and Bioengineering*, *9*(1), 467–508. doi:10.1146/annurev.bb.09.060180.002343 PMID:6994593

Talsma, H., Van Steenbergen, M. J., Borchert, J. C., & Crommelin, D. J. (1994). A novel technique for the one-step preparation of liposomes and nonionic surfactant vesicles without the use of organic solvents. Liposome formation in a continuous gas stream: The 'Bubble' method. *Journal of Pharmaceutical Sciences*, *83*(3), 276–280. doi:10.1002/jps.2600830303 PMID:8207668

Thewalt, J. L., & Bloom, M. (1992). Phosphatidylcholine: Cholesterol phase diagrams. *Biophysical Journal*, *63*(4), 1176–1181. doi:10.1016/S0006-3495(92)81681-8 PMID:19431848

Torchilin, V. (2012). *Liposomes in drug delivery. In Fundamentals and Applications of Controlled Release Drug Delivery* (pp. 289–328). Springer. doi:10.1007/978-1-4614-0881-9_11

Torchilin, V. P. (2010). Passive and active drug targeting: Drug delivery to tumors as an example. *Drug Delivery*, 3–53. PMID:20217525

van Hoogevest, P., & Wendel, A. (2014). The use of natural and synthetic phospholipids as pharmaceutical excipients. *European Journal of Lipid Science and Technology*, *116*(9), 1088–1107. doi:10.1002/ejlt.201400219 PMID:25400504

Vemuri, S., & Rhodes, C. (1995). Preparation and characterization of liposomes as therapeutic delivery systems: A review. *Pharmaceutica Acta Helvetiae*, *70*(2), 95–111. doi:10.1016/0031-6865(95)00010-7 PMID:7651973

Vo, T. N., Kasper, F. K., & Mikos, A. G. (2012). Strategies for controlled delivery of growth factors and cells for bone regeneration. *Advanced Drug Delivery Reviews*, *64*(12), 1292–1309. doi:10.1016/j.addr.2012.01.016 PMID:22342771

Weissig, V. (2010). *Liposomes: Methods and protocols* (Vol. 2). Humana Press USA.

Williams, K. J., Werth, V. P., & Wolff, J. A. (1984). Intravenously administered lecithin liposomes: A synthetic antiatherogenic lipid particle. *Perspectives in Biology and Medicine*, *27*(3), 417–431. doi:10.1353/pbm.1984.0031 PMID:6374607

Yamauchi, H., Yano, T., Kato, T., Tanaka, I., Nakabayashi, S., Higashi, K., & Yamada, H. et al. (1995). Effects of sialic acid derivative on long circulation time and tumor concentration of liposomes. *International Journal of Pharmaceutics*, *113*(2), 141–148. doi:10.1016/0378-5173(94)00188-B

Yarmolenko, P. S., Zhao, Y., Landon, C., Spasojevic, I., Yuan, F., Needham, D., & Dewhirst, M. W. et al. (2010). Comparative effects of thermosensitive doxorubicin-containing liposomes and hyperthermia in human and murine tumours. *International Journal of Hyperthermia*, *26*(5), 485–498. doi:10.3109/02656731003789284 PMID:20597627

Zimmermann, T. S., Lee, A. C., Akinc, A., Bramlage, B., Bumcrot, D., Fedoruk, M. N., & John, M. et al. (2006). RNAi-mediated gene silencing in non-human primates. *Nature*, *441*(7089), 111–114. doi:10.1038/nature04688 PMID:16565705

KEY TERMS AND DEFINITIONS

Amphiphile: This term describes a molecule having a hydrophilic terminal polar group attached to a hydrophobic portion. The latter may be a long chain like that present in phospholipids or a small molecule like a hydrophobic amino acid.

Bilayer: A two-molecule thick film comprising amphiphilic molecules with the polar hydrophilic portion oriented towards the aqueous phase on the outside and hydrophobic segments facing each other on the inside is called as a bilayer.

Bilayer Curvature: A mechanical property of the bilayer that defines the magnitude of bending of a bilayer caused by work done to deform the same is called bilayer curvature. bilayers can be bent in two planes and therefore possess two principal curvatures which can be combined into a sum defined by mean curvature 'h' or a product defined by Gaussian curvature 'k'.

Double Liposomes: Double liposomes are specially designed liposomes for oral delivery consisting of smaller liposomes enclosed in lipid bilayers, the latter providing protection to the inner liposomes against enzymatic degradation. double liposomes can be prepared by a modified glass-filter method.

EPR Effect (Enhanced Permeation and Retention Effect): The ability of a nanosystem to passively accumulate into tumours/infarcts/inflamed areas due to leaky vasculature (enhanced permeation) and reside in the same owing to poor lymphatic drainage (improved retention) is called enhanced permeation and retention effect.

Immunologic Adjuvant: A substance which enhances the immune response to an antigen but does not confer any immunity by itself is called as immunologic adjuvant. Examples include Freund's adjuvant, lipid A, and a few muramyl peptides.

Ligands: Small molecules which may be carbohydrate /lipid /protein in nature that recognise and interact with specific receptors present on cells of interest and used for actively targeting delivery systems to such cells are called ligands. Examples of ligands include antibodies, vitamins, hormones, lipid/carbohydrate/protein based small molecules.

Mesophase: A mesophase is defined as an 'intermediate' phase or a subphase of a liquid crystalline material and is formed due to changes in one, two or three dimensional order of a liquid crystalline material.

Off-Target Toxicity: Manifestation of adverse effects owing to clinical activity of the drug on unintended organs/tissues which may be biologically related/unrelated to the target of interest is called off-target toxicity.

Section 3
Niosomes

Chapter 4
Non-Ionic Surfactant Vesicles (Niosomes) as New Drug Delivery Systems

Abbas Pardakhty
Kerman University of Medical Sciences, Iran

ABSTRACT

Lipid vesicular systems composed of hydrated amphihiles with or without bilayer inducing agents such as cholesterol. On the basis of used amphiphilic molecule different nomenclature are used as liposomes, ufasomes and niosomes. Nonionic surfactants with mono-, di- or trialkyl chains form niosomes which are lipid vesicles with more chemical stability in comparison with phospholipids of liposomes. Both hydrophobic and hydrophilic chemicals can be encapsulated in niosomes as a new drug delivery system. This drug carrier system could have administered via injection, oral, pulmonary, vaginal, rectal, ophthalmic, nasal or transdermal routes with penetration enhancing potential. This chapter presents a detailed explain about niosome forming components, methods of preparation and routes of administration. Many examples for drug delivery potential of niosomes are also available in this review. Vaccine adjuvant and genetic substances vector capabilities are not given here.

INTRODUCTION

There are versatile lists of amphiphilic compounds for production of lipid vesicles which on the basis of used amphiphiles or structural compounds, different nomenclature has been used such as liposomes (Kaminskas et al. 2012), niosomes (Moazeni et al. 2010; Akbari et al. 2013), ufasomes (Patel et al. 2011), ethosomes (Liu et al. 2012), eliposomes (Lattin et al. 2012) and so on. In lipid vesicular systems, polar headgroups of amphiphilic molecules are oriented into aqueous compartments and their lipophilic parts form bilayer membranes. Niosomes are bilayer vesicles composed mainly of hydrated non-ionic surfactants in addition to, in many cases, cholesterol (CHOL) or its derivatives (Pardakhty and Moazeni 2013). Cosmetic industry was the place for the first account of niosome production (Handjani-Vila et Al. 1979) after which a large number of niosome applications in drug, vaccine and gene delivery have been

DOI: 10.4018/978-1-5225-0751-2.ch004

explored. While most niosomes are in the nano or sub-micron (colloidal) size range, not many authors used the “nanoniosome” or “nanovesicle” titles in their published articles due to introduction the new nanotechnology related phrases during the few recent years. Niosomes are capable to encapsulate both hydrophilic and lipophilic substances which the first ones usually are entrapped in vesicular aqueous core or adsorbed on the bilayer surfaces, and lyophobic molecules are encapsulated by their partitioning into the lipophilic domain of the bilayers. Incorporation of charged molecules into non-ionic surfactant vesicles forms charged or hybrid niosomes (Sennato et al. 2008). Vesicles can be also prepared from the mixed cationic and anionic surfactant systems such as cetyltrimethylammonium bromide and sodium lauryl sulfate (CTAB-SLS) (Aiello et al. 2010). These types of vesicles are presented as “cat-anionic” or “catanionic” vesicles. Catanionic vesicles can also be formed from electrostatic interaction between an ionized drug, such as diclofenac (Zhao et al. 2013) or alprenolol (Dew et al. 2012) and a positively/negatively charged surfactant.

Non-ionic surfactants have more chemical stability against oxidation and are less thermo-labile in comparison to phospholipids, the main constituent of liposomes (Fang et al. 2001; Tarekegn et al. 2010) thus less significant care in handling and storage are needed. Furthermore, greater versatility and lower cost make this type of vesicles more attractive in drug, gene and vaccine delivery (Florence 1993). From the pharmaceutical manufacturing stand of view the superiority of niosomes is simple methods required for industrialized and large–scale production of them without the use of pharmaceutically unacceptable solvents (Sahin 2007). In this chapter the most important aspects of niosomes and drug delivery potentials will be reviewed. Application of niosomes as gene or vaccine delivery tools will not discussed in this chapter.

Amphiphiles (Surfactants)

Following the application of some forms of energy such as mechanical or heating, the formation of niosomes is a self-assembly process due to high interfacial tension between aqueous medium and the lipophilic alkyl chain(s) resulted in the association of non-ionic surfactant monomers into vesicles (Uchegbu and Vyas 1998). Concurrently, the hydrophilic headgroups of amphiphilic molecules make water mediated interactions counter the previous formed force, finally result in bilayer formation. The energy required to form vesicles with amphiphile molecules has three contributors related to the surface energy, the mechanical energy due to overpressure and the chemical potential excess (Manconi et al. 2005).

Formation of niosomes needs at the first step to an amphiphilic molecule, but in many cases the presence a wedge shaped molecule such as CHOL is essential to turn the micellar structure of surfactant aggregates to bilayer arrangement (Pozzi et al. 2009). The lipophilic moiety of amphiphile molecule may be contain one (Varshosaz et al. 2003), two (Okahata et al. 1981)or three (Yoshioka et al. 1994; Jain and Vyas 1995; Jain et al. 2005)alkyl or perfluoroalkyl(Zarif et al. 1994)groups or in some cases a single steroidal group(Echegoyen et al. 1988).

Amino acid-based surfactants (Guedj et al. 1994; Polidori et al. 1994), glycolipids (Polidori et al. 1997) and crown ether compounds (Echegoyen, Hernandez et al. 1988; Darwish and Uchegbu 1997; Muzzalupo et al. 2007; Paolino et al. 2007)were used to form niosomes in aqueous hydration media. More recently gemini surfactants, composed of two amphiphilic molecules connected to each other by a spacer, were also used to form niosomes (Muzzalupo et al. 2008; Paolino et al. 2008) (Figure 1).

The flexibility of compounds capable for vesicle forming is due to different and various polar head groups attached to saturated or unsaturated alkyl chain(s) composed of 12 to 18 carbon atoms (C_{12}-C_{18}).

Figure 1. α,ω-trioxyethylene-bis(sodium 2-dodecyloxy-propylenesulfonate), an anionic gemini surfactant, used for preparation of niosomes
Muzzalupo et al. 2008.

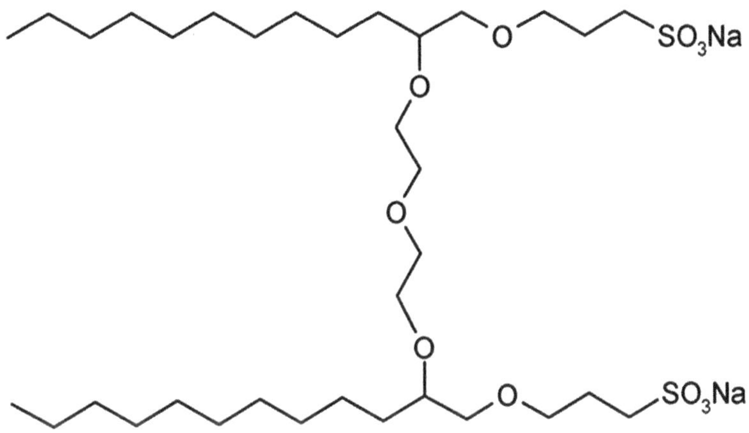

However, here the main non-ionic surfactant classes used for niosome production will be presented which are alkyl ethers, alkyl esters, alkyl amides andsome other amphipathic compounds such as fatty acids.

Alkyl Ethers

Surfactant I (polyglyceryl-3 cethyl ether) has one n-alkyl chain and was the first amphihpile used for niosomes preparation (Handjani-Vila, Ribier et al. 1979). This amphiphile has been used for preparation of niosomes encapsulating adriamycin (Rogerson et al. 1987) and diclofenac sodium (Türker et al. 2005). Özer et al. (Özer et al. 2013) showed diclofenac sodium niosomes formulated by Surfactant I/ CHOL could bear different γ-radiation doses.

Hofland et al. (1992); Hofland et al. (1993); Hofland et al. *1994) reported the formation of a series of vesicles composed of n-alkyl polyoxyethylene ether surfactants(C*n*EO*m*) mainly designed for topical delivery of therapeutic compounds. Van Hal et al. (van Hal et al. 1996)used C*n*EO*m*, in which the number of oxyethylene units (*m*) ranged from 3 to 7 and the number of carbon atoms (*n*) ranged from 12 to 18, in order to obtain a systematic variation in length of alkyl chain and headgroup. They showed without CHOL in C_nEO_3 surfactants the vesicle formation was probable by sonication method but increasing the polyoxyethylene units to C_nEO_7 put an end to vesicle formation. Bouwstra et al (Bouwstra et al. 1997) also reported the vesicle forming ability of $C_{14}EO_5$ and $C_{16}EO_5$ in the absence of CHOL. Pardakhty et al. (2007) prepared vesicles composed of $C_{16}EO_2$ (Brij® 52), $C_{18}EO_2$ (Brij 72), $C_{18}EO_{10}$ (Brij 76), $C_{9=9}EO_2$ (Brij 92) and $C_{9=9}EO_{10}$ (Brij 97) without any added CHOL by film hydration method. In contrast with their results, Suwakul et al. (Suwakul et al. 2006)reported the lack of niosome formation with the mentioned surfactants in the absence of CHOL. This is maybe caused by different used methods for preparation of vesicles and unlike encapsulated drug's nature; Suwakul's group utilized direct sonication of molten lipids, in addition to use of propylthiouracil, a lyophobic drug which interact with bilayer formation ability of the applied surfactants and even made the bilayer less accommodating for CHOL molecules (Suwakul, Ongpipattanakul et al. 2006).While we used film hydarttion method with a water soluble molecule, insulin(Pardakhty, Varshosaz et al. 2007).

Various lipophilic drugs such as cycloslporin-A(Niemiec et al. 1995; Waranuch et al. 1998), erythromycin (Jayaraman et al. 1996), estradiol (Hofland, van der Geest et al. 1994), finasteride (Tabbakhian et al. 2005; Tabbakhian et al. 2006) minoxidil (Balakrishnan et al. 2009), tretinoin (Manconi et al. 2002; Manconi et al. 2003; Manconi et al. 2006), triamcinolone acetonide (Sankar et al. 2013), and some water soluble ones like α-interferon (Niemiec, Ramachandran et al. 1995), cimetidine (Lieb et al. 1994), and recombinant human granulocyte-macrophage colony stimulating factor (rhGM-CSF) (Memisoğlu et al. 1997),were encapsulated in C_nEO_m containing vesicles. All the mentioned vesicular formulations were formulated for topical delivery to stratum corneum, follicular (pilosebaceous units) and the other parts of the dermis. Hofland, van der Geest et al. (1994) studied permeation of estradiol from C_nEO_m niosomes. They showed that direct contact between niosomes and skin was imperative to exert the highest effect on drug transport. This effect even reported when pretreatment of the skin withnon-occlusive C_nEO_m niosomes enhanced the iontophoretic transport of R-apomorphine through human abdominal skin (Li et al. 2001). Hydroxychloroquine niosomes composed of Brij 98/CHOL were also formulated for topical management of oral lichen planus (Bendas et al. 2013).

Alkyl Esters

Among the alkyl esters, the most important and frequently used surfactants are sugar esters. These surfactants contain a sugar group as the polar headgroup of the amphiphilic molecule. The sugar moieties can be sucrose, glucose, sorbitan, methyl glucose, mallitol, or other sugars. The hydroxyl moieties of the sugars are partially esterified with alkyl chains. Kiwada et al. (KIWADA et al. 1985; Kiwada et al. 1985)used alkyl glycosides for preparation of vesicles and Schenk et al. (Schenk et al. 1989)worked on vesicles of sucrose ester surfactants. Sucrose cocoate, a mixture of fatty acid sucrose esters, was used for vesicle formation and encapsulation of sulfadiazine or diclofenac, both for topical delivery in nanoniosome forms (Tavano et al. 2010). Manconi et al. (Manconi et al. 2006)also reported the formation of niosomes composed of decylpolyglucoside with or without CHOL entrapping methylene blue as a hydrophilic model compound.

Sorbitanmono esters (Span®) can be known as the basic and the most widely applied surfactants used for niosome preparations (Figure 2). Many articles could be found in literature about using sorbitan ester niosomes for entrapping different compounds with various physicochemical and therapeutic properties such as acetazolamide (Guinedi et al. 2005; Aggarwal et al. 2007), acyclovir(Attia et al. 2007), insulin (Khaksa et al. 2000; Ning et al. 2005), methotrexate (Chandraprakash et al. 1990; Chandraprakash et al. 1992), doxorubicin (Uchegbu et al. 1995; Uchegbu et al. 1996); vincristine (Parthasarathi et al. 1994), hydroxycamptothecin (Shi et al. 2006; Hong et al. 2009), vasoactive intestinal peptide (Dufes et al. 2004) and salicylic acid (Junyaprasert et al. 2008).

Generally, by increasing the hydrocarbon chain length from C_{12} to C_{18} and also more rigidity in bilayers by saturation of hydrophobic chain (stearate vs. oleate) in sorbitan esters vesicles, the encapsulation of water soluble molecules such as insulin (Varshosaz, Pardakhty et al. 2003), colchicine (Hao et al. 2002), salicylic acid and p-hydroxyl benzoic acid (Hao and Li 2010) or poorly soluble compounds such as flurbiprofen (Mokhtar et al. 2008)will be increased. Sorbitan esters can form vesicles in the presence or absence of molecules which operate co-operatively to form bilayer membranes; for instance, Span 60 with C_{18} mono-alkyl chain has been used for vesicle formation alone (Varshosaz et al. 2003), with CHOL (Suwakul, Ongpipattanakul et al. 2006) or CHOL/cholesteryl poly-24-oxyethylene ether (Solulan C24)

Figure 2. Dark field microscopy photomicograph of Leishmania major recombinant gp63 (r-GP63) multilamellar vesicles (MLVs) containing Span 60/cholesterol (70:30 molar ratio); magnification 40×40, bar = 5 µm

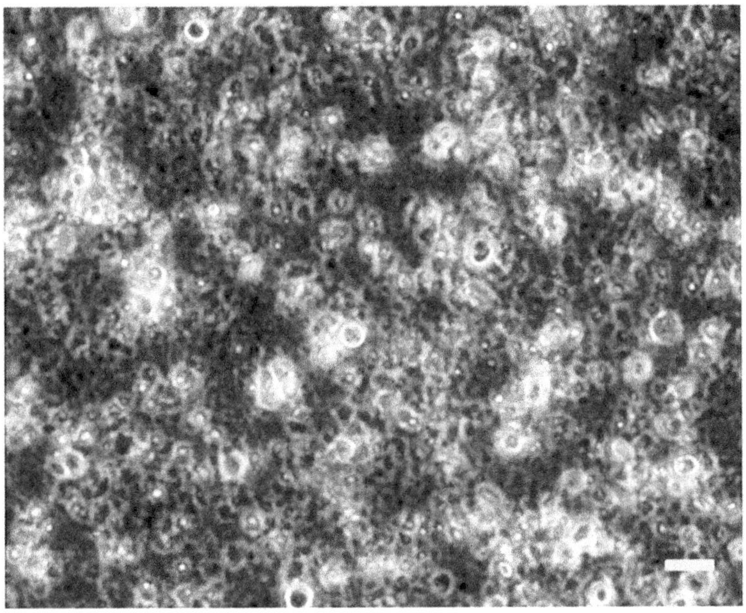

(Uchegbu, Double et al. 1995). Kato et al. prepared temperature-sensitive fusogenic niosomes composed of Span 80 alone, or with CHOL (Kato et al. 2008).

Shi, Fang et al. (2006) used different poly (methoxypolyethyleneglycol cyanoacrylate-co-n-hexadecyl cyanoacrylate) (PEG-PHDCA) acted as surface modification materials, Span 60 and CHOLto encapsulate hydroxycamptothecin in "stealth nanoniosomes". The tumor inhibition rate of PEG5000-PHDCA niosomes (92.5 nm) at a dose of 2 mg/kg was five times that of drug injection at 4 mg/kg. Used PEG was likely to fold on the surface of the niosomes due to its compressibility, which is favorable for niosomes to prevent aggregation and improve its ability to evade macrophages uptake (Shi, Fang et al. 2006). Hong et al. (Hong, Zhu et al. 2009) modified the stealth nanoniosomes by coupling periodate-oxidated transferrin to terminal amino group of PEG to produce the active targeting vesicles with average diameters of 116 nm. Compared with injected free drug/non-stealth and stealth niosomes, transferrin holding PEG-PHDCA niosomes demonstrated the strongest cytotoxicity to three carcinomatous cell lines (KB, K562 and S180cells), the greatest intracellular uptake especially in nuclei, the highest tumor concentration and largest are under the intratumoral hydroxycamptothecin concentration curve, as well as the most powerful anti-tumoractivity with the inhibition rate of 71% against S180 tumor in mice.

Yoshioka, Sternberg et al. (1994) studied the vesicle forming ability of sorbitan monoesters and a sorbitan triester (Span 85). Sorbitan tri-stearate (Span 85) was also utilized for rifampicin niosome preparation (Jain and Vyas 1995). Increasing the amount of CHOL led to decrease in the entrapment efficiency of rifampicin due to rigidity increase of niosomal bilayers following CHOL content increment (Baillie et al. 1985).

Even though the polyoxyethylene sorbitan esters (Tween®) are more soluble and have higher hydrophilic lipophilic balance (HLB) values in comparison to sorbitan esters, this class of surfactants have been used for vesicle preparation in combination with sufficient amount of CHOL (Carafa et al. 1998; Di Marzio et al. 2011; Di Marzio et al. 2012). Carafa et al. (2006) reported the formation of pH sensitive nanoniosomes made from polxoxyethylene sorbitan mono-laurate (Tween 20), CHOL and its derivative, cholesteryl hemisuccinate, as pH-sensitive molecule. More recently a novel class of compounds based on Tween 20 surfactant bearing different pH-sensitive head groups (i.e., glycine, N-methyl-glycine, N,N-dimethyl-glycine) were used successfully for delivery of Na calcein, a carboxylic fluorescent dye, to human hepatoblastoma (HepG2) cell line (Masotti et al. 2010). Di Marzio et al. (Di Marzio, Marianecci et al. 2011) studies suggest that the Tween 21/CHOL nanovesicle is also a pH-sensitive system. The pH-sensitivity and more bilayer fluidity of Tween 21 vesicles could be related to the lower content of counter ions and associated waters of hydration near the head groups, bearing only 4 PEG units, in comparison with Tween 20, bearing 20 PEG units.

Nano size niosomes composed of polyoxyethylene sorbitan monostearate (Tween 61) and CHOL were used for encapsulation of azelaic acid and its derivatives (Panyosak et al. 2009), diclofenac diethylammonium (Manosroi et al. 2008), glucose (Manosroi et al. 2008), and rice bran extract (Manosroi et al. 2012). Manosroi et al. (2010) reported the entrapment enhancement of three peptides including bacitracin, insulin and bovine serum albuminin neutral, anionic and cationic Tween 61 niosomes.

Utilizing of combination of sorbitan esters and their polyethoxylated derivatives has led to stable and efficient vesicles encapsulating of ciprofloxacin (Moazeni, Gilani et al. 2010)with low cytotoxicity against alveolar human carcinoma cell line (A549) suggesting a good aerosol drug delivery system. Combinations of different Spans and Tweens with CHOL were also successfully utilized to encapsulate ciprofloxacin in nanoniosomes for enhance intracellular delivery of this flouroquinolone (Akbari, Abedi et al. 2013; Akbari et al. 2015); the high physical stability of the prepared niosomes shown as little size change during the storage may be was due to the steric stabilization of vesicles following the incorporation of polyoxyethylene bearing surfactants, Tweens, in the formulations. Desai and Finlay (Desai and Finlay 2002) demonstrated the potential of encapsulating all-trans-retinoic acid in niosomes composed of Span 20 or Span 60 with Tween 80 and delivering it as an inhaled aerosol by nebulization. Such a combination, even though without CHOL and in the presence of Span 80/Tween 80/PEG 6000/water has been experimented for vesicle forming ability by transformation of lamellar liquid crystal structure to vesicular ones enable for encapsulation both hydrophilic (ribavirin) and hydrophobic (ibuprofen) substances (Liu and Guo 2007). Devaraj et al. (2002) prepared different niosomal formulations in which a combination of polysorbates (Tweens), polyglyceryl-3-diisostearate and different fatty alcohols used for vesicle formation and encapsulation of anti-inflammatory drug, ketorolac. Combination of Span 20 or Tween 20/ polyglycero-6-oleate was also used for stable nano size niosomes enable to encapsulate three model peptide or proteins (Cortesi et al. 2007). Span and Tween niosomes were also used for encapsulation of poorly water soluble antifungal drug, itraconazole (Alomrani et al. 2015). Rat abdominal skin permeation studies showed Span niosomes had enhancement penetration of itraconazole compared to its solution; however, it was less in magnitude than that of Tweens.

Alkyl Amides

Zarif, Gulik-Krzywicki et al. (1994) studied the supramolecular assemblies or vesicles produced by applying alkyl galactosides and glucosides incorporating amino acid spacers. They also reported the formation of perfluoralkyl glycolipid-based vesicles (Zarif 2002). Uchegbu (Uchegbu 1998)reported the formation of nanoniosomes composed of palmitoyl muramic acid/CHOL/Solulan C24 which were loaded with doxorubicin by the use of ammonium sulfate gradients. The biodistribution of prepared 200 nm vesicles in male Balb/c mice after i.v. administration were found to avoid liver uptake but not splenic uptake when compared to drug loaded Span 60 niosomes. N-palmitoylglucosamine (NPG) niosomes were also prepared by sonication of NPG/ Span 60/CHOL/ Solulan C24 which had a z-average mean diameter of 164 nm (Dufes et al. 2000).

Other Amphiphilic Compounds

Many other compounds with surfactant-like behavior have been used for vesicle formation; for example, long chain fatty acids such as oleic acid can be used for vesicle formation which usually named as unsaturated fatty acid vesicles or 'ufasomes' (Gebicki and Hicks 1973). Intranasal lyophilized gels containing ufasomes were prepared from oleic acid to circumvent the low and erratic absorption of orally administrated cinnarizin (Salama and Aburahma 2015).

Covalently bound alkyl amino acids with efficient amphiphilic properties have been used for vesicle formation (Neumann et al. 1987).

Gopinath et al. (2004) utilized one ascorbic acid derivative, ascorbyl palmitate, for vesicle formation and *in vitro* transdermal delivery of azidothymidine by these vesicles which named as 'aspasomes'. Conacher et al. (2001) has also developed drug delivery vehicles called 'bilosomes', which are vesicles prepared from bile salts such as deoxycholate for oral immunization with peptide and protein antigens.

BILAYER INDUCING AGENTS

Cholesterol

The most common additive found in niosomal systems is cholesterol (CHOL) which is known to abolish the gel to liquid phase transition of liposomal and niosomal systems, resulting in less leakiness of the vesicles and improved niosomes stability (Junyaprasert, Teeranachaideekul et al. 2008). Surface pressure measurements on monolayers of nonionic surfactant/CHOL mixtures demonstrated a condensing effect of CHOL as evidenced by the decrease in the effective area per molecule as the CHOL content of the monolayer increased. This effect might have attributed to the accommodation of CHOL in the molecular cavities formed by surfactant monomers assembled into vesicles and is responsible for the observed decreased permeability of CHOL-containing membranes compared to CHOL free membranes (Devaraj et al. 2002). CHOL is used to complete the hydrophobic moiety of high HLB single alkyl chain non-ionic surfactants for vesicle formation (Masotti, Vicennati et al. 2010). In general, it has been found that a molar ratio of 1:1 between CHOL and non-ionic surfactants is an optimal ratio for the formulation of physically stable niosomal vesicles (Nasseri 2005). Some reports denote the formation of monohydrate or anhydrous CHOL crystals among the surfactant/CHOL bilayers (Caracciolo et al. 2008). The minimum amount of CHOL required to form vesicles without evoking surfactant aggregates or other irregular structures depended on the type of surfactant and it's HLB (van Hal, Bouwstra et al. 1996; Uchegbu and Vyas 1998).

Other Bilayer Inducing Agents

Non-ionic surfactant vesicles have been formed with different lipid compositions without CHOL. In Table 1, a complete list of these compounds was presented. The resultant vesicles showed different physicochemical behaviors; for example, polyhedral niosomes were formed from systems containing $C_{16}G_2$ (hexadecyl diglycerol ether) and Solulan C24 alone, while cholesterol-containing systems formed spherical vesicles (Arunothayanun et al. 2000).

Methods of Niosome Preparation

Generally, there are two classes of niosome or liposome preparation methods; the first set includes dissolving the whole lipids in organic solvent(s) for molecular level mixing of the bilayer constituents, then removing the organic solvent and hydration of formed lipid thin films or surfaces by an aqueous medium. The second series of vesicle formulation comprises the direct mixing of lipids and hydration medium, usually in high elevated temperature, which have omitting the hazardous effect of trace residuals of organic solvents on entrapped substance or biologically applied environments.

Detailed preparation methods which use organic solvents are presented here:

1. **Thin Film Hydration (Hand Shaking):** In this method all lipids are dissolved in an organic solvent, typically chloroform. The solvent is evaporated under reduced pressure and the hydration phase containing water soluble components is added at a temperature higher than phase transition temperature of used surfactants (Figure 3). This is the most common method of niosome preparation and for instance was reported for encapsulating of nimesulidea (Shahiwala and Misra 2002).
2. **Reverse-Phase Evaporation:** Vesicle forming ingredients are dissolved in chloroform/diethyl ether and water in oil emulsion is formed by sonication of two phase's mixture. The organic solvent(s) is evaporated in a rotary evaporator and the resultant viscous niosomal suspension is diluted by adding aqueous phase. This technique was reported for preparation of acetazolamide niosomes (Guinedi, Mortada et al. 2005).

Table 1. Different compounds utilized for niosome preparation in the absence of cholesterol

Bilayer Additives	Used Surfactant	Encapsulated Compound	Reference(s)
Soybean phosphatidylcholine	Span 80	------	(Kato, Walde et al. 2008)
PEG 400	Span 80	Ribavirin or ibuprofen	(Hua and Liu 2007)
PEG 6000	Tween 80/Span 80	Hemoglobin	(Liu et al. 2007)
PEG 6000	Tween 80/Span 80	Ribavirin or ibuprofen	(Liu and Guo 2007)
Poly-24-oxyethylene cholesteryl ether (Solulan C24)	Hexadecyl diglycerol ether (C16G2)	5(6)-carboxyfluorescein	(Arunothayanun, Bernard et al. 2000)
Fatty alcohols (C12, C14, C16, C18, and C16+18)	Tween 20, 40, 60, 80	Ketorolac tromethamine	(Devaraj, Parakh et al. 2002)
Absolute ethanol	Span 20, 40, 60, 80	Flurbiprofen (proniosome)	(Mokhtar, Sammour et al. 2008)

Figure 3. Thin film hydration (hand shaking) for preparation of MLV niosomes

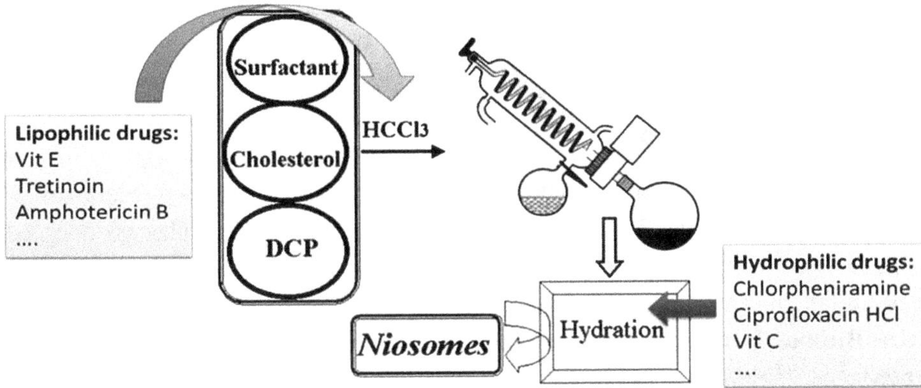

3. **Ether Injection:** Lipids are dissolved in diethyl ether and slowly injected into the preheated aqueous phase (about 60°C) by a needle. Under this condition, the organic solvent is evaporated and niosomal suspension is formed as used for entrapment of some newly synthesized beta-blockers (Piplani, Kumar et al. 2015).
4. **Dehydration Rehydration Method:** The prepared vesicles are freeze dried (lyophilized) and then rehydrated by appropriate aqueous dehydration rehydration (DRV) medium (Tafreshi and Mirdamadi 2015). We used this method for encapsulation of N, N-diethyl-meta-toluamide, as an insect repellant, in niosomes (Amanatfard et al. 2015).
5. **Solvent Evaporation from Double Emulsion Droplets:** By using a microfluidic flow focusing device to form the double emulsion (monodisperse water–oil–water emulsion droplets) following by organic solvents evaporation from the oil shells, giant vesicles are created (Foster et al. 2010).
6. Comprehensive lipid vesicle preparation techniques without need to use an organic solvent are described below:
7. **Heating and Sonication of Lipids:** A mixture of vesicle forming lipids is melted in a glass test tube. The pre-warmed aqueous phase containing the drug is then added to the molten lipid. The mixture is immediately sonicated at elevated temperature in an ultrasonic bath followed by vortexing. This method was used for encapsulation of propylthiouracil (Suwakul, Ongpipattanakul et al. 2006).
8. **Homogenization of Lipids:** Initially, a combination of lipids and absolute ethanol is heated in tightly sealed glass vials in water bath (55–60°C). To each of the formed transparent solutions, the specified amount of drug containing hot distilled water (55–60°C) is added while warming in the water bath till a clear or translucent proniosomal solution is obtained. By addition an appropriate buffer, niosomes are formed and processed with a high-pressure homogenizer. Niosomes of tenofovir, an anti-HIV drug, were formulated by this technique (Zidan et al. 2011).
9. **Lamellar Liquid Crystal (LLC) Transformation:** This method is based on the microstructure and transformation of surfactant/polymer mixtures such as Tween 80, poly(ethylene glycol) (PEG) 6000, Span 80 and water which are vortex mixed to prepare the LLC at specific mass ratio (Liu and Guo 2007). PEG aqueous solution is then added to the LLC and the samples are mixed by sonicating to prepare niosomes.

10. **Heating (Mozafari) Method:** This method involves the hydration of the lipid vesicle components in an aqueous medium followed by the heating of these components, in the presence of glycerol (3% v/v), up to *c.*120°C (Pardakhty and Moazeni 2013).
11. **Application of Super Critical CO_2 ($scCO_2$):** Lipids and aqueous phase containing drug are added into the view cell and the temperature is raised to 50°C. CO_2 gas is introduced into the view cell and pressure and temperature in the view cell are maintained at 200 bar and 50±1°C, respectively. The pressure was released after 30 min and the niosomal dispersion is obtained (Manosroi, Chutoprapat et al. 2008). Rapid expansion of supercritical solution (RESS)-based process coupled with a gas ejector again uses $scCO_2$ in elevated temperature to change the dissolved surfactant into multilamellar or unilamellar niosomes (Wagner and Rizvi 2015).
12. **Inert Gas Bubble:** Introduction of inert gas (N_2) bubbles into a coarse dispersion of non-hydrated lipids produces stable lipid vesicular dispersions with a mean particle size in the range between 0.2 and 0.5 µm (Talsma et al. 1994).
13. **Microfluidic Hydrodynamic Focusing:** Surfactant mixture dissolved in a water miscible solvent such as isopropyl alcohol and aqueous phase are vigorously mixed in microchannels under high hydrodynamic pressure (Lo et al. 2010). The resultant nanoscaled niosomes had narrower size distributions in comparison with traditional methods.
14. **Electroformation of Vesicles:** This procedure is based on swelling of membrane-forming lipid deposit on an electrode assisted by applied alternating electric fields to generate vesicles in aqueous solutions of the amphiphilic molecules (Okumura and Iwata 2011). The resulting giant vesicles of 30–50 µm, some as large as 100 µm, were formed with the standard setup.

Niosomes as New Drug Delivery Systems

Niosomes are currently used as versatile drug delivery systems with many pharmaceutical applications. Various routes for niosome administration are available which in this section some examples for therapeutic medicines incorporated in such vesicular systems are listed. In transdermal route of drug administration, many vesicles have been derived from proniosomal formulations which were more stable and appropriate dosage forms for topical application.

Nasal Route

Nasal mucosa offers advantages to deliver drugs to brain via olfactory route thus provides rapid onset of drug action and hence faster therapeutic effect (Ravouru et al. 2013; Illum 2015). Niosomes of sumatriptan succinate were prepared and evaluated for nasal absorption using an ex vivo animal model, showing 78.1% of the drug absorption (Gayathri Devi and Udupa 2000). Folic acid, a water soluble vitamin, showing difficulty in crossing blood-brain barrier (BBB), was successfully encapsulated in niosomes and administered through nasal cavity of rats (Ravouru, Kondreddy et al. 2013).

Ophthalmic Route

There are some problems of conventional ocular therapy, such as short residence time, loss of drug through nasolacrimal drainage, impermeability of corneal epithelium and frequent instillation (Guinedi,

Mortada et al. 2005). To overcome these limitations, colloidal drug delivery systems, such as niosomes, have been evaluated.

Aggarwal et al. (Aggarwal et al. 2004)prepared acetazolamide-loaded Span 60/ CHOL niosomes and evaluated their intraocular pressure (IOP) lowering potential in adult male rabbits. Results of the study indicated that it was possible to develop a safe (as indicated by corneal toxicity studies) and physiologically active topical niosomal formulation of acetazolamide relative in efficiency to the newer local carbonic anhydrase inhibitor, dorzolamide. Selected acetazolamide niosomal formulations composed of Span 60/ CHOL were tested for their intraocular pressure lowering activity on normotensive albino rabbits and the results were compared with that of plain niosomes and acetazolamide solution (1%) prepared using polyethylene glycol 400 (7%, v/v) and propylene glycol (53%, v/v) (Guinedi, Mortada et al. 2005). Multilamellar acetazolamide niosomes formulated with Span 60/CHOL in a 7:4 molar ratio were found to be the most effective and showed prolonged decrease in IOP.

Niosomes prepared by reverse phase evaporation (REV) method loaded with acetazolamide were coated with 0.05% Carbopol934P in order to increase the retention time of the drug in the eye of New Zealand albino rabbits (Aggarwal, Pal et al. 2007). Microdialysis method for determination of drug levels in aqueous humor showed a significant broadening of peak time and concentration extent for the bioadhesive coated niosomal formulation. Similar results were reported for brimonidine tartrate, an α2-adrenergic agonist indicated in open angle glaucoma, when entrapped in Span 60/CHOL niosomes (Prabhu et al. 2010).

The potential ocular irritancy and/or damaging effects of niosomal formulations containing gentamicin sulfate were evaluated by observing them for any redness, inflammation, or increased tear production, upon application to the eyes of albino rabbits (Abdelbary and El-gendy 2008); no sign of irritation for all tested niosomal formulations.

Conjunctival and corneal tolerability assessment of ocular naltrexone niosomes on the hen's egg test-chorioallantoic membrane (HET-CAM) and bovine corneal opacity and permeability (BCOP) models showed good ocular tolerability and minimal ocular tissue irritation (Abdelkader et al. 2010; Abdelkader et al. 2011; Abdelkader et al. 2012).

Atenolol (Abu Hashim et al. 2014), cyclopentolate (Perini et al. 1996), ganciclovir (Mutha et al. 2013), ofloxacin (Gupta et al. 2010), pilocarpine (Sheena et al. 1997), prednisolone (Gaafar et al. 2014), some newly synthesized beta blockers (Piplani, Kumar et al. 2015), tacrolimus (Li et al. 2014) andtimolol (Kaur et al. 2010) were also successfully entrapped in niosomes and evaluated for ophthalmic drug delivery.

Oral Route

The delivery of peptide and protein therapeutic agents to the systemic circulation through oral administration is hindered by numerous barriers, including proteolytic enzymes, sharp pH gradients and low epithelial permeability (Lee and Yamamoto 1989). Niosomes could be used to overcome these barriers and improve protein absorption following oral delivery. Yoshida et al. (Yoshida et al. 1992) investigated oral delivery of 9-desglycinamide-8-arginine vasopressin entrapped in niosomes in an *in vitro* intestinal loop model and reported that stability of peptide increased significantly. Animals treated with oral niosome-encapsulated insulin (100 IU/Kg) showed decreased levels of blood glucose and elevated serum insulin, which in the case of Brij 92 vesicles, hypoglycemic effect was significant ($P< 0.05$) (Pardakhty et al. 2011). More recently, Span 60/CHOL/N-trimethyl chitosan (TMC) niosomal nanostructure has been used to enhance insulin permeability through Caco-2 cell monolayer 4-fold, compared with insulin alone (Moghassemi et al. 2015).

Niosomes also could be used for improvement of botanical extract oral absorption and distribution; the in vivo distribution study of *Ginkgo biloba* extract nano-vesicles composed of Tween 80/Span 80/ CHOL showed that the flavonoid glycoside content in heart, lung, kidney, brain, and blood of rats treated with niosomal carrier system was greater than those treated with the oral *Ginkgo biloba* extract tablet (Jin et al. 2013).

Di Marzio et al. (Di Marzio et al. 2013)prepared polysorbate 20 nano-niosomes for oral delivery of unstable or poorly soluble compounds by film hydration associated with sonication in order to reduce the size down to sub-micron range. These vesicles were stable in different pH and in simulated gastro-intestinal media with high mucoadhesion properties.

Niosomes could be used to enhance the aqueous solubility of poorly soluble compounds, thus improving their oral bioavailability. *In vivo* study on rats revealed five-time increment in bioavailability of ganciclovir after oral administration of Span60/CHOL (3:2 molar ratio) as compared with tablet (Akhter et al. 2012). Sezgin-Bayindir et al. (2015) formulated candesartan cilexetil-loaded niosomes and mixed niosomes with promising water solubility and bile solution stability promotion of entrapped compound. Developed niosomal griseofulvin improved the oral bioavailability and maintained therapeutic level of drug for a longer period of time as compared to free griseofulvin in albino rats (Jadon et al. 2009). Acyclovir (Attia, El-Gizawy et al. 2007), carvedilol (Arzani et al. 2015), celecoxib (Nasr 2010), gliclazide (Tamizharasi et al. 2009), paclitaxel (Bayindir and Yuksel 2010), piroxicam (Abdallah et al. 2011) and tenofovir disoproxil fumarate (Kamboj et al. 2014)are some drugs which their oral bioavailabilities were enhanced after encapsulation in niosomal formulations. Cationic niosomes were also used for improving oral bioavailability and lung targeting efficiency afteroral or intravenous administration of azithromycin in rats, respectively (Non-Lecithoid 2014).

Parenteral Route

Many researchers used parenteral route of administration such as intramuscular injection of luteinizing hormone releasing hormone (LHRH) vesicles (Arunothayanun et al. 1999) and subcutaneous injection of norfloxacin niosomes (Abdelaziz et al. 2015) for evaluation of prepared drug delivery systems. However, anticancer therapy and brain targeting are two main goals which could be used for effective niosomal drug delivery and here would be focused on.

Anticancer chemotherapy by using vesicular systems have many benefits such as reduced organ toxicity (O'brien et al. 2004), enhanced antineoplastic efficacy (ElBayoumi and Torchilin 2009), prolonged circulation of vesicular carriers (Cosco et al. 2009)and less mortality in patients (Hamilton et al. 2002). Gude et al. (2002) prepared cisplatin-loaded niosomes and investigated them for antineoplastic activity in experimental metastatic model of B16F10 melanoma. Theophylline and its combination effect with free cisplatin and niosomal cisplatin were also carried out in the same model. Treatment with niosomal cisplatin (1 mg/kg) and combination of the same with theophylline (15 mg/kg) showed significant reduction in the number of lung nodules as compared to untreated control as well as with free cisplatin (1 mg/kg).

Carboplatin was incorporated into niosomes and the therapeutic efficacy of prepared vesicles against S-180 lung neoplasm model was evaluated (Lu et al. 2003). Antitumor effect was increased and differed significantly ($p<.05$) compared with the original drug of the same dose. Cisplatin-loaded niosomes (CP-NMs) were prepared under optimized conditions with Span 40 and cholesterol and their anticancer efficacy was tested in rabbits bearing VX2 sarcoma (Yang et al. 2013). The rabbits locally injected with the CP-NMs gave significantly superior results of inhibition of tumor growth, much lower mortality and improved results of body weight change and inhibition of tumor metastasis to inguinal lymph nodes and liver compared to those treated in the same way with the drug solution.

The blood–brain barrier (BBB) is the most important barrier impeding drug transport into the brain via the blood circulation (Chen and Liu 2012). Many attempts have been done to overcome this barrier for effective drug delivery into brain such as administration of lipid vesicles; both conventional niosomes or niosomal surface decorated with a targeting agent, such as N-palmitoylglucosamine (NPG), permit an enhanced drug delivery to brain parenchyma (Paolino et al. 2011). Niosomal formulation functionalized with NPG loaded with doxorubicin was intravenously injected in rats for reducing drug accumulation in heart and increasing brain concentration of drug (Bragagni et al. 2012). I.v. injection of vasoactive intestinal peptide (VIP)-loaded glucose-bearing niosomes to mice confirmed the presence of intact VIP in brain after administration of VIP-loaded niosomes, but not after administration of VIP solution (Dufes, Gaillard et al. 2004).

A niosomal formulation, functionalized with NPG, was also developed as potential brain targeted delivery system for an endogenous neuropeptide, dynorphin-B (Bragagni et al. 2014); i.v. administration of dynorphin-B optimized niosomal formulation to mice (100 mg/kg) showed a pronounced antinociceptive effect, significantly higher ($P< 0.05$) than that given by i.v. administration of the simple solution of the peptide.

Recently, Span-Tween 60/CHOL niosomes of ascorbic acid and α-tocopherol were i.v. administered in male rats with cerebral ischemia-reperfusion induced by middle cerebral artery occlusion for 30 min (Varshosaz, Taymouri et al. 2014); *in vivo* results showed that the used niosomes had more neuroprotective effects against cerebral ischemic injuries than free ascorbic acid.

Pulmonary Route

Pulmonary administration of drug-loaded vesicles may represent an interesting approach for both the targeting of drugs to lungs and the improvement of the passage of drugs through the mucus barrier and hence of their intracellular uptake (Carafa, Di Marzio et al. 2006). One of most targeted lung diseases for colloidal drug delivery is tuberculosis, due to emersion of Mycobacterium multi-, single- and extensive-drug resistance infections in humans (Garg et al. 2015). Jain and Vyas (Jain and Vyas 1995) injected micron-sized rifampicin-loaded niosomes through the caudal vein into albino rats. More than 60% of the drug was localized in the lungs after 3 h. Rifampicin niosomes attained substantially higher drug concentrations in thoracic lymph nodes when administered through the intraperitoneal (i.p.) route suggesting compartmentalization of the drug took place in the lymphous tissue when administered through this route of administration (Jain et al. 2006).

However, for pulmonary route of administration, promising results were obtained after biological evaluation of selected pyrazinamide niosomal formulations on guinea pigs infected with *Mycobacterium tuberculosis* (El-Ridy et al. 2011). Encapsulation of ethambutol hydrochloride in niosomal formulations for the treatment of tuberculosis also showed higher efficacy and safety compared with the free drug (El-Ridy et al. 2015). The organ distribution pattern of rifampicin (Mullaicharam and Murthy 2004) and gentamicin sulfate (Mullaicharam and Murthy 2006)from niosomes was also studied in albino rats; after intratracheal administration of niosomal-entrapped drugs, a 145-time and 27-time increase in drug accumulation capacity of rifampicin and gentamicin niosomes to free drug solution in lungs was observed, respectively. Mehta and Jindal (Mehta and Jindal 2013) used Tyloxapol, a biocompatible surfactant, for preparation of nano-sized niosomes with high encapsulation efficiencies of antituberculosis drugs (rifampicin, isoniazid and pyrazinamide).

Topical Route

The ability of a particle to diffuse through the *stratum corneum* (for particles of the same charge) depends mainly on its size and viscoelastic properties (Babu et al. 2009). Niosomal bilayers could fuse in *stratum corneum*, the main barrier impeding drug transport through human skin (Hofland, van der Geest et al. 1994), resulting to penetration enhancing effect of lipid vesicular systems both for water soluble or insoluble compounds. Alvi et al. (Alvi et al. 2011)reported that vesiculization of 5-FU not only improved the topical delivery, but also enhanced the cytotoxic effect of 5-FU in actinic keratosis and non-melanoma skin carcinoma. There are many clinical applications of topical niosomes and proniosomes for treatment of acne, cutaneous inflammation, cutaneous leishmaniasis, hair loss and alopecia, local anesthesia, psoriasis, skin and nail fungal infections, vitiligo and whitening effect (Rahimpour and Hamishehkar 2012; Hamishehkar et al. 2013; Rahimpour et al. 2015). Proniosomes are liquid crystalline-compact niosomal hybrid that can be hydrated to form niosomal dispersion instantly before use (Rahimpour, Kouhsoltani et al. 2015).

Asadi et al. (Asadi et al. 2012) prepared and evaluated topical anti-leishmanial effect of paromomycin niosomes in balb/C mice model with promising results. Non-steroidal anti-inflammatory drugs such as acelofenac (Nasr et al. 2008; Solanki et al. 2010; Srinivas et al. 2010), diclofenac(Raja et al. 1994; Manosroi et al. 2008; Özer, Turker et al. 2013), flurbiprofen (Reddy and Udupa 1993; Mokhtar, Sammour et al. 2008),indomethacin (Noori 2012), ketorolac (Alsarra et al. 2005), meloxicam (El-Menshawe and Hussein 2013) andpiroxicam (Solanki et al. 2007; Chandra and Sharma 2008; AHMED et al. 2013)have been formulated as niosomal or proniosomal formulation for enhancement of drug transport through skin after transdermal route of administration.

Minoxidil is a lipophilic drugs approved by FDA for topical use in androgenic alopecia. For increasing skin latency and penetration, many reports are available for niosomal encapsulation and application of minoxidil (Mura et al. 2007; Balakrishnan, Shanmugam et al. 2009; Mura et al. 2009; Mura et al. 2011; Mali et al. 2013). Recently, by a randomized and controlled double-blind clinical trial, we endorsed the superiority and better efficacy of minoxidil niosomes in comparison to conventional formulation (Shamsi Meymandi et al. 2014). Manosroi et al. reported in vivo hair growth promotion activity of gel containing niosomes loaded with the *Oryza sativa* bran fraction (Manosroi et al. 2012). The *in vitro* permeation, skin retention and hair follicular transport of finasteride were reported by Tabbakhian et al. (Tabbakhian, Daneshamouz et al. 2005; Tabbakhian, Tavakoli et al. 2006).

A combination of iontophoresis and vesicular entrapment have been used for transdermal transport enhancement of, finasteride (Prasanthi and K Lakshmi 2013), isosorbide dinitrate (Jain et al. 2011) and triamcinolone acetonide (Sankar, Babu et al. 2013).

Vaginal Route

Ning et al. (Ning, Guo et al. 2005) prepared insulin-loaded Span 40 and 60 niosomes and investigated the hypoglycemic effects and insulin concentrations after vaginal administration of vesicles to rats in comparison to subcutaneous administration of insulin solution. The same research group developed alternative formulations (liposomes/niosomes) for the vaginal administration of clotrimazole to provide sustained and controlled release of appropriate drug for local vaginal therapy, were evaluated as delivery vehicles (Ning et al. 2005). The prepared liposomes/niosomes were incorporated into 2% carbopol gel, and the systems were evaluated for drug stability in phosphate-buffered saline (pH 7.4) and simulated vaginal fluid at 37 ± 1°C.

Zidan and Habib prepared tenofovir niosomal gel to overcome the low permeability of this antiretroviral drug through mucosal membranes. Vesicular size, shape and surface charge, drug entrapment efficiency, *in vitro* release, and skin permeation were used to assess the gels. In addition, their biological performance on *Lactobacillus crispatus* viability and mucoadhesion to porcine vaginal tissue was also assessed with promising results.

CONCLUSION

Niosomes are widely used by research scientists for improving drug pharmacokinetic, targeting, and penetration through biological membranes. Intracellular delivery of therapeutic compounds, enhancing the stability and solubility of vast range of chemical compounds and reducing the toxic effect of some active therapeutic agents are also utilized by niosomal drug delivery. This lipid vesicular system are also widely used in cosmetic industry and can be used for vaccine and gene delivery.

REFERENCES

Abdallah, M. H., Omaima, A., Sammour, H., Ghamry, E., & Mohammed, E. (2013). Design and development of piroxicam-entrapped niosomes as an oral drug delivery system. *International Journal of Advances in Pharmaceutical Research*, *4*(6), 205–215.

Abdelaziz, A. A., Elbanna, T. E., Sonbol, F. I., Gamaleldin, N. M., & El Maghraby, G. M. (2015). Optimization of niosomes for enhanced antibacterial activity and reduced bacterial resistance: in vitro and in vivo evaluation. *Expert Opinion on Drug Delivery, 12*(2).163-180.

Abdelbary, G., & El-gendy, N. (2008). Niosome-encapsulated gentamicin for ophthalmic controlled delivery. *AAPS PharmSciTech*, *9*(3), 740–747. doi:10.1208/s12249-008-9105-1 PMID:18563578

Abdelkader, H., Ismail, S., Hussein, A., Wu, Z., Al-Kassas, R., & Alany, R. G. (2012). Conjunctival and corneal tolerability assessment of ocular naltrexone niosomes and their ingredients on the hen's egg chorioallantoic membrane and excised bovine cornea models. *International Journal of Pharmaceutics*, *432*(1-2), 1–10. doi:10.1016/j.ijpharm.2012.04.063 PMID:22575752

Abdelkader, H., Ismail, S., Kamal, A., & Alany, R. G. (2010). Preparation of niosomes as an ocular delivery system for naltrexone hydrochloride: Physicochemical characterization. *Die Pharmazie-An International Journal of Pharmaceutical Sciences*, *65*(11), 811–817. PMID:21155387

Abdelkader, H., Ismail, S., Kamal, A., & Alany, R. G. (2011). Design and evaluation of controlled-release niosomes and discomes for naltrexone hydrochloride ocular delivery. *Journal of Pharmaceutical Sciences*, *100*(5), 1833–1846. doi:10.1002/jps.22422 PMID:21246556

Abu Hashim, I. I., El-dahan, M. S., Yusif, R. M., Abd-ElGawad, A. E. H., & Arima, H. (2014). Potential use of niosomal hydrogel as an ocular delivery system for atenolol. *Biological & Pharmaceutical Bulletin*, *37*(4), 541–551. doi:10.1248/bpb.b13-00724 PMID:24694602

Aggarwal, D., Garg, A., & Kaur, I. P. (2004). Development of a topical niosomal preparation of acetazolamide: Preparation and evaluation. *The Journal of Pharmacy and Pharmacology*, *56*(12), 1509–1517. doi:10.1211/0022357044896 PMID:15563757

Aggarwal, D., Pal, D., Mitra, A. K., & Kaur, I. P. (2007). Study of the extent of ocular absorption of acetazolamide from a developed niosomal formulation, by microdialysis sampling of aqueous humor. *International Journal of Pharmaceutics*, *338*(1), 21–26. doi:10.1016/j.ijpharm.2007.01.019 PMID:17300885

Ahmed, A. M., Ghourab, M. M., Shedid, S. G., & Qushawy, M. K. (2013). Optimization of piroxicam niosomes using central composite design. *International Journal of Pharmacy and Pharmaceutical Sciences*, *5*(3), 229–236.

Aiello, C., Andreozzi, P., La Mesa, C., & Risuleo, G. (2010). Biological activity of SDS-CTAB catanionic vesicles in cultured cells and assessment of their cytotoxicity ending in apoptosis. *Colloids and Surfaces. B, Biointerfaces*, *78*(2), 149–154. doi:10.1016/j.colsurfb.2010.02.013 PMID:20347276

Akbari, V., Abedi, D., Pardakhty, A., & Sadeghi-Aliabadi, H. (2013). Ciprofloxacin nano-niosomes for targeting intracellular infections: An in vitro evaluation. *Journal of Nanoparticle Research*, *15*(4), 1–14. doi:10.1007/s11051-013-1556-y

Akbari, V., Abedi, D., Pardakhty, A., & Sadeghi-Aliabadi, H. (2015). Release Studies on Ciprofloxacin Loaded Non-ionic Surfactant Vesicles. *Avicenna Journal of Medical Biotechnology*, *7*(2), 69–75. PMID:26140184

Akhter, S., Kushwaha, S., Warsi, M. H., Anwar, M., Ahmad, M. Z., Ahmad, I., & Ahmad, F. J. et al. (2012). Development and evaluation of nanosized niosomal dispersion for oral delivery of Ganciclovir. *Drug Development and Industrial Pharmacy*, *38*(1), 84–92. doi:10.3109/03639045.2011.592529 PMID:21726136

Alomrani, A. H., Al-Agamy, M. H., & Badran, M. M. (2015). In vitro skin penetration and antimycotic activity of itraconazole loaded niosomes: Various non-ionic surfactants. *Journal of Drug Delivery Science and Technology*, *28*, 37–45. doi:10.1016/j.jddst.2015.04.009

Alsarra, I. A., Bosela, A., Ahmed, S., & Mahrous, G. (2005). Proniosomes as a drug carrier for transdermal delivery of ketorolac. *European Journal of Pharmaceutics and Biopharmaceutics*, *59*(3), 485–490. doi:10.1016/j.ejpb.2004.09.006 PMID:15760729

Alvi, I. A., Madan, J., Kaushik, D., Sardana, S., Pandey, R. S., & Ali, A. (2011). Comparative study of transfersomes, liposomes, and niosomes for topical delivery of 5-fluorouracil to skin cancer cells: Preparation, characterization, in-vitro release, and cytotoxicity analysis. *Anti-Cancer Drugs*, *22*(8), 774–782. doi:10.1097/CAD.0b013e328346c7d6 PMID:21799471

Amanatfard, A., Khazaeli, P., Pardakhty, A., Najafi, M. L., & Mohammadi, A. (2015). Preparation and characterization of physicochemical properties of N, N-diethyl-meta-toluamide niosomes. *International Journal of Pharmaceutical Investigation*, *5*(4), 259–265. doi:10.4103/2230-973X.167691 PMID:26682196

Arunothayanun, P., Bernard, M. S., Craig, D., Uchegbu, I., & Florence, A. (2000). The effect of processing variables on the physical characteristics of non-ionic surfactant vesicles (niosomes) formed from a hexadecyl diglycerol ether. *International Journal of Pharmaceutics*, *201*(1), 7–14. doi:10.1016/S0378-5173(00)00362-8 PMID:10867260

Arunothayanun, P., Turton, J. A., Uchegbu, I. F., & Florence, A. T. (1999). Preparation and in vitro/in vivo evaluation of luteinizing hormone releasing hormone (LHRH)-loaded polyhedral and spherical/tubular niosomes. *Journal of Pharmaceutical Sciences*, *88*(1), 34–38. doi:10.1021/js980286u PMID:9874699

Arzani, G., Haeri, A., Daeihamed, M., Bakhtiari-Kaboutaraki, H., & Dadashzadeh, S. (2015). Niosomal carriers enhance oral bioavailability of carvedilol: Effects of bile salt-enriched vesicles and carrier surface charge. *International Journal of Nanomedicine*, *10*, 4797. PMID:26251598

Asadi, A. P., Moshafi, M., & Sharifi, M. I. (2012). Preparation and in vivo administration of paromomycin niosomes in balb/c mice. *Research in Pharmaceutical Sciences*, *7*(5), S373.

Attia, I. A., El-Gizawy, S. A., Fouda, M. A., & Donia, A. M. (2007). Influence of a niosomal formulation on the oral bioavailability of acyclovir in rabbits. *AAPS PharmSciTech*, *8*(4), 206–212. doi:10.1208/pt0804106 PMID:18181527

Babu, S., Fan, C., Stepanskiy, L., Uitto, J., & Papazoglou, E. (2009). Effect of size at the nanoscale and bilayer rigidity on skin diffusion of liposomes. *Journal of Biomedical Materials Research. Part A*, *91*(1), 140–148. doi:10.1002/jbm.a.32197 PMID:18770522

Baillie, A., Florence, A., Hume, L., Muirhead, G., & Rogerson, A. (1985). The preparation and properties of niosomes--non-ionic surfactant vesicles. *The Journal of Pharmacy and Pharmacology*, *37*(12), 863–868. doi:10.1111/j.2042-7158.1985.tb04990.x PMID:2868092

Balakrishnan, P., Shanmugam, S., Lee, W. S., Lee, W. M., Kim, J. O., Oh, D. H., & Choi, H. G. et al. (2009). Formulation and in vitro assessment of minoxidil niosomes for enhanced skin delivery. *International Journal of Pharmaceutics*, *377*(1), 1–8. doi:10.1016/j.ijpharm.2009.04.020 PMID:19394413

Bayindir, Z. S., & Yuksel, N. (2010). Characterization of niosomes prepared with various nonionic surfactants for paclitaxel oral delivery. *Journal of Pharmaceutical Sciences*, *99*(4), 2049–2060. doi:10.1002/jps.21944 PMID:19780133

Bendas, E. R., Abdullah, H., El-Komy, M. H., & Kassem, M. A. (2013). Hydroxychloroquine niosomes: A new trend in topical management of oral lichen planus. *International Journal of Pharmaceutics*, *458*(2), 287–295. doi:10.1016/j.ijpharm.2013.10.042 PMID:24184035

Bouwstra, J. A., van Hal, D. A., Hofl, H. E., & Junginger, H. E. (1997). Preparation and characterization of nonionic surfactant vesicles. *Colloids and Surfaces. A, Physicochemical and Engineering Aspects*, *123*, 71–80. doi:10.1016/S0927-7757(96)03800-9

Bragagni, M., Mennini, N., Furlanetto, S., Orlandini, S., Ghelardini, C., & Mura, P. (2014). Development and characterization of functionalized niosomes for brain targeting of dynorphin-B. *European Journal of Pharmaceutics and Biopharmaceutics*, *87*(1), 73–79. doi:10.1016/j.ejpb.2014.01.006 PMID:24462793

Bragagni, M., Mennini, N., Ghelardini, C., & Mura, P. (2012). Development and characterization of niosomal formulations of doxorubicin aimed at brain targeting. *Journal of Pharmacy & Pharmaceutical Sciences*, *15*(1), 184–196. doi:10.18433/J3230M PMID:22365096

Caracciolo, G., Pozzi, D., Caminiti, R., Marianecci, C., Moglioni, S., Carafa, M., & Amenitsch, H. (2008). Effect of hydration on the structure of solid-supported Niosomal membranes investigated by in situ energy dispersive X-ray diffraction. *Chemical Physics Letters*, *462*(4-6), 307–312. doi:10.1016/j.cplett.2008.07.094

Carafa, M., Santucci, E., Alhaique, F., Coviello, T., Murtas, E., Riccieri, F., & Torrisi, M. et al. (1998). Preparation and properties of new unilamellar non-ionic/ionic surfactant vesicles. *International Journal of Pharmaceutics*, *160*(1), 51–59. doi:10.1016/S0378-5173(97)00294-9

Carafa, M. L., Marzio, D., Marianecci, C., Cinque, B., Lucania, G., Kajiwara, K., & Santucci, E. et al. (2006). Designing novel pH-sensitive non-phospholipid vesicle: Characterization and cell interaction. *European Journal of Pharmaceutical Sciences*, *28*(5), 385–393. doi:10.1016/j.ejps.2006.04.009 PMID:16797946

Chandra, A. & Sharma, P. (2008). Proniosome based drug delivery system of piroxicam. *African Journal of Pharmacy and Pharmacology, 2*(9),184-190.

Chandraprakash, K., Udupa, N., Umadevi, P., & Pillai, G. (1990). Pharmacokinetic evaluation of surfactant vesicle-entrapped methotrexate in tumor-bearing mice. *International Journal of Pharmaceutics*, *61*(1-2), R1–R4. doi:10.1016/0378-5173(90)90056-A

Chandraprakash, K., Udupa, N., Umadevi, P., & Pillai, G. (1992). Formulation and evaluation of Methotrexate niosomes. *Indian Journal of Pharmaceutical Sciences*, *54*, 197–197.

Chen, Y., & Liu, L. (2012). Modern methods for delivery of drugs across the blood–brain barrier. *Advanced Drug Delivery Reviews*, *64*(7), 640–665. doi:10.1016/j.addr.2011.11.010 PMID:22154620

Conacher, M., Alexander, J., & Brewer, J. M. (2001). Oral immunisation with peptide and protein antigens by formulation in lipid vesicles incorporating bile salts (bilosomes). *Vaccine*, *19*(20), 2965–2974. doi:10.1016/S0264-410X(00)00537-5 PMID:11282208

Cortesi, R., Esposito, E., Corradini, F., Sivieri, E., Drechsler, M., Rossi, A., & Menegatti, E. et al. (2007). Non-phospholipid vesicles as carriers for peptides and proteins: Production, characterization and stability studies. *International Journal of Pharmaceutics*, *339*(1), 52–60. doi:10.1016/j.ijpharm.2007.02.024 PMID:17395411

Cosco, D., Paolino, D., Muzzalupo, R., Celia, C., Citraro, R., Caponio, D., & Fresta, M. et al. (2009). Novel PEG-coated niosomes based on bola-surfactant as drug carriers for 5-fluorouracil. *Biomedical Microdevices*, *11*(5), 1115–1125. doi:10.1007/s10544-009-9328-2 PMID:19507033

Darwish, I. A., & Uchegbu, I. F. (1997). The evaluation of crown ether based niosomes as cation containing and cation sensitive drug delivery systems. *International Journal of Pharmaceutics*, *159*(2), 207–213. doi:10.1016/S0378-5173(97)00289-5

Desai, T., & Finlay, W. (2002). Nebulization of niosomal all-trans-retinoic acid: An inexpensive alternative to conventional liposomes. *International Journal of Pharmaceutics*, *241*(2), 311–317. doi:10.1016/S0378-5173(02)00245-4 PMID:12100858

Devaraj, G., Parakh, S., Devraj, R., Apte, S., Rao, B., & Rambhau, D. (2002). Release studies on niosomes containing fatty alcohols as bilayer stabilizers instead of cholesterol. *Journal of Colloid and Interface Science*, *251*(2), 360–365. doi:10.1006/jcis.2002.8399 PMID:16290741

Dew, N., Edwards, K., Eriksson, J., Edsman, K., & Björk, E. (2012). Gel formulations containing catanionic vesicles composed of alprenolol and SDS: Effects of drug release and skin penetration on aggregate structure. *Colloids and Surfaces. B, Biointerfaces*, *89*(10), 53–60. doi:10.1016/j.colsurfb.2011.08.022 PMID:21958537

Di Marzio, L., Esposito, S., Rinaldi, F., Marianecci, C., & Carafa, M. (2012). Polysorbate 20 vesicles as oral delivery system: In-vitro characterization. *Colloids and Surfaces. B, Biointerfaces*, *104*, 200–206. doi:10.1016/j.colsurfb.2012.10.036 PMID:23314494

Di Marzio, L., Marianecci, C., Petrone, M., Rinaldi, F., & Carafa, M. (2011). Novel pH-sensitive non-ionic surfactant vesicles: Comparison between Tween 21 and Tween 20. *Colloids and Surfaces. B, Biointerfaces*, *82*(1), 18–24. doi:10.1016/j.colsurfb.2010.08.004 PMID:20832262

Dufes, C., Gaillard, F., Uchegbu, I. F., Schatzlein, A. G., Olivier, J. C., & Muller, J. M. (2004). Glucose-targeted niosomes deliver vasoactive intestinal peptide (VIP) to the brain. *International Journal of Pharmaceutics*, *285*(1-2), 77–85. doi:10.1016/j.ijpharm.2004.07.020 PMID:15488681

Dufes, C., Schätzlein, A., Tetley, L., Gray, A., Watson, D., Olivier, J., & Uchegbu, I. et al. (2000). Niosomes and polymeric chitosan based vesicles bearing transferrin and glucose ligands for drug targeting. *Pharmaceutical Research*, *17*(10), 1250–1258. doi:10.1023/A:1026422915326 PMID:11145231

Echegoyen, L. E., Hernandez, J. C., Kaifer, A. E., Gokel, G. W., & Echegoyen, L. (1988). Aggregation of steroidal lariat ethers: The first example of nonionic liposomes (niosomes) formed from neutral crown ether compounds. *Journal of the Chemical Society. Chemical Communications*, *12*(12), 836–837. doi:10.1039/c39880000836

El-Menshawe, S. F., & Hussein, A. K. (2013). Formulation and evaluation of meloxicam niosomes as vesicular carriers for enhanced skin delivery. *Pharmaceutical Development and Technology*, *18*(4), 779–786. doi:10.3109/10837450.2011.598166 PMID:21913880

El-Ridy, M. S., Abdelbary, A., Nasr, E. A., Khalil, R. M., Mostafa, D. M., El-Batal, A. I., & Abd El-Alim, H. S. (2011). Niosomal encapsulation of the antitubercular drug, pyrazinamide. *Drug Development and Industrial Pharmacy*, *37*(9), 1110–1118. doi:10.3109/03639045.2011.560605 PMID:21417612

El-Ridy, M. S., Yehia, S. A., Kassem, M. A. E. M., Mostafa, D. M., Nasr, E. A., & Asfour, M. H. (2015). Niosomal encapsulation of ethambutol hydrochloride for increasing its efficacy and safety. *Drug Delivery*, *22*(1), 21–36. doi:10.3109/10717544.2013.868556 PMID:24359403

ElBayoumi, T. A., & Torchilin, V. P. (2009). Tumor-targeted nanomedicines: Enhanced antitumor efficacy in vivo of doxorubicin-loaded, long-circulating liposomes modified with cancer-specific monoclonal antibody. *Clinical Cancer Research*, *15*(6), 1973–1980. doi:10.1158/1078-0432.CCR-08-2392 PMID:19276264

Fang, J. Y., Hong, C. T., Chiu, W. T., & Wang, Y. Y. (2001). Effect of liposomes and niosomes on skin permeation of enoxacin. *International Journal of Pharmaceutics*, *219*(1-2), 61–72. doi:10.1016/S0378-5173(01)00627-5 PMID:11337166

Florence, A. (1993). Nonionic surfactant vesicles: preparation and characterization. *Liposome technology 2*,157-176.

Foster, T., Dorfman, K. D., & Davis, H. T. (2010). Giant biocompatible and biodegradable PEG–PMCL vesicles and microcapsules by solvent evaporation from double emulsion droplets. *Journal of Colloid and Interface Science*, *351*(1), 140–150. doi:10.1016/j.jcis.2010.05.020 PMID:20627256

Gaafar, P. M., Abdallah, O. Y., Farid, R. M., & Abdelkader, H. (2014). Preparation, characterization and evaluation of novel elastic nano-sized niosomes (ethoniosomes) for ocular delivery of prednisolone. *Journal of Liposome Research*, *24*(3), 204–215. doi:10.3109/08982104.2014.881850 PMID:24484536

Garg, T., Rath, G., Murthy, R. R., Gupta, U. D., Vatsala, P. G., & Goyal, A. K. (2015). Current nanotechnological approaches for an effective delivery of bioactive drug molecules to overcome drug resistance tuberculosis. *Current Pharmaceutical Design*, *21*(22), 3076–3089. doi:10.2174/138161282166615053 1163254 PMID:26027577

Gayathri Devi, S., & Udupa, N. (2000). Niosomal Sumartriptan Succinate For Nasal Administration. *Indian Journal of Pharmaceutical Sciences*, *62*(6), 479–486.

Gebicki, J., & Hicks, M. (1973). Ufasomes are stable particles surrounded by unsaturated fatty acid membranes. *Nature*, *243*(5404), 232–234. doi:10.1038/243232a0 PMID:4706295

Gopinath, D., Ravi, D., Rao, B., Apte, S., Renuka, D., & Rambhau, D. (2004). Ascorbyl palmitate vesicles (Aspasomes): Formation, characterization and applications. *International Journal of Pharmaceutics*, *271*(1), 95–113. doi:10.1016/j.ijpharm.2003.10.032 PMID:15129977

Gude, R., Jadhav, M., Rao, S., & Jagtap, A. (2002). Effects of niosomal cisplatin and combination of the same with theophylline and with activated macrophages in murine B16F10 melanoma model. *Cancer Biotherapy & Radiopharmaceuticals*, *17*(2), 183–192. doi:10.1089/108497802753773801 PMID:12030112

Guedj, C., Pucci, B., Zarif, L., Coulomb, C., Riess, J., & Pavia, A. (1994). Vesicles and other supramolecular systems from biocompatible synthetic glycolipids with hydrocarbon and/or fluorocarbon chains. *Chemistry and Physics of Lipids*, *72*(2), 153–173. doi:10.1016/0009-3084(94)90099-X PMID:7954977

Guinedi, A. S., Mortada, N. D., Mansour, S., & Hathout, R. M. (2005). Preparation and evaluation of reverse-phase evaporation and multilamellar niosomes as ophthalmic carriers of acetazolamide. *International Journal of Pharmaceutics*, *306*(1-2), 71–82. doi:10.1016/j.ijpharm.2005.09.023 PMID:16263229

Gupta, N., Srivastava, V., Saxena, S., & Pandey, A. (2010). Formulation and evaluation of non-ionic surfactant vesicles for ocular delivery of ofloxacin, *International Journal of Life Science and Pharma Reviews*, (7), 413-418.

Hamilton, A., Biganzoli, L., Coleman, R., Mauriac, L., Hennebert, P., Awada, A., & de Valeriola, D. et al. (2002). A phase I clinical and pharmacokinetic study of polyethylene glycol liposomal doxorubicin (Caelyx, Doxil) at a 6-week interval in patients with metastatic breast cancer. *Annals of Oncology*, *13*(6), 910–918. doi:10.1093/annonc/mdf157 PMID:12123337

Hamishehkar, H., Rahimpour, Y., & Kouhsoltani, M. (2013). Niosomes as a propitious carrier for topical drug delivery. *Expert Opinion on Drug Delivery*, *10*(2), 261–272. doi:10.1517/17425247.2013.746310 PMID:23252629

Handjani-Vila, R. M., Ribier, A., Rondot, B., & Vanlerberghie, G. (1979). Dispersions of lamellar phases of non-ionic lipids in cosmetic products. *International Journal of Cosmetic Science*, *1*(5), 303–314. doi:10.1111/j.1467-2494.1979.tb00224.x PMID:19467076

Hao, Y., & Li, K. (2010). Entrapment and release difference resulting from hydrogen bonding interactions in niosome. *International Journal of Pharmaceutics*, *403*(1-2), 245–253. doi:10.1016/j.ijpharm.2010.10.027 PMID:20971171

Hao, Y., Zhao, F., Li, N., Yang, Y., & Li, K. (2002). Studies on a high encapsulation of colchicine by a niosome system. *International Journal of Pharmaceutics*, *244*(1-2), 73–80. doi:10.1016/S0378-5173(02)00301-0 PMID:12204566

Hofland, H., Bouwstra, J., Verhoef, J., Buckton, G., Chowdry, B., Ponec, M., & Junginger, H. (1992). Safety Aspects of Non-ionic Surfactant Vesicles: A Toxicity Study Related to the Physicochemical Characteristics of Non-ionic Surfactants. *The Journal of Pharmacy and Pharmacology*, *44*(4), 287–294. doi:10.1111/j.2042-7158.1992.tb03608.x PMID:1355538

Hofland, H. E., van der Geest, R., Bodde, H. E., Junginger, H. E., & Bouwstra, J. A. (1994). Estradiol permeation from nonionic surfactant vesicles through human stratum corneum in vitro. *Pharmaceutical Research*, *11*(5), 659–664. doi:10.1023/A:1018963910260 PMID:8058633

Hofland, H. E. J., Bouwstra, J. A., Gooris, G. S., Spies, F., Talsma, H., & Junginger, H. E. (1993). Non-ionic surfactant vesicles: A study of vesicle formation, characterization, and stability. *Journal of Colloid and Interface Science*, *161*(2), 366–376. doi:10.1006/jcis.1993.1479

Hong, M., Zhu, S., Jiang, Y., Tang, G., & Pei, Y. (2009). Efficient tumor targeting of hydroxycamptothecin loaded PEGylated niosomes modified with transferrin. *Journal of Controlled Release*, *133*(2), 96–102. doi:10.1016/j.jconrel.2008.09.005 PMID:18840485

Hua, W., & Liu, T. (2007). Preparation and properties of highly stable innocuous niosome in Span 80/PEG 400/H 2 O system. *Colloids and Surfaces. A, Physicochemical and Engineering Aspects*, *302*(1), 377–382. doi:10.1016/j.colsurfa.2007.02.068

Illum, L. (2015). Intranasal Delivery to the Central Nervous System. In *Blood-Brain Barrier in Drug Discovery: Optimizing Brain Exposure of CNS Drugs and Minimizing Brain Side Effects for Peripheral Drugs*.

Jadon, P. S., Gajbhiye, V., Jadon, R. S., Gajbhiye, K. R., & Ganesh, N. (2009). Enhanced oral bioavailability of griseofulvin via niosomes. *AAPS PharmSciTech*, *10*(4), 1186–1192. doi:10.1208/s12249-009-9325-z PMID:19856107

Jain, C., & Vyas, S. (1995). Preparation and characterization of niosomes containing rifampicin for lung targeting. *Journal of Microencapsulation*, *12*(4), 401–407. doi:10.3109/02652049509087252 PMID:8583314

Jain, C., Vyas, S., & Dixit, V. (2006). Niosomal system for delivery of rifampicin to lymphatics. *Indian Journal of Pharmaceutical Sciences*, *68*(5), 575–583. doi:10.4103/0250-474X.29622

Jain, S., Chaudhari, & Swarnakar. (2011). Preparation and characterization of niosomal gel for iontophoresis mediated transdermal delivery of isosorbide dinitrate. *Drug Delivery and Translational Research*, *1*(4), 309-321.

Jain, S., Singh, P., Mishra, V., & Vyas, S. P. (2005). Mannosylated niosomes as adjuvant-carrier system for oral genetic immunization against hepatitis B. *Immunology Letters*, *101*(1), 41–49. doi:10.1016/j.imlet.2005.04.002 PMID:15869802

Jayaraman, S. C., Ramachandran, C., & Weiner, N. (1996). Topical delivery of erythromycin from various formulations: An in vivo hairless mouse study. *Journal of Pharmaceutical Sciences*, *85*(10), 1082–1084. doi:10.1021/js960040u PMID:8897275

Jin, Y., Wen, J., Garg, S., Liu, D., Zhou, Y., Teng, L., & Zhang, W. (2013). Development of a novel niosomal system for oral delivery of Ginkgo biloba extract. *International Journal of Nanomedicine*, *8*, 421. doi:10.2147/IJN.S37984 PMID:23378764

Junyaprasert, V., Teeranachaideekul, V., & Supaperm, T. (2008). Effect of charged and non-ionic membrane additives on physicochemical properties and stability of niosomes. *AAPS PharmSciTech*, *9*(3), 851–859. doi:10.1208/s12249-008-9121-1 PMID:18636334

Kamboj, S., Saini, V., & Bala, S. (2014). Formulation and characterization of drug loaded nonionic surfactant vesicles (niosomes) for oral bioavailability enhancement. *The Scientific World Journal*. PMID:24672401

Kaminskas, L. M., McLeod, V. M., Kelly, B. D., Sberna, G., Boyd, B. J., Williamson, M., & Porter, C. J. et al. (2012). A comparison of changes to doxorubicin pharmacokinetics, antitumor activity, and toxicity mediated by PEGylated dendrimer and PEGylated liposome drug delivery systems. *Nanomedicine; Nanotechnology, Biology, and Medicine*, *8*(1), 103–111. doi:10.1016/j.nano.2011.05.013 PMID:21704192

Kato, K., Walde, P., Koine, N., Ichikawa, S., Ishikawa, T., Nagahama, R., & Omokawa, M. et al. (2008). Temperature-sensitive nonionic vesicles prepared from Span 80 (sorbitan monooleate). *Langmuir*, *24*(19), 10762–10770. doi:10.1021/la801581f PMID:18720959

Kaur, I. P., Aggarwal, D., Singh, H., & Kakkar, S. (2010). Improved ocular absorption kinetics of timolol maleate loaded into a bioadhesive niosomal delivery system. *Graefes Archive for Clinical and Experimental Ophthalmology*, *248*(10), 1467–1472. doi:10.1007/s00417-010-1383-0 PMID:20437246

Khaksa, G., Souza, R. D., Lewis, S., & Udupa, N. (2000). Pharmacokinetic study of niosome encapsulated insulin. *Indian Journal of Experimental Biology*, *38*(9), 901–905. PMID:12561948

Kiwada, H., Niimura, H., Fujisaki, Y., Yamada, S., & Kato, Y. (1985). Application of synthetic alkyl glycoside vesicles as drug carriers. I. Preparation and physical properties. *Chemical & Pharmaceutical Bulletin*, *33*(2), 753–759. doi:10.1248/cpb.33.753 PMID:4017121

Kiwada, H., Niimura, H., & Kato, Y. (1985). Tissue distribution and pharmacokinetic evaluation of the targeting efficiency of synthetic alkyl glycoside vesicles. *Chemical & Pharmaceutical Bulletin*, *33*(6), 2475–2482. doi:10.1248/cpb.33.2475 PMID:4064206

Lattin, J., Belnap, D., & Pitt, W. (2012). Formation of Liposomes as a drug delivery vehicle. *Colloids and Surfaces. B, Biointerfaces*, *89*, 93–100. doi:10.1016/j.colsurfb.2011.08.030 PMID:21962853

Lee, V. H., & Yamamoto, A. (1989). Penetration and enzymatic barriers to peptide and protein absorption. *Advanced Drug Delivery Reviews*, *4*(2), 171–207. doi:10.1016/0169-409X(89)90018-5

Li, G. L., Danhof, M., & Bouwstra, J. A. (2001). Effect of elastic liquid-state vesicle on apomorphine iontophoresis transport through human skin in vitro. *Pharmaceutical Research*, *18*(11), 1627–1630. doi:10.1023/A:1013098902260 PMID:11758773

Li, Q., Li, Z., Zeng, W., Ge, S., Lu, H., Wu, C., & Xu, Y. et al. (2014). Proniosome-derived niosomes for tacrolimus topical ocular delivery: In vitro cornea permeation, ocular irritation, and in vivo anti-allograft rejection. *European Journal of Pharmaceutical Sciences*, *62*, 115–123. doi:10.1016/j.ejps.2014.05.020 PMID:24905830

Lieb, L. M., Flynn, G., & Weiner, N. (1994). Follicular (pilosebaceous unit) deposition and pharmacological behavior of cimetidine as a function of formulation. *Pharmaceutical Research*, *11*(10), 1419–1423. doi:10.1023/A:1018939805601 PMID:7855045

Liu, T., & Guo, R. (2007). Structure and transformation of the niosome prepared from PEG 6000/Tween 80/Span 80/H2O lamellar liquid crystal. *Colloids and Surfaces. A, Physicochemical and Engineering Aspects*, *295*(1), 130–134. doi:10.1016/j.colsurfa.2006.08.041

Liu, T., Guo, R., Hua, W., & Qiu, J. (2007). Structure behaviors of hemoglobin in PEG 6000/Tween 80/Span 80/H2O niosome system. *Colloids and Surfaces. A, Physicochemical and Engineering Aspects*, *293*(1), 255–261. doi:10.1016/j.colsurfa.2006.07.053

Liu, Y. S., Wen, C. F., & Yang, Y. M. (2012). Development of ethosome-like catanionic vesicles for dermal drug delivery. *Journal of the Taiwan Institute of Chemical Engineers*, *43*(6), 830–838. doi:10.1016/j.jtice.2012.06.008

Lo, C. T., Jahn, A., Locascio, L. E., & Vreeland, W. N. (2010). Controlled self-assembly of monodisperse niosomes by microfluidic hydrodynamic focusing. *Langmuir*, *26*(11), 8559–8566. doi:10.1021/la904616s PMID:20146467

Lu, B., Zhang, J., & Yang, H. (2003). Nonphospholipid vesicles of carboplatin for lung targeting. *Drug Delivery*, *10*(2), 87–94. doi:10.1080/713840364 PMID:12746054

Mali, N., Darandale, S., & Vavia, P. (2013). Niosomes as a vesicular carrier for topical administration of minoxidil: formulation and in vitro assessment. *Drug Delivery and Translational Research, 3*(6), 587-592.

Manconi, M., Sinico, C., Fadda, A., Vila, A., Figueruelo, J., & Molina, F. (2005). Thermodynamical aspects regarding the formation of self-assembly decylpolyglucoside structures. *Colloids and Surfaces. A, Physicochemical and Engineering Aspects*, *270*, 124–128. doi:10.1016/j.colsurfa.2005.05.051

Manconi, M., Sinico, C., Valenti, D., Lai, F., & Fadda, A. (2006). Niosomes as carriers for tretinoin III. A study into the in vitro cutaneous delivery of vesicle-incorporated tretinoin. *International Journal of Pharmaceutics*, *311*(1-2), 11–19. doi:10.1016/j.ijpharm.2005.11.045 PMID:16439071

Manconi, M., Sinico, C., Valenti, D., Loy, G., & Fadda, A. (2002). Niosomes as carriers for tretinoin. I. Preparation and properties. *International Journal of Pharmaceutics*, *234*(1-2), 237–248. doi:10.1016/S0378-5173(01)00971-1 PMID:11839454

Manconi, M., Valenti, D., Sinico, C., Lai, F., Loy, G., & Fadda, A. (2003). Niosomes as carriers for tretinoin. II. Influence of vesicular incorporation on tretinoin photostability. *International Journal of Pharmaceutics*, *260*(2), 261–272. doi:10.1016/S0378-5173(03)00268-0 PMID:12842345

Manconi, M., Vila, A., Sinico, C., Figueruelo, J., Molina, F., & Fadda, A. (2006). Theoretical and experimental evaluation of decypolyglucoside vesicles as potential drug delivery systems. *Journal of Drug Delivery Science and Technology*, *16*(2), 141–146. doi:10.1016/S1773-2247(06)50021-8

Manosroi, A., Chutoprapat, R., Abe, M., & Manosroi, J. (2008). Characteristics of niosomes prepared by supercritical carbon dioxide (scCO2) fluid. *International Journal of Pharmaceutics*, *352*(1-2), 248–255. doi:10.1016/j.ijpharm.2007.10.013 PMID:18036754

Manosroi, A., Chutoprapat, R., Abe, M., Manosroi, W., & Manosroi, J. (2012). Transdermal absorption enhancement of rice bran bioactive compounds entrapped in niosomes. *AAPS PharmSciTech*, *13*(1), 323–335. doi:10.1208/s12249-012-9751-1 PMID:22258804

Manosroi, A., Jantrawut, P., & Manosroi, J. (2008). Anti-inflammatory activity of gel containing novel elastic niosomes entrapped with diclofenac diethylammonium. *International Journal of Pharmaceutics*, *360*(1-2), 156–163. doi:10.1016/j.ijpharm.2008.04.033 PMID:18539416

Manosroi, A., Khanrin, P., Werner, R., Götz, F., Manosroi, W., & Manosroi, J. (2010). Entrapment enhancement of peptide drugs in niosomes. *Journal of Microencapsulation*, *27*(3), 272–280. doi:10.3109/02652040903131293 PMID:20113169

Manosroi, A., Ruksiriwanich, W., Manosroi, W., Abe, M., & Manosroi, J. (2012). In Vivo Hair Growth Promotion Activity of Gel Containing Niosomes Loaded with the Oryza sativa Bran Fraction (OSF3). Advanced Science Letters, 16(1),222-228.

Masotti, A., Vicennati, P., Alisi, A., Marianecci, C., Rinaldi, F., Carafa, M., & Ortaggi, G. (2010). Novel Tween® 20 derivatives enable the formation of efficient pH-sensitive drug delivery vehicles for human hepatoblastoma. *Bioorganic & Medicinal Chemistry Letters*, *20*(10), 3021–3025. doi:10.1016/j.bmcl.2010.04.010 PMID:20427183

Mehta, S., & Jindal, N. (2013). Formulation of tyloxapol niosomes for encapsulation, stabilization and dissolution of anti-tubercular drugs. *Colloids and Surfaces. B, Biointerfaces*, *101*, 434–441. doi:10.1016/j.colsurfb.2012.07.006 PMID:23010052

Memisoğlu, E., Oner, F., Ayhan, A., Basaran, I., & Hincal, A. (1997). In vivo evaluation for rhGM-CSF wound-healing efficacy in topical vehicles. *Pharmaceutical Development and Technology*, *2*(2), 171–180. doi:10.3109/10837459709022622 PMID:9552443

Moazeni, E., Gilani, K., Sotoudegan, F., Pardakhty, A., Najafabadi, A. R., Ghalandari, R., & Jamalifar, H. et al. (2010). Formulation and in vitro evaluation of ciprofloxacin containing niosomes for pulmonary delivery. *Journal of Microencapsulation*, *10*, 1–10. PMID:20681747

Moghassemi, S., Parnian, E., Hakamivala, A., Darzianiazizi, M., Vardanjani, M. M., Kashanian, S., & Omidfar, K. et al. (2015). Uptake and transport of insulin across intestinal membrane model using trimethyl chitosan coated insulin niosomes. *Materials Science and Engineering C*, *46*, 333–340. doi:10.1016/j.msec.2014.10.070 PMID:25491995

Mokhtar, M., Sammour, O. A., Hammad, M. A., & Megrab, N. A. (2008). Effect of some formulation parameters on flurbiprofen encapsulation and release rates of niosomes prepared from proniosomes. *International Journal of Pharmaceutics*, *361*(1-2), 104–111. doi:10.1016/j.ijpharm.2008.05.031 PMID:18577437

Mullaicharam, A., & Murthy, R. (2004). Lung accumulation of niosome-entrapped rifampicin following intravenous and intratracheal administration in the rat. *Journal of Drug Delivery Science and Technology*, *14*(2), 99–104. doi:10.1016/S1773-2247(04)50020-5

Mullaicharam, A., & Murthy, R. (2006). Lung accumulation of niosome-entrapped gentamicin sulfate follows intravenous and intratracheal administration in rats. *Journal of Drug Delivery Science and Technology*, *16*(2), 109–113. doi:10.1016/S1773-2247(06)50016-4

Mura, S., Manconi, M., Sinico, C., Valenti, D., & Fadda, A. M. (2009). Penetration enhancer-containing vesicles (PEVs) as carriers for cutaneous delivery of minoxidil. *International Journal of Pharmaceutics*, *380*(1), 72–79. doi:10.1016/j.ijpharm.2009.06.040 PMID:19589377

Mura, S., Manconi, M., Valenti, D., Sinico, C., Vila, A. O., & Fadda, A. M. (2011). Transcutol containing vesicles for topical delivery of minoxidil. *Journal of Drug Targeting*, *19*(3), 189–196. doi:10.3109/1061186X.2010.483516 PMID:20446805

Mura, S., Pirot, F., Manconi, M., Falson, M., & Fadda, A. M. (2007). Liposomes and niosomes as potential carriers for dermal delivery of minoxidil. *Journal of Drug Targeting*, *15*(2), 101–108. doi:10.1080/10611860600991993 PMID:17365280

Mutha, S., Patil, S., & Bhosale, A. (2013). Thermoreversible niosomal gel as a potential ophthalmic drug delivery system for Ganciclovir. *Indo American Journal of Pharmaceutical Research*, *3*(11), 1990–9201.

Muzzalupo, R., Nicoletta, F. P., Trombino, S., Cassano, R., Iemma, F., & Picci, N. (2007). A new crown ether as vesicular carrier for 5-fluoruracil: Synthesis, characterization and drug delivery evaluation. *Colloids and Surfaces. B, Biointerfaces*, *58*(2), 197–202. doi:10.1016/j.colsurfb.2007.03.010 PMID:17434295

Muzzalupo, R., Tavano, L., Trombino, S., Cassano, R., Picci, N., & La Mesa, C. (2008). Niosomes from [alpha],[omega]-trioxyethylene-bis (sodium 2-dodecyloxy-propylenesulfonate): Preparation and characterization. *Colloids and Surfaces. B, Biointerfaces*, *64*(2), 200–207. doi:10.1016/j.colsurfb.2008.01.026 PMID:18378125

Nademi, M., Mozaffari, A., & Farrokhabadi, A. (2011). A New Self Healing Method in Composite Laminates Using the Hollow Glass Fiber. *Key Engineering Materials*, *471*, 548–551. doi:10.4028/www.scientific.net/KEM.471-472.548

Nasr, M. (2010). In vitro and in vivo evaluation of proniosomes containing celecoxib for oral administration. *AAPS PharmSciTech*, *11*(1), 85–89. doi:10.1208/s12249-009-9364-5 PMID:20058106

Nasr, M., Mansour, S., Mortada, N. D., & Elshamy, A. (2008). Vesicular aceclofenac systems: A comparative study between liposomes and niosomes. *Journal of Microencapsulation*, *25*(7), 499–512. doi:10.1080/02652040802055411 PMID:18608811

Nasseri, B. (2005). Effect of cholesterol and temperature on the elastic properties of niosomal membranes. *International Journal of Pharmaceutics*, *300*(1-2), 95–101. doi:10.1016/j.ijpharm.2005.05.009 PMID:16006080

Neumann, R., Ringsdorf, H., Patton, E. V., & O'Brien, D. F. (1987). Preparation and characterization of long chain amino acid and peptide vesicle membranes. *Biochimica et Biophysica Acta (BBA)-. Biomembranes*, *898*(3), 338–348. doi:10.1016/0005-2736(87)90075-7

Niemiec, S. M., Ramachandran, C., & Weiner, N. (1995). Influence of nonionic liposomal composition on topical delivery of peptide drugs into pilosebaceous units: An in vivo study using the hamster ear model. *Pharmaceutical Research*, *12*(8), 1184–1188. doi:10.1023/A:1016268027854 PMID:7494832

Ning, M., Guo, Y., Pan, H., Chen, X., & Gu, Z. (2005). Preparation, in vitro and in vivo evaluation of liposomal/niosomal gel delivery systems for clotrimazole. *Drug Development and Industrial Pharmacy*, *31*(4-5), 375–383. doi:10.1081/DDC-54315 PMID:16093203

Ning, M., Guo, Y., Pan, H., Yu, H., & Gu, Z. (2005). Niosomes with sorbitan monoester as a carrier for vaginal delivery of insulin: Studies in rats. *Drug Delivery*, *12*(6), 399–407. doi:10.1080/10717540590968891 PMID:16253956

Noori, A. P. (2012). Preparation, characterization and anti-inflammatory evaluation of indomethacin niosomes in carrageenan inflammation model. *Research in Pharmaceutical Sciences*, *7*(5), S381.

O'brien, M., Wigler, N., Inbar, M., Rosso, R., Grischke, E., Santoro, A., & Ackland, S. et al. (2004). Reduced cardiotoxicity and comparable efficacy in a phase III trial of pegylated liposomal doxorubicin HCl (CAELYX™/Doxil®) versus conventional doxorubicin for first-line treatment of metastatic breast cancer. *Annals of Oncology*, *15*(3), 440–449. doi:10.1093/annonc/mdh097 PMID:14998846

Okahata, Y., Tanamachi, S., Nagai, M., & Kunitake, T. (1981). Synthetic bilayer membranes prepared from dialkyl amphiphiles with nonionic and zwitterionic head groups. *Journal of Colloid and Interface Science*, *82*(2), 401–417. doi:10.1016/0021-9797(81)90382-9

Okumura, Y., & Iwata, Y. (2011). Electroformation of Giant Vesicles and Electrode Polarity. *Bulletin of the Chemical Society of Japan*, *84*(10), 1147–1149. doi:10.1246/bcsj.20110097

Özer, A., Turker, S., Çolak, S., Korkmaz, M., Kiliç, E., & Özalp, M. (2013). The effects of gamma irradiation on diclofenac sodium, liposome and niosome ingredients for rheumatoid arthritis. *Interventional Medicine and Applied Science*, *5*(3), 122–130. doi:10.1556/IMAS.5.2013.3.5 PMID:24265902

Panyosak, A., Manosroi, J., Rojanasakul, Y., & Manosroi, A. (2009). Safety assessment of azelaic acid and its derivatives entrapped in nanovesicles. *Human and Experimental Toxicology*, *28*(6-7), 387–392. doi:10.1177/0960327109105164 PMID:19755450

Paolino, D., Cosco, D., Molinaro, R., Celia, C., & Fresta, M. (2011). Supramolecular devices to improve the treatment of brain diseases. *Drug Discovery Today*, *16*(7), 311–324. doi:10.1016/j.drudis.2011.02.006 PMID:21335100

Paolino, D., Cosco, D., Muzzalupo, R., Trapasso, E., Picci, N., & Fresta, M. (2008). Innovative bola-surfactant niosomes as topical delivery systems of 5-fluorouracil for the treatment of skin cancer. *International Journal of Pharmaceutics*, *353*(1-2), 233–242. doi:10.1016/j.ijpharm.2007.11.037 PMID:18191509

Paolino, D., Muzzalupo, R., Ricciardi, A., Celia, C., Picci, N., & Fresta, M. (2007). In vitro and in vivo evaluation of Bola-surfactant containing niosomes for transdermal delivery. *Biomedical Microdevices*, *9*(4), 421–433. doi:10.1007/s10544-007-9046-6 PMID:17252206

Pardakhty, A., & Moazeni, E. (2013). Nano-niosomes in drug, vaccine and gene delivery: A rapid overview. *Nanomedicine Journal*, *1*(1), 1–12.

Pardakhty, A., Moazeni, E., Varshosaz, J., Hajhashemi, V., & Najafabadi, A. R. (2011). Pharmacokinetic study of niosome-loaded insulin in diabetic rats. *DARU Journal of Pharmaceutical Sciences*, *19*(6), 404. PMID:23008685

Pardakhty, A., Varshosaz, J., & Rouholamini, A. (2007). In vitro study of polyoxyethylene alkyl ether niosomes for delivery of insulin. *International Journal of Pharmaceutics*, *328*(2), 130–141. doi:10.1016/j.ijpharm.2006.08.002 PMID:16997517

Parthasarathi, G., Udupa, N., Umadevi, P., & Pillai, G. (1994). Niosome encapsulated of vincristine sulfate: Improved anticancer activity with reduced toxicity in mice. *Journal of Drug Targeting*, *2*(2), 173–182. doi:10.3109/10611869409015907 PMID:8069596

Patel, D., Jani, R., & Patel, C. (2011). Ufasomes: A vesicular drug delivery. *Systematic Reviews in Pharmacy*, *2*(2), 72. doi:10.4103/0975-8453.86290

Perini, G., Saettone, M., Carafa, M., Santucci, E., & Alhaique, F. (1996). Niosomes as carriers for ophthalmic drugs: In vitro/in vivo evaluation. *Bollettino Chimico Farmaceutico*, *135*(2), 145. PMID:8791827

Piplani, P., Kumar, P., Rohilla, A., Singla, S., & Kaur, I. P. (2015). Development and evaluation of an ocular niosomal delivery system for some newly synthesized Beta blockers. *Asian Journal of Biomedical and Pharmaceutical Sciences*, *4*(40), 8–17. doi:10.15272/ajbps.v4i40.634

Polidori, A., Braun, O., Mora, N., & Pucci, B. (1997). Synthesis of polymerizable double-chain glycolipids derived from Tris. Polymerization in aqueous media. Preliminary investigation of their colloidal behavior. *Tetrahedron Letters*, *38*(14), 2475–2478. doi:10.1016/S0040-4039(97)00413-9

Polidori, A., Pucci, B., Riess, J. G., Zarif, L., & Pavia, A. A. (1994). Synthesis of double-chain glycolipids derived from aspartic acid: Preliminary investigation of their colloidal behavior. *Tetrahedron Letters*, *35*(18), 2899–2902. doi:10.1016/S0040-4039(00)76654-8

Pozzi, D., Caminiti, R., Marianecci, C., Carafa, M., Santucci, E., De Sanctis, S. C., & Caracciolo, G. (2009). Effect of cholesterol on the formation and hydration behavior of solid-supported niosomal membranes. *Langmuir*, *26*(4), 2268–2273. doi:10.1021/la9026877 PMID:19761205

Prabhu, P., Koland, M., Vijaynarayan, K., Harish, N., Ganesh, D., Charyulu, R., & Satynarayana, D. (2010). Preaparation and evaluation of niosomes of Brimonidine tartrate as ocular drug delivery system. *Journal of Pharmaceutical Research and Health Care*, *2*(4), 293–301.

Prasanthi, D., & Lakshmi, K. (2013). Iontophoretic transdermal delivery of finasteride in vesicular invasomal carriers. *Pharmaceutical Nanotechnology*, *1*(2), 136–150. doi:10.2174/2211738511301020009

Rahimpour, Y., & Hamishehkar, H. (2012). Niosomes as Carrier in Dermal Drug Delivery, Recent Advances in Novel Drug Carrier Systems. Current Pharmaceutical Design, 21(20), 2883-2891.

Raja, N., Pillai, G., Udupa, N., & Chandrashekar, G. (1994). Anti-inflammatory activity of niosome encapsulated diclofenac sodium in arthritic rats. *Indian Journal of Pharmacology*, *26*(1), 46.

Ravouru, N., Kondreddy, P., Korakanchi, D., & M, H. (2013). Formulation and evaluation of niosomal nasal drug delivery system of folic acid for brain targeting. *Current Drug Discovery Technologies*, *10*(4), 270–282. doi:10.2174/15701638113109990031 PMID:23863098

Reddy, D. N., & Udupa, N. (1993). Formulation and evaluation of oral and transdermal preparations of flurbiprofen and piroxicam incorporated with different carriers. *Drug Development and Industrial Pharmacy*, *19*(7), 843–852. doi:10.3109/03639049309062986

Rogerson, A., Cummings, J., & Florence, A. T. (1987). Adriamycin-loaded niosomes: Drug entrapment, stability and release. *Journal of Microencapsulation*, *4*(4), 321–328. doi:10.3109/02652048709021824 PMID:3504513

Sahin, N. O. (2007). Niosomes as nanocarrier systems. *Nanomaterials and Nanosystems for Biomedical Applications,* 67-81.

Salama, A. H., & Aburahma, M. H. (2015). Ufasomes nano-vesicles-based lyophilized platforms for intranasal delivery of cinnarizine: Preparation, optimization, ex-vivo histopathological safety assessment and mucosal confocal imaging. *Pharmaceutical Development and Technology*, 1–10. doi:10.3109/10837450.2015.1048553 PMID:25996631

Sankar, V., Babu, E., Siram, K., Penmetsa, S. D., Kabila, B., Srinavas, C. R., & Rai, R. (2013). Formulation and Clinical Evaluation of Triamcinolone Acetonide Niosomes: Effect of Iontophoresis on the Permeation Across Skin. *Pharmaceutical Nanotechnology*, *1*(4), 282–289. doi:10.2174/22117385113016660008

Schenk, P., Ausborn, M., Bendas, F., Nuhn, P., Arndt, D., & Meyer, H. W. (1989). The preparation and characterization of lipid vesicles containing esters of sucrose and fatty acids. *Journal of Microencapsulation*, *6*(1), 95–103. doi:10.3109/02652048909019906 PMID:2715918

Sennato, S., Bordi, F., Cametti, C., Marianecci, C., Carafa, M., & Cametti, M. (2008). Hybrid niosome complexation in the presence of oppositely charged polyions. *The Journal of Physical Chemistry B*, *112*(12), 3720–3727. doi:10.1021/jp0775449 PMID:18307334

Sezgin-Bayindir, Z., Antep, M. N., & Yuksel, N. (2015). Development and Characterization of Mixed Niosomes for Oral Delivery Using Candesartan Cilexetil as a Model Poorly Water-Soluble Drug. *AAPS PharmSciTech*, *16*(1), 108–117. doi:10.1208/s12249-014-0213-9 PMID:25204859

Shahiwala, A., & Misra, A. (2002). Studies in topical application of niosomally entrapped nimesulide. *Journal of Pharmacy and Pharmaceutical Sciences*, *5*(3), 220–225.

Shamsi Meymandi, S., Amiri, R., Aflatunian, M., & Pardakhty, A. (2014). Comparison of the efficacy of niosomal minoxidil with conventional minoxidil in the treatment of androgenetic alopecia: A randomized, controlled, double-blind clinical trial. *Dermatology and Cosmetic*, *5*(2), 53–60.

Sheena, I., Singh, U., Aithal, K., & Udupa, N. (1997). Pilocarpine β-cyclodextrin Complexation and Niosomal Entrapment. *Pharmacy and Pharmacology Communications*, *3*(8), 383–386.

Shi, B., Fang, C., & Pei, Y. (2006). Stealth PEG-PHDCA niosomes: Effects of chain length of PEG and particle size on niosomes surface properties, in vitro drug release, phagocytic uptake, in vivo pharmacokinetics and antitumor activity. *Journal of Pharmaceutical Sciences*, *95*(9), 1873–1887. doi:10.1002/jps.20491 PMID:16795003

Solanki, A., Parikh, J., & Parikh, R. (2010). Preparation, characterization, optimization, and stability studies of aceclofenac proniosomes. *Iranian Journal of Pharmaceutical Research*, 237–246.

Solanki, A. B., Parikh, J. R., & Parikh, R. H. (2007). Formulation and optimization of piroxicam pro niosomes by 3-factor, 3-level Box-Behnken design. *AAPS PharmSciTech*, *8*(4), 43–49. doi:10.1208/pt0804086 PMID:18181547

Srinivas, S., Kumar, Y. A., Hemanth, A., & Anitha, M. (2010). Preparation and evaluation of niosomes containing aceclofenac. *Digest Journal of Nanomaterials and Biostructures*, *5*(1), 249–254.

Suwakul, W., Ongpipattanakul, B., & Vardhanabhuti, N. (2006). Preparation and characterization of propylthiouracil niosomes. *Journal of Liposome Research*, *16*(14), 391–401. doi:10.1080/08982100600992542 PMID:17162580

Tabbakhian, M., Daneshamouz, S., Tavakoli, N., & Jaafari, M. R. (2005). Influence of liposomes and niosomes on the in vitro permeation and skin retention of finasteride. *Indian Journal of Pharmaceutical Sciences*, *1*(3), 119–130.

Tabbakhian, M., Tavakoli, N., Jaafari, M. R., & Daneshamouz, S. (2006). Enhancement of follicular delivery of finasteride by liposomes and niosomes 1. In vitro permeation and in vivo deposition studies using hamster flank and ear models. *International Journal of Pharmaceutics*, *323*(1-2), 1–10. doi:10.1016/j.ijpharm.2006.05.041 PMID:16837150

Tafreshi, S.-H., & Mirdamadi, S. (2015). Survey Study of Lipid Effect on Nisin Nanoliposome Formation and Application in Pasteurized Milk as a Food Model. *Applied Food Biotechnology*, *3*(2), 7–14.

Talsma, H., Van Steenbergen, M. J., Borchert, J. C., & Crommelin, D. J. (1994). A novel technique for the one-step preparation of liposomes and nonionic surfactant vesicles without the use of organic solvents. Liposome formation in a continuous gas stream: The 'Bubble' method. *Journal of Pharmaceutical Sciences*, *83*(3), 276–280. doi:10.1002/jps.2600830303 PMID:8207668

Tamizharasi, S., Dubey, A., Rathi, V., & Rathi, J. (2009). Development and characterization of niosomal drug delivery of gliclazide. *Journal of Young Pharmacists*, *1*(3), 205. doi:10.4103/0975-1483.57065

Tarekegn, A., Joseph, Palani, Zacharia, & Ayenew. (2010). Niosomes in targeted drug delivery some recent advances. *Int j pharm sci res, 29*(1), 9.

Tavano, L., Muzzalupo, R., Cassano, R., Trombino, S., Ferrarelli, T., & Picci, N. (2010). New sucrose cocoate based vesicles: Preparation, characterization and skin permeation studies. *Colloids and Surfaces. B, Biointerfaces*, *75*(1), 319–322. doi:10.1016/j.colsurfb.2009.09.003 PMID:19782543

Türker, S., Erdoğan, S., Ozer, A., Ergün, E., Tuncel, M., Bilgili, H., & Deveci, S. (2005). Scintigraphic imaging of radiolabelled drug delivery systems in rabbits with arthritis. *International Journal of Pharmaceutics*, *296*(1-2), 34–43. doi:10.1016/j.ijpharm.2005.02.017 PMID:15885453

Uchegbu, I. (1998). The biodistribution of novel 200-nm palmitoyl muramic acid vesicles. *International Journal of Pharmaceutics*, *162*(1), 19–27. doi:10.1016/S0378-5173(97)00408-0

Uchegbu, I., Double, J., Kelland, L., Turton, J., & Florence, A. (1996). The activity of doxorubicin niosomes against an ovarian cancer cell line and three in vivo mouse tumour models. *Journal of Drug Targeting*, *3*(5), 399–409. doi:10.3109/10611869608996831 PMID:8866659

Uchegbu, I., Double, J., Turton, J., & Florence, A. (1995). Distribution, metabolism and tumoricidal activity of doxorubicin administered in sorbitan monostearate (Span 60) niosomes in the mouse. *Pharmaceutical Research*, *12*(7), 1019–1024. doi:10.1023/A:1016210515134 PMID:7494796

Uchegbu, I. F., & Vyas, S. P. (1998). Non-ionic surfactant based vesicles (niosomes) in drug delivery. *International Journal of Pharmaceutics*, *172*(1-2), 33–70. doi:10.1016/S0378-5173(98)00169-0

van Hal, D. A., Bouwstra, J. A., van Rensen, A., Jeremiasse, E., de Vringer, T., & Junginger, H. E. (1996). Preparation and characterization of nonionic surfactant vesicles. *Journal of Colloid and Interface Science*, *178*(1), 263–273. doi:10.1006/jcis.1996.0114 PMID:10479441

Varshosaz, J., Pardakhty, A., Hajhashemi, V.-I., & Najafabadi, A. R. (2003). Development and physical characterization of sorbitan monoester niosomes for insulin oral delivery. *Drug Delivery*, *10*(4), 251–262. doi:10.1080/drd_10_4_251 PMID:14612341

Varshosaz, J., Taymouri, Pardakhty, Asadi-Shekaari, & Babaee (2014). *Niosomes of Ascorbic Acid and α-Tocopherol in the Cerebral Ischemia-Reperfusion Model in Male Rats*. BioMed Research International.

Wagner, M. E., & Rizvi, S. S. (2015). Novel method of niosome generation using supercritical carbon dioxide part I: Process mechanics. *Journal of Liposome Research*, (0): 1–13. doi:10.3109/08982104.2015.1088868 PMID:25945392

Waranuch, N., Ramachandran, C., & Weiner, N. D. (1998). Controlled topical delivery of cyclosporin-A from nonionic liposomal formulations: Mechanistic aspects. *Journal of Liposome Research*, *8*(2), 225–238. doi:10.3109/08982109809035528

Yang, H., Deng, A., Zhang, J., Wang, J., & Lu, B. (2013). Preparation, characterization and anticancer therapeutic efficacy of cisplatin-loaded niosomes. *Journal of Microencapsulation*, *30*(3), 237–244. doi:10.3109/02652048.2012.717116 PMID:23272761

Yoshida, H., Lehr, C.-M., Kok, W., Junginger, H., Verhoef, J., & Bouwstra, J. (1992). Niosomes for oral delivery of peptide drugs. *Journal of Controlled Release*, *21*(1), 145–153. doi:10.1016/0168-3659(92)90016-K

Yoshioka, T., Sternberg, B., & Florence, A. (1994). Preparation and properties of vesicles (niosomes)of sorbitan monoesters (Span 20, 40, 60, and 80) and a sorbitan triester (Span 85). *International Journal of Pharmaceutics*, *105*(1), 1–6. doi:10.1016/0378-5173(94)90228-3

Zarif, L. (2002). Elongated supramolecular assemblies in drug delivery. *Journal of Controlled Release*, *81*(1), 7–23. doi:10.1016/S0168-3659(02)00010-X PMID:11992674

Zarif, L., Gulik-Krzywicki, T., Riess, J. G., Pucci, B., Guedj, C., & Pavia, A. A. (1994). Alkyl and perfluoroalkyl glycolipid-based supramolecular assemblies. *Colloids and Surfaces. A, Physicochemical and Engineering Aspects*, *84*(1), 107–112. doi:10.1016/0927-7757(93)02680-D

Zhao, L., Liu, J., Zhang, L., Gao, Y., Zhang, Z., & Luan, Y. (2013). Self-assembly properties, aggregation behavior and prospective application for sustained drug delivery of a drug-participating catanionic system. *International Journal of Pharmaceutics*, *452*(1-2), 108–115. doi:10.1016/j.ijpharm.2013.04.072 PMID:23644346

Zhong, M., Feng, Y., Liao, H., Hu, X., Wan, S., Zhu, B., & Zhang, J. et al. (2014). Azithromycin cationic non-lecithoid nano/microparticles improve bioavailability and targeting efficiency. *Pharmaceutical Research*, *31*(10), 2857–2867. doi:10.1007/s11095-014-1382-7 PMID:25208873

Zidan, A. S., & Habib, M. J. (2014). Maximized Mucoadhesion and Skin Permeation of Anti-AIDS-Loaded Niosomal Gels. *Journal of Pharmaceutical Sciences*, *103*(3), 952–964. doi:10.1002/jps.23867 PMID:24464823

Zidan, A. S., Rahman, Z., & Khan, M. A. (2011). Product and process understanding of a novel pediatric anti-HIV tenofovir niosomes with a high-pressure homogenizer. *European Journal of Pharmaceutical Sciences*, *44*(1), 93–102. doi:10.1016/j.ejps.2011.06.012 PMID:21726640

Section 4
Pharmacosomes

Chapter 5
Vesicular Drug Delivery Systems:
A Special Emphasis on Pharmacosomes

Preeti Khulbe
Jaipur National University, India

ABSTRACT

Pharmacosomes are the colloidal dispersions of drugs covalently bound to lipids and may exist as ultrafine vesicular, micellar or hexagonal aggregates, depending on the chemical structure of the drug lipid complex. The term pharmacosomes is explicitly used to describe the zwitterion, amphiphilic stoichiometric complexes of polyphenolic compounds with phospholipids. The system is formed by linking a drug (pharmakon) to a carrier (soma), they are called pharmacosomes. Pharmacosomes can pass through biomembranes efficiently and possess advantages over the use of other vesicular systems such as transferosomes liposomes and noisome. Pharmacososmes are design to avoid the unusual problems associated with the liposomal entrapment of polar drug molecules like low drug incorporation, leakage and solubility. This chapter includes the basic introduction, applications, method of preparation, characterisation, advantages, some research experiences and future prospects of pharmacosomes.

INTRODUCTION

Pharmacosomes are the novel drug delivery system in which drugs are covalently bound to lipids and exist as vesicular, micellar or hexagonal aggregates, according to the chemical structure of the drug lipid complex. The term pharmacosomes is used to describe the zwitterion, amphiphilic stoichiometric complexes of polyphenolic compounds with phospholipids. The pharmacosomes are formed by linking a drug (pharmakon) to a carrier (soma). Pharmacosomes can be able to cross the biomembrane efficiently and having lots of advantages other vesicular systems such as liposomes, niosome and transferosomes.

Pharmacosomes possess better biopharmaceutical properties of the drug resulting in improved bioavailability. Till date various pharmacosomes containing formulations of non-steroidal anti-inflammatory drugs, proteins, cardiovascular and antineoplastic drugs have been prepared. By the development of

DOI: 10.4018/978-1-5225-0751-2.ch005

pharmacosomes the drugs absorption can improve and gastrointestinal toxicity can minimise. Pharmacosomes can interact with biomembranes and perform better transfer of drugs. By this interaction the phase transition temperature of bio membrane can changed, and membrane fluidity is improved, leading to enhanced permeation. Pharmacosomes can reduce problems associated with the entrapment of polar molecules like low drug incorporation, solubility and leakage.

Amphiphilic drug lipid complexes or pharmacosomes may have approach for maximizing therapeutic efficacy of the drugs by improving the bioavailability (mprovement in solubility in gastro-intestinal fluid and permeation across the biomembrane).

According to Langer (1998) drug delivery can be achieved via drug's formulation, and it involves drug-device combination or medical devices products. Drug delivery is a concept integrated with dosage form and route of administration. Kumar (2008) described drug delivery refers to formulations, technologies, approaches and systems for delivering a pharmaceutical compound in the body when needed to achieve its therapeutic. It can perform scientific site-targeting within the body, or it can facilitate systemic pharmacokinetics; it is concerned with quantity and duration of drug release.

Wang (2008) coated that currently the development of targeted delivery is in progress, in which the drug shows its effect only in the target site of the body and sustain release in which the drug is released over a period of time in a predetermined manner. In case of targeted delivery, the formulation must avoid the host's defence mechanisms and reaches the site of action. There are many sustained release formulations such as liposomes, microspheres, drug loaded biodegradable and drug polymer conjugates.

Park (1997) and Bertrand et al., (2011) show drug delivery technologies works by modifying drug release profile, and its absorption, distribution metabolism and elimination for improving products efficacy and safety, as well as patient compliance. Drug release is from: diffusion, degradation, swelling, and affinity-based mechanisms. Some common routes of administration include the preferred non-invasive peroral, topical, transmucosal and other systems such as nasal, buccal, and inhalation routes. Park and Mersny, (2000) discuss that as peptide and protein, antibody, vaccine and gene based drugs, in general might be susceptible to enzymatic degradation or cannot be absorbed into the systemic circulation properly due to charge issues and molecular size to be therapeutically effective. For this reason many protein and peptide drugs delivered by injection or a nanoneedle. For example, many immunizations for delivery of protein drugs and are delivered done by injection.

In case of carrier mediated drug delivery system Juliano, (1980) suggested that it is a powerful technique for the treatment of various diseases. The therapeutic index of conventional and novel drugs is increased via the increase of specificity by the use of drug targeting to a particular cell or intracellular compartment, the management of release kinetics, the active agent or a combination of the above. Nanoparticles (NPs) were announced as drug carriers from about 30 years ago and have been growing day by day, mainly because of its stability, high loading capabilities and improved physicochemical properties. The pathophysiology of tumours may passive accumulation of NPs at sites of action upon intravenous injection. NPs with long circulation times are more effective in reaching tumour tissue. Langer and Goldberg (1983) supported that in addition to systemic administration, localized drug release may be achieved using macroscopic drug depots close to the target site. Among maximum systems considered for this, in situ-forming biomaterials in response to environmental stimuli have gained considerable attention, because of non-invasive character, less side effects with systemic administration and good controlled bio-distribution.

Wang and Recum (2011) said that in the past years, almost all formulators focused on the development of novel drug delivery system. The novel drug delivery system must fulfil two criteria. One is to deliver the drug at a rate directed by the needs of the body, over the period of treatment. The second, should channel the active entity to the site of action. Conventional dosage forms are unable to meet these goals and are being achieved by attention either on drug distribution of drug into a carrier system, modifying molecular drug construct, or by restraining drug release in the environment to show assigned distribution profile.

Gregoriadis (1977) shows that the method of drug delivery can have a significant effect on its efficacy. Many drugs have an optimum concentration range within which maximum benefit is derived, and concentrations above or below this range can be toxic or produce no therapeutic benefit at all. And the very slow progress in the efficacy of the treatment of severe diseases, has gave a growing need for a multidisciplinary approach to the delivery of therapeutics to targets in tissues.

According to this ideas on controlling the pharmacodynamics, pharmacokinetics, non-specific toxicity, bio-recognition, and efficacy of drugs has been generated. These new techniques often called drug delivery systems (DDS), are based on interdisciplinary approaches that combine polymer science, bio-conjugate chemistry, and molecular biology. Goyal et al., (2005) discuss that any drug delivery system may be defined as a system comprising of: a) drug formulation, b) medical device or dosage form/technology to carry the drug inside the body c) mechanism for the release conventional drug delivery involves the formulation of the drug into a suitable form, such as a compressed tablet for oral administration or a solution for intravenous administration.

This type dosage forms have been found to have serious limitations in terms of higher dosage required, lower effectiveness, toxicity and adverse side effects. New drug delivery systems have been developed to overcome the limitation of the conventional drug delivery systems. Sharma (1977) shows in his article that these systems can be called as controlled drug release systems and targeted drug delivery systems. The therapeutic benefits of these new systems include:

- Increased efficacy of the drug site specific delivery,
- Decreased toxicity/side effects,
- Increased convenience,
- Shorter hospitalization,
- Viable treatments for previously incurable diseases,
- Potential for prophylactic applications,
- Lower healthcare costs - both short and long term,
- Better patient compliance.

There is no uniform and established definition of drug delivery systems. According to Fraley et al., (1981) it is assumed to be based on two basic parameters: Route of entry and Dosage form. Any member of the Cartesian product of is defined as a drug delivery system. Such a definition implies that there are a vast number of members in this group. Many of them may not even be feasible, while many others may not be relevant.

Biju and Jin (2006) supported that many drug delivery systems are under development due to minimize drug to, prevent harmful side-effects, to reduce drug loss and to increase drug bioavailability. Lieberman (1998) and Kaur (2002) said that among drug carriers one can name, micro particles, soluble polymers made of biodegradable natural and synthetic polymers or non-biodegradable, microcapsules, cell ghosts, lipoproteins, liposomes, and micelles. The carriers can be made slowly degradable, stimuli-reactive (e.g., pH- or temperature-sensitive), and even targeted (e.g., by conjugating them with specific antibodies against certain characteristic components of the area of interest). Targeting is any ability of the dosage form to direct the drug-loaded system to the site of interest. Two major mechanisms can be given to distinguish for addressing the desired sites for drug release: passive and active targeting. The passive targeting is the accumulation of chemotherapeutic agents in solid tumors by which enhanced vascular permeability of tumor tissues compared with healthy tissue occurs. A strategy that could allow active targeting involves the surface functionalization of drug carriers with ligands that are selectively recognized by receptors on the surface of the cells of interest. Because ligand-receptor interactions is always highly selective, these allow a more specific targeting of the site of interest.

Development of controlled drug release biodegradation are important for the development of successful formulations was described by Jain (2003) and Volkering (1993) already discussed that good release mechanisms involve: desorption of surface-bound adsorbed drugs; diffusion (in the case of nanocapsules) through the carrier wall; diffusion through the carrier matrix; carrier matrix erosion; and a combined erosion diffusion process. The delivery mode can be the difference between a drug's failure and its success, the choice of a drug is always influenced by the way the formulation is administered. Sustained release of a drug involves polymers that release the drug at a predetermined rate due to diffuse out the polymer or by degradation of the polymer throughout the time. One of the method is pulsatile release which often preferred for drug delivery, as it somewhat like the way by which the body naturally produces hormones. It is done by the use of drug-carrying polymers which respond to specific stimuli, e.g., changes in pH (Krusic, Ilic & Filipovic, 2009) or temperature (Ilic-Stojanovic et al., 2012; Ilic-Stojanovic, et al., 2013), exposure to light (Kashyap et al., 2005).

For many years, researchers appreciated the benefits of nanotechnology for giving improvements in drug delivery and drug targeting. By Lawrence (1994) improving delivery techniques that can reduce toxicity and enhances efficacy gives great potential benefits to patients, and start new markets for drug delivery systems and pharmaceutical companies. Chiranjeevi et al., (2013) said that some good approaches to drug delivery are being focused on crossing particular physical barriers, for example the blood brain barrier, for the betterment of target the drug and improve its effectiveness; or on finding alternative and routes for the delivery of protein drugs other than via the gastro-intestinal tract, where degradation can occur.

Vesicular systems are extremely useful carrier systems in various fields. From many years, vesicular systems have been investigated as a useful drug delivery system, due to their flexibility to be used for varied desirable purposes. As there are some drawbacks, the vesicular delivery systems still play an important role in the drug targeting, and the controlled delivery of many drugs. Researchers from whole world continue to efforts in improving the vesicular system by making them steady in nature, in order to prevent leaching of contents, oxidation, and their uptake by natural defence mechanisms.

Pharmacosomes

According to Kumar (2012) pharmacosomes are a type of novel drug delivery carrier system, in which the dispersions of colloids containing drugs covalently bound to lipids. Depending upon the drug–lipid complex chemical structure they may exist as vesicular, micellar, or hexagonal aggregates. This is an effective tool to achieve desired therapeutic goals in drug targeting and controlled release of drug.

Colloidal drug carrier systems such as micellar solutions, vesicle and liquid crystal dispersions, as well as nanoparticle dispersions containing small particles of 10–400 nm diameter has great effect as drug delivery systems. By Gangwa, Singh, Goel & Nath (2011) when developing these formulations, the goal is to obtain systems with optimized drug loading and release properties, long shelf-life and low toxicity. The incorporated drug participates in the microstructure of the system, and may even influence it due to molecular interactions, especially if the drug possesses amphiphilic properties and can be mesophilic too.

Any drug having a free carboxyl group or an active hydrogen atom (–OH, NH_2) can be suitable (with or without a spacer group) to the hydroxyl group of a lipid molecule, by this formulating an amphiphilic prodrug, which will give facilitated membrane, tissue, or cell wall transfer, in the organism. The drug's having a certain cut-off molecular weight can be formulated as pharmacosomes but it should has active functional groups to the formation of vesicle-forming amphiphilic molecule. Gupta et al., (2011) said that a prodrug having amphiphilic properties are converted to pharmacosomes upon dilution with water. The conjugate of drug with carrier forms a compound, amphiphilic in nature. The aqueous solution of these amphiphiles surprisingly gives concentration dependent aggregation, which differs from most polar or ionic molecules. The amphiphile at low concentration can dispersed in the monomer state. When the monomer are added a critical micelle concentration is reached, and it gives dramatic changes in the concentration dependence of many parameters of drugs, such as surface tension, electrical conductivity and osmotic pressure. The further enhancement in monomers may lead to variety of structures i.e. micelles of spherical or rod like or disc shaped or bilayered vesicles or cubic or hexagonal phases depending upon physiochemical interactions and thermodynamic variables of amphiphile. Kavitha et al., (2012) showed in her research that the prodrug conjoins hydrophilic and lipophilic properties thereby acquiring amphiphilic characteristics thus reduces interfacial tension, and, at higher concentrations, exhibit mesomorphic behaviour. Because of a decrease in interfacial tension, the contact area increases, therefore increasing bioavailability.

Pharmacosomes are defined as colloidal dispersions of drugs covalently bound to lipids and may exist as ultrafine vesicular, micellar or hexagonal aggregates, depending on the chemical structure of drug-lipid complex. (Pavan Kumar, Subhashis Debnath, Niranjan Babu, 2013).

According to Ajay Semalty et al (2009) pharmacosomes can improve the water solublity of diclofenac, its pharmacosomes (phospholipid complex) have been prepared and evaluated for physicochemical analysis. This improvement in water solubility in prepared pharmacosomes may result in improved dissolution and lower gastrointestinal toxicity.

In the study conducted by Amandeep Kaur, Neha Sharma and S.L. Harikumar (2013) ketoprofen–phospholipid complex (pharmacosomes) were prepared by a simple and reproducible method. According to this article physicochemical investigations showed that ketoprofen formed a complex with phospholipids with better solubility and dissolution profile.

Pharmacosomes impart better biopharmaceutical properties to the drug, resulting in improved bioavailability. Pharmacosomes have been formulated for various non-steroidal anti-inflammatory drugs, proteins, cardiovascular and antineoplastic drugs. Developing the pharmacosomes of the drugs has been found to improve the absorption and minimize the gastrointestinal toxicity. The idea for the development of the vesicular pharmacosome is based on surface and bulk interactions of lipids with drug. The different membranes in body contain phosphatidylcholine, phosphatidyl-ethanolamine, ceramides and sphingomyeline. These resemble lipid prodrugs in physicochemical structure. Therefore, it can be expected that pharmacosomes can interact with biomembranes enabling a better transfer of active ingredient. This interaction can also change the phase transition temperature of biomembranes, thereby improving the membrane fluidity leading to enhanced permeation. Pharmacosomes are designed to avoid the usual problems associated with the liposomal entrapment of polar drug molecules like low drug incorporation, leakage and poor stability.

According to D. Nagasamy Venkatesh et al (2014) pharmacosomes for cellular targeting, may be concluded that pharmacosomes are promising delivery system for poorly soluble drugs and can also improve the biopharmaceutical properties of biologically active phytoconstituents such as flavones, glycosides, xanthones, and so on.

Pharmacosomes is used as ensure proficiency and it can be for ordained on the grounds that medication itself in conjugation with lipids structures vesicles. Since the drug formulations covalently joined, mismatch because of spillage of medication, does not occur. Be that as it may, mismatch may happen by hydrolysis. There is no issue of medication consolidation. Encaptured volume and medication bilayer connections don't impact entanglement effectiveness, if pharmacosome starts appearing. These pharmacosomes again have brilliant impact on entanglement proficiency in the event of liposomes. The lipid is in liposomes chooses its chain ease, which impacts the rate of medication discharge, and physical solid of the framework. Notwithstanding, in pharmacosomes, layer ease relies on the stage move temperature of the medication lipid complex, yet it doesn't influence discharge rate since the medication is covalently bound. The pharmacosome discharges the drug by hydrolysis (counting enzymatic). Phospholipid exchange/trade is diminished, and solubilisation is low. The physicochemical solidness of the pharmacosome relies on the physicochemical properties of the medication lipid complex. Because of their amphiphilic conduct, such frameworks permit, after pharmaceutical, a various exchange through the lipophilic film framework or tissue, through cell dividers piggyback endocytosis and exocytosis. Their dissolution speed into medication particle depending on an extraordinary expansion the size and practical gatherings of medication atom, the chain length of the lipids, and the spacer. These can be differed moderately definitely for advanced in vivo pharmacokinetics. This is effective as given orally, topically, additional or intravascularly. They help an extended bioavailability, lessen treatment cost and give controlled and it is focused on arrival of medications.

By P. H. Sharma, P. V. Powar, S. S. Sharma (2014) the approach of pharmacosomes has successfully improved the therapeutic performance of various drugs i.e. pindolol maleate, bupranolol hydrochloride, taxol, acyclovir, etc.

Pharmacosomes of Ketoprofen was formulated by Mali Kamalesh et al (2014) conventional solvent evaporation technique to increase the solubility and bioavailability in different media with minimizing the GI disturbance. Two different ratio of drug: phosphatidylcholine (PC) in 1:1 and 1:2 were used to form pharmacosomes. Drug content was found to be 93.28% (w/w) for Ketoprofen phospholipid complex (1:1) and 85.44% (w/w) Ketoprofen-phospholipid complex (1:2). Ketoprofen phospholipid complex (1:1) showed better solubility profile than Ketoprofen-phospholipid complex (1:2).

A Semalty (2011) uses pharmacosomes as drug delivery, to improve the water solubility, bioavailability and minimize the gastrointestinal toxicity of aceclofenac. Aceclofenac was complexed with phosphatidylcholine (80%) in two different ratios (1:1 and 2:1) using conventional solvent evaporation technique.

The great advantages of pharmacosomes are it may be minimize drug degradation and diminised the toxicity (GIT) reported by vijay singh (2014).

Micelles

According to Vaizoglu (1986) micelles fashioned by self-assembly of amphiphilic block copolymers (5-50 nm) in aqueous solutions area unit of nice interest for drug delivery applications. The medication may be physically entrapped within the core of block copolymer micelles and transported at concentrations which will exceed their intrinsic water- solubility. Moreover, the hydrophilic blocks will form hydrogen bonds with the liquid surroundings and form a good shell round the micellar core. As a result, the contents of the hydrophobic core are effectively protected against chemical reaction and enzymatic degradation. Additionally, the corona could stop recognition by the RES and thus preliminary elimination of the micelles from the blood. A final feature that creates amphiphilic block copolymers engaging for drug delivery applications is that the proven fact that their chemical composition, total relative molecular mass and block length ratios may be simply modified, that permits management of the dimensions and morphology of the micelles. Functionalization of block copolymers with cross linkable groups will increase the soundness of the corresponding micelles and improve their temporal management. Substitution of block copolymer micelles with specific ligands could be a terribly promising strategy to a broader vary of sites of activity with a way higher selectivity.

Liposomes

Liposomes are a variety of vesicles that consist either of the many, few or simply one lipid bilayers. The polar character of the liposomal core permits polar drug molecules to be encapsulated. Amphiphilic and lipophilic molecules are solubilized at intervals the lipid bilayer per their affinity towards the phospholipids. Participation of nonionic surfactants rather than phospholipids within the bilayer formation ends up in niosomes. Channel proteins is incorporated while not loss of their activity at intervals the hydrophobic domain of vesicle membranes, acting as a size-selective filter, solely permitting passive diffusion of little solutes like ions, nutrients and antibiotics. Thus, medication that are encapsulated in an exceedingly nanocage-functionalized with channel proteins are effectively protected against premature degradation by chemical process enzymes. The drug molecule, however, is able to diffuse through the channe, driven by the concentration distinction between the inside and also the exterior of the nanocage.

Dendrimers

Dendrimers area unit nanometer-sized, extremely branched and monodisperse macromolecules with symmetrical design. They incorporates a central core, branching units and terminal useful groups. The core beside the interior units, confirm the atmosphere of the nanocavities and consequently their solubilizing properties, whereas the external teams the solubility and chemical behaviour of those polymers. Targeting effectiveness is full of attaching targeting ligands at the external surface of dendrimers, whereas their stability and protection from the mononuclear phagocyte System (MPS) is being achieved by functionalization of the dendrimers with polyethylene glycol chains (PEG).

Liquid Crystals

Liquid Crystals mix the properties of each liquid and solid states. Vaizoglu, (1986) in his research showed that they were created to make completely different geometries, with various polar and non-polar layers (i.e., a lamellar phase) wherever liquid drug solutions will be enclosed. Liquid crystals were divided into thermotropic, lyotropic and metallotropic phases. Thermotropic and lyotropic liquid crystals (LCs) incorporates organic molecules. Thermotropic LCs exhibit a phase transition into the liquid-crystal section as temperature phase. Lyotropic LCs exhibit section transitions as a function of each temperature and concentration of the liquid-crystal molecules during a solvent (typically water). Metallotropic LCs are composed of each organic and inorganic molecules; their liquid-crystal transition depends not solely on temperature and concentration, however additionally on the inorganic-organic composition ratio.

Examples of liquid crystals will be found each within the natural world and in technological applications. Most contemporary electronic displays use liquid crystals. Lyotropic liquid-crystalline phases are abundant in living systems. As an example, several proteins and cell membranes are liquid crystals. Other well-known samples of liquid crystals are solutions of soap and varied related detergents, also because the mosaic virus.

Nanoparticles

Nanoparticles (including nanospheres and nanocapsules of size 10-200 nm) are within the solid state and are either amorphous or crystalline. Pansuriya, (n.d.) said that they're able to adsorb and/or encapsulate a drug, therefore protecting it against chemical and enzymatic degradation. Nanocapsules are vesicular systems during which the drug is confined to a cavity encircled by a unique polymer membrane, whereas nanospheres are matrix systems during which the drug is physically and uniformly spread. Nanoparticles as drug carriers may be fashioned from each biodegradable polymers and non-biodegradable polymers. In recent years, biodegradable polymeric nanoparticles have attracted goodish attention as potential drug delivery devices in sight of their applications within the controlled unharness of medication, in targeting specific organs / tissues, as carriers of DNA in gene medical care, and in their ability to deliver proteins, peptides and genes through the per oral route.

Transferosomes

A transfer some may be an extremely convertible, stress-responsive complicated mixture. The shape most well-liked by researchers and pharmacologists is an ultra-deformable vesicle possessing an liquid core enclosed by the complicated lipid bilayer.

Transferosomes provide a flexible delivery concept for improving the steadiness still because the potential to be used with a good vary of active compounds. They're (quasi) constancy, that makes the vesicle membrane ultra-flexible, and thus, the vesicles are extremely deformable that squeeze through pores within the stratum less than tenth part of their own diameter once applied below non-occlusive conditions. Thus, even sizes up to 200–300 nm will penetrate intact skin. It's primarily owing to the outstanding sturdy membrane ability that enables the transferosomal vesicles to reside a confining pore, and so permeate that pore. However the low viscosity of transfeorsomal suspensions constrains its application in percutaneous delivery owing to its cumbersome use. Biocompatible gels having weak interactions with surfactants have already been explored to switch the rheological behaviour of the transferosomal suspension. Thus, the incorporation of the transfeorsomal suspension into the gel matrix may end up in a very transferosomal gel which can be additional relevant for percutaneous application.

Most of the medicine, notably chemotherapeutic agents, have shown to possess narrow therapeutic window, and their clinical use is proscribed. Thus, their therapeutic effectiveness is also redoubled by incorporating them in an advantageous manner. Sadly, at this time no obtainable drug delivery system behaves ideally, however sincere attempts are created to attain them through numerous novel approaches in drug delivery.

Pharmacosomes By Muller-Goymannet & Hamann (1991) bearing distinctive advantages over liposome and niosome vesicles and are function an alternative to traditional vesicles.

(Prasanthi, 2010 and Choudhary, 2012) said that novel drug delivery won't to minimize the side effects and maintain comparatively potent levels of drug within the body. The carriers or chemical derivatization could facilitate to localize the drug action spatially in diseased tissue or organ or adjacent tissues. Differing kinds of pharmaceutical carriers like particulate, polymeric, organic compound and cellular are present. Advances are created within the space of vesicular drug delivery. Resulting in the development of systems that enable drug targeting, and also the sustained and controlled release of typical medicines. Pharmacosomes is one in every of the necessary milestones during this series because the carrier has a large variety of benefits over the opposite vesicular carrier system.

According to (Nilesh, 2007) the term pharmacosomes is expressly wont to describe the zwitterion - complexes of polyphenolic compounds with phospholipids. These are the lipoid based mostly drug delivery systems that are fittingly detailed because the mixture dispersions of medication having a covalent, static or hydrogen bonding with lipids deliver with phospholipids. These are the lipoid based mostly drug systems that are fittingly detailed because the colloidal dispersions of medication having a valence, being amphiphilic compounds facilitate membrane, tissue or plasma membrane transfer within the organism. Any drug possessing a full of life hydrogen atom (cool, oil, etc.) will be esterified to the lipoid, with or while not spacer chain that powerfully result in associate degree amphiphilic compound Pharmacosomes being amphiphilic compounds facilitate membrane. Tissue, or plasma membrane transfer within the organism. By Patel (2011)Theamphiphilic characters facilitate pharmacosomes to scale back surface tension and at higher concentrations exhibit an active behaviour.

Advantages of Pharmacosomes over Other Vesicular Systems

- The pharmacosomes bearing benefits blessings over liposome and niosome vesicles have come up as potential various to conventional vesicles by Peng (2005).
- The limitations of transferosomes are often overcome by the "pharmacosome" approach.
- Different varieties of supermolecule primarily based vesicular systems are developed currently days for many applications within the controlled and targeted drug delivery.
- Pharmacosomes bearing unique benefits over liposomes in conjunction with niosomes are emerged as potential various to traditional vesicles. These are the amphiphilic phospholipid complexes of medicine that having active hydrogen that bind to phospholipids. They supply an economical technique for delivery of drug directly to the positioning of infection additionally as reduction of drug toxicity with no adverse effects in conjunction with low price of medical aid.
- They facilitate for improved biopharmaceutical properties to the drug, leading to improved bioavailability, particularly just in case of poorly soluble medication.
- The pharmacosomes are created for many applications like non-steroidal anti-inflammatory medication, proteins, cardiovascular and antineoplastic medication. Interaction of pharmacosomes leads to modification within the phase transition temperature of biomembranes improves membrane facility and increased permeation discussed by Peng (2012).
- Volume of inclusion doesn't influence defence efficiency.

- No loss of drug happen because the drug is covalently coupled to carrier.
- Drugs are often delivered directly into the positioning of inflation.
- Drug release from pharmacosomes is by chemical reaction.
- There is not any would like of removing the free, untrapped drug from the formulation.
- According to Ping, Jin & Dawei (2005) improves the bioavailability of strictly water soluble medication.
- The degradation velocity of active drug molecule depends on the dimensions and functional cluster of drug molecule.
- Reduction in adverse effects.
- They will meet up with the biomembrane expeditiously.

Limitations of Pharmacosome

- By (Pozansky,1983) a compound is synthesised looking on the amphiphilic nature.
- They need superficial also as mass drug lipid interaction.
- Covalent variety of bond is needed to limit drug leak.
- Pharmacosomes are vulnerable to get amalgamate, aggregate, or hydrolyze by chemicals on storage.

Salient Features of Pharmacosomes

- The physical and chemical traits of the conjugate management the steadiness of the entire system said by Kumar (2011).
- As they encompass each water affectionate and fat liking properties, they need a simple passing through the plasma membrane, walls, or tissues either by the action of endocytosis or exocytosis.
- The rate of degradation depends on size nature of useful cluster present within the drug molecule fatty acid chain length in lipids, presence, or absence of spacer. All these factors will be varied to optimize *in vivo* pharmacokinetic behaviour.
- They will be administered via topical oral extra- or intravascular route.
- Pharmacosomes are appropriate for incorporating each hydrophilic and lipophilic drugs. The solution in water of those amphiphiles exhibits concentration dependent aggregation.
- Entrapment potency isn't solely, as a result of drug itself in conjugation with lipid forms vesicles and covalently coupled along.
- Unlike liposomes, there's no need of following the tedious, time intense step for removing the free unentrapped drug from the formulation.
- Since the drug is covalently coupled, loss because of leak of drug, doesn't occur. However, loss could occur by hydrolysis.
- Encaptured volume and drug bilayer interactions don't Influence entrapment potency, just in case of pharmacosomes described by Ritika (2012).
- The physicochemical, stability of the pharmacosome depends upon the physical and chemical properties of the drug lipid.
- Due to their amphiphilic behavior, such systems enable, once medication, a multiple transfer through the lipophilic membrane system or tissue, through cellular walls piggyback endocytosis and exocytosis, suggested by Bansal (n.d.)

Comparison between Liposomes, Transferosomes, and Pharmacosomes

In liposomes incorporation of drug within the liquid or macromolecule phase of a combination of lipid wherever the physicochemical properties of the carrier and unleash of drug are functions of various lipids used. Loss of drug through escape could occur. According to Seema, (n.d) and Poste (1983) just in case of pharmacosomes covalent binding of a drug to a lipid wherever the ensuing compound is that the carrier and therefore the active compound at a similar time. The chemistry properties depend upon drug still because the lipid. No leakage, since drug is covalently certain however loss of drug by hydrolysis is feasible.

Poznansky (1983) said that the limitations of transfeorsomes will be overcome by the "pharmacosome" approach. The prodrug conjoins hydrophilic and lipophilic properties, and thus acquires amphiphilic characters. Kind of like alternative forming parts, it had been found to scale back interfacial surface tension and at higher concentrations exhibits mesomorphic behavior. These are outlined as colloidal dispersions of medicine covalently absolute to lipids, and will exist as ultrafine vesicular, micellar, or hexagonal aggregates, looking on the chemical structure of drug-lipid advanced. Several constraints of varied classical drug delivery systems, like issues of drug incorporation, escape from the carrier, or lean period of time, shelf life avoided by the pharmacosome approach. The thought for the event of the vesicular pharmacosome, is predicated on surface and bulk interactions of lipids with drug. Any drug possessing an active atom (-COOH, -OH, $-NH_{2,}$ etc) will be esterified to the lipid, with or while not spacer chain. Synthesis of such a compound is also guided in such some way that powerfully results in an amphiphilic compound, which can facilitate membrane, tissue, or semipermeable membrane transfer, within the organism.

Material of Pharmacosomes

- **Lipid:** Bangham (1955) described that lipid or lecithin or phosphatidylcholine is that the chief molecular building block of cell membranes. Phospholipids are the medication yield amphiphilic merchandise that renders phospholipids water soluble and also the drug lipid soluble.
- **Drug:** Any drug possessing an effective atom (-COOH,-OH,$-NH_2$ etc.) is esterified to the lipid, with or while not spacer chain, resulting in amphiphilic complexes. Synthesis of such a compound could also be guided in such how that powerfully lead to an amphiphilic compound, which can facilitate membrane, tissue, or plasma membrane transfer, within the organism.
- **Solvents:** For the preparation of Pharmacosomes, according to Mayer (1985)the solvents ought to have high purity and volatile in nature. A solvent with intermediate polarity is chosen for pharmacosome preparation.

Method for Preparation of Pharmacosomes

In general four methods have been employed to prepare pharmacosomes:

- **Handshaking Method:** By Kremer (1977) in the handshaking methodology, the dried film of the drug lipid complicated (with or without egg lecithin) is deposited in a very spherical bottom flask and upon association with aqueous medium without delay provides a vesicular suspension. Within the ether injection technique, an organic resolution of the drug lipid complex is injected slowly into the hot liquid medium whereby the vesicles are without delay fashioned.

At low concentration the amphiphiles exists within the chemical compound state. Batzre (1973) said that additional increase in monomers might cause kind of structures i.e. micelles of spherical rod like or disc formed type or isometric or form shape. Compared the result of diglyceride prodrug on interfacial surface tension, with the result created by a standard detergent dodecylamine hydrochloride and found similar impact on lowering of surface tension. Above the critical particle concentration, the prodrug exhibits mesomorphic lyotropic behavior, and assembles in supramolecular structures.

- **Ether Injection Technique:** In this technique, by Deamer (1978) the drug lipoid advanced is dissolved in an organic solvent. This mixture is then slowly injected into a heated liquid agent, leading to the formation of vesicles. The state of amphiphiles depends on the concentration. Once the concentration is a smaller amount amphiphilies introduced a chemical compound state however because the concentration is inflated, form of structures could be shaped, that is spherical cylindrical, disc, cubic, or hexagonal type. Then study of the comparative impact of prodrug of diglyceride a customary wetting agent, dodecylamine hydrochloride on the interfacial surface tension. It absolutely was finished that higher than the critical micellar concentration, long cylinders were ascertained in hexagonal arrangement, and prodrug exhibited liquid-crystalline part, exhibiting massive molecular structures.
- **Supercritical Fluid Process:** This is said by Deamer (1976) that (Solution increased dispersion by complex supercritical fluid) Drug and lipoid complicated are dissolved in a very supercritical fluid of carbon dioxide, then combine into nozzle intermixture chamber.
- **Anhydrous Co-Solvent Evaporation Method:** Schieran (1978) said that the concerns glacial acetic acid at that time agitates the mixture to get clear liquid. Free dried long at condenser temperature. Then resultant complex flushed with nitrogen and keep at 40°C.
- **Other Approaches:** Kim (1981) suggested that another approach for manufacturing pharmacosomes is to include a hydrophobic drug into a polymer invented from a glycol and aspartic acid by-product leading to formation of a biodegradable micelle drug conjunct. Being a water soluble conjunct of drug the possibilities of precipitation of drug on dilution are reduced.

A changed technique involving diluted lyotropic liquid crystals of amphiphilic medication was employed for developing nonsteroidal anti-inflammatory drug based mostly pharmacosomes.

Characterisation of Pharmacosomes

- **Complex Determination:** According to Batalle Memorial Inst., (1979) with the assistance of Fourier transform infrared spectroscopy, the formation of the complex or the conjugate will be determined by correlating spectrum discovered in complicated sample therewith of separate constituents and additionally with their mixture.
- **Stability of Pharmacosomes:** In this correlation of the spectrum at varied points of time within the solid state with spectrum of a dispersion in water consisting of tiny particles were examined, once the product has been lyophilized, is employed to evaluate the steadiness of the system.

- **Solubility:** The modification in solubility caused by complexation will be evaluated using shake flask technique. In this technique, two phase, that is, one octanol and aqueous phase is used, and constant shaking equilibrium is maintained at a temperature of 37°C for one day. The liquid section is separated and so concentration is determined using ultraviolet of high performance liquid chromatography technique.
- **Drug Lipid Compatibility:** Arnardottir (1995) said that differential scanning measuring could be a thermo analytical technique used to see drug lipid compatibility and their interactions if any thermal response is studied exploitation separate samples and heating them in an exceedingly sample pan that is closed. The gas is purged, and the temperature is maintained in an exceedingly definite vary with a selected heating rate.

Lipid-based formulations may be used to increase drug absorption by increasing solubilization, enhancing permeability, reducing drug metabolism by inhibiting hepatic enzymes, and rising transport via the inhibition of effluence transporters and an increase of particle production. The pharmaceutical and medicine implications of evaluating drug-lipid miscibility in solid lipid nanoparticles. The miscibility of a drug and excipient is found to be dependent upon the unit interactions shaped between the drug (solute) and excipient (solvent). Miscibility will be an important part for the formulation stability of (solid lipid nanoparticles) SLN. Mixed glycerides, like glycerylmonooleate (GMO), function a well-liked solvent for poorly water soluble medication. GMO could be a waxy, long-chain glyceride helpful in formulating liquid dosage forms. Sorbitan fatty acids (Spans) have similar physical properties to GMO. These polar oils, additionally referred to as co-surfactants, promote miscibility because of the presence of radical teams. Co-surfactants decrease interfacial surface tension between two immiscible elements to enhance thermodynamic stability and therefore, miscibility.

- **Crystalline State Measurement:** Most of the present solids are found to possess definite crystalline shapes which might be recognized simply. These are in massive size as a result of these are shaped terribly slowly, therefore particles get enough time to induce correct position within the crystal structure. Some crystalline therefore lipids are so tiny that seem to be amorphous. However on examination beneath a hard microscope they additionally seen to possess an explicit crystalline form. Such solids are referred to as small crystalline solids. (Korenbrot, 1977) proposed that the crystalline nature of drug may be determined using X -ray diffraction technique. The general combined intensity of all reflection peaks is projected by space beneath curve of X-ray powder diffraction pattern that specifies the specimen attributes.
- **Scanning Electron Microscopy/Transmission Electron Microscopy:** These techniques may be used for finding out the surface order of pharmacosomes. The purity grades of the lipid being employed and few variables discovered throughout operation (method of preparation, vacuum appointed, and move speed) alter the form and size of pharmacosomes discussed by Razin (1972) says that pharmacosomes are formed of greasy nature if prepared using lower purity grades of lipids resulting in massive aggregate formation and those fabricated using lipids of over 90% purity grade show status to degradation because of oxidation, that complicated stability. So, 80% purity grade is that the usually used phospholipid grade.

Applications of Pharmacosomes

- By Hargreaves (1978) pharmacosomes have potential drug delivery system for prolonged result in tissue and liver targeting.
- Solubility of diclofenac was increased by diclofenac pharmacosomes and additionally improved drug release.
- The phase transition temperature of pharmacosomes within the vesicular and micellar state might have important influence on their interaction with biomembranes sanctioning a stronger transfer of active ingredient. This interaction results in modification in phase transition temperature of biomemebranes thereby improve the membranes thinness resulting in enhance permeations.
- By (Huang, 1969) pharmacosomes may improve the speed of permeation by improving the membrane fluidity.
- The transition temperature of vesicles within the kind of vesicles and micelles may cause an apparent impact on vesicular interaction with biomembrane, thus improving the transfer of drug across membrane.
- Pharmacosomes are amphiphilic lipid core system which may also be used for the event of novel ophthalmic dosage forms. In this amphiphilic prodrug once diluted with tear, it modify tissue layer drug transport and release profile.
- Pharmacosomes have achieved a new level by enhancing therapeutic effects of many medicine like beta blocker pindolol, taxol, bupranolo acid derivative, cytarabin, Amoxicillin, dermatan sulphate, and so on.
- Pharmacosomes have greater degree of selectivity for action on specific target cells and bigger stability. They're building particles of capable in transporting of biological substances.
- Plasma protein in blood absorb pharmacosomes and interfere with interaction erythrocytes and reduce hemolytic method.
- Pharmacosomes may be used for liver targeting as they increase the solubility within the gall salts. There's a discount in drug dose due to higher absorption of active phytoconstituents.
- Pharmacosomes gives a synergistic hepatoprotective effect with phytosomes, besides acting as a carrier. Pharmacosomes could also be employed in cosmetic business because of their improved skin penetration and high lipid profile.

Stability Comparison of Some Effective Vesicular Systems

Liposomes have been the nice candidates for increasing the solubility of poorly soluble medicine, Bangham (1974). However the soundness issue of liposomes remains an area that is enclosed by variety of issues due the formation of ice crystals in liposomes, the next instability of bilayers results in the escape of entrapped material. The physical instability is another drawback featured by liposomes. The oxidation of cholesterol and phospholipids conjointly results in the formulation instability. Chemical instability primarily indicates hydrolysis and oxidation of lipids. Hydrolysis detaches the hydrophobic chains of ester bonds. Oxidation is a lot of probably due to the presence of unsaturated chains. Adding antioxidants to the liposome formulation will typically defend the lipids from oxidation. The cationic liposomes may be stable at 4°C (refrigerator) for an extended amount of time if they're properly sterilized. Liposomes in plasma are vulnerable to aggregation and exhibit the destabilization of liposomes is due to the lipid exchange between the liposomes and high density lipoproteins (HDLs).

Niosomes

Niosome may be a non-ionic surfactant-based vesicle (biology and chemistry) (Rosieret al., 1979). Niosomes are shaped mostly by non-ionic surfactant and cholesterol incorporation as an excipient. Alternative excipients can also be used. Niosomes have more penetrating capability than the previous preparations of emulsions. They're structurally similar to liposomes in having a bilayer, however, the materials used to prepare niosomes build them more stable and thus niosomes provide more blessings over liposomes. Niosomes structure may be measured by microscopic examination. They represent of non-ionic surfactant of the alkyl group or dialkylpolyglycerol ether category and cholesterol with consequent hydration in liquid media. The wetting agent molecules tend to orient themselves in such the way that the hydrophilic ends of the non-ionic surfactant purpose outward, whereas the hydrophobic ends face one another to create the bilayer.

The niosomes even being superior than liposomes have various stability issues related to them like physical stability of fusion, aggregation, alleviation and escape on storage. The chemical reaction of encapsulated medicine that limits the period of time of the dispersion is additionally a problem for nisomes.

The in vitro release profile was fitted by Sunil Kamboj, Vipin Saini, and Suman Bala (2014) to various release kinetics models to predict the release mechanism of drug from the niosomes and the results revealed that all the formulations were best explained as zero order release. The results of in vivo study revealed more than two fold increase in oral bioavailability by niosomal vesicles compared with the plane solution in same dose. So the prepared niosomal vesicles could be the promising drug delivery system for controlled release.

According to Dina Fathalla, A. Abdel-Mageed, F. Abdel-Hamid and M. Ahmed (2014) aceclofenac loaded niosomes were prepared using reverse phase evaporation technique. The effects of concentration of non-ionic surfactant, cholesterol and concentration of drug on the encapsulation efficiency were studied. The in-vivo anti-inflammatory activity of the selected niosomal gel formulation was significantly higher and more sustained than the corresponding non-niosomal gel formulation containing free drug. The results suggest that the niosome-containing gels are promising formulations for sustained local delivery of aceclofenac.

Gaafar PM, Abdallah OY, Farid RM, Abdelkader H (2014) reported novel nano-sized elastic niosomes (ethoniosomes) composed of Span 60: cholesterol (7:3 mol/mol) and ethanol, for ocular delivery of prednisolone acetate (Pred A) and prednisolone sodium phosphate (Pred P). These ethoniosomes were prepared with the thin film hydration (TFH) and ethanol injection (EI) methods, characterized for percentage entrapment efficiency (% EE), size, zeta potential, morphology, elasticity, in vitro release and physical stability. Moghassemi S, Hadjizadeh A (2014) surveyed and discussed the recent, rapidly growing reported studies along with their theoretical principals is required for the fully understanding and exploring the great potential of this approach.

Entrapment efficiency isn't solely high however predetermined, as a result of drug itself in conjugation with lipids forms vesicles. It's no time-consuming steps for removing the free, unentrapped drug from the formulation. Since the drug is covalently coupled, loss because of escape of drug, doesn't happen (Gunter et al,1982).

Ethosomes

Ethosomes are the foremost advances in vesicle research. Ethosomes are soft vesicles made from phospholipids and ethanol (in higher quantity) and water, commented by Pidgeon,(1986). Ethosomes are non-invasive delivery carriers that modify medicine to reach the deep skin layers and/or the circulation. Ethosomes are soft, malleable vesicles composed chiefly of phospholipids (phosphatidyl choline, phosphatidyl serine, and phosphatitidic acid), ethanol (relatively high concentration) and water. These "soft vesicles" represents novel vesicular carrier for increased delivery through skin. The soft, malleable vesicles tailored for increased delivery of active agents. The size of ethosomes may be modulated to vary anyplace from 30 nm to a number of microns. Though ethosomal systems are conceptually subtle, they're characterised by simplicity in their preparation, safety and efficaciousness that may extremely expand their application. Ethosomal systems were rather more economical at delivering a fluorescent probe to the skin in terms of amount and depth than either liposomes or hydro alcoholic resolution. Ethosomes provides variety of vital advantages together with raising the drug's efficaciousness, enhancing patient compliance, comfort and reducing the entire value of treatment. Ethosomes were appropriate for numerous applications at intervals the prescribed drugs, biotechnology, veterinary, cosmetic and nutraceutical markets. Increased delivery of bioactive molecules through the skin and cellular membranes by suggests that of an ethosomal carrier opens varied challenges and opportunities for the analysis and future development of novel improved therapies. Ethosomes are lipid vesicles containing phospholipids, alcohol (ethanol and isopropyl alcohol) in comparatively high concentration and water. Ethosomes has initiated a replacement space in vesicular analysis for transdermic drug delivery which may give higher skin permeation and stability than liposomes. Application of ethosomes provides the benefits like improved entrapment and physical stability.

Transdermal administration could be a better option as dermal route could provide relatively consistent systemic drug levels for prolonged period of time, avoid GI related issues, and improve patient compliance because of non-invasive nature and less frequent dose regime. In recent times, ethosomes have attracted considerable attention for their opportunity to enhance dermal/transdermal delivery of a number of bioactive agents (R. Rakesh and K. R. Anoop, 2012). Ethosomes enhance permeation of drugs with its ethanol effect and show lipid perturbation. By adding penetration enhancer in ethosomes such as propylene glycol act by solvation of keratin within the stratum corneum and oleic acid endorses phase separation by declining melting temperature of ceramides; both have good penetration along with ethosomes formulation (Sudhakar & Narayan, 2014). Vijayakumar K.S et al (2014) formulated and Gliclazide ethosomal gel in order to increase bioavailability and reduce side effects by achieving transdermal drug delivery. Ethanol increased lipid fluidity of ethosomes result increased skin permeability.

Ethosomes easy to permeate inside deep layer which fused with skin lipids and release the drug layer of skin reparted by V. Sujatha, T. Vishnuvaravidyadhar, M.Parvathi & Suryaprakash Reddy (2014)

Transferosomes

Hope *et al,* (1985) said that transferosomes square measure with chemicals unstable due to their predisposition to aerophilous degradation. Purity of natural phospholipids is another criterion militating against stability of transferosomes as drug delivery vehicles. These square measure a lot of elastic than the quality liposomes and so square measure used as a unique carrier for effective transdermic drug delivery. Transfersomes square measure with chemicals unstable due to their predisposition to aerophilous degradation, lack of purity of the natural lipide comes within the approach of adoption of transfersomes as drug delivery vehicles sixty.

Transfersomal vesicular system was employed for the topical administration of capsaicin in experimental rats., the better tolerance of prepared vesicular formulation in biological system further enlightens the suitability of the transfersomal vesicle to be used as a novel carrier system for the topical administration of such highly irritant substance by Sarwa KK, Mazumder B, Rudrapal M & Verma VK (2014).

Ahmed TA (2014) aimed to study the effect of different processing and formulation parameters on the preparation of sildenafil (SD) transfersomes utilizing the Plackett-Burman design. The significant variables could be optimized again to produce smaller vesicle size that could increase SD permeation from transdermal delivery systems loaded drug optimized transfersomes. D. Nagasamy Venkatesh, K. Kalyani, K. Tulasi, V. Swetha Priyanka, S. K. Abid Ali, H. C. Kiran (2014) uses ultra-deformable vesicles. Which can provide the novelsolution for the transport related problems. They are free from the rigid nature of conventional vesicle and can transport even the large molecules. They work on number of mechanisms working together to provide an excellent carrier system for the drug transport.

Herbosomes

The effectiveness of any herbal medication relies on the delivery of effective level of the therapeutically active compounds (Biju, 2009). Herbosomes are recently introduced herbal formulations that are higher absorbed and as a result turn out higher bioavailability and actions than the traditional botanical extracts. Herbal excipients are non-toxic and compatible so there use may be more significant in pharmaceutical formulation. There are several herbal extracts having wonderful bioactivity *in vitro* however less *in vivo* thanks to their poor macromolecule solubility and improper size of the molecule or each, that lead to poor absorption and bioavailability of seasoning extract or constituents from seasoner extract and that they destroyed within the viscus fluids once taken. Chemical bonds area unit shaped between phosphatidylcholine molecule and phytoconstituent, therefore the herbosomes show higher stability profile with considerable drug defense.

Sphingosomes

Sphingolipid are now days used for the preparation of stable liposomes, called sphingosomes. Higher price of sphingolipid hinders the preparation and use of those vesicular systems. They show higher stability as compared to liposomes though they need low defense effectivity. Sphingosomes solve the most important disadvantage of vesicle system (liposomes, niosomes) like less stability, less *in vivo* circulation time, low tumour loading effectivity just in case of cancer therapy.

Cubosomes

Cubosomes have higher chemico-physical stability and easy producible (Doijad, 2009). They're the great choice with several benefits over liposomes, manufacture of cubosomes on an oversized scale embodied issue due to their viscosity. Kaiser studied the result of different electrolyte media on physical and chemical stability of bupranolol hydrochloride pharmacosomes. Yang et.al. Found that cubosomes diacylprodrug initially forms giant vesicles, which diminish in size and eventually kind micelles. They shows that slow mechanics are essential demand for lipoid on bimembrane so as to confirm stability to the lipid bilayer and stop the speedy exchange of lipids between membranes of living cells.

Impoved Drug Properties with Pharmacosomes

Bupranolol hydrochloride the prodrug consisting of β-blocker bupranolol that is covalently bounded to 1, 3-dipalmioyl-2-succinyl-glycerol. The ensuing prodrug was amphipathic and dispersed without delay in water higher than 30°C forming a smectic lamellar phase.

1-β-D-arabinofuranosylcytosine

(MacCoss et al., 1982) synthesized varied amphipathic liponucleotideprodrugs, 1-β-D-arabinofuranosylcytosine 5'- diacylglycerols (containing either dimyristoyl, dipalmitoyldistearoyl free carboxylic acid side chains) and determined the aggregation and morphological characteristics of their sonicated dispersions to change in temperature. The sonication at low temperature gave turbid solutions containing massive bilayer sheets on rising the transition temperature.

The sonication at low temperature gave muddy solutions containing large bilayer sheets. On rising the temperature, a transition temperature and act as a promising drug-targeting system for the treatment of central nervous system disorders. In another study, didanosine pharmacosomes were prepared and therefore the *in vivo* behavior in rats was investigated. The study discovered liver targeting and sustained release result in rats once i.v. administration. The study found that there was targeting within the respiratory organ and spleen which drug elimination from the target tissues was slow. The pharmacosomes ready from the lipophilic diglyceride derivative of the drug (pindolol), increased the plasma concentrations of the drug 3 to 5 folds higher compared with its free form. Moreover, the administration of pharmacosomes semiconductor diode to a lower excretory organ clearance. The pharmacosomes as building particles characterised by high degree of selectivity (acting on track cells). These are capable of delivering varied biologically active substances as well as biopolymers (nucleic acid and proteins).

Aceclofenac

Semalty, A., Semalty, M., Rawat, B. S., Singh, D., & Rawat, M. S. M. (2010). optimized development and analysis of pharmacosomes of aceclofenac and located the drug content 88% (w/w) for aceclofennac lipoid complex (1:1), 03% (w/w) aceclofenac lipoid complicated (2:1). Solubility of aceclofenac pharmacosome was found to be over the aceclofenac, during this study the free aceclofenac showed a complete of solely 69% drug unleash at the top of 4 hourr dissolution study whereas aceclofenac pharmacosome (1:1) showed 79.78% and aceclofenac pharmacosome (2:1) showed 17% at the top of 4hr dissolution study.

Diclofenac

Semalty, A., Semalty, M., Rawat, B. S., Singh, D., & Rawat, M. S. M. (2009) studied development of diclofenacpharmacosome and physicochemical analysis for drug solubility, *in vitro* dissolution study, drug content, surface morphology, crystallinity and section transitions behavior. Water solubility of diclofenac pharmmacosome was found to be 22.1 μ/ml as compared to 10.5 μ/ml of diclofenac. Drug release of diclofenac pharmacosome was 87.8% as compared to 60.4% of diclofenac at the end of 10 hour dissolution study and therefore the drug content of diclofenac pharmacosome was found to be 96.2+/-1%. In SEM, pharmacosomes of diclofenac were found to be disc formed. XPRD analysis and DSC thermograms proved the formation of phospholipid complex66.

Ibuprofen

The improvement in bioavailability similarly as minimisation of GI toxicity of free ibuprofen would be achieved by pharmacosome approach. The pharmacosome of ibuprofen would be ready by conjugation of free ibuprofen with phosphatidylcholine (80%) in 2 totally different molar ratios. The water solubility of ibuprofen pharmacosome (1:1) and ibuprofen pharmacosome (2:1) were found to be 1.63 mg/ml and 1.26 mg/ml severally, far better than free ibuprofen showing solubility 0.212 mg/ml. The free ibuprofen showed solely 67.96% drug release at the top of four hour dissolution study whereas ibuprofen pharmacosome (1:1) showed 79.97% and ibuprofen pharmacosome (2:1) showed 77.03% at the top of four hour dissolution study. Therefore the solubility and dissolution of ibuprofen will be increased by pharmacosome formulation that might additionally minimize the GI toxicity.

Phytosomes/ Pharmacosomes

A unique Drug Delivery System for herbal medication pharmacosomes normally called phytosome, are drug-phospholipid complexes having active ingredients of the herb and might be able to develope the suspension, emulsion, syrup, lotion, gel, cream, liquid small dispersion, pill, capsule, powder, granules and chewable pill. Plants specifically Silybum marianum, gingko, and ginseng showed higher effectivity than typical herbal formulations. Additionally, the clinical trials of phytosomes have shown enhanced bioavailability compared to traditional herbal formulations usually containing polyphenols and flavonoids in humans. Researchers incontestable enhanced bioavailability of polyphenol phytosome preparations (curcumin, silybin, catechins and proanthocyanidin) and this result was thanks to the intermolecular bonding between individual polyphenol molecules and one or additional molecules of the phospholipid phosphatidylcholine. Phytosomal herbal drug delivery systems are mainly used: i) to deliver general inhibitor (mainly polyphenols, flavonoid and terpenoid components), ii) helpful in treatment of the unwellness like blood pressure, cancer, skin condition and iii) helps in protective the brain lining. Gastro retentive drug formulations (GRDFs) are particularly effective in delivery of sparingly soluble and insoluble medication as they supply continuous controlled administration of those medication at the absorption site. additionally to tablet and capsules these dose forms these are also helpful for delivering medication incorporated into vesicular systems like liposomes, nanoparticles, proteinoid microspheres and pharmacosomes, etc

For Opthalmic Applications

By (Ganesan, 1984) delivery to the internal components of the eye still remains difficult due to the anatomical and protecting structure of the eye. The freshly developed particulate and vesicular systems like liposomes, pharmacosomes and discomes are helpful in delivering the drug for an extended extent and useful in reaching the circulation. The pharmacosomes show greater shelf stability.

Research Update on Pharmacosomes

Several studies show that pharmacosomes are able to enhance the dissolution ability of the poorly soluble nonsteroidal anti-inflamatory medication. The solubility of the diclofenac pho sphatidylcholine (80%) was enhanced. Aceclofenac loaded pharmacosomes ready through solvent evaporation technique showed a release rate of 79.78% at the top of 4hrs. aspirin and Naringenin loaded pharmacosomes also pictured similar results. more studies by Garcia et al., (1998) on dioleylphosphatidylcholine (DOPC) and Orudis KT (KP) showed solubility improvement ability of the pharmacosomes. The permeation of the drug across the skin was additionally increased within the complex once assayed by in vitro transdermic absorption by employing a flow-through diffusion cell. Muller-Goymann and Hamann, (1991) developed fenoprofen pharmacosomes employing a changed technique that concerned diluting lyotropic liquid crystals of amphiphilic medication.

JIN Yi-Guang et al., (2006) developed the charged nm acyclovir succinyl group monostearate pharmacosomes by the tetrahydrofuran injection technique. Transmission electron microscope and laser scattering technique were used for the analysis of the advanced shaped. Terribly weak impact of action and heating were found on the steadiness of the pharmacosomes whereas freezing and freeze noncontinuous the Pharmacosome structure. *In vivo*, pharmacosomes were found absorbed by the plasma proteins within the blood thereby reducing the haemolytic reaction. Meihua Han et al., developed 20(S)-Protopanaxadiol (Ppd) pharmacosome by straightforward thin film-dispersion preparation properties were found to be stable. Tube shaped pharmacosomes of 5′-cholesterylsuccinyl-dideoxyinosine (CS-ddI) were devoloped by means that of THF injection technique by Ping, Jin &Dawei (2005). CS-ddI and ddI in plasma and tissues were determined with the assistance of HPLC. Half life of CS-ddI in plasma of rat was found to be 7.64 min, CS-ddI got focused in liver quickly when intravenous administration, there was additionally some concentration in lung and spleen; its elimination from target tissues was found slow because the half-life of CS-ddIin liver was 10 d. Zhang et al. (2005) found mean particle size of 3',5'-dioctanoyl-5-fluoro-2'-deoxyuridine pharmacosomes (DO-FudR-PS), with drug loading of 29.02% and entrapment potency of 96.62%. They additionally reported that the concentration of FUdR in numerous tested organs was quite high once determined by reversed phase high performance liquid chromatography when i.v. administration of DO-FUdR-PS and FUdR. Few researchers have additionally reported that the isoniazid pharmacosomes have improved porosity and macrophage targeting. Shi et al. showed a replacement insulin–phospholipid advanced by an anhydrous co-solvent lyophilization technique. Compared with native insulin, the physicochemical properties of insulin modified significantly. When it was combined with phospholipids, it shows the improved lipophilicity, and contributes to the improved oral absorption of insulin.

In the year 2013 ketoprofen–phospholipid advanced (pharmacosomes) were ready by a straight forward and reproducible technique. The physicochemical investigations showed that ketoprofen combined with phospholipids with higher solubility and dissolution profile. (Egbaria, 1990) said the lipid complex of ketoprofen is also of potential use for improving bioavailability. Because the lipid complexes have additionally been reported to reduce the GI toxicity of the medication, the lipid advanced of ketoprofen may be helpful or minimizing the GI toxicity of ketoprofen.

The pharmacosomes is also developed for different NSAIDs with poor bioavailability and GI aspect effects. Thus, the developed pharmacosomes appear to be potential candidate as an oral controlled drug delivery system during this era of novel and controlled drug delivery systems. The developed formulations are expected to enhance the patient compliance, kind higher dosage regimen and supply optimum maintenance medical aid to rheumatoid arthritis patients.

Pharmacosomes are amphiphilic lipid vesicular systems containing phospholipid complexes with a possible to enhance bioavailability of poorly water soluble further as poorly lipophilic medication. Aceclofenac was complexed with phosphatidylcholine (80%) in different ratios (1:1 and 2:1) exploitation standard solvent evaporation technique to enhance the water solubility, bioavailability and minimize the gastrointestinal toxicity of aceclofenac. Pharmacosomes so ready were subjected to solubility and drug content analysis, scanning electron microscopy, differential scanning calorimetry, X ray powder diffraction and *in vitro* dissolution study. Pharmacosomes of aceclofenac were found to be disc formed with rough surface in scanning microscopy. Drug content was found to be 91.88% (w/w) for aceclofenac lipid complex (1:1) and 89.03% (w/w) aceclofenac-phospholipid complex (2:1). Differential scanning calorimetric thermograms and X ray powder diffraction datas confirmed the formation of lipid complex. Solubility and dissolution profile of the ready advanced was found to be far better than aceclofenac

In the area of solubility improvement, many issues are encountered. A completely unique approach supported lipid drug delivery system has evolved, pharmacosomes. Pharmacosomes are mixture, nanometric size micelles, and vesicles or is also within the kind of polygon assembly of mixture drug dispersions connected covalently to the phospholipid. They act as befitting carrier for delivery of medicine quite exactly as a result of their distinctive properties like little size, amphiphilicity, active drug loading, high entrapment potency, and stability. They help in controlled release of drug at the location of action as well as in reduction in cost of medical aid, drug leak and toxicity, multiplied bioavailability of poorly soluble medication, and restorative effects. There has been advancement within the scope of this delivery system for variety of medicine used for inflammation, heart diseases, cancer, and protein delivery along with a large range of herbal medication. Hence, pharmacosomes open new challenges and opportunities for improved novel vesicular drug delivery system.

Gangwar, Singh, Goel &Nath (2011) said that pharmacosome is also outlined as a neutral molecule possessing each positive and charge, water-loving and fat-loving properties, and an optimum quantitative relation of polyphenol with phospholipids in a very advanced kind. The medication are present in a dispersion kind in these lipoidal drug delivery system conjugated by electron combine sharings and electricity forces or by forming a bond with lipids. These lipid conjugated vesicles might exist as mixture, nanometric size micelles, vesicles or is also within the kind of hexagonal assembly enjoying a useful hydrogen atom banking upon the design of the advanced. The drug molecule with a free radical or useful atom like amino, hydroxyl group teams, is converted to an organic compound with the help of the hydroxyl group moiety of the lipid, leading to the formation of a prodrug. A spacer chain might or might not be used for this purpose. The prodrug possesses each hydrophilic and lipophilic properties. Despite these properties, prodrugs have the potential to reduce interfacial surface tension, increase the area of contact, and therefore improve bioavailability. They aid the deportation through the cell wall, cell wall, and tissues. If the concentration is multiplied beyond a level, it should exist in an intermediate state between liquid and crystal. On contact with water, these prodrugs assemble into one or multiple layers leading to the formation of pharmacosomes. This method is developed by keeping the surface properties further because the bulk properties of the drug-lipid conjugate in consideration.

CONCLUSION

Vesicular systems are investigated as a significant drug delivery system due to their flexibility to be tailored for diverse desirable functions. Pharmacosomes are one in all the novel drug delivery system having varies benefits over others. Pharmacosomes isn't only having high entrapment potency however it may be predetermined, as a result of drug itself in conjugation with lipids forms vesicles. Not like liposomes there's no want of following the tedious time consuming step for removing the free, unentrapped drug from the formulation. In spite of bound drawbacks fusion and aggregation, pharmacosomes still play a crucial role within the selective targeting, and also the controlled delivery of varied medicine. Since the drug is covalently connected, loss thanks to leak of drug doesn't occur. However, loss might occur by chemical reaction. These factors on the opposite hand have nice influence of drug release, and physical stability of the system. There's no drawback of drug incorporation and drug bilayer interactions don't influence defences potency, just in case of pharmacosome.

The drug is free from pharmacosome by hydrolysis on defense potency just in case of liposomes. The lipid composition in liposomes decides its membrane fluidity. However, in pharmacosomes membrane fluidity depends upon the phase transition temperature of the drug lipoid complex, however it will have an effect on release rate since the drug is covalently bound. Because of their amphiphilic behavior, such systems enable, when medication, a multiple, transfer through the oleophilic membrane system or tissue through cellular walls piggyback endocytosis and exocytosis. They assist in achieving inflated bioavailability, cut back the value of medical aid and supply controlled still as targeted unharness of drug. The rise in solubility of drug within the complex may be explained by the solubilisation resulted from the formation of particle within the medium and by the amorphous characteristics of the complicated.

The pharmacosomes of NSAIDs like diclofenac and acelofenac have already developed. Thus, the developed pharmacosomes appear to be potential candidate as a drug delivery system during this era of novel and controlled drug delivery system. Pharmacosomes have large potential in rising the drug delivery just in case of each natural and artificial active constituents. Current analysis trends cellular targeting using different approaches like PEGylation, biotinylation, so forth. It is going to be all over that pharmacosomes are novel delivery system and may additionally improve the biopharmaceutical properties of medicine.

REFERENCES

Arnardottir, H. B., Sveinsson, S. L., & Kristmundsdottir, T. (1995). The use of a high intensity ultrasonic processor equipped with a flow cell in the production of reverse-phase liposomes. *International Journal of Pharmaceutics*, *117*(2), 237–241. doi:10.1016/0378-5173(94)00356-A

Bangham, A. D., Hill, M. V., & Miller, N. G. (1974). Methods in cell biology. *The Journal of Membrane Biology*, *1*, 1–68.

Bangham, A. D., Standish, M. M., & Watkins, J. G. (1955). Diffusion of univalent ions across the lamellae of swollen phospholipids. *Journal of Molecular Biology*, *13*(1), 238–252. doi:10.1016/S0022-2836(65)80093-6 PMID:5859039

Bangham, A. D., Standish, M. M., & Watkins, J. G. (1965). The action of steroids and streptolysin S on the permeability of phospholipid structures to cations. *Journal of Molecular Biology*, 213–238. PMID:5859040

Bansal,S.(n.d.) A Comparative Review On Vesicular Drug Delivery System and Stability Issues. *International Journal of Research in Pharmacy and Chemistry*, *4*, 704.

Bartlett, G. R. J. (1959). Purification of polysaccharide-protein conjugate vaccines by ultrafiltration with ammonium sulfate solutions. *The Journal of Biological Chemistry*, *234*, 466. PMID:13641241

Batzre, S., & Korn, E. D. (1973). Single bilayer liposomes prepared without sonication. *Biochimica et Biophysica Acta*, *298*(4), 1015–1019. doi:10.1016/0005-2736(73)90408-2 PMID:4738145

Bertrand, N., & Leroux, J. C. (2011). The journey of a drug carrier in the body: An anatomo-physiological perspective. *Journal of Controlled Release*, *161*(2), 152–163. doi:10.1016/j.jconrel.2011.09.098 PMID:22001607

Biju, S. S., Taleganokar, S., Misra, P. R., & Khar, R. K. (2006). Vesicular systems: An overview. *Indian Journal of Pharmaceutical Sciences*, *68*(2), 141–153. doi:10.4103/0250-474X.25707

Biju, S.S., Talegaonkar, S., & Mishra, P.R., Khar & K.R. (2009). Vesicular System: An overveiw. *Indian Journal of Pharmaceutical Sciences*, *71*(4), 421–427. PMID:20502548

Brooks, C. J. W., Machachlan, J., Cole, W. J., & Lawric, T. D. V. (1984). Vesicular system.*International Symposium, 349*.

Chiranjeevi, G., Muthukumaran, M., & Krishnamoorthy, B. (2013). A review on potency of vesicular systems in targeting drug delivery. *Research Journal of Pharmaceutical Biological Chemical Sciences*, *4*(2), 156–170.

Choudhary, N., & Sekhon, B. S. (2012). An overview of advances in the standardization of herbal drugs. *Journal of Pharmaceutical Education and Research*, *2*, 2.

Cullins, P. R., & Hope, M. J. (1986). Biochemistry of lipid and membrane. Benzain/Cumning.

Deamer, D. W., & Ann, N. Y. (1978). Preparation and properties of ether-injection liposomes. National Academy of Sciences, 308, 250.

Deamer, D. W., & Bangham, A. D. (1976). large voume liposomes by anether vaporisation method. *Biochimica et Biophysica Acta*, *443*, 629. PMID:963074

Doijad, R. C., Bhambere, D. S., Fakirappa, M. V., & Deshmukh, N. V. (2009). Formulation and characterization of vesicular drug delivery system for Anti-HIV drug. *Journal of Global Pharma Technology*, *1*, 94–100.

Egbaria, K., & Weiner, N. D. (1990). Liposomes as a topical drug delivery system. *Advanced Drug Delivery Reviews*, *5*(3), 287–300. doi:10.1016/0169-409X(90)90021-J

Fraley, R., Wyatt, J. P., & Papahadjopoulus, D. (1981). Liposomes: From Physical Structues to Therapeutics Applications. Elsevier.

Ganesan, M. G., Weiner, N. D., Flynn, G. I., & Ho, N. F. H. (1984). Influence of liposomal drug entrapment on percutaneous absorption. *International Journal of Pharmaceutics*, *20*(1-2), 139–154. doi:10.1016/0378-5173(84)90225-4

Gangwar, M., Singh, R., Goel, R. K., & Nath, G. (2011). Recent Advances In Various Emerging Vescicular Systems: An Overview. *Asian Pacific Journal of Tropical Biomedicine*, *33*, 848.

Goldberg, E. P. (1983). *Local chemo- and immunotherapy by intratumor drug injection: opportunities for polymer-drug compositions. In Targeted Drugs* (p. 312). New York: Wiley.

Goyal, P., Goyal, K., Kumar, S. G., Singh, A., Katare, O. P., & Mishra, D. N. (2005). Liposomal drug delivery systems: Clincal applications. *Acta Pharmaceutica (Zagreb, Croatia)*, *55*, 1–25. PMID:15907221

Gregoriadis, G. (1977). Targeting of drugs. *Controlled drug delivery. Nature*, *265*(5593), 407–411. doi:10.1038/265407a0 PMID:834290

Gunter, K. K., Gunter, T. E., Jarkowski, A., & Rosier, R. N. (1982). evidence for more than one calcium ion transport mechanism in mitochondria. *Analytical Biochemistry*, *110*, 123.

Gupta, S., Singh, R. P., Lokwani, P., Yadav, S., & Gupta, S. K. (2011). Vesicular system as targeted drug delivery system: An overview. *International Journal of Pharmacy and Technology*, *3*(2), 987–1021.

Hargreaves, W. R., & Deamer, D. W. (1978). Evidence against the partially and cost effectiveness of gram positive culture. *Biochemistry*, *17*, 3759. doi:10.1021/bi00611a014 PMID:698196

Hope, M. J., Bally, M. B., Webb, G., & Cullis, P. R. (1985). Production of large unilamellar vesicles by a rapid extrusion procedure. *Biochimica et Biophysica Acta*, *812*(1), 55–65. doi:10.1016/0005-2736(85)90521-8 PMID:23008845

Huang, C. H. (1969). Studies on phosphatidylcholine vesicles. Formation and physical characteristics. *Biochemistry*, *8*(1), 344–352. doi:10.1021/bi00829a048 PMID:5777332

Jain, N. K. (2003). Advances. In *Controlled and Novel Drug Delivery* (p. 276). New Delhi, India: CBS Publishers.

Jin, Y., Tong, L., Ai, P., Li, M., & Hou, X. (2006). Self-assembled drug delivery systems: Properties and in vitro/in vivo behavior of acyclovir self-assembled nanoparticles (SAN). *International Journal of Pharmaceutics*, *309*(1), 199–207. doi:10.1016/j.ijpharm.2005.11.025 PMID:16377106

Jin, Y., Tong, L., Ai, P., Li, M., & Hou, X. (2006). Self-assembled drug delivery systems- Properties and in vitro-in vivo behavior of acyclovir self-assembled nanoparticles. *International Journal of Pharmaceutics*, *309*(1–2), 199–207. doi:10.1016/j.ijpharm.2005.11.025 PMID:16377106

Jin, Y., Tong, L., Ai, P., Li, M., & Hou, X. (2006). Self-assembled drug delivery systems- Properties and in vitro-in vivo behavior of acyclovir self-assembled nanoparticles. *International Journal of Pharmaceutics*, *309*(1–2), 199–207. doi:10.1016/j.ijpharm.2005.11.025 PMID:16377106

Juliano, R.L. (1980). Controlled delivery of drugs: an overview and prospectus. *Drug Delivery Systems: Characteristics and Biomedical Application,* 310.

Kaur, & Kanwar, M. (2002). Ocular Preparations: The Formulation Approach. *Drug Development and Industrial Pharmacy, 28*(5), 473–493.

Kavitha, D., Sowjanya, J., & Shankar, P. (2012). Pharmacosomes: An Emerging Vesicular System. *International Journal of Pharmaceutical Sciences Review and Research*, *5*(3), 168–171.

Kim, S., & Martin, G. M. (1981). A method for the preparation of liposomes, a pack for use therein and a composition for use in preparing a liposomal material. *Biochimica et Biophysica Acta*, *646*, 4.

Korenbrot, J. I. (1977). Structural and spectroscopic characteristics of BR in air-water interface films. *Annual Review of Physiology*, *39*, 17.

Kremer, J. M., Eskai, M. W., Pathmamanoharan, G., & Wiersema, P. H. (1977). Renal biopsy specimens from patients with rheumatoid arthritis. *Biochemistry*, *16*, 3932. doi:10.1021/bi00636a033 PMID:901761

Kumar, D. P., & Arnab, D. (2012). Pharmacosomes: A potential vesicular drug delivery system. *International Research Journal of Pharmacy*, *3*(3), 102–105.

Kumar, R. (2008). Enzymatic Hydrolysis of Cellulosic Biomass Solids Prepared by Leading Pretreatments and Identification. Handbook of Particulate Drug Delivery, 2.

Kumar, R. (2011). Vesicular System-Carrier for Drug Delivery. *Pelagia Research Library Der Pharmacia Sinica*, *2*(4), 192–202.

Langer, R. (1983). Implantable controlled release systems. *Pharmacology & Therapeutics*, *21*(1), 35–51. doi:10.1016/0163-7258(83)90066-9 PMID:6353438

Langer, R. (1998). Drug delivery and targeting. *Nature*, *392*, 5–10. PMID:9579855

Lawrence, M. J. (1994). Surfactant systems: Their use in drug delivery. *Chemical Society Reviews*, *23*(6), 417–424. doi:10.1039/cs9942300417 PMID:7867669

Lieberman, H. A., Rieger, M. M., & Banker, G. S. (1998). *Pharmaceutical Dosage Forms: Disperse Systems*. London: Informa Healthcare.

Mayer, L. D., Hope, M. J., Cullis, P. R., & Janoff, A. S. (1985). Solute distributions and trapping efficiencies observed in freeze-thawed multilamellar vesicles. *Biochimica et Biophysica Acta*, 817–193. PMID:4005257

Muller-Goymann, C. C., & Hamann, H. J. (1991). Pharmacosomes: Multilamellar vesicles consisting of Pure Drug. *European Journal of Pharmaceutics and Biopharmaceutics*, *37*, 113–117.

Nilesh. (2007). *Pharmacosomes*. Retrieved from farmavita.net

Ogihara, U., Sasaki, T., Toyama, H., Odak, S. M., & Nishigori, H. (1997). Pharmacosomes: An emerging vesicular system. *Cancer Detection and Prevention*, *21*(6), 56–62.

Pansuriya, M., Gupta, A., & Gadhvi, V. (n.d.). Pharmacosomes: A Novel Vesicular System. *GTC.*

Park, K. (1997). *Controlled Drug Delivery: Challenges and Strategies.* Washington, DC: American Chemical Society.

Park, K., & Mersny, R.J. (2000). Controlled drug delivery: present and future. *Controlled Drug Delivery: Designing Technology for the Future,* 2–13.

Patel, V., & Agrawal, Y. K. (2011). Current Status and Advanced Approaches In Ocular Drug Delivery System. *Journal of Global Trends In Pharmaceutical Sciences*, *2*(2), 131–148.

Peng, F. Y., Qin, Z., Bin, W., Ming, Y., & Mu-Sheng, W. (2012). Process optimization by response surface design and characterization study on geniposidepharmacosomes. *Pharmaceutical Development and Technology*, *17*(1), 94–102. doi:10.3109/10837450.2010.516439 PMID:20919929

Pidgeon, C., Hunt, A. H., & Dittrich, K. (1986). Formation of multilayered vesicles from water/organic-solvent (W/O) emulsions: Theory and practice. *Pharmaceutical Research*, *3*(1), 23–34. doi:10.1023/A:1016316730560 PMID:24271353

Ping, A., Jin, Y., & Dawei, C. (2005). Preparation and In Vivo Behavior of DidanosinePharmacosomes in Rats. *Chinese Journal of Pharmaceuticals*, *3*, 227–235.

Poste, G., Kirsch, R., & Koestler, T. (1983). Liposomes Technology. CRC Press Inc.

Poznansky, M. J., & Juliano, R. L. (1983). Liposome targeting in vivo: Problems and opportunities. *Pharmacological Reviews*, *36*, 277. PMID:6395142

Prajapati, S. K., Kumar, S., Sahu, V. K., & Prakash, G. (2012). Proniosomal gel of flurbiprofen: Formulation and evaluation. *Journal of Drug Delivery & Therapeutics*, *2*, 105–114.

Prasanthi,N.L., Manikiran,S.S., Rama Rao, N.(2010) Pharmacosomes: An Alternative Carrier System for Drug Delivery. *The Pharma Review*, 93-96.

Razin, S. (1972). Physiology of michoplasm: Advance in microbiology. *Biochimica et Biophysica Acta*, *265*, 241. doi:10.1016/0304-4157(72)90004-4 PMID:4555471

Ritika, S.L., & Aggarwal G.H. (2012). Formulation Tactics for the Delivery of Poorly Soluble Drugs. *International Journal of Physical Therapy and Rehabilitation,* 915-919.

Rosier, R. N., Gunter, T. E., Tucker, D. A., & Gunter, K. K. (1979). A rapid method for separating small vesicles from suspension. *Analytical Biochemistry*, *120*, 113. PMID:474964

Schieran, H., Rudolph, S., Fiukelstein, M., Coleman, P., & Weisman, G. (1978). Comparison of large unilamellar vesicles prepared by a petroleum ether vaporization method with multilamellar vesicles: ESR, diffusion and entrapment analyses. *Biochimica et Biophysica Acta*, *646*, 4.

Seema, M., & Jadhav, P.M. (n.d.). Novel Vesicular System: An Overview. *Journal of Pharmaceutical Sciences,* 193-202.

Sharma, P., Tyrell, D. A., & Ryman, B. T. (1977). Use of ordination and other multivariate descriptive methods to study. *Biochemical Society Transactions*, *5*, 1146. doi:10.1042/bst0051146 PMID:913809

Volkering, F. (1995). Influence of Nonionic Surfactants on Bioavailability and Biodegradation of Polycyclic Aromatic Hydrocarbons. *Applied and Environmental Microbiology*, *61*(5), 1699–1705. PMID:16535016

Wang, N. X., & Recum, H. A. (2011). Affinity-Based Drug Delivery. *Macromolecular Bioscience*, *11*(3), 321–332. doi:10.1002/mabi.201000206 PMID:21108454

Section 5
Transfersomes and Protransfersomes

Chapter 6
Transfersomes and Protransfersome:
Ultradeformable Vesicular System

Bhushan Rajendra Rane
P. S. G. V. P. Mandal's College of Pharmacy, India

Nayan Ashok Gujarathi
P. S. G. V. P. Mandal's College of Pharmacy, India

ABSTRACT

Vesicular system brings several possible advantages over conventional route of drug delivery system. Formulation of system to administered via transdermal is an attractive option because this route is suitable and safe. Transfersomes is one of vesicular system which possesses a single chain surfactant as it offers ultra deformation property which provides better penetration. Vesicles of hydrophobic and hydrophilic moieties can be formulated together and as a result can deliver drug molecules with wide range of solubility. Problems of drug leakage and low entrapment could be overcome in this system. Materials which are widely used in the formulation of it are various phospholipids, surfactants, alcohol, dye and buffering agent. These systems can deform up to 5 times lesser than its original size to pass through narrow constriction without showing drug leakage. These are more flexible and adjustable than that of liposomes thus can be used to carry drugs across the biological membrane, such as skin. It can act as a carrier for wide variety of drugs.

INTRODUCTION

History

The German company IDEA AG firstly introduced transfersome vesicular system and it is the registered trademark of this company which is being used as proprietary drug delivery technology. Gregor Cevc defined the term transfersome and described the concept related to it in broad sense (Cevc, 1991). Transfersome is an ultradeformable, highly flexible and stress-responsive, complex system. The name

DOI: 10.4018/978-1-5225-0751-2.ch006

means "carrying body", and is derived from the Latin word 'transferre', meaning 'to carry across', and the Greek word 'soma', for a 'body' (Walve et al., 2011). Transfersomes are ultradeformable vesicles; possess an aqueous core which is surrounded by the composite lipid bilayer. Transfersomes are interdependent of their composition and shape; it makes the system as self-regulating and self-optimizing. Thus, it is ready to cross various barriers of skin very efficiently. It targets drug via non-invasive route to specific site as well as releases the later in sustained manner to show therapeutic effect (Nanda et al., 2005). Transfersomes have stability problems, to overcome stability problem the more stable vesicular system is developed in relation to transport of drug, molecules, proteins and other drug moieties via transdermal route, this new vesicular system is called as Pro-transfersome. Pro-ultraflexible lipid vesicles called as pro-transfersomes, they possess better stability in comparison to transfersome vesicular systems they have ability to absorb water from the different layers of skin. Pro-transfersomes are more stable than conventional vesicular systems (Gupta et al., 2011).

In the new era, the vesicular type of approach have been used as an option because of their wide applications such as membrane biology, diagnostic techniques, immunology, and nowadays genetic technology thus promoted as a best system for sustained release and controlled release of drug through transdermal route, as it has number of advantages such as biodegradation, lack of toxicity, encapsulating capacity for hydrophilic as well as lipophilic molecules, prolonging the existence of drug in the body by encapsulating drug in vesicular system. It also offers the advantage of targeting of drug to specific organs and tissues, it reduces the toxicity of drug and most important it increases drug bioavailability. Vesicles because of their unique structure have a capacity to entrap both the types of drugs such as lipophilic, hydrophilic, amphiphilic and charged hydrophilic drugs. Transfersome and pro-transfersome is a vesicular system in which an aqueous filled core surrounded by lipids and surfactant arranges it into bilayer system. The concentration of aqueous system is increased, and then multi concentric bilayers can be formed. Entrapment of hydrophilic drugs into the internal aqueous environment while other drug of amphiphilic, lipophilic nature finds a place into bilayered wall and the hydrophobic forces as well as electrostatic forces are involved in it (Bain et al., 1993).

Transdermal route is convenient and safe route of administration so it is best approach to deliver the drug at specific site. Transfersomes and pro-transfersomes have number of advantages in comparison to conventional routes such as these avoid first pass metabolism, predetermined and longer duration of activity, reducing side effects, use of lesser half-life drugs, improving pharmacological response, drug levels fluctuation is avoided, variations in inter-and intra-patient is reduced, and lastly the patient compliance is improved (Cevc et al., 1997). Now research is oriented towards applying physical and chemical approaches in order to raise the drug transfer through skin, the approaches available are as follows:

1. By using penetration enhancers,
2. Enhancers,
3. Iontophoresis,
4. Sonophoresis, and
5. Vesicular carriers such as lipid vesicles and niosomes (Chapman and Walsh, 1998).

Transfersomes and pro-transfersomes were formulated with the main objective to deliver the drug into or through skin in order to show therapeutic response at predetermined rate. Transfersomes and pro-transfersomes are ultradeformable vesicles and it takes advantage of phospholipid as composition material to carry drug. These are more elastic in nature in comparison to other vesicle systems (e.g. liposomes) and thus suitable to deliver the drug via transdermal route. It is very difficult to penetrate drug through skin which can be overcome in transfersomes and pro-transfersomes by squeezing themselves along into deeper region of stratum corneum as shown in Figure 1. These are self-adaptable in nature and also have property of ultradeformation, thus it can enter into skin by changing shape and size as well as due to the mechanical stress from the surrounding. Flexibility of transfersomes and pro-transfersomes membrane is achieved by mixing suitable surface-active components in the proper ratios (Bain et al., 1993). The chances of complete vesicle rupture in the skin are minimized due to flexible nature of such vesicles. It allows them to follow the natural water gradient across the epidermis, when applied under non-occlusive condition.

Skin as a Barrier

The skin is the largest tissue of human body. It has large surface area thus acts as a protective barrier against various influences such as microbial, mechanical, external, chemical, and physical factors. Skin also offers their best property of easy accessibility. Because of this, skin delivery has potential application in drug delivery. Drug penetration through the skin is achieved with main objective to deliver the drug to treat skin infections or deliver the various drugs through stratum corneum to target at specific sites and to reach the systemic circulation. It is a challenging task to deliver the drug via skin to specific region to treat disease. Physiological study reveals that skin is made up of four noticeable layers i) stratum corneum, ii) epidermal layer, iii) dermal layer and iv) subcutaneous layer. Stratum corneum is the outer part of the skin and is made up of broad matrix of size 10-15 µm of dehydrated and dead keratolytic cells. It is surrounded by lipid layers which have high order, thus it provide a barrier. Transfersomes vesicles resize their shape easily and so rapidly, by adjusting lipid bilayer component to the surrounding stress experienced by system. The fundamental structure of these vesicles is broadly similar to liposomes. But the transfersomes and pro-transfersomes differ from the conventional vesicles mainly by their soft nature, ultradeformable property, and adjustability. When applied via transdermal route it searches 'pores' present into the different layers of skin or different pathways in the skin through which it enters carrying drug molecule. Onwards it gets deformed without losing their vesicular contents. Self-regulating and self-optimizing property is because of their local composition and shape (Chapman and Walsh, 1998). They are more elastic and more flexible than the other vesicular systems such as liposomes and thus suitable for skin penetration (Fry et al., 1978). Each colloidal carrier overcomes barriers of

Figure 1. Schematic diagram of penetration pathway for conventional and ultra-deformable vesicles

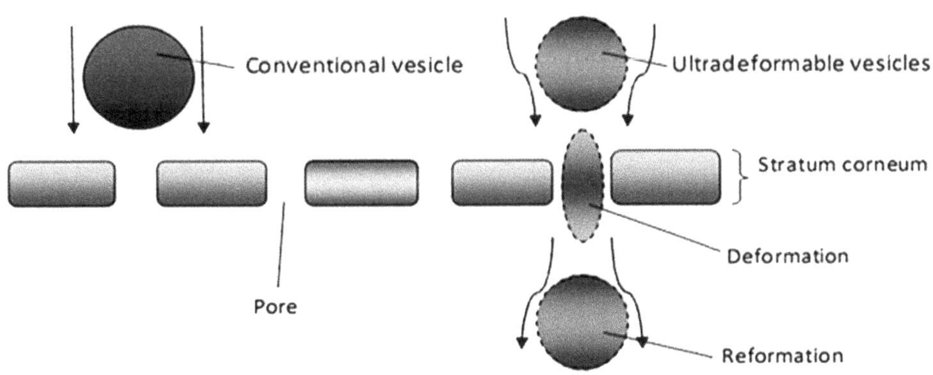

skin, to deliver the drug into deeper region of skin. The carrier releases drug to their targeted tissue in predetermined manner upto certain depth of skin regions. The depth and extent of the drug targeting is controlled by the nature of carrier and their composition. Metabolic degradation of embedded drug can be avoided in transfersomes and pro-transfersomes, it act as reservoir, which releases drug very slowly and in sustained manner (Cevc, 1991).

Transfersomes and pro-transfersomes can enter the stratum corneum (SC) via two routes:

1. Intracellularly and
2. Transcellularly, both have different bilayer properties (Schatzlein and Cevc, 1995; Panchagnula 1997).

Both possible routes for the drug penetration through human skin i.e. intracellular and transcellular are as shown in Figure 1.

The self-optimizing deformability nature of transfersomes and pro-transfersomes system is able to adapt ambient stress which allows the system to change their shape reversibly when it passes through the narrow pores of skin. The components show membrane deformation property, while the less deformable molecules are diluted at site of great stress. These vesicles are able to permit highly flexible particles to enter through skin and then to pass through the different available pores rapidly and efficiently (Bain et al., 1993).

Necessity of Transfersomes for Skin Delivery

Transfersomes are phospholipids colloidal vesicles having self-optimized and ultra-flexible membrane properties which is best for the transdermal drug delivery. Transfersomes have ability to deliver the drug in reproducible manner either into or through the skin, which depend on method of application with greater efficiency. Elasticity of transfersomes is more than the liposomes and thus suitable to penetrate various drugs through skin. Transfersomes and pro-transfersomes squeeze themself into SC; this mechanism can be well understood from the Figure 2. Flexible property of transfersome and pro-transfersomes is optimized by mixing suitable surfactants in the suitable ratios with phospholipids (Cevc et al., 1997).

The flexible property reduces the risk of vesicle breakage in the SC. Transfersomes and pro-transfersomes when applied under non-occlusive condition it follow natural water gradient across the skin layer epidermis. Bangham discovered liposomes in 1963, since then vesicular systems have attracted increasing attention (Cevc et al., 1997). It has been reported that classic liposomes have less penetration ability and CSLM studies confirmed that liposomes are remained into upper part of SC; unable to go deeper into granular layer of epidermis. The drug release rate into skin via transdermal route and targeting to specific site can be achieved by the modification of the compositions of transfersome and pro-transfersome or surface properties

Advantages

These are able to deform upto 5 to 10 times less than their own size and ability to pass through narrow pores (Gamal et al., 1999).

- They have high encapsulation ability, which will be upto 90% in case of lipophilic drug.
- Ultradeformability gives better penetration property for vesicles.

Figure 2. Optical diagram transfersome

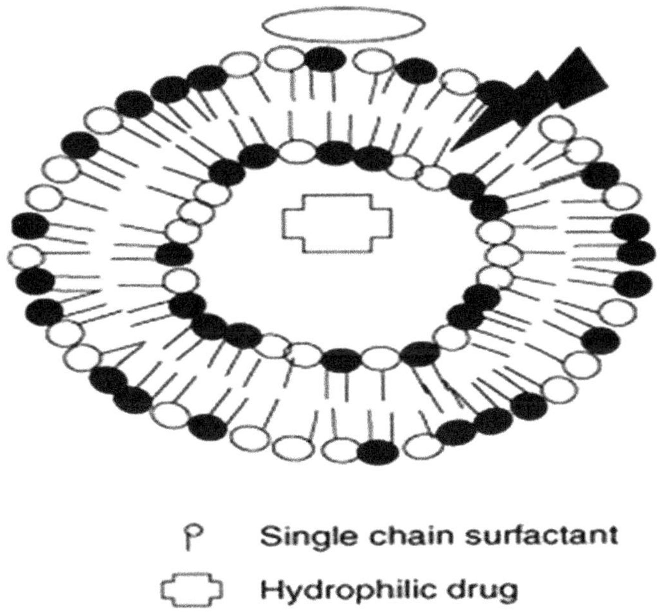

- Suitable carrier for all type of drugs which have wide variety of molecular weight such as anesthetic, analgesic, sex hormone, corticosteroids, insulin, anticancer, albumin and gap junction protein.
- Easy to incorporate hydrophilic and hydrophobic drugs together into it.
- It acts as reservoir for drug which releases drug in sustained manner.
- Transfersomes and pro-transfersomes useful not only for systemic treatment but also to deliver the drug topically.
- Their composition is same as that of liposomes thus it possesses biodegradability and biocompatibility.
- Metabolic degradation of drug is avoided during encapsulation.
- Easy to formulate.
- Drug molecules which have wide range of solubility can be encapsulated.

Salient Features

Transfersomes and pro-transfersomes are useful not only for systemic treatment but also to deliver the drug topically. It can be able to deform up to 5 to 10 times less than their own size and ability to pass through narrow pores. They have high encapsulation ability, which will be up to 90% in case of lipophilic drug. Ultradeformable property of it gives better penetration property for vesicles. It is a suitable carrier for all type of drugs which have wide variety of molecular weight such as anesthetic, analgesic, sex hormones, corticosteroids, insulin, anticancer, albumin and gap junction protein. It is easy to incorporate hydrophilic and hydrophobic drugs together into it, also act as reservoir for drug which releases drug into sustained manner. Their composition is same as that of liposomes thus it possesses biodegradability and biocompatibility also the metabolic degradation of drug is avoided during encapsulation. It is easy to formulate transfersomes and pro-transfersomes due to their simple method of preparation. Drug molecules which have wide range of solubility can be encapsulated (Cevc et al., 1996; Gamal et al., 1999).

Limitations

- Due to oxidative degradation and predisposition property they are chemically unstable.
- Stability of transfersomes and pro-transfersomes depend on purity of natural phospholipids.
- This vesicular system is not cost effective (Gompper and Kroll, 1995; Jain, 2001).

Composition and Mechanism

A simple lipid vesicle is lipid bilayered formed by the mechanism of self-assembly of phosphatidyl choline (amphiphilic) in aqueous solvents. Flexibility and permeability of system can be increased by the addition of bilayer softening component (such as an amphiphilic drug or a biocompatible surfactant). Transfersomes and pro-transfersomes can acquire their shape very rapidly and easily, by adjusting concentration of each bilayer contents to the limited stress practiced by the bilayer results into greater permeability and flexibility, as shown in Figure 3.

Figure 3. Diagrammatic representation of routes of penetration through the stratum corneum (intercellularly and transcellularly)

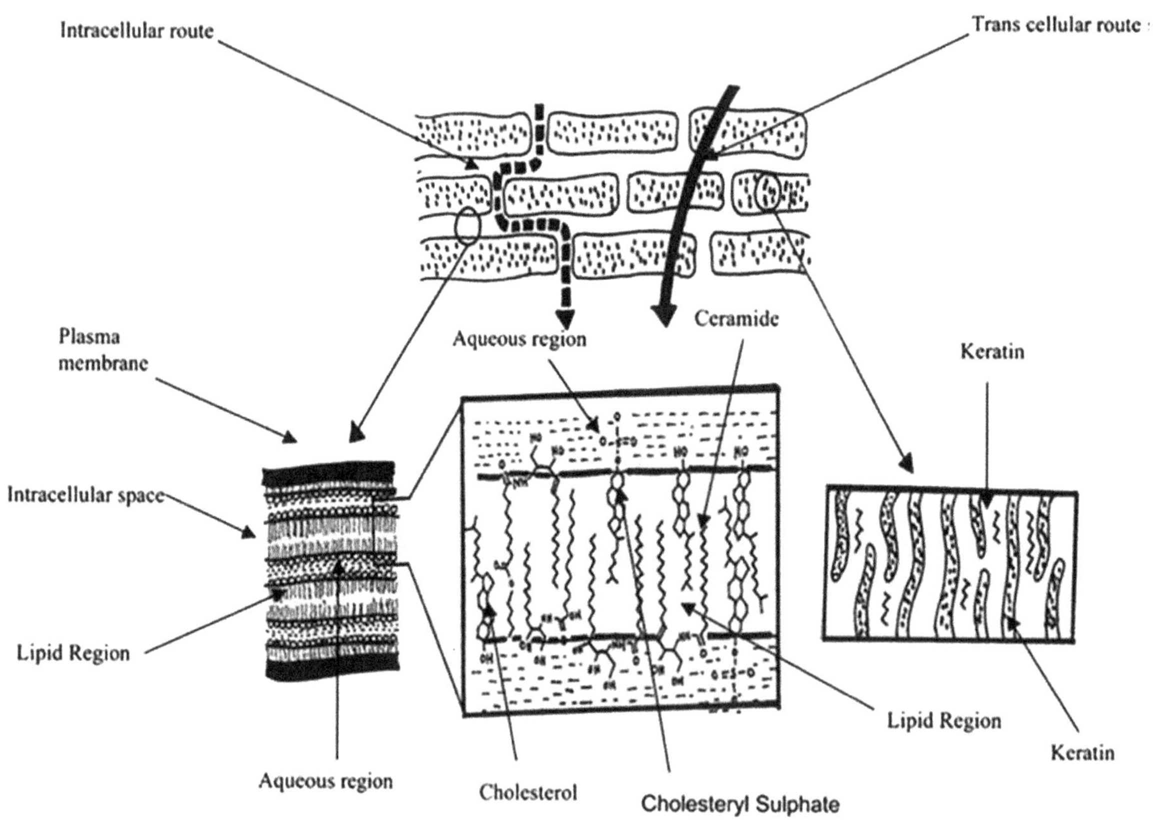

The basic structure of transfersomes and pro-transfersomes is like classic liposome, still it differs from liposome by soft nature, ultradeformable property and better adjustable nature of system membrane (Elsayed et al., 2006).

Other important property of transfersomes and pro-transfersomes is their strong bilayered deformation ability with ability to bind with skin moisture and retain water. Transfersomes and pro-transfersomes have extra deformable property and contain high amount of hydrophilic molecules, such vesicles avoid dehydration. Such process may entail a transport process related to but not the same with forward osmosis. On an open biological surface (such as non-occluded skin) if transfersomes and pro-transfersomes vesicle are applied, then due to their properties it leads to deeper movement into skin barrier and move more deeper towards the water containing strata to acquire their hydration. Skin barrier penetration of transfersomes and pro-transfersomes is due to reversible bilayered ultradeformation but the vesicle integrity of transfersomes and pro-transfersomes and the skin barrier layer properties along with water gradient of skin not changed (Jain et al., 1998).

It is very difficult to diffuse drug through the barriers of skin, still the transfersomes and pro-transfersomes find and put in force their own way through the layers. The transfersomes and pro-transfersomes are useful in the delivery of various drug molecules which depend on the ability of carrier to carry drug deeper into skin SC; subsequently the drug releases from depot, release of drug from their carrier allows binding to their target after it diffuses from the reservoir. The transport of drug into subcutaneous layer is by the process of endocytosis (Jain, 2001) i.e. transfersomes and pro-transfersomes vesicle is taken up by cell or at an intra-cellular action site it may also involve fusion of the lipid bilayer of carrier.

Pro-transfersomes also have ultraflexible nature and its mechanism of action to release and transport the drug molecules through the skin is similar to transfersome vesicular approach. The difference is that they can able to absorb water from the skin layers. Because of this reason pro- transfersomes have more stability in comparison to transfersomes. Pro-transfersomes also have better skin penetration property to deliver the drug at the site of action in comparison to other traditional vesicular systems such as niosomes, liposomes etc. For transdermal delivery of the drug it is better to formulate gel system of pro-transfersomes to achieve desired effect rapidly. Some of the contraceptive in order to stop ovulation process can be delivered through transdermal route such as norgestrol and observed results show effective contraception, increased stability and high encapsulation efficiency of drug (Jain et al., 2001).

Tendency of Penetration

Transport driving force magnitude plays an important role in penetration; as we know that:

Flow = Area x force x Permeability.

where, Force is Trans-barrier and permeability is barrier

Thus, the lipid flow across the skin by chemically driven forces always decreases interestingly when minor amount of lipids in a suspension is added instead of lipid solution (Jain, 2001) (see Figure 4).

Materials and Methods

Transfersomes and pro-transfersomes are formulated by using materials various lipid (phospholipids), surfactants, dye, alcohol, buffering agent as well as some other additives. The materials used in the

Figure 4. Mechanism of penetration of transfersomes

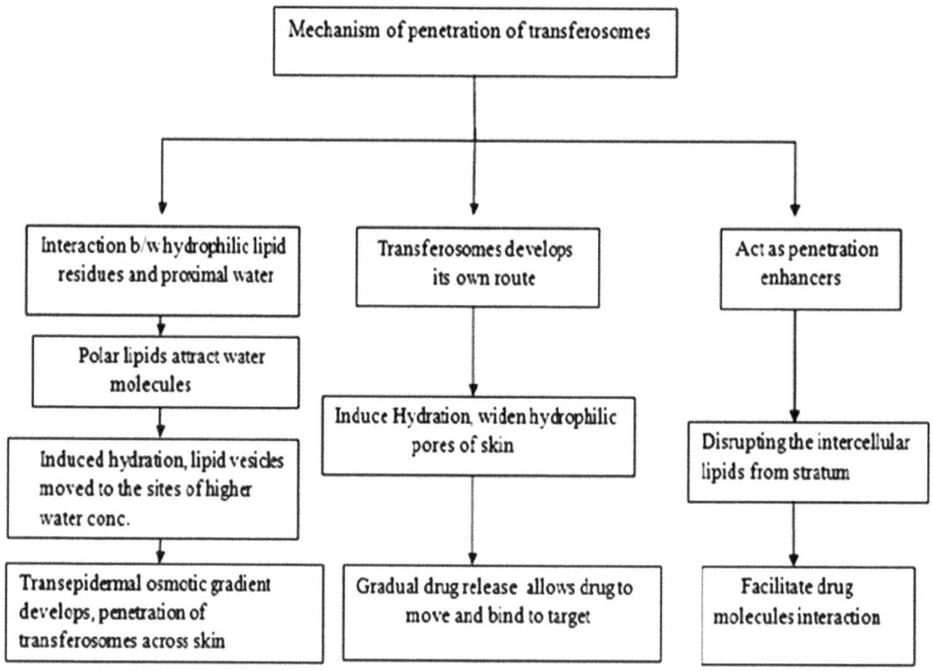

preparation of transfersomes and pro-transfersomes are mentioned in Table 1 (Cevc et al., 1997; Wearner et al., 1988; Gamal et al., 1999; Maghraby et al., 1998; Paul and Cevec, 1998)

General Method

Method for the preparation of transfersomes and pro-transfersomes is similar to method for preparation of liposome, it consist of two steps:

1. A thin lipid film is hydrated in suitable medium and then shift it for sonication to obtain desired size;

Table 1. Different ingredients used in preparation of transfersomes and pro-transfersomes

Ingredients	Material	Role
Lipids (Phospholipids)	Egg phosphatidyl choline, Soya phosphatidyl choline, dipalmitoyl phosphatidyl choline	For formation of vesicles
Surface active agents	Sod.cholate,Sod.deoxycholate,Tween -80,Span-80	To impart flexibility
Primary alcohols	Methanol, Ethanol	Solvent
Buffering agent	pH 6.4 saline phosphate buffer	Hydrating medium
Chemical Dye	Nile-red, Rhodamine-DHPE, Fluorescein-DHPE, Rhodamine-123	For Confocal Scanning Laser Microscopy study

2. Previously sonicated vesicles are shifted for homogenizer and by extrusion through a polycarbonate membrane get suitable size vesicles.

Suitable concentration of phospholipids and surfactant were dissolved in organic solvent of volatile nature (chloroform, methanol). Due to escaping tendency of organic solvent it leaves the mixture and evaporated at 50 °C in case of dipalmitoyl phosphatidyl choline (PC) or above the lipid transition temperature or room temperature for pure PC vesicles by using rotary flash evaporator. The mixture is kept under vacuum for overnight to remove traces of solvent (see Figure 5)

Thin Film Hydration Method

In this method phospholipids and surfactant are dissolved in suitable volatile organic solvent such as chloroform-Methanol and thin film is prepared. Above the lipid transition temperature or at 50 °C using rotary evaporator the organic solvent is evaporated. The dispersion is kept under vacuum for overnight to remove final traces of solvent. Saline phosphate buffer of pH 6.4 is added to hydrate stack of film and subsequently kept for rotation at 60 rpm for 1 hour at the mentioned temperature; kept at room temperature for 2 hours till the swelling of vesicles is completed. Afterwards to obtain the desired vesicles of small size the dispersion is sonicated using a bath sonicator at 50 °C or at room temperature for 30 min or sonicated using probe sonicator at 40 °C for 30 min. Lastly a sandwich of 200 and 100 nm polycarbonate membranes (Fry et al., 1978; Paul et al., 1995) is used to homogenize the sonicated vesicles by manual extrusion.

Figure 5. Method of preparation of transfersomes

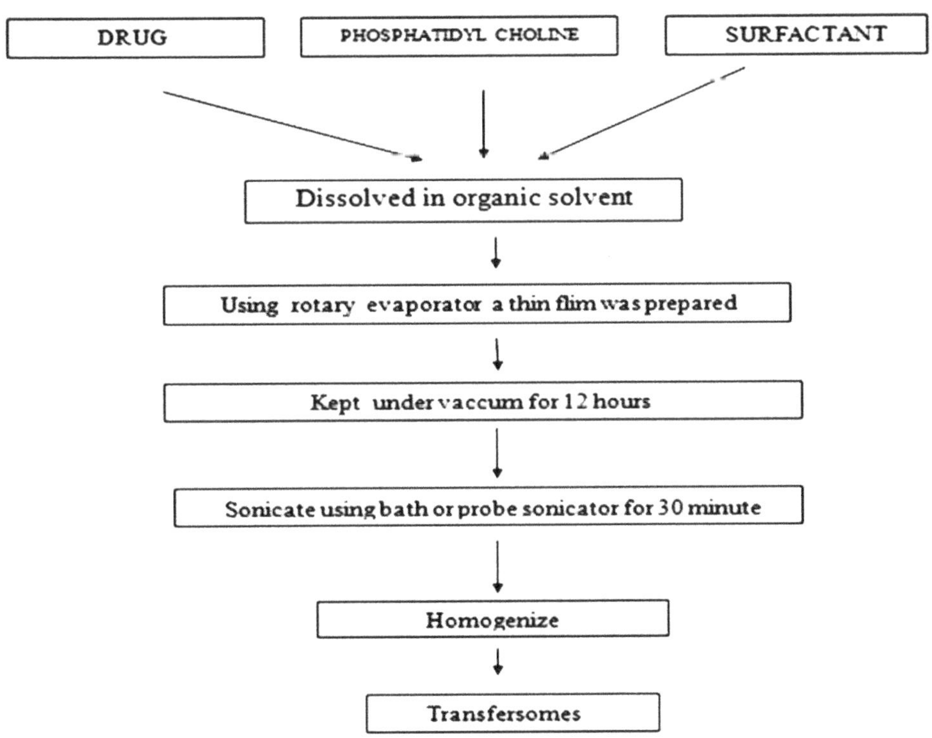

Modified Hand Shaking, Lipid Film Hydration Technique (Planas et al., 1992)

Drug molecule, phosphatidyl choline (Lecithin) and other additives such as edge activator are dissolved in chloroform: Ethanol (1:1) mixture, the mixture of organic solvent is removed by evaporation by using rotary flash evaporator or by hand shaking at 43 °C (above lipid transition temperature). A stack of thin lipid film was formed at the inner wall of container. The obtained stack of thin film is kept overnight under vacuum for complete removal of traces of solvent. The phosphate buffer (pH 7.4) is added to re-hydrate the film with the hand shaking for 15 minutes at mentioned temperature. The vesicle of desired size is obtained by placing previously obtained sample for homogenization.

How to Optimize the Formulation Containing Transfersomes and Pro-Transfersomes

The numbers of process variables are responsible to obtain the best ultradeformable transfersomes and pro-transfersomes which can affect the properties of vesicular system. The method for the preparation of transfersome is accordingly checked, optimized and then validated (Rand and Parsegian, 1989). The different process variables during preparation of vesicular system such as,

1. Phosphatidyl choline/Lecithin,
2. Ratio of surfactants added,
3. Solvent effect,
4. Effect of different surfactants,
5. Medium used for hydration.

By selecting encapsulation efficiency of drug the system can be optimized. Once the method is optimized the other process variables kept constant while preparing transfersomes and pro-transfersomes vesicular system.

Evaluation Parameters

The characterization of transfersomes and pro-transfersomes is generally similar to liposomes, niosomes and micelles (Nanda et al., 2005; Jain et al., 1998)

- **Entrapment Efficiency:** The entrapment efficiency is the percentage amount of drug entrapped in the formulation. Percentage entrapment of prepared formulation is determined by separating the entrapped drug by use of various techniques such as (mini-column) centrifugation method. The % entrapment efficiency is calculated by the following formula:

Entrapment efficiency= (amount of drug entrapped/ total amount of drug added) x 100.

- **Diameter of Vesicle:** Photon correlation spectroscopy or dynamic light scattering (DLS) method is used to determine vesicle diameter. Distilled water is used for the preparation of samples and filtered through a membrane filter (0.2 mm) and filtered saline used to dilute upto certain dilution ratio to measure the size of vesicle (Gamal et al., 1999).

- **Number of Vesicle/mm^3:** Number of vesicles / mm^3 is an important characterization parameter of system to check quality as well as for the composition and other process variables. Transfersome system (without sonication) diluted upto five times with 0.9% of NaCl solution and observed with optical microscopy by using haemocytometer.

Confocal Scanning Laser Microscopy Study (CSLM)

Electron microscopy and conventional light microscopy have problem of sectioning, fixation and staining of the skin samples, so these methods are unable to interpret the results accurately even examination of the structures are incompatible with the above techniques; the recent tool Confocal Scanning Laser Microscopy (CSLM) is the best option for it. Fluorescence markers of lipophilic nature are used to for transfersomes and pro-transfersomes confirmation. When the light falls on such sample, emission of fluorescent light by used markers which have numerous uses as mentioned below:

1. To investigate the mechanism of transfersomes and pro-transfersomess penetration across the skin.
2. To determine organization of the skin, architecture and shape of the skin
3. To compare the different penetration pathways
4. To differentiate the mechanism of penetration in between transfersomes and pro-transfersomes with liposomes, Niosomes and micelles.

Fluorescence markers for CSLM study are as follows:

1. Nile red.
2. Rhodamine-DHPE(1,2-dihexadecanoyl-sn-glycero-3ogisogietgabikanube-N-Lissa -mineTmrhodamine B sulfonyl), triethanolamine salt).
3. Fluorescein-DHPE(1,2-dihexadecanoyl-sn-glycero-3-phosphoethanolamine-N-(5-fluoresdenthiocarbamoyl), triethylammonium salt).
4. NBD-PE (1, 2-dihexadecanoyl-sn-glycero-3-phosphoethanolamine-N-(7-nitro-Benz-2- oxa-1, 3-diazol-4-yl) triethanolamine salt).

Measurement of Permeability or Degree of Deformation

Measurement of permeability is the one of most important and unique parameter in the evaluation of transfersomes and pro-transfersomes. Pure water is taken as standard to study the degree of deformation for transfersomes and pro-transfersomes sample.

Transfersomes and pro-transfersomes suspension is passed through a multiple number of pores of size ranges from 50 nm and 400 nm as per according to sample. Note down the particle size and size distributions when it passes through filter pores by using dynamic light scattering (DLS) measurements.

- **Measurement of Turbidity:** Nephelometer is used for the measurement of turbidity sample in aqueous solution.
- **Surface Charge and Charge Density:** Zeta sizer is used for the measurement of surface charge and charge density of transfersomes and pro-transfersomes sample.

- **Penetration Ability:** Fluorescence microscopy is used for penetration ability of transfersomes and pro-transfersomess.
- **Percent Drug Content:** The % amount of drug is estimated by using sophisticated instruments such as ultra pressure high performance liquid chromatography (UPLC) which have UV detector, column oven, auto sampling system, pump, and software operating program for analysis.
- **Occlusion Study:** It is reported that the occlusion of skin is more; the permeation of drug is increased in case of our traditional topical preparations, while occlusion effect shows negative impact on the ultradeformable vesicles. The driving force for the movement of transfersomes and pro-transfersomes vesicle through the skin is hydrotaxis i.e. movement in the direction of water for deeper permeation. Hydration forces are influenced by occlusion as it avoids the evaporation of water from skin.
- **In Vitro Drug Release:** To determine the rate of permeation rate in vitro drug release is calculated. Sample of transfersomes and pro-transfersomes suspension is incubated at 32 °C and at various time intervals aliquot quantity of samples are withdrawn to estimate the amount of drug which is released after minicolumn centrifugation process. The % amount of in vitro drug release is calculated from initial amount of drug added as 100% and drug released after each time interval.
- **Skin Deposition Study:** After completion of permeation study (24 hours), sample is subjected for skin deposition study. Wash the skin surface five times by using Et-OH (ethanol): PBS (Phosphate buffer solution) pH 7.4 in 1:1 ratios, subsequently wash with distilled water in order to remove excess amount of drug from the skin surface. Cut the skin into small pieces further the tissue is homogenized with Et-OH: PBS pH 7.4 (1:1 ratio) and kept at room temperature for 6 hr. Later on shake it for 5 minutes and centrifuge at 5000 rpm for 5 minutes, the drug content was checked after suitable dilutions with phosphate buffer solution.
- **Stability Study:** The % drug entrapment is calculated and recorded for prepared formulation. Optimized formulation is stored in sealed glass ampoules different storage conditions such as at 4 °C ± 2 °C (refrigeration temperature), 25 °C ± 2 °C (room temperature), and 37 ± 2 °C (body temperature) for the period of 3 months. After each month the samples from each ampoule is analyzed and amount of drug leak from the vesicular system is note down. The amount of % drug loss is calculated after each month by taking initial entrapped drug as 100%.
- **In Vivo and Kinetic Study of Transfersome:** Transfersomes reach into the deeper part of skin layer after penetration through the surface of skin and dermal layers. After dermis region vesicular system is washed out, via the lymph in lymphatic system, into the blood stream latter throughout the body, if applied at normal conditions. Thus transfersome vesicles can reach to all body tissues which are accessible to the liposomes injected subcutaneously. The velocity of carrier penetration and the speed of drug (re) distribution are responsible for the kinetics of action of an epi-cutaneously applied agent. The chief factors in this process are carrier in-flow, carrier accumulation at the targets site and carrier elimination.

The volume of the suspension medium is responsible for penetration-driving force. The suspension additional volume must have to evaporate from the skin surface to establish the water activity gradient. Less solvent suspension is favorable to establish water gradient. The rate of carrier penetration through the surface and layers of skin is determined by activation energy for ultradeformable vesicle of transfersomes and pro-transfersomes. Rate of penetration is one of driving force which also plays a key role in kinetics of transfersomes and pro-transfersomes. Therefore, it explains on own accord that why the skin occlusion or diluted suspensions reduces the process of penetration. Lymphatic flow affect the carrier elimination from the sub cutis, sometimes general anesthesia or other factor may be affects lymphatic flow. It is reported that not more than 10% of the cardiac blood flow pass through one gram of living skin tissue, no evidence is found for the lymph.

The use of number of carriers influences the rate of drug distribution by affecting the rate of vehicle degradation and/or filtration in the lymphatic system. The type of drug and formulation administration is influenced by the lag between the time of application and the time of drug appearance in the body. In case of local analgesics the skin penetration lag amounts upto 15 minutes are detected right under the skin permeability barrier, while in case of molecules measured in the blood compartment or less rapidly exchanging molecules have lag time in between 2 to 6 hours which totally depend on composition of drug formulation. Less rapidly exchanging molecules such as molecules unable to diffuse from the carriers have more lag time. The physicochemical properties of the transfersomes and pro-transfersomes suspension controls kinetics of vesicle penetration into and across the skin. In the direct biological assays in which vesicle system associated drugs exert their action directly under the skin surface best reveals the kinetics of the transfersomes and pro-transfersomes penetration through the intact skin. Lidocaine loaded vesicles (local analgesics) are useful for determining the vesicles kinetics of penetration; corresponding subcutaneous injection is used as control. The animal's sensitivity to pain was then measured as a function of time at the treated site after each application.

If liposomes or simple lidocaine solution are applied via dermal route then they never caused any analgesic effect; It is necessary to achieve significant pain suppression by injecting such agents. But if we applied the lidocaine loaded transfersomes and pro-transfersomes, they show more analgesic effect which will be observed after the 15 minutes of application and the marked analgesic effect is still observed after very long time. In precise manner it is clear that kinetics of transfersomes and pro-transfersomes penetration through the skin are affected by various factors such as application condition or dosage form, drug carrier interaction, applied dose and skin characteristics (Planas and Cevec, 1992).

Ultra Deformable Vesicular System vs. Other Vesicular and Carrier Systems

Transfersomes and pro-transfersomes are differentiated from other vesicular system by their most important ultradeformable property; as this vesicular system is lipid bilayered vesicle like that of other vesicular systems such as, liposomes, niosomes, pharmacosomes etc. Transfersomes and pro-transfersomes have best property of more flexibility and adaptability which differentiate transfersomes and pro-transfersomes from other vesicular systems or commonly used liposomes. The ultradeformable nature of transfersomes and pro-transfersomes allows these to deform at the site of application to compress themselves even through the tiny pores which are smaller than their own size. The very high flexibility of the transfersomes and pro-transfersomes membrane is just because of combining at least two lipophilic/amphiphilic components like phosphatidyl choline. The resulted high degree of deformation allows transfersomes and pro-transfersomes to penetrate and cross the skin spontaneously; such kind of deeper penetration is achieved by the high hydrophilicity at the surface of transfersomes and pro-transfersomes which enforces to search for the surrounding of high water content activity.

The high penetration ability or penetration potential of the transfersomes and pro-transfersomes is not a result of stratum corneum fluidization by the surfactant because other micelle suspension contains more amount of surfactant than that of transfersomes and pro-transfersomes (Phosphatidyl Choline/ Sodium cholate 65/35 w/w %, respectively). Ultimately the increased penetration of transfersomes and pro-transfersomes as a result of solubilization of lipid present in the skin, so the authors expect same from or an even better penetration performance of the surfactant micelles. But the higher level of surfactant concentration in the micelles does not show the efficient penetration of material transport through or into the skin. As these mixed micelles stay on the upper part of the stratum corneum of skin even they are applied non-occlusively (Walve et al., 2011).

Mixed micelles are less sensitive to the trans-epidermal water activity gradient than that of transfersomes and pro-transfersomes. Transfersomes and pro-transfersomes are differentiated from the mixed micelles by basic two features:

1. A transfersome and pro-transfersome is normally by one to two orders of magnitude (in size) greater than standard lipid micelles.
2. Each vesicular transfersome and pro-transfersome contains a water filled core whereas a micelle is just a simple fatty droplet.

Micelles unable to carry and transfer fat-soluble agent and water while transfersomes and pro-transfersomes can have such application, mixed micelles can only transfer or incorporate substances having lipoid nature (Gompper and Kroll, 1995; Wearner et al., 1998). Label the mixed lipid micelles, liposomes and transfersomes and pro-transfersomess by using fluorescent markers and measured by the confocal scanning laser microscopy study (CSLM) in the intact murine skin to differentiate the penetration ability of all these carrier systems (Schatzlein and Cevc, 1998) and to propose the distribution profiles of these all vesicular systems. Out of all these vesicular systems the ultradeformable vesicles of transfersomes and pro-transfersomes penetrate through the stratum corneum and enter into epidermal layer in major quantity. It was reported that the mixed lipid micelles, liposomes are limited to the outer layer of the skin which have horny nature, while the intercellular seals and cellular packing are already compromised by the desquamation process. It is clear that vesicles of pure lipid or mixed micelles appear to access only the low-resistance pathways and thus able to reach upto the lower stratum corneum not in the deeper region of skin or get penetrated into the viable part of the skin in considerable quantity (see Table 2).

Table 2. Differentiation of various vesicles

Vesicular System	Merits	Demerits
Liposome	Biocompatible, Biodegradable	Stability issue, less penetration property
Pro-liposome	Greater stability than liposomes, Phospholipid vesicle	Also have less penetration property leads to aggregation and fusion of vesicles at the site of application
Niosome (Jain et al., 2006)	Improved stability due to use of non-ionic surfactants	Not efficient skin penetration
Pro-niosomes	Greater stability, in situ conversion into noisome	Deeper skin penetration problem
Transfersomes (Prajapati et al. 2011)	Ultradeformable with high stability, high penetration property due to high deformability, biodegradable and biocompatible, Incorporate low and high molecular weight drugs, Penetration into deeper skin regions.	None
Iontophoresis	Intermediate size charged molecule with increased penetration	Charged drugs can be penetrated

Walve et al., 2011.

APPLICATION OF TRANSFERSOMES AND PRO-TRANSFERSOMESS

Transfersomes and pro-transfersomes have wide variety of applications in the targeting of drug and other molecules through the transdermal route. Ultradeformable vesicle system is used as carrier for the delivery of peptides and transport of proteins. It is very difficult to transport big and large biogenic molecules such as body Proteins and peptide into the body, when administered through oral route; because such molecules shows it is complete degradation in the gastrointestinal tract. Parenteral route is best route of choice to administer these biogenic molecules into body. The number of options and ways are developed to tackle such kind of problems (Hofland et al., 1994) but transfersomes and pro-transfersomes are the best and suitable approach for the delivery of all kind of molecules into body. In case of suspension of protein, it is observed that bioavailability of the molecule delivered via dermal route in the form of transfersomes and pro-transfersomes is similar to that of drug administered via subcutaneous injection (Sachan et al., 2013; Shaw et al., 1999; Walve et al., 2011; Bai et al., 2001)

Pro-transfersomes can be used as better non parenteral delivery for transport of anticancer drugs such as cisplatin with site specific and improved drug action. It opens the options for treatment of skin cancer through transdermal route (Gupta et al. 2011).

The protein preparation in the form of transfersomes applied repetitively through epi-cutaneous route it induces strong immune response; for example, transfersomes of the bovine serum albumin (adjuvant immunogenic). The number of challenges in the path when the drug is delivered through dermal route; but advantageous thing is that the proteo-transfersomes preparations are active immunologically through transfersomes administration in comparison to system administered through parenteral route.

Transfersomes are also used as a carrier for number of molecules have high or low molecular weight, also for the hydrophilic and lipophilic drugs, likewise for naturally occurring protein interferons having antiproliferive, antiviral and some immunomodulatory effects, such as leukocytic derived interferon-α (INF-α). Ultradeformable nature of transfersomes and pro-transfersomes allows them to deliver the drug at specific site through various transport routes and these have ability to release the drug in controlled manner with increased stability in case of labile drugs. It is reported that the transfersome vesicular formulation of interferon-α and interleukin-2 potential shows best results via dermal route. For immune therapy delivery of IL-2 and INF- α in the form of transfersomes show better results in adequate concentration (Kombath et al., 2012).

Other applications of transfersomes and pro-transfersomes for the delivery of different molecules are as follows:

1. **Insulin Delivery:** It is non-invasive approach to deliver insulin in the form of transfersomes with increased therapeutic response; as it is clear that insulin is large molecular weight peptide bond linked amino acid. Subcutaneous route is commonly used route for the delivery of insulin which is not convenient and patient incompliance. Preparation of transfersulin (insulin transfersomes) by encapsulating insulin into vesicle system conquers the all problems in relation to delivery of insulin. After 1.5 to 3 hours hypoglycemic effect is observed during application of insulin transfersome through skin in case of diabetic patient, which is depend on the composition of vesicular system as carrier.
2. **Corticosteroid Delivery:** The class corticosteroid of drugs can be delivered via dermal route by preparing it into transfersomes vesicular system. Vesicular system imparts the site specificity and safety of corticosteroid drugs delivery into the deeper part of skin; by optimizing prescribed amount

of drug which is applied through the transdermal route. Low amount of dose is required for the delivery of corticosteroids in the form of transfersomes in the certain kind of skin treatments.

3. **Peptides Delivery and Targeting of Proteins:** Transfersomes possess ultradeformable nature which is utilized for the transport of peptides and targeting of boy proteins. Parenteral route is best route of choice to administer these biogenic molecules into body. The number of options and ways are developed to tackle such kind of problems but transfersome is the best and suitable approach for the delivery of all kind of molecules into body. In case of suspension of protein it is observed that bioavailability of the molecule delivered via dermal route in the form of transfersome is similar to that of drug administered via subcutaneous injection.
4. **Interferon Delivery:** Transfersomes also used as a carrier for number of molecules have high or low molecular weight, also for the hydrophilic and lipophilic drugs, likewise for naturally occurring protein interferons having antiproliferive, antiviral and some immunomodulatory effects, such as leukocytic derived interferon-α (INF-α). Ultradeformable nature of transfersomes allows themself to deliver the drug at specific site through various transport routes and it have ability to release the drug in controlled manner with increased stability in case of labile drugs. It is reported that the transfersome vesicular formulation of interferon-α and interleukin-2 potential shows best results via dermal route. For immune therapy delivery of IL-2 and INF- α in the form of transfersomes show better results in adequate concentration.
5. **Anticancer Drugs Delivery:** Vesicular approach of deformation property can be used for the delivery of anticancer drug such as methotrexate which applied through transdermal route; the response obtained is more positive in comparison to methotrexate administered through other system. Recently this technology is suitable for treatment of skin cancer.
6. **Anesthetic Delivery:** Anesthesia is important before minor and major surgeries; ultradeformable vesicular system is new approach for topical anesthesia with positive results within few minutes under some conditions. Longer anesthesia is observed in comparison to subcutaneous bolus injection.
7. **In Delivery of Non-Steroidal Anti-Inflammatory (NSAIDs) Drugs:** Most of the drugs falls in the category of non-steroidal anti-inflammatory have numerous gastrointestinal tract side effects with desired pharmacological response. Such kind of problems overcomes by formulating ultra-deformable vesicles to apply through dermal route. Literature gives an idea for such issues in case of drugs ketoprofen and salt form of diclofenac. The marketed transfersome formulation of ketoprofen is launched by company SwissMedic in 2007 with name Diractin and now available in Switzerland. Some of the formulations based under the same technology by IDEA AG, are in clinical development and expected to launch in market.
8. **Herbal Molecules Delivery:** Ultradeformable vesicular system has ability to penetrate deeper into skin towards stratum corneum and able to transport the nutrients via dermal route for active functioning of skin. It is reported that capsaicin transfersome shows better absorption than that of capsaicin (pure).

Among the all applications of transfersomes the most important applications is immunization via transdermal route by use of soluble protein loaded transfersomes, also in case of integral membrane protein, gap junction protein, human serum albumin; for all mentioned molecules administration is not through parenteral route which is painful.

Transfersomes and pro-transfersomes look up for better site specificity and safety of drug molecules of corticosteroid delivery through skin by optimizing the epi-cutaneously administered drug dose (Trotta et al., 2004; Dubey et al., 2006; Xiao et al., 2006; Matthias et al., 2009) (see Table 3).

CONCLUSION

Transfersomes and pro-transfersomes are recent technology which is optimized with an aim to transport and deliver different molecules at specific site via transdermal route. Basically transfersomes and pro-transfersomes is an ultradeformable vesicular system to target drug molecules through dermal way. Basic composition of this vesicular system is commonly used phospholipid such as phospatidyl choline with other surfactants and additives. It is prepared by simple techniques of hand shaking and evapora-

Table 3. Different drugs and their results after transfersome formulation

Drug	Result
Norgesterol (Jain et al., 1998)	Greater transdermal flux
Tamoxifen (Bhatia et al., 2004)	Greater transdermal flux
Oestradiol (Maghraby et al., 1998)	Improved transdermal flux
Topical analgesic and anesthetic agent (Tetracaine, lignocain) (Planas et al., 1992)	Best approach for the non-parenteral treatment of local pain in comparison to other modes of administration.
Corticosteroids Hydrocortisone Triamcinolone acetonide (Cevc et al., 1997)	Improved safety of drug with their site specific nature. Shows better pharmacological response in case of vesicular system at low dose. Used in both local and systemic delivery.
Soluble proteins (Paul et al., 1995) Gap junction proteins Human serum albumin (Paul and Cevec., 1998) Integral membrane protein (Paul et al., 1995)	Allows non-invasive immunization via skin. Quantity of Ab titer is same or even slightly higher than other parenteral injection.
Interferon-α Interleukin-2 (Hafer et al., 1999)	Efficient delivery Controlled release. No issue of stability.
Insulin (Cevc et al., 1998)	More entrapment of drug. Transportation of moiety through skin is more than half of their original amount. Non parenteral route of drug administration
Curcumin (Patel et al., 2009; Saraf et al., 2011)	Better permeation for anti-inflammatory activity
Indinavir sulfate (Sheo et al., 2010;Jalon et al. 2001)	Improved influx for activity against AIDS
Ketoprofen (Matthias et al., 2009)	Improved penetration for anti-inflammatory activity
Capsaicin	Improved passage through skin
Colchicine	Improved passage through skin
Vincristine	Improved drug entrapment and skin permeation
Methotrexate (Trotta et al., 2004)	Improved transdermal flux
Stavudine (Sheo et al.,2010)	Improved the in vitro skin delivery of Stavudine for antiretroviral activity
Tetanus toxoid (Gupta et al., 2005)	Immunization via dermal route.

tion like that of liposomes. It has ability to deliver large as well as low molecular weight molecules at specific site via transdermal route. It is a technology by which easy to incorporate hydrophilic as well as lipophilic drug by entrapment for the better therapeutic response. Drug and other molecules such as insulin, interferon, interleukins, corticosteroids and number of NSAIDs can be delivered via transdermal route. In comparison to other conventional systems transfersomes and pro-transfersomes show increased entrapment efficiency and site specificity. Transfersomes and pro-transfersomes can deliver drug via different intracellular and trans-cellular route through intact skin with increased penetration into deeper part of skin.

Transfersomes and pro-transfersomes are able to deliver the drug at specific site through via transdermal route by an external stress due to water gradient; so these ultradeformable vesicles used to carry the drug and other molecules across the different layers of skin as barrier. Transfersomes and pro-transfersomes have ability to pass through very small pores of size 100 nm; so this is best way of drug delivery in comparison to painful injections. This system can transfer more amounts of drug / unit time through the biological barriers such as skin in comparison to other topical systems; so the drug systemic availability is normally more than other approaches. Radio labeled phospholipids in the form of transfersomes and pro-transfersomes have better bio-distribution into deeper region of skin and it is same after an epi-cutaneous application or subcutaneous injection of the preparations within 1 day. In future, transfersomes and pro-transfersomes will be the best vesicular approach to deliver different kind of molecules to achieve desired therapeutic effect via transdermal route; when it is used under normal application conditions. Now It is an opportunity for the researchers of new era to modify new techniques for the preparation of transfersomes and pro-transfersomes with an aim to deliver the large molecules through intact skin to cure all the kind of infections and diseases by specific site targeting.

REFERENCES

Bai, B. V., Wertz, P. W., Junginer, H. E., & Bouwstra, J. A. (2001). Elasticity of vesicles assessed by electron microscopy and extrusion measurement. *International Journal of Pharmaceutics*, *217*, 13–2. doi:10.1016/S0378-5173(01)00576-2 PMID:11292538

Benson, H. A. (2006). Transfersomes for transdermal drug delivery. *Expert Opinion on Drug Delivery*, *3*(6), 727–737. doi:10.1517/17425247.3.6.727 PMID:17076595

Bhatia, A., & Kumar, R. (2004). Tamoxifen in topical liposomes: Development, characterization and in-vitro evaluation. *Journal of Pharmaceutical Sciences*, *7*(2), 252–259. PMID:15367383

Cevc, G. (1991). Isothermal lipid phase. *Transitions Chemistry and Physics of Lipids*, *57*(2-3), 293–299. doi:10.1016/0009-3084(91)90082-M PMID:2054910

Cevc, G., Blume, G., & Schatzlein, A. (1997). Transfersomes-mediated transepidermal delivery improves the regiospecificity and biological activity of corticosteroids in vivo. *Journal of Controlled Release*, *45*, 211–226. doi:10.1016/S0168-3659(96)01566-0

Cevc, G., Blume, G., Sehatzlein, A., Gebauer, D., & Paul, A. (1996). The skin- a pathway for systemic treatment with patches and lipid-based agent carriers. *Advanced Drug Delivery Reviews*, *18*(3), 349–378. doi:10.1016/0169-409X(95)00091-K

Chapman, S. J., & Walsh, A. (1990). Desmosomes and desquamation: An ultrastructural study of adult pig epidermis. *Archives of Dermatological Research*, *282*(5), 304–310. doi:10.1007/BF00375724 PMID:2221982

Dubey, V., Mishra, D., Asthana, A., & Jain, N. K. (2006). Transdermal delivery of a pineal hormone: Melatonin via elastic liposomes. *Biomaterials*, *27*(18), 3491–3496. doi:10.1016/j.biomaterials.2006.01.060 PMID:16513163

Elsayed, M. M., Abdallah, O. Y., & Nagar, V. F. (2006). Deformable liposomes and ethosomes: Mechanism of enhanced skin delivery. *International Journal of Pharmaceutics*, *322*(1-2), 60–66. doi:10.1016/j.ijpharm.2006.05.027 PMID:16806755

Fry, D. W., White, J. C., & Goldman, I. D. (1978). Rapid separation of low molecular weight solutes from liposomes without dilution. *Journal of Analytical Biochemistry*, *90*(2), 809–815. doi:10.1016/0003-2697(78)90172-0 PMID:727510

Gamal, M., Maghraby, M., Williams, A. C., & Barry, B. W. (1999). Skin delivery of oestradiol from deformable and traditional liposomes- Mechanistic studies. *The Journal of Pharmacy and Pharmacology*, *51*(10), 1123–1134. doi:10.1211/0022357991776813 PMID:10579683

Gompper, G., & Kroll, D. M. (1995). Driven transport of fluid vesicles through narrow pores. *Physical Review E: Statistical Physics, Plasmas, Fluids, and Related Interdisciplinary Topics*, *52*(4), 4198–4211. doi:10.1103/PhysRevE.52.4198 PMID:9963891

Gupta, P. N., Mishra, V., Singh, P., Rawat, A., Dubey, P., Mahor, S., & Vyas, S. P. (2005). Tetanus toxoid-loaded transfersomes for topical immunization. *The Journal of Pharmacy and Pharmacology*, *57*(3), 295–301. doi:10.1211/0022357055515 PMID:15807984

Gupta, V., Agrawal, R., & Triwedi, P. (2011). Reduction in cisplatin genotoxity in non-target cells of mice by protrasfersome gel formulation used for management of cutaneous squamous cell carcinoma. *Acta Pharmaceutica (Zagreb, Croatia)*, *61*, 63–71. doi:10.2478/v10007-011-0004-8 PMID:21406344

Hafcr, C., Goblc, R., Dccring, P., Lchmcr, A., & Breut, J. (1999). Formulation of interleukin-2 and Interferon-a containing ultradeformable carriers for potential transdermal application. *Journal of Anticancer Research*, *19*(2c), 1505–1512. PMID:10365133

Heather, A., & Benson, E. (2005). Transdermal drug delivery: Penetration enhancement techniques. *Current Drug Delivery*, *2*(1), 23–33. doi:10.2174/1567201052772915 PMID:16305405

Hofland, H., Bootstrap, J. A., Spies, F., Gooris, G., & Nagelkerke, J. F. (1994). Liposomes as carriers for topical and transdermal delivery. *Journal of Pharmaceutical Sciences*, *83*(9), 1189–1203. doi:10.1002/jps.2600830902 PMID:7830230

Jain, C. P., Vyas, S. P., & Dixit, V. K. (2006). Niosomal system for delivery of rifampicin to lymphatics. *International Journal of Pharmaceutics*, *68*, 57–58.

Jain, N. K. (2001). *Advances in controlled and novel drug delivery*. New Delhi: CBS Publishers and Distributers.

Jalon, G. E., Ygartua, P., & Santoyo, S. (2001). Topical application of acyclovir-loaded microparticles: Quantification of the drug in porcine skin layers. *Journal of Controlled Release*, *75*(1-2), 191–197. doi:10.1016/S0168-3659(01)00395-9 PMID:11451509

Kombath, R., Minumula, S., Sockalingam, A., Subadhra, S., Parre, S., Reddy, T. & David, B. (2012). Critical issues related to transfersomes – Novel vesicular system. *Acta Sci Pol Tech Aliment*, 67-82.

Maghraby, E. I., Williams, M., & Barry, B. W. (1998). Optimization of deformable vesicles for epidermal delivery of oestradiol. *The Journal of Pharmacy and Pharmacology*, *50*(S9), 146. doi:10.1111/j.2042-7158.1998.tb02346.x

Matthias, R., Egbert, J., Priscilla, M., Stefan, M., Ulrich, V., & Ilka, R. (2009). Efficacy of epicutaneous diractin® (ketoprofen in transfersome® gel) for the treatment of pain related to eccentric muscle contractions. *Drug Des Devel Ther*, *3*, 143–149. PMID:19920930

Maurya, S., Aggarwal, S., Tilak, V., Dhakar, R., Singh, A., & Maurya, G. (2010). Enhanced transdermal delivery of indinavir sulfate via transfersomes. *IJCP*, *1*(06), 1–7.

Nanda, A., Nanda, S., Dhall, M., & Rao, R. (2005). Transferosomes: A novel ultradeformable vesicular carrier for transdermal drug delivery. *Drug Delivery Technology*, *5*(8), 59–64.

Panchagnula, R. (1997). Transdermal delivery of drugs. *Indian Journal of Pharmacology*, *29*, 140–156.

Patel, R., Singh, S., Singh, S., Sheth, N., & Gendle, R. (2009). Development and characterization of curcumin loaded transfersome for transdermal delivery. *Journal of Pharm Sci Res*, *1*(4), 71–80.

Paul, A., & Cevec, G. (1998). Non-invasive administration of protein antigens epicutaneous with bovin serum albulmine. *Vaccine Research*, *4*, 145–164.

Paul, A., Cevec, G., & Bachhavat, B. K. (1995). Transdermal immunization with large proteins by means of ultradeformable drug carriers. *European Journal of Immunology*, *25*(12), 3551–3524. doi:10.1002/eji.1830251248 PMID:8566048

Planas, M., Gonzalez, P., Rodriguez, S., Sanchez, G. & Cevc, G. (1992). Noninvasive percutaneous induction of topical analgesia by a new type of drug carrier, and prolongation of local pain insensitivity by anesthetic liposomes. *Anesthia Analoge*, 615-621.

Prajapati, S. T., Patel, C. G., & Patel, C. N. (2011). Transfersomes: A vesicular carrier system for transdermal drug delivery. *Asian J Biochemical Pharma Res*, *1*(2), 507–524.

Rand, R. P., & Parsegian, V. A. (1989). Hydration forces between phospholipid bilayers. *Biochimica et Biophysica Acta*, *988*(3), 351–377. doi:10.1016/0304-4157(89)90010-5

Sachan, R., Parashar, T., Singh, V., Singh, G., Tyagi, S., Patel, C., & Gupta, A. (2013). Drug carrier transfersomes: A novel tool for transdermal drug delivery system. *IJRDPLS*, *2*(2), 309–316.

Saraf, S., Jeswani, G., Deep Kaur, C., & Saraf, S. (2011). Development of novel herbal cosmetic cream with curcuma longa extract loaded transfersomes for anti-wrinkle effect. *African J Pharm Pharmacol*, *5*(8), 1054–1062.

Schatzlein, A., & Cevc, G. (1995). *Skin penetration by phospholipids vesicles, transfersomes as visualized by means of the confocal scanning laser microscopy, in characterization, metabolism, and novel biological applications*. Champaign, IL: AOCS Press.

Schatzlein, A., & Cevc, G. (1998). Non-uniform cellular packing of the stratum corneum and permeability barrier function of intact skin: A high-resolution confocal laser scanning microscopy study using highly deformable vesicles (Transfersomes). *The British Journal of Dermatology*, *138*(4), 583–598. doi:10.1046/j.1365-2133.1998.02166.x PMID:9640361

Sheo, D., Shweta, A., Ram, C., Ghanshyam, M., Girish, K., & Sunil, K. (2010). Transfersomes- a novel vesicular carrier for enhanced transdermal delivery of stavudine: Development, characterization and performance evaluation. *Journal of Scientific Speculations and Res*, *1*(1), 30–36.

Trotta, M., Peira, E., Carlotti, M., & Gallarate, M. (2004). Deformable liposomes for dermal administration of methotrexate. *International Journal of Pharmaceutics*, *270*(1-2), 119–125. doi:10.1016/j.ijpharm.2003.10.006 PMID:14726128

Walve, J., Bakliwal, S., Rane, B., & Pawar, S. (2011). Transfersomes: A surrogated carrier for transdermal drug delivery system. *IJABPT*, *2*(1), 204–213.

Wearner, R. R., Myers, M. C., & Taylor, D. A. (1988). Electron probe analysis of human skin: Determination of the water concentration profile. *The Journal of Investigative Dermatology*, *90*(2), 218–224. doi:10.1111/1523-1747.ep12462252 PMID:3339263

Section 6
Biosimilars

Chapter 7
Biosimilars:
Concept and Regulation

Anil K. Sharma
Delhi Institute of Pharmaceutical Sciences and Research, India

Raj K. Keservani
Rajiv Gandhi Proudyogiki Vishwavidhyalaya, India

Rajesh K. Kesharwani
National Institute of Technology, Warangal, India

ABSTRACT

Biosimilars are a new class of drugs, which are derived from live organism through the recombinant DNA technology. These are recently introduced in the pharmaceutical field for the preparation of drug to prevent or control the diseases. Patients with diabetes and renal failure may already be receiving biosimilar epoetin and may receive same insulin in coming years. The main aim of present article is to introduce the fundamentals of biologics and to explain how they are different and what these differences mean for pharmacists.

INTRODUCTION

Biosimilars also called follow-on biologics are biological medical products, whose active moieties are generated from a living organism via recombinant DNA or controlled gene expression methods. These terms are used to portray officially approved ensuing types of innovator biopharmaceutical products designed by a different sponsors following patent and exclusivity expiry of the innovator's product (Nick, 2012). The definition of biosimilars by different regulatory authorities is as follows:

1. **The World Health Organization:** A biotherapeutic product, which is similar in terms of quality, safety and efficacy to an already licensed reference biotherapeutic product (WHO, 2009).
2. **The European Medicines Agency:** A biological medicine that is generated to be comparable to an existing biological medicine (the 'reference medicine'). Upon approval, a biosimilar's variance

DOI: 10.4018/978-1-5225-0751-2.ch007

and any deviation between it and its reference medicine will have to be shown not to affect safety or effectiveness (EMA, 2012).

3. **The U.S. Food and Drug Administration:** A biological product that is remarkably comparable to a U.S. licensed reference biological product notwithstanding minor differences in clinically inactive components and for which there are no clinically meaningful divergence between the biological product and the reference product in specifications of the safety, purity and potency of the product (USFDA, 2012).

The use of biotechnology to develop medicines is rapidly growing and it is estimated that biological medicines are likely to become the biggest selling medicinal products by 2016 (Pharmacophorum, 2012). Global Industry Analysts Inc. (GIA) has forecasted that biosimilars market around the world is expected to achieve $18 billion by 2017 (GIAI, 2012). Driven by the passing by the US Congress of the 2010 Biologics Price Competition and Innovation Act (BPCI), it is also suggested that the US will go beyond Europe during analysis period to become globally largest market for biosimilars in the near future.

Biotechnology uses proteins, enzymes, antibodies and other substances that are produced in the human body to create biological medicines. Living organisms are also used in the production of these medicines, including plant and animal cells, bacteria and viruses. Biological medicines are much more complex than conventional medicines, which are comparatively simpler chemical molecules (APG, 2011). Since 2006, 13 biosimilars have been granted marketing authorizations in the EU (EBE-EFPIA, 2006) and the use of these presents challenges for clinical practice that are different to those that relate to conventional generic medicines.

All biotechnology products, including biosimilars have different starting materials and manufacturing processes, which means they have different characteristics that may not be detectable in conventional clinical trials such as rare adverse drug reactions, especially events that are immune mediated. This key difference has influenced the current legislative framework for biosimilars, which treats biosimilars differently to conventional generic medicines (EBE-EFPIA 2006). Biosimilars present a different set of challenges as compared with conventional generics. Further market approval for biosimilars is much complicated. The intricacy of biopharmaceuticals renders it hard to circumvent heterogeneity among batches from the same manufacturer and between the same products from different manufacturers (Crommelin et al., 2005). Moreover, it is not easy to ascertain therapeutic equivalence of biosimilars with reference products and compounds used in clinical trials (Roger, 2006; Chirino and Mire-sluis, 2004; Locatelli, 2006).

Need of Biosimilars

Medicinal products generated by biotechnology make an essential part of medicaments available to patients nowadays. They represent about 6% of the pharmaceuticals presently marketed and account for more than 9% of gross pharmaceutical expenses (IMS Health, 2009). More significantly, one third of products in the pipeline are derived biotechnologically. A number of main biotechnology derived medicines are, or will soon go off patent (Mellstedt et al., 2007). This brings up competition to the market, which facilitates patient reach to safe, effective and more affordable biotechnology-derived products. The prices of the innovator products would remain artificially high in absence of competition. At the same time, fair competition will serve to trigger research for new medicines.

The scene in the US where more than 50% of medicines utilized are generic medicines reinforces this fact. At the same time, more and more new innovator medicines are developed in US than anywhere else in the world (Zanotech, 2007; BMI, 2008). Another imperative cause for introducing biosimilar medicines is, of course, that the scientific base for biosimilar development and technology lies to take approval and bring these new medicines to the market. Consequently, a legal framework has been set up in Europe in order to govern development and approval of biosimilars.

Medicinal Product Derived from Biologicals

Biological medicines (also known as biopharmaceuticals) are made up of proteins viz. - hormones (growth hormones, insulins, erythropoietins), enzymes that are produced in the human body, or monoclonal antibodies as well as blood products, immunological products such as sera and vaccines, allergens and advanced technology products.

Biotechnology employs living systems (plant or animal cells, bacteria, viruses and yeast) and modern technologies to develop biological medicines to cure diseases and genetic disorders in humans. Many, but not all biologicals are made exploiting genetically modified cells (CIP, 2013).

Difference between Chemical and Biosimilar Drug

The principal differentiation among the chemical and biosimilar drugs are given in Table 1 (Paul, 2012).

Size and Structure

Drug are small low molecular compounds (<1000 Da) and active in a definite conformation against the diseases. Biological products have larger sizes and more complex structures and the range varies from 4000 Da for non-glycosylated proteins to more than 140,000 Da for monoclonal antibodies (Lanthier et al., 2008).

Recombinant-protein drugs fold into three-dimensional structures that have four distinct levels. Amino acids form linear arrangement of polypeptide with the help of peptide covalent bonds between

Table 1. Difference between chemical and biosimilar drug

S. N.	Chemical Drug	Biosimilar Drug
1.	It is produced by chemical synthesis	It is produced by living cell cultures
2.	Low Mol.wt.	High Mol.wt.
3.	Chemical drug has well-defined structure	Biological drug has complex, heterogeneous structure
4.	They are generally process-independent	They are strongly process-dependent
5.	It is thoroughly characterized	Impossible to entirely characterize the molecular composition and heterogeneity
6.	They are stable	Unstable, sensitive to external conditions
7.	They are often non-immunogenic	Immunogenic

the amino group of one amino acid and the carboxyl group of the next, which is referred to as the primary structure of proteins.

Stability

Small molecules tend to follow Arrhenius behavior (thermally dependent molecular motion) and thus have predictable stability based on acceleration studies. In contrast, the biological activity and function of proteins are highly dependent on their unique 3 dimensional conformation, which is the reason, that biologicals are much less stable than small-molecule compounds (Schellekens, 2005).

Pharmacokinetic Differences

Chemical drugs have higher oral bioavailability, as biologics (usually proteins) which will be degraded by proteases. These have the property to rapidly diffuse across the cell membranes and reached to intracellular sites of action inside the cell. Therefore, biologic drugs have been used as an injection form to human bodies and required high purity and safety.

Pharmacological Mechanisms

Chemotherapeutic compounds show their pharmacological activity via inhibiting or inducing the enzymatic or protein function via binding with the active or allosteric sites e.g. tamoxifen, a small-molecule drug, used as standard endocrine chemotherapeutic agent for the treatment of steroid hormone receptor-positive breast cancer.

It can competitively bind to estrogen receptors of tumor cells and also on other normal cells of tissue and inhibit or decrease the synthesis of DNA or inhibition of estrogen effect together with the cell proliferation of tumor cells. The pharmacological effect and mechanisms of biologic products are varying from those of drugs. Hormones have been used to treat the disease and show pharmacological effects via the alleviation of deficiencies. For example, for the treatment of diabetes, biosynthetic human insulin is commonly used to treat and fulfill the insulin deficiency, and in case of growth disorder of children and adult human growth hormone is used (Los et al., 2007).

Safety

The conventional therapeutic drugs are usually considered to have a higher toxicity in comparison to biologicals. Such therapeutics may affect the function of other enzyme or protein by binding to its active site and cause toxicity or off-target effects; many anticancer drugs target both normal and cancerous cells and show toxic effects in form of non-proper growth and metabolic functions. During metabolism of such anti-cancerous drug, it may get converted into toxic metabolites and leading to carcinogenesis and mutagenesis. In contrast, biologic products have less toxicity, but for human safety an important issue that needs to be considered is immunogenicity. For example, there is an increase in the number of cases of Ab-mediated pure red cell aplasia (PRCA) associated with one specific formulation of epoetin-distributed outside the USA (Schellekens, 2003).

Table 2. Marketed products of biosimilars and their uses

S. N.	Product Name	Biological Name	Manufacturer	Uses
1.	Tevagrastim	Filgrastim	Aspen Pharmacare P/L	Myelosuppressive or myeloablative chemotherapy used to treat the disease neutropenia, the mobilization of peripheral blood progenitor cells in normal volunteers has been used to treat patients infected with HIV and allogenic cell therapy.
2.	Nivestim	Filgrastim (rbe)	Hospira P/L	Myelosuppressive or myeloablative chemotherapy used to treat the disease neutropenia, the mobilization of peripheral blood progenitor cells in normal volunteers has been used to treat patients infected with HIV and allogenic cell therapy.
3.	Zarzio	Filgrastim (rbe)	Sandoz P/L	Myelosuppressive or myeloablative chemotherapy used to treat the disease neutropenia, the mobilization of peripheral blood progenitor cells in normal volunteers has been used to treat patients infected with HIV and allogenic cell therapy.
4.	Novicrit	Epoetin lambda (rch)	Novartis Pharm. Aust. P/L	Treatment of anaemia in chronic renal failure, non-myeloid malignancies or enable/augment pre-elective surgery blood donations to minimize allogenic blood transfusions.

Marketed Products and Uses of Biosimilars

Currently different company manufactured biosimilar drugs for the diverse diseased conditions, but some of available marketed product are given in Table 2 (Roger, 2010; BMP, 2014).

The biosimilar products market is segmented into recombinant peptides, recombinant non-glycosylated proteins and, recombinant glycosylated proteins. The recombinant non-glycosylated proteins market is further divided in insulin, granulocyte colony-stimulating factor (G-CSF), human growth hormone and, interferons, whereas the recombinant glycosylated proteins market belongs to erythropoietin, monoclonal antibodies, and follitropin. Recombinant peptide is divided into Calcitonin and Glucagon. Monoclonal antibody production is one of the fastest growing and lucrative markets for drug manufacturer companies, for future investment to develop mAb at a large scale and is also an estimated CAGR of 41.9% from 2013 to 2018.

From the current data, it is found that about eight biologic mAb drugs are expected to become off-patent products from 2013 to 2018. Some drugs are going to lose their patent protection within few years are Rituxan/mAbThera, Remicade, Herceptin, Humira, Avastin, Synagis, Erbitux, and Lucentis. The RituximAb, InfliximAb, and AdalimumAb are three most targeted products for biosimilars because of their huge sales all over the world and approvals for multiple indications. Due to high scope and response of mAbs use many generic drug manufacturer key industries have been started to work on the manufacturing and clinical trial activities and about 50 biosimilar mAbs are in the pipeline for future use. Alone a Switzerland based company Bioexpress Therapeutic has 16 biosimilar products of mAbs in the pipeline. Many other companies have started to invest their money in the development and production of mAbs are Celltrion (South Korea), Zydus-Cadila (India), GeneTechno Science (Japan), Biocon (India), and Samsung Biologics (South Korea). Among all the mAbs, insulin alone will be the fastest growing segment and is estimated to grow at a Compound Annual Growth Rate (CAGR) of 35.6% from 2013 to 2018.

The growth is attributed to the rise in incidences of diabetes, ongoing patent expirations of biologic drugs such as Lantus, Humalog, and Novorapid, and the cost effectiveness of the biosimilars of insulin.

Other factors that drive the global market are the rise in the number of off-patented biologic drugs, rise in incidences of chronic disorders, growing pressure to cut healthcare expenditure, rise in aging populations, and government support and initiatives.

Across countries, China and India are considered attractive destinations for R&D outsourcing of foreign biosimilar manufacturing companies that look to reduce their growing R&D costs and increase the number of drug applications and approvals. Both the countries are expected to grow at the fastest CAGR of 30.2% and 29% from 2013 to 2018. Factors responsible for the high growth rate in India and China are the lack of government regulations with regards to the approval of biosimilars, the low Intellectual Property (IP) protection of biologic compounds in China, semi regulatory environment to approve biosimilars in India, and low manufacturing costs, that have enabled domestic manufacturers to market the generic version of biologic compounds at a low price.

Sandoz has emerged as the market leader in the global market and is likely to maintain this leadership position in the coming years. Sandoz entered the biosimilars market in 2006, with the launch of Omnitrope (human growth hormone)-a biosimilar drug-in the European market. Sandoz's biosimilar product offerings include Zarzio (G-CSF), Omnitrope (Human Growth Hormone), and Binocrit (epoeitin-alpha). Thus, the broad product portfolio enables the company to gain a competitive advantage over other players in the market. The company focuses on strengthening their market position by significantly investing in research and development activities. It has a robust biosimilar pipeline with about 10 drugs.

Teva, another major player, has the capability to provide a stiff competition to Sandoz. In 2000 Teva entered the biosimilars market by setting up a clear long term biosimilar strategy. Since then Teva has undergone several acquisitions and agreements with contract manufacturing organizations as well as various strategic alliances to strengthen their manufacturing unit and R&D capabilities. Other notable players are Hospira (U.S.), Dr. Reddy's Laboratories (India), Biocon Ltd. (India), Mylan (U.S.), Biopartners (Switzerland), Amgen (U.S.), and Intas Biopharmaceultical Ltd. (India).

Recently Ranbaxy has launched India's first biosimilar of inflictimAb drug, INFIMAB™. This product is being introduced in the Indian market through a licensing partnership with EPIRUS Biopharmaceuticals, Inc. a US and Swiss-based biopharmaceutical company focused on the global development and commercialization of biosimilar monoclonal antibodies. The innovator reference product is currently marketed for the treatment of inflammatory diseases including rheumatoid arthritis, Crohn's Disease, ankylosing spondylitis, ulcerative colitis, psoriatic arthritis and psoriasis.

Patient Safety of Biosimilars

Patient safety is most important for any drug development protocol or process and in case of biosimilar it is very crucial. Biosimilars are more complex and any minute changes in the structure can cause very drastic effect and harm for the human body and even of foremost concern for the development of all medicines, but biosimilars raise safety issues after those of chemical drugs. This is because biosimilars are more structurally intricate drugs than chemical drugs, and even small deviation by their manufacturer may lead to undetected changes in the biological makeup of the product. These changes can in turn influence the safety and effectiveness of the product. (Johnson, 2008).

Products that lost patent shield few years back, such as human insulin, still do not have a biosimilar in Western Europe or the US. However, biosimilars approvals have gained acceleration in Europe recently. The so-called first wave that started losing patent protection in the past years is now a crowded zone. For example, India itself has minimum of 13 companies that hunt EPO (erythropoietin), which is the precursor to darbepoeitin. Three of them are preparing for entry to Europe. EPOs from Sandoz and Teva, the world first and second, respectively in biosimilars, are previously there.

Approval Pathways for Biologic and Biosimilar Medicines

Innovator companies and biosimilar manufacturers must submit robust data to demonstrate a product's efficacy and safety profile prior to grant of marketing authorization by regulators such as the U.S. Food and Drug Administration (FDA) or the European Medicines Agency (EMA)/European Commission (EC). Elaborate analytical chemistry, manufacturing and control (CMC), non-clinical and clinical proofs are likely desired for the relevant therapeutic area (EMA, 2012; USFDA 2012). A decision on how detailed clinical data is required depends on each individual case. However, the quantum of clinical efficacy and safety data will be somewhat lesser for a biosimilar than the original biologic (Niederwieser and Schmitz, 2011). The 2012 draft FDA biosimilar guidance provides a list of factors that a sponsor should consider while assessing the similarity of its proposed products including: (USFDA, 2012).

- Expression system,
- Manufacturing process,
- Physicochemical properties,
- Functional activities,
- Receptor binding and immunochemical properties,
- Impurities,
- Characterization of the reference product and reference standards,
- Characterization of the finished drug product,
- Stability.

REGULATORY MODELS FOR BIOSIMILARS

A number of countries have regulatory committee set up for monitoring and approval of biosimilar products and amongst them European Union has the latest framework in this order. Canada's regulatory authority is not yet finalized but is already in parlance. World Health Organization together with US and Japan is trying to establish the regulatory authority and also set the global standard, monitor the selection of biosimilar products for public use. These are few facts which are broadly under discussion. There are mainly two levels which are used to analyze various approaches, First, protocol or style which is based on mainly safety concerns e.g. whether they require additional clinical data, within reason, for the approval of a biosimilar, prerequisites for post-marketing safety studies, the standard they adopt for interchangeability, etc., Second, the manner in which such frameworks deal with different intellectual property issues (including questions concerning patents and data exclusivity).

In general, it can be illustrious that like the abbreviated process for generic drugs, these frameworks tend to assess biosimilars based on how they compare to the original biologic (in terms of quality, safety and efficacy rather than on their individual worth, although this is partially correct for the two US proposals. Besides, the frameworks tend to determine the necessary clinical studies based on the scientific differences between the biosimilar and the original biologic. This may attribute to improve the efficiency at the clinical stage without sacrificing public safety.

European Union (EU)

European Union (EU) has taken first time initiative and developed regulatory authority to monitor the production of biosimilars by making amendment to the article 10(4) of Human Medicine Directive (2001/83/EC) EU's Code by Directive 2004/27/EC in the year 2004. This amendment helps to get approval for such biologics which are similar to the natural. However, the legislation confers a wide margin of prudence to the Committee for Medicinal Products for Human Use (CHMP) of the European Medicines Agency (EMEA) to develop product class-specific guidelines that decide the level of nonclinical and clinical testing that will be essential. Since 2006, EMEA has issued guidelines encompassing several types of recombinant proteins, including insulin, granulocyte-colony stimulating factor (G-CSF), somotropin and erythropoietin, low-molecular weight heparins (EMEA, 2009). Hitherto, EMEA has allowed about 13 biosimilars, all versions of Somatropin, Epoetin alfa, Epoetin zeta or Filgrastim (Perry, 2009).

Safety Standards

EMEA's product class-specific guidelines (as well as the primary EU legislation) assist to lay down a bare minimum standard for safety in the approval of biosimilars. They explicitly require the outcome of preclinical and clinical tests, although they differ as to the level of testing- for somatropin, the guideline suggests at least 1 clinical trial, while for erythropoietins at least two are needed (Tsang and Kracov, 2008). EMEA has brought unique guidelines for immunogenicity determination and for cases in which changes are made to the manufacturing process post approval. Further, all the products authorized so far are subject to post-marketing safety surveillance. As mentioned in preceding sections, with reference to whether a biosimilar is interchangeable or spontaneously substitutable, although the decision is a national competency, EMEA has asserted that biosimilars cannot be considered similar to original biologics. Accordingly, 15 member states have either banned automatic substitution of biosimilars for original biologics (i.e. UK, Germany, Sweden, Spain and the Netherlands) or need of physician to prescribe by brand name (i.e. Greece, Austria, Czech Republic) (Stanley, 2008). The standard for employing the same International Nonproprietary Name (INN) as the reference biologic remains imprecise at the European level. Biosimilars are essential to have a diverse trade name, but do not need a different INN. Consequently, in practice some biosimilars use the reference drug's INN, while others do not.

World Health Organization (WHO)

World Health Organization WHO has formulated an outline of general ideology as part of its "Biological Standardization Process" that seeks to oversee the scientific aspects of biosimilars approval (Kang, 2009). The WHO plans to decide it subsequent to a public discussion. To help in the standardization process, WHO defines a biosimilar, which it labels a "similar biological product" (SBP), as a biotherapeutic product claimed to be similar in terms of quality, safety and efficacy to an existing licensed reference biotherapeutic product (RBP), which must have been licensed by national regulatory authorities on the basis of a full registration dossier. However, WHO emphasizes that its framework is indiscriminate and will exclusively applicable to well established biologics. The WHO framework reinforces the argument for high standards of safety based on scientific justification. In particular, it seeks to diminish clinical requirements, but recognizes that minimum of one clinical study will be required for a biosimilar to be approved, especially to test its immunogenicity (Kang, 2009).

Canada

Canada is also in the process of framing regulations that permit the approval of biosimilars, which it pronounces "subsequent entry biologics" (SEBs), in the Food and Drugs Act. Although the regulations have not yet been finalized, the first biosimilar, Omnitrope, has already been permitted (Sandoz, 2009). Like WHO, Canada's approach with reference to safety resembles that of EMEA, but goes further than EMEA in addressing intellectual property discussions.

Noteworthy in case of Canada's biosimilar framework is its suppleness in the biosimilar applicant's choice of which original biologic it chooses as its reference; dissimilar to the other major frameworks, the original biologic may be one that has not been official and marketed in Canada. This approach has been presented so that the size of this market might not discourage biosimilar applicants. However, Health Canada (Canada's department of health) suggests using those original biologics that have been approved by jurisdictions with which it has "an established relationship".

Safety Standards

Health Canada needs "comparative clinical trials in order to exhibit the resemblance in efficacy and safety profiles between the SEB and reference biologic" (Nyarko, 2009). However, like the EMEA and WHO guidelines, the quantum of clinical testing will be on the basis of difference in biosimilar and original biologic. It is still quite gloomy that how this will appear in vague, with Omnitrope as the only example (its application involved the results of at least 1 clinical trial).

Further, a post-marketing safety approach, the "Risk Management Plan", is necessary as part of the biosimilar application and "Periodic Safety Update Reporting" will in addition be mandatory. The Health Canada will not take the decision with regard to interchangeability; it is to be taken at the provincial stage. Though in this way, Health Canada is fundamentally similar to EMEA, it takes a rather atypical policy approach. Specially, there is no clear proclamation that a biosimilar cannot be considered identical to the original biologic. Fairly, Health Canada emphasizes that (1) approval of a biosimilar does not point towards the automatically substitution with the original; and (2) if a body is to compose a decision on interchangeability, this should be based on suitable scientific and clinical data.

United States (US)

Representative of how multifarious the discussion has been in the US, in the last Congress meeting five proposals for an abbreviated biologics process were introduced, but were never fully argued. Of the 3 bills floored in the current Congress, 2 are cohort bills in the House and the Senate (H.R. 1427 and S. 726), introduced by Representative Waxman (D-CA) and Senator Schumer (D-NY), respectively as a little modified forms of an old proposal. The third is the proposal Representative Eshoo (D-CA) has reintroduced from the last Congress (H.R. 1548). The approaches of the Waxman/Schumer and Eshoo proposals in taking care of the challenges presented by biosimilars vary considerably, especially on safety and intellectual property issues.

Safety Standards

The Waxman/Schumer scheme is unclear on the fundamental safety principles prerequisite for approval and on how much competence it will give to the FDA to lay down these standards, mostly product-specific requirements. This is correct regarding clinical testing ordinarily, but exclusively for testing of immunogenicity.

On the contrary, the Eshoo proposal requires non-clinical as well as clinical studies and while it permits the FDA to relinquish them if it finds them uncalled for, it may only do so if it has published extremely specific guidelines on immunogenicity.

If the FDA is authorized to take the decision on interchangeability, the Eshoo would only allow it when the biosimilar applicant can produce clinical data (based on FDA guidelines) which points that the biosimilar "can be expected to produce the same clinical result as the reference product in any given patient for each condition of use prescribed" (H.R. 1548).

India

The government of India, Department of Biotechnology (DBT) and Central Drugs Standard Control Organization (CDSCO), have published guidelines for an abbreviated pathway for biosimilars registration in June 2012. India's guidelines are similar to EU and U.S. guidelines in many aspects, including the recommendation of a stepwise approach to demonstrating biosimilarity, starting with extensive quality characterization comparing the "similar biologic" against the reference biologic. The reference product should be an innovator product licensed in India or, if it is not yet registered in India, it should have been licensed and widely marketed for four years in the innovator's country of origin in a jurisdiction with a well-established regulatory framework.

India's generic-driven domestic biopharmaceuticals industry has created a strong foundation for biosimilars development, and Indian companies are positioned to become major players in the global biosimilars market. By the time its biosimilars regulatory pathway was issued in 2012, India had already approved more than 25 products designated as 'similar biologics'. (Generic & Biosimilar Initiative 2012) A number of Indian companies are well ahead of their regional competitors. Ranbaxy Ltd, for example, announced plans to launch at least three biosimilar cancer products in India by 2015 (biosimilarnews.com 2012).

Biologics and the Emergence of Biosimilars

Biologics are nothing but recombinant DNA-derived products, therapeutic proteins and oligonucleotides, which includes hormones, monoclonal antibodies, cytokine and growth factors. These biologics are used for the treatment of various diseases including inflammatory disease (rheumatoid arthritis, Crohns disease etc), cancer, and infectious disease. The biologics producing industries are growing rapidly due to high demands of new biologics and expiry of many key patents. According to Walsh in 2010, prior to four and half year to late 2010, alone within the European Union and/or the United States, 58 approvals has been sent and among them about 40% were new biologics; and around 50% of the remaining approvals were biosimilars and reformulated existing products. Dr. Reichert in 2010 mentioned that Monoclonal antibodies are the most rapidly growing class of biologic medicine and since 2007 every year 40 new biologics are enters for clinical trials.

Human Embryonic Kidney (HEK) cells are commonly used for transient expression; however, there may be instances where a stable cell line may be advantageous. Generation of stable, high producing HEK cell lines is described in the second research article by Song et al (Song et al., 2011), where a combination of Fluorescence-activated cell sorting (FACS) and Clonpix has facilitated the development of a clonal selection method for isolating HEK293 cell lines with high specific productivity.

Analytical Techniques

Demonstration of comparability between a candidate biosimilar and innovator product includes analytical studies for structural characterization and for evaluation of physicochemical properties as per International Conference on Harmonization of standards (ICH) guidelines. Poly acrylamide gel electrophoresis (PAGE) is an analytical method that has a long history of application in protein analysis (Laemmli, 1970) and has been a principal analytical technique since the earliest days of recombinant protein expression (Goeddel et al., 1979; Lee 1984). PAGE separates proteins by hydrodynamic radius (size and shape) and is a qualitative assay.

Capillary zone electrophoresis (CZE) provides an alternative method for analyzing proteins to PAGE that has the advantage of being automated and better suited to conformance with method qualification and validation. CZE separates proteins by a combination of hydrodynamic radius, friction and charge. CZE was demonstrated to be superior in separating charge isoforms of EPO (i.e. differing in the number of sialic residues) compared with PAGE/IEF blotting (Park et al., 2009).

High performance liquid chromatography (HPLC) has become an invaluable workhorse for analysis of proteins. It is compatible with a range of separation methodologies, is amenable to validation and with automation can be used to process large numbers of samples with minimal labor input. Reverse phase High performance liquid chromatography (RP-HPLC) is able to separate proteins on the basis of their surface polar-apolar amino acid side chains. This technique is especially suited to separating folding isomers and can be used to assess refolding reactions as well as monitoring product purity and determining product heterogeneity. Cation exchange High performance liquid chromatography (CEX-HPLC) separates proteins according to charge, can separate glycoforms and can identify chemical modifications such as deamidation and cleavage reactions. EPO biosimilars analysed by CEX-HPLC demonstrate diverse isotypes (Heavner et al., 2007) and its use for analyzing monoclonal antibodies (mAbs) is also well established (Roshkova, 2009).

Analytical ultracentrifugation (AUC) is able to provide a higher degree of confidence in aggregation analysis compared with alternative methods, and is an excellent method for validation of SEC or AF4 analytical assays used in routine analysis; however, AUC has the disadvantage of being time consuming and expensive to acquire (Liu et al., 2006). Even with simple non-glycosylated proteins it is necessary to have an understanding of the levels of chemical modification between an innovator and biosimilar product. Jiang et al. used peptide mapping with liquid Chromatography Mass spectrometry (LC-MS) of three sources of human growth hormone, and identified different levels of oxidation of methionine residues, deamidation of asparagines and cleavage at two sites between an innovator, a biosimilar and a counterfeit product (Jiang et al., 2009).

There are a range of different types of cell-based bioassays. For proteins that have an endocrine function most bioassays are based on stimulating growth factor-dependent cell lines or natural cell lines that respond to the therapeutic protein via receptor binding and signal transduction, perhaps measured through increases in intracellular cyclic adenosine monophosphate (cAMP). In the case of EPO, the

32D cell line, made dependent on EPO by the introduction of the EPO receptor gene, can be utilized, and cell proliferation can be monitored by measuring radio-labelled thymidine uptake (Greenberger et al., 1983; Elliott et al., 2004).

Elucidation of conformational epitopes is more complex and may incorporate synthesizing muteins of the protein of interest, and testing for binding. Conformational and linear epitope mapping for EPO has been reported, and the data used for modelling recombinant human EPO structure (Elliott et al., 1996). Differential scanning Calorimetry (DSC) or the combination of a spectroscopic technique with Peltier temperature control with a linear upward thermal scan can be used to determine the thermal stability of a protein in a given formulation. Each method can measure the transition temperature (Tm) where the protein unfolds. The Tm value can be used to rank thermal stability of proteins (Weiss et al., 2009).

FDA Approach Regarding the Use of Biosimilar Drugs

FDA was given the authority to approve biosimilars, including interchangeable, to maintain safety, efficacy, and quality of biosimilar products (Hodgson 2009; WHO 2009). Biologics Price Competition and Innovation Act of 2009 authorize the FDA to oversee an "abbreviated pathway" for approval of biologics that are "biosimilar" to already approved products.

Pharmacovigilance of Biosimilars

Pharmacovigilance is particularly concerned with adverse drug reactions. Recently, pharmacovigilance concerns have been widened to include innovator product and biosimilars. Clinical trials and post-authorization pharmacovigilance are considered essential to guarantee the product's safety and efficacy over time. Pharmacovigilance, as part of a comprehensive risk management programme, will need to include regular testing for consistent manufacturing of the drug (Locatelli et al., 2006). To improve patient safety through enhanced pharmacovigilance, Novartis supports the recent initiative in the EU to review and improve the pharmacovigilance system of medicinal products in Europe. In addition, valid pharmacovigilance procedures should be mandatory for all products of a certain category (e.g.- bio-pharmaceutical) and not depend on whether the relevant brand is an innovator product or a biosimilar product (http://www.corporatecitizenship.novartis.com).

Biosimilars in Clinical Practice

Despite the comparability of biosimilars to the innovator product, clinicians and health care workers should be aware of some of the issues that have emerged during the development and approval of these products, which highlight the challenges of biosimilars. The use of biosimilars is essentially a change in clinical management (Mellstedt et al., 2008).

The Role of Hospital Pharmacists

It is of utmost importance that the hospital pharmacist is aware that the innovator products and biosimilars are not interchangeable, because patients must be carefully monitored if their treatment is changed between products. Moreover, patient welfare is foremost and for pharmacists, the knowledge that biosimilars are not generics, and the possible implications for clinical outcomes when products are switched, will help ensure patient safety (Schellekens et al., 2008).

Systematic checklists have been proposed for the evaluation of biopharmaceuticals coming on to the market, which have provided additional reassurance for the pharmacist. For example, the Pharmacy Checklist for Retacrit (epoetin zeta) provides information on manufacturing, protein and product formulation, batch consistency, supply reliability, good handling practice, clinical efficacy, and clinical safety and tolerability (Hospira symp on assessing biosimilars. http://www.thepharmaletter.com/file/89334/hospira-symp-on-assessing-biosimilars.html.). The successful introduction of EU biosimilar erythropoietins, such as Retacrit gives hospital pharmacists the opportunity to reduce costs and improve the treatment of patients with anemia.

Biosimilar as Granulocyte Colony Stimulating Factor

Biosimilars are approved biologics with comparable quality, safety, and efficacy to a reference product for which patent protection has expired. Biosimilar regulatory approval is provided on the basis of a robust comparability exercise demonstrating similarity with the original product, rather than on the need to show a positive risk-benefit assessment per se, which it is assumed has already been proven. Similarity must be demonstrated through biochemical characterization (purity, chemical identity, i.e., primary, secondary, and tertiary protein structure and receptor on–off kinetics); biologic activity in vitro, if applicable; and clinical similarity for at least one indication (Bonig et at., 2015).

Biosimilars of recombinant human granulocyte–colony-stimulating factor (rHuG-CSF), based on the original filgrastim product (Neupogen), have been available for more than 5 years now and are widely used in Europe. Four biosimilars of filgrastim have been approved by the EMA, these being Zarzio/Filgrastim Hexal (Sandoz Biopharmaceuticals), Tevagrastim/Ratiograstim (Teva), Nivestim (Hospira), and Grastofil (Stada). In many countries, use of biosimilar filgrastim products now exceeds that of the original (Bonig et al., 2015).

In addition to these "true" biosimilars, copies of original products are available in some less highly regulated markets, such as parts of South America, India, and South-East Asia. These copies of biopharmaceuticals cannot, however, be considered to be biosimilars, as they have not been approved through a stringent regulatory process (Roger and Goldsmith 2008; KDIGO 2012). These biologic copies can differ widely in composition, do not always meet self-declared specifications, exhibit considerable batch-to-batch variation, and may lack adequate clinical data to show comparability (Schellekens 2009). This difference is beginning to be noted in more recent treatment guidelines, which recommend that only "true" biosimilar products should be used (i.e., those that have received approval by official regulatory bodies) (KDIGO 2012).

FUTURE PROSPECTS

For any drug development strategy, efficiency and cost effectiveness is biggest challenge. And in case of biosimilars this is more important aspects in comparison to marketed drugs. As biosimilar products are very intricate molecules, factors such as the robustness of the manufacturing process, structural similarity to the parent molecule, level of understanding of the mechanism of action, quality of pharmacodynamic assays used, exhibited comparability in pharmacokinetics and immunogenicity, amount and features of clinical information and the innovator's experience with the parent product, requires to be evaluated critically prior to marketing approval of biosimilars.

Till date there is no single authority or controllers which take care of biosimilar products nomenclature, labeling, acceptability over worldwide, so there is urgent need to create such body. Physician should take care of safety concern and understand the difference between drugs and biosimilar products is very essential before giving to patient. Before marketing of biosimilars, every information should be clearly given to healthcare professional, doctors and users or patients in documented form. Clinicians require broad information on biosimilars, and biopharmaceuticals ordinarily, to make conversant treatment decisions. Approvals of biosimilar products should continue to be dealt with on a case-by-case basis.

CONCLUSION

The importance and frequent use of biologics shows its therapeutic applications and since past three decades biologics are in developing stage. More new biologic products are still in the pipeline for approval from the different authorities all over the world. The development of the biosimilars in UK and biologics in USA has been increased due to the expiry of patent protection. Biosimilar and biologics are not generic or small compounds/drugs, rather it is highly complex and product of modern biotechnology approach. Many companies are not following the proper guidelines before the use of such products for the treatment of disease. The biggest challenge to use such product should be take care for selection of patient and passes with all the necessary clinical trials. However, biosimilars are not the only way to meet the needs of the population for expensive biological products. A country must be able to effectively develop technology to meet its needs and thus grow and leverage the competitiveness of its industry in the country and the world in order to facilitate economic and social progress.

REFERENCES

APG. (2011). *Procurement and prescribing practices for biologics in the UK*. APG.

Biosimilars Market Product (BMP) [Recombinant Non-Glycosylated Proteins (Insulin, Filgrastim, Somatropin), Glycosylated (Monoclonal Antibodies, Erythropoietin), Peptides (Glucagon, Calcitonin)] & Application (Oncology, Blood Disorders) - Global Forecast to 2018. (n.d.). Retrieved from http://www.marketsandmarkets.com/Market-Reports/biosimilars-40.html

Biosimilarsnews.com. (2012). *Ranbaxy will boost biosimilar business*. Retrieved from www.biosimilarnews.com/ranbaxy-will-boost-biosimilar-business

Bonig, H., Becker, P. S., Schwebig, A., & Turner, M. (2015). Biosimilar granulocyte–colony-stimulating factor for healthy donor stem cell mobilization: Need we be afraid. *Transfusion*, *55*(2), 430–539. doi:10.1111/trf.12770 PMID:24965197

Business Monitor International. (2008). First Biosimilar Submitted for Approval. In BMI Industry Insights—Pharma and Healthcare, Asia.

Chirino, A. J., & Mire-Sluis, A. (2004). Characterizing biological products and assessing comparability following manufacturing changes. *Nature Biotechnology*, *22*(11), 1383–1391. doi:10.1038/nbt1030 PMID:15529163

Consensus Information Paper (CIP). (2013). *What you need to know about Biosimilar Medicinal Products*. CIP.

Crommelin, D. J., Bermejo, T., Bissig, M., Damiaans, J., Krämer, I., Rambourg, P., & Tredree, R. (2005). Pharmaceutical evaluation of biosimilars: Important differences from generic low-molecular weight pharm. *Eur J Hosp Pharm Sci*, *1*, 11–17.

Declerck, P. J. (2012). Biologicals and biosimilars: A review of the science and its implications. *Generics and Biosimilars Initiative Journal*, *1*(1), 13–16. doi:10.5639/gabij.2012.0101.005

EBE-EFPIA. (2006). *Position Paper: Inapplicability of automatic substitution rules to biotechnology products, including biosimilar medicinal products: recommendation for addressing unique safety concerns*. Author.

Elliott, S., Egrie, J., Browne, J., Lorenzini, T., Busse, L., Rogers, N., & Ponting, I. (2004). Control of rHuEPO biological activity: The role of carbohydrate. *Experimental Hematology*, *32*(12), 1146–1155. doi:10.1016/j.exphem.2004.08.004 PMID:15588939

Elliott, S., Lorenzini, T., Chang, D., Barzilay, J., Delorme, E., Giffin, J., & Hesterberg, L. (1996). Fine structure epitope mapping of antierythropoietin monoclonal antibodies reveals a model of recombinant human erythropoietin structure. *Blood*, *87*, 2702–2713. PMID:8639886

EMEA. (2009). *Scientific Guidelines for Human Medicines*. Retrieved from http://www.emea.Europa .eu/ htms /human/humanguidelines/multidiscipline.htm

European Biopharmaceutical Enterprises (EBE). (n.d.). *Biosimilars*. EBE.

European Medicines Agency (EMA). (2012). *Questions and Answers on biosimilar medicines (similar medicinal products)*. European Medicines Agency. Retrieved from http://www.ema.europa.eu/ema/index.jsp?curl=pages/special_topics/document_listing/document_listing_000318.jsp

European Medicines Agency (EMA). (n.d.). *Guideline on similar biological medicinal products containing biotechnology-derived proteins as active substance: quality issues (revision 1)*. European Medicines Agency - Europa.

Generics and Biosimilars Initiative. (2012). *India releases draft similar biologic guidelines*. Retrieved from www. gabionline.net/layout/set/print/guidelines/india-releases-draft-similar-biologic-guidelines

Global Industry Analysts Inc. (GIAI). (2012). *Biosimilars – a global strategic business report*. GIAI.

Goeddel, D. V., Heyneker, H. L., Hozumi, T., Arentzen, R., Itakura, K., Yansura, D. G., & Seeburg, P. H. (1979). Direct expression in *Escherichia coli* of a DNA sequence coding for human growth hormone. *Nature*, *281*(5732), 544–548. doi:10.1038/281544a0 PMID:386136

Greenberger, J. S., Sakakeeny, M. A., Humphries, R. K., Eaves, C. J., & Eckner, R. J. (1983). Demonstration of permanent factor-dependent multipotential (erythroid/neutrophil/basophil) hematopoietic progenitor cell lines. *Proceedings of the National Academy of Sciences of the United States of America*, *80*(10), 2931–2935. doi:10.1073/pnas.80.10.2931 PMID:6574462

H.R. 1548 (112th Congress), Title I (a)(4)(A)(i)(II).

Heavner, G. A., Arakawa, T., Philo, J. S., & Labrenz, S. (2007). Protein isolation from biopharmaceutical formulations cannot be used for comparative studies: Follow-up to ''A case study using Epoetin Alfa fromEpogen and EPREX. *Journal of Pharmaceutical Sciences*, *96*(12), 3214–3225. doi:10.1002/jps.20993 PMID:17721976

Hodgson, J. (2009). WHO guidelines presage US biosimilars legislation? *Nature Biotechnology*, *27*(11), 963–965. doi:10.1038/nbt1109-963a PMID:19898430

Hospira Symp on Assessing Biosimilars. (2015). Retrieved from http://www.corporatecitizenship.novartis.com/downloads/businessconduct/Novartis_Perspective_Pharmacovigilance_for_Biosimilars.pdf

ICH Q6B Note for guidance on specifications: test procedures and acceptance criteria for biotechnological/biological products (CPMP/ICH/365/96).

Jiang, H. T., Wu, S. L., Karger, B. L., & Hancock, W. S. (2009). Mass spectrometric analysis of innovator, counterfeit, and follow-on recombinant human growth hormone. *Biotechnology Progress*, *25*(1), 207–218. doi:10.1002/btpr.72 PMID:19224592

Johnson, P. E. (2008). Implications of biosimilars for the future. *American Journal of Health-System Pharmacy*, *65*(Supplement 6). PMID:18591711

Kang, H. N. (2009). *WHO Guideline on Evaluation of Similar Biotherapeutic Products: The Next Steps*. Presented at the EGA 7th Symposium on Biosimilar Medicines.

Kidney Disease Improving Global Outcomes (KDIGO) AnemiaWork Group. (2012). KDIGO clinical practice guideline for anemia in chronic kidney disease. *Kidney International. Supplement*, *2*, 279–335.

Laemmli, U. K. (1970). Cleavage of structural proteins during assembly of head of bacteriophage T4. *Nature*, *227*(5259), 680–685. doi:10.1038/227680a0 PMID:5432063

Lanthier, M., Behrman, R., & Nardinelli, C. (2008). Economic issues with follow-on protein products. *Nature Reviews. Drug Discovery*, *7*(9), 733–737. doi:10.1038/nrd2636 PMID:18654570

Lee, H. S. (1984). Cloning and expression of human erythropoietin in *Escherichia coli. Proceedings of the National Academy of Sciences of the United States of America*, *81*(9), 2708–2712. doi:10.1073/pnas.81.9.2708 PMID:6371819

Liu, J., Andya, J. D., & Shire, S. J. (2006). A critical review of analytical ultracentrifugation and field flow fractionation methods for measuring protein aggregation. *The AAPS Journal*, *8*(3), E580–E589. doi:10.1208/aapsj080367 PMID:17025276

Locatelli, F., & Roger, S. (2006). Comparative testing and pharmacovigilance of biosimilars. *Nephrology, Dialysis, Transplantation*, *21*(Suppl 5), v13–v16. doi:10.1093/ndt/gfl475 PMID:16959789

Los, M., Roodhart, J. M., & Voest, E. E. (2007). Target practice: Lessons from phase III trials with bevacizumAb and vatalanib in the treatment of advanced colorectal cancer. *The Oncologist*, *12*(4), 443–450. doi:10.1634/theoncologist.12-4-443 PMID:17470687

Mellstedt, H., Niederwieser, D., & Ludwig, H. (2008). The challenge of biosimilars. *Ann Omol.*, *19*, 411–419. PMID:17872902

Nick, C. (2012). The US Biosimilars Act: Challenges Facing RegulatoryApproval. *Pharm Med.*, *26*(3), 145–152. doi:10.1007/BF03262388

Niederwieser, D., & Schmitz, S. (2011). Biosimilar agents in oncology/haematology: From approval to. *European Journal of Haematology*, *86*(4), 277–288. doi:10.1111/j.1600-0609.2010.01566.x PMID:21175852

Niederwieser, H. D., & Ludwig, H. (2007). The challenge of biosimilars. *Annals of Oncology*, *19*(3), 411–419. doi:10.1093/annonc/mdm345 PMID:17872902

Nyarko, K. A. (2009). *Regulatory Approach for Subsequent Entry Biologics in Canada, Health Canada*. Presented at the PMDA 3rd International Symposium on Biologics.

Park, S. S., Park, J., Ko, J., Chen, L., Meriage, D., Crouse-Zeineddini, J., & Kerwin, B. A. et al. (2009). Biochemical assessment of erythropoietin products from Asia versus Epoetin alfa manufactured by Amgen. *Journal of Pharmaceutical Sciences*, *98*(5), 1688–1699. doi:10.1002/jps.21546 PMID:18781649

Perry, G. (2009). *Biosimilar Medicines: Towards Global Development and Monoclonal Antibodies*. Presented at the 7th EGA Annual Symposium on Biosimilar Medicines, EGA.

Pharmaphorum. (2012). *Biosimilars 2012 – what does the current landscape look like?* Author.

Reichert, J. M. (2010). Metrics for antibody therapeutics development. *mAbs*, *2*, 695–700.

Roger, S. D. (2010). Biosimilars: Current status and future directions. *Expert Opinion on Biological Therapy*, *10*(7), 1011–1018. doi:10.1517/14712591003796553 PMID:20384525

Roger, S. D., & Goldsmith, D. (2008). Biosimilars: It's not as simple as cost alone. *Journal of Clinical Pharmacy and Therapeutics*, *33*(5), 459–464. doi:10.1111/j.1365-2710.2008.00942.x PMID:18834359

Roger, S. D. (2006). Biosimilars: How similar or dissimilar are they? *Nephrology (Carlton, Vic.)*, *11*(4), 341–346. doi:10.1111/j.1440-1797.2006.00594.x PMID:16889575

Roshkova, A. (2009). Quantitative analysis of monoclonal antibodies by cationexchange chromatofocusing. *Journal of Chromatography. A*, *1216*(32), 5989–5994. doi:10.1016/j.chroma.2009.06.045 PMID:19560777

Sandoz. (2009). *Sandoz Canada receives approval for recombinant human-growth hormone Omnitrope, the first Subsequent Entry Biologic in Canada*. Sandoz.

Schellekens, H. (2003). Relationship between biopharmaceutical immunogenicity of epoetin alfa and pure red cell aplasia. *Current Medical Research and Opinion*, *19*(5), 433–434. doi:10.1185/030079903125002072 PMID:13678481

Schellekens, H. (2005). Follow-on biologics: Challenges of the next generation. *Nephrology, Dialysis, Transplantation*, *20*(4), 31–36. PMID:15827057

Schellekens, H. (2009). Biosimilar therapeutics- what do we need to consider? *NDT Plus*, *2*(Supplement 1), 27–36. doi:10.1093/ndtplus/sfn177 PMID:19461855

Schellekens, H., Lisman, J., & Bols, T. (2008). Biosimilars in clinical practice – the challenges for hospital pharmacists. *EJHPP Practice.*, *14*, 32–33.

Song, M., Raphaelli, K., Jones, M. L., Aliabadi-Zadeh, K., Leung, K. M., Crowley, D., & Chin, D. Y. (2011). Clonal selection of high producing, stably transfected HEK293 cell lines utilizing modified, high-throughput FACS screening. *Journal of Chemical Technology and Biotechnology (Oxford, Oxfordshire)*, *86*(7), 935–941. doi:10.1002/jctb.2618

Tsang, L., & Kracov, D. (2008). Biosimilars, developments in the EU and US. In *PLC Life Sciences Handbook* (pp. 17-21). Academic Press.

U.S. Food and Drug Administration (USFDA). (2012). Guidance for Industry: Quality considerations in demonstration biosimilarity to a reference protein product. Washington, DC: U.S. Food and Drug Administration.

U.S. Food and Drug Administration. (2015). *Guidance for Industry. Scientific Considerations in Demonstrating Biosimilarity to a Reference Product. Draft Guidance*. U.S. Food and Drug Administration. Retrieved from http://www.fda.gov/downloads/DrugsGuidanceComplianceRegulatoryInformation/Guidances/UCM291128.pdf

Walsh, G. (2010). Biopharmaceutical Benchmarks. *Nature Biotechnology*, *28*(9), 917–924. doi:10.1038/nbt0910-917 PMID:20829826

Weiss, W. F. IV, Young, T. M., & Roberts, C. J. (2009). Princples, approaches, and challenges for predicting protein aggregation rates and shelf life. *Journal of Pharmaceutical Sciences*, *98*(4), 1247–1277. doi:10.1002/jps.21521 PMID:18683878

World Health Organisation (WHO). (2009). *Expert Committee on Biological standardization. Guidelines on evaluation of similar biotherapeutic products (SBPs)*. Retrieved from http://www.who.int/biologicals/areas/biological_therapeutics/BIOTHERAPEUTICS_FOR_WEB_22APRIL2010.pdf

Zenotech Builds Pipeline of 'Generic' Monoclonals. (2007). *Scrip*, (3237), 10.

Section 7
Liquid Crystals

Chapter 8
Liquid Crystalline System: A Novel Approach in Drug Delivery

Nayan Ashok Gujarathi
P. S. G. V. P. Mandal's College of Pharmacy, India

Bhushan Rajendra Rane
P. S. G. V. P. Mandal's College of Pharmacy, India

Raj K. Keservani
Rajiv Gandhi Proudyogiki Vishwavidhyalaya, India

ABSTRACT

Liquid crystalline system is a thermodynamically stable phase which is characterized by anisotropy. Liquid Crystals (LCs) are also termed as mesophase as they exhibit isotropic properties and liquid like behavior under some conditions (alter in temperature and concentration). Liquid crystals are influenced by number of parameters includes concentration, temperature, pH, and presence of salt. Liquid crystals are divided on the basis of shape of the molecules into two groups one is calmitic and other is discotic. A range of liquid crystalline phase (called mesophases) can be categorized by their sort of arrangement. The alignment of fragments in liquid crystalline phases is extensive on the molecular scale. Liquid crystal technology has a most important influence on several areas of pharmacy science and engineering, as well as device technology. As a novel type of drug delivery system, liquid crystals are explored and examined, definitely achieve mounting significance in industrial and scientific purposes.

INTRODUCTION

History

The physical and chemical characteristic of different derivative of cholesterol was determined in 1888. The credit goes to Friedrich Reinitzer, a physiologist in Botany from Austria, presently serving in Karl-Ferdinands-Universität. Derivatives of cholesterol now classified as a material called as cholesteric liquid crystal. Formerly, scientists have been revealed diverse color effect, obtained by cooling derivative of

DOI: 10.4018/978-1-5225-0751-2.ch008

cholesterol at little higher than the freezing point, but did not related it with a novel observable fact. Reinitzer supposed that change in color of cholesteryl benzoate derivatives is not the major unusual trait (Figure 1).

Reinitzer introduce that the manner in which cholesteryl benzoate melts differs from other compound, bears double melting points. It melts into a cloudy liquid at 144-145 °C, and then it melts again from the hazy liquid to clear fluid at 177-178 °C. This phenomenon is reversible, he wrote to Otto Lehmann on March 14, 1888, seeking help from a physicist. They exchange scientific material and test models. Lehmann observed the intermediary hazy fluid, and report that there is existence of crystallites. Von Zepharovich, colleague of Reinitzer's Viennese, also added that the intermediate "liquid" was crystalline. Reinitzer offered his outcomes, with acknowledgment to Lehmann and von Zepharovich in the meeting at Vienna Chemical Society on May 3, 1888, (Reinitzer & Friedrich, 1888).

Still that moment, Reinitzer has invented and explained three main characters of cholesteric liquid crystal (Otto Lehmann specified this term in 1904): a) Double melting points are existed b) ability to reflect circular polarized light and c) capability to rotate the polarization direction of light.

Reinitzer did not trail studying liquid crystals further, following his accidental discovery. The investigation was sustained by Lehmann, comprehends that he has met a novel observable fact and be in a situation to examine it: he become specialist in the field of crystallography and microscopy during his postdoctoral years. Lehmann initiated an orderly study started from cholesteryl benzoate then followed by associated materials that displays the double melting phenomenon. The facility of hot stage provided in microscope (sample holder in contact with heater) helps to scan the material at high temperature and also make observations in polarized light. Predominantly the crystals observed in microscope persuaded Lehmann that he was came across a frozen material in the intermediate cloudy phase which shows clearly sustained flow. He had published his results in the literature by the end of august 1889 (Lehman, 1889).

After Lehmann, the German chemist Daniel Vorländer continued and extensively prolonged his work up to his retirement in 1935, during his course of study he synthesize number of liquid crystal. While the liquid crystal, was not admired throughout the world among researchers from different region, so the material remained silent for next research with more scientific curiosity (Sluckin et al., 2004).

Definition (Gennes & Prost, 1993; Chandrasekhar, 1993)

A liquid crystal is a thermodynamically stable phase existing in the range of temperature between the solid and isotropic liquid phase, which is characterized by anisotropy. But a three-dimensional crystal

Figure 1. Structure of cholesteryl benzoate molecule

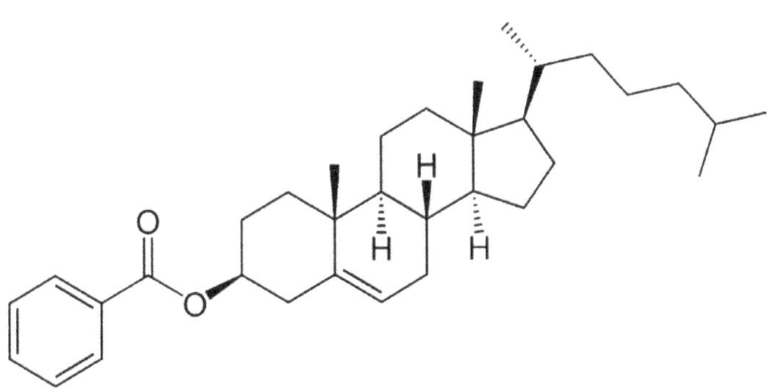

lattice remained absent. The term mesophase was coined due to existence of liquid crystal in between two phases.

In some situation, liquid crystals occupy a state in which they reveal isotropic, fluid like behavior. It means a little long range ordering. However, in next situation, they occupy one or more phases with prominent anisotropic structure and long range ordering though still possess a capacity to flow.

Liquid crystals are typically elongated organic molecules with an uneven distribution of electrical charges along their axes (dipole). This gives rise to a special physical characteristic to which liquid crystals owe their name: between the crystalline and liquid states they exhibit a further state of aggregation, namely the liquid crystalline or mesophase. In liquid crystalline phase the fragments are allied parallel to each other but are able to rotate about their long axes.

Anisometric molecular shape is a prerequisite for the development of LC's phases, which is usually linked with a distinct anisotropy of the polarizability. The molecules which have ability to create liquid crystalline phases are known as Mesogens. The latter may or may not be excipients e.g. surface active agents. Drug compounds themselves may accomplish the prerequisite for the liquid crystal formation, having anisometric molecular shape such as the salts of organic acids or bases (Miller-Goymann, 2004), are given in Table 1.

The liquid crystalline phase was attained either by increasing the temperature called as thermotropic liquid crystals or by adding a solvent called as lyotropic liquid crystals being initially started from the crystalline state. The deviation in temperature can leads to a phase transition between various phases of not only thermotropic liquid crystals, but it also affects lyotropic liquid crystals.

In liquid crystal displays, it has found wide scope which specifically based on the optical property of molecules (LC's) in existence or lack of an electric field. The liquid crystalline molecules show the alignment with direction of electric field and alter the polarization of light in a positive way.

The order of mesophase is widely based on the molecular scale however it may not be broaden to the macroscopic scale similar to that of solid conventional crystals. The order of crystal's in mesophase is fixed in one dimension however in next dimension there may be a wide disarrangement of molecules of LC's.

Liquid crystals are classified on the basis of molecular shape into two groups:

Table 1. Liquid crystal formation by drugs

Drug	Type of Liquid Crystal
Arsphenamine	Nematic
Disodium cromoglicinate	Nematic (Hexagonal)
Nafoxidine hydrochloride	Lamellar – Hexagonal, Cubic
Fenoprofen	Lamellar
Ibuprofen	Lamellar
Flurbiprofen	Lamellar
Diclofenac	Lamellar
Peptide Hormone (LH-RH analogue)	Lamellar

1. Calamitic liquid crystal, which possess rod like fragments with alignment in the path of the longer axis of the fragment while
2. Discotic liquid crystals are made up of flat shaped entity. These flat shaped crystals having order in the path of the shorter axis of the fragment.

Figure 2 shows the classification of the crystalline system.

Phases of Liquid-Crystals

The different types of mesophases were distinguished on the basis of nature of ordering. The molecules in the phase, when aligned in any kind of ordered pattern, can be characterized by positional order. If the molecules in the phase are mostly pointing in the same direction then can be specified by their orientation order, and however order of fragments may be either short range (for entity which are in close vicinity) or long range (extend to larger, occasionally macroscopic magnitude). At high temperature number of the thermotropic liquid crystals possesses an isotropic phase. It means that high temperature will ultimately impel them into a classical liquid phase distinguished by isotropic and random molecular arrangement, and fluid like run behavior. At the same time a prominent anisotropic orientation in structure as well as short-range point of reference, having capability to flow, might be dwelled by one or more phases of liquid crystals at lower temperature (Gennes & Prost, 1993; Chandrasekhar, 1993).

The orientation of molecules is widespread in liquid crystalline phases. This ordering extend to the intact field magnitude, that might be on the scale of micrometers, while generally cannot be widen to the macroscopic order as usually takes place in conventional crystalline solid. But many systems might be utilized to implement a single ordered structure in a macroscopic mesogen sample such as an applied electric field or the use of boundaries. The molecules of liquid crystalline phase was basically disordered in two directions and only in one dimension the ordering might be extended in a liquid crystal phase (Table 2) (Dierking, 2003; Collings & Hird, 1997).

Figure 2. Classification of liquid crystalline system

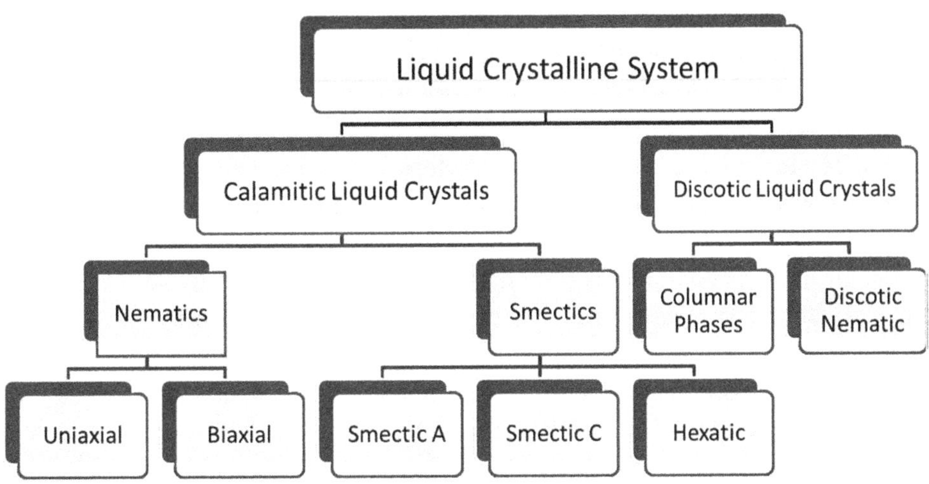

Table 2. Mesophase classifications and characteristics

Mesophase Classification	Phase Transition	Mesogen Characteristics	Mesophase Characteristics	Example
		Thermotrpic		
Smectic	Temperature	Rigid part with one/ two flexible aliphatic chains	Layered structure, Viscous fluid	Cholesteryl esters
Nematic			Thread like structure, less viscous	
Cholesteric			Twisted or helical structure, more fluid with colour	
		Lyotropic		
Lamellar	Concentrations	Amphiphilic molecules (Surfactants)	Stack bilayer	Phospholipid
Cubic			Balls like	
Hexagonal			Cylinder like micelles	

Thermotropic Liquid Crystal

The transformation in phase of thermotropic liquid crystal depends upon change in temperature. A fine ordering of molecules in liquid crystal phase gets disordered with increase in temperature due to thermal motion to an extent level thus converts the phase into a conventional isotropic liquid. In contrast, the liquid crystalline phase will form conventional solid crystals at too low temperature (Gennes & Prost, 1993; Chandrasekhar, 1993). A variety of smectic and nematic liquid crystal phases were exhibited by a particular type of mesogen molecule with rise in temperature e.g. para-azoxyanisole (Shao & Zerda, 1998).

A derivative of cholesterol, $C_{27}H_{46}O$ is a basic composition of commonly occurring thermotropic liquid crystalline systems. The cholesteric derivatives (cholest-5, 6-en-3β-R) are made up of 27 carbon atoms and have 17 of these carbon atoms linked together in a manner so as to figure a jagged, which was not simply collapsed nucleus or frame. The 17 carbon atoms were held mutually in three six-numbered rings and one five-numbered ring; a prototype that is quasiplanar. There exist a side chains three in numbered at one side of the structure, out of which two side chains are build up by only one carbon atom. The 17β substituent consists of a eight carbon atoms chain. The chains were projected above the flat surface of the framework. An R group is attached in the 3β position, at the reverse end of the framework and was projected out of the flat surface. The 3β substituent extends the molecular long axis and favours mesophase formation. The mesophase is formed by cholesteric derivatives only when the substituents are in the 3β position, and when rings A and B are quasiplanar. The 17β side chain is not a critical feature for the preservation of cholesteric properties (Figure 3) (Tai & Lee, 1990).

The two type of liquid crystal phases were naturally demonstrated by cholesteryl esters: i) smectic mesophase and ii) cholesteric mesophase. The smectic mesophase is characterized by a little cloudy and glutinous state which exhibit central cone like texture with an affirmative signal of birefringence under a polarizing microscope. The cholesteric mesophase become visible at elevated temperature in comparison to smectic mesophase and is also little cloudy in nature. However, it is more liquify than

Figure 3. Chemical structure of cholesterylesters (R= C_xH_y, number of carbons: 1 to 20+, number of double bonds: 0 to 3)

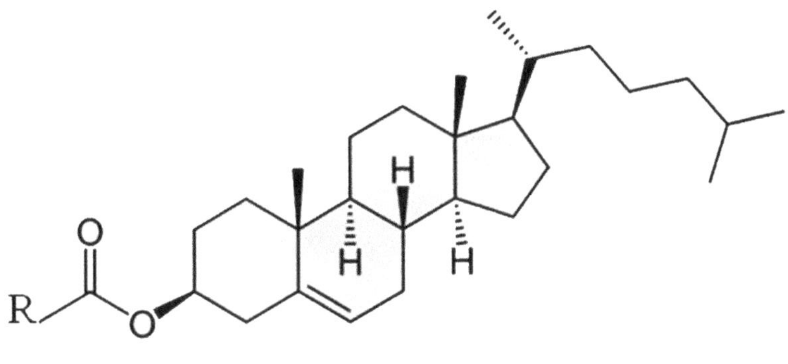

the smectic phase and frequently long range twisted or helical structure shows a variety of colors. This type of mesophase when observed under microscope displayed focal-conic textures along with a negative sign of birefringence.

On the basis of thickness determination, found to be 17 Å of the sterol region of saturated esters nearer to the 16.5-18 Å thickness of absolute length of cholesterol molecule, it is specified that the sterol axes exist almost regular to the smectic planes. A monounsaturated series of the cholesterol region exhibit only 14 Å thickness and it indicates that the sterol axis is slanted about 54° with reference to the smectic phase. Hence, a saturated chain materializes as smectic A liquid crystal (fragments in line of axis normal to the smectic plane), whereas the unsaturated chain referred as smectic C liquid crystal (fragments in line of axis tilted with reference to smectic plane).

The ordering of molecules in the ring of cholesteryl esters is seems to be an essential characteristic of mesophases, and a ring ordering at higher degree is distinguishing feature of the configuration of a cholesteric phase. In fact, an isotropic liquid phase transformation (with double the usual entropy) of cholesteric lipids was revealed by calorimetry studies on dicholesteryl esters. Thus indicates that the interaction of steroid rings is essential in ordering the cholesteric phase.

Histologically or submicrosopically, cholesteryl ester droplets exhibit a range of normal and pathological cellular fragments. Hence, the droplets of cholesteryl esters had been illustrated in neural tissue former to nerve myelination. Lipoprotein moieties responsible for transport of cholesterol in the blood to and from the tissues are characterized by the existence of a cholesteryl ester rich core (Figure 4).

Figure 4. Thermotropic liquid crystals (with the increase of temperature): (a) crystal; (b) smectic; (c) nematic; (d) liquid

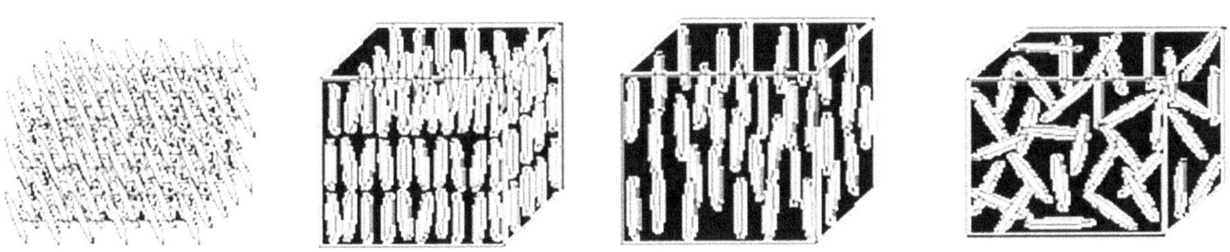

Phase Transition between States

The temperature at which the crystal lattice collapses is called as either melting point or the transition point, while temperature at which the true liquid is obtained has been referred to as the clarification point, clearing point, transition point, or melting point.

The transitions from the completely ordered solid crystal through the smectic and nematic structures to the true liquid may be outlined as follows (Brown & Shaw, 1957):

1. **Three-Dimensional Crystal:** Apart from vibration, the centers of gravity of all lattice units are fixed; rotations are not possible.
2. **Crystal with Rotating Molecules:** The centers of gravity of all lattice units are fixed; rotation about one or more axes is possible. Example: butyl halides.
3. **Smectic Structure:** The centers of gravity of the units (fragments) are movable in two dimensions; rotation in relation to one axis is permitted.
4. **Nematic Structure:** The centers of gravity of the units (molecules) are movable in three dimensions; rotation in relation to one axis is permitted.
5. **True Liquid:** The centers of gravity of the units are mobile in three directions; rotation about three axes perpendicular to one another is possible.

One can distinguish a stable smectic phase, forms by strong chain-chain interaction, as in the situation of esters group with long space between the first double bond and the terminal ester moiety. On the other hand, if ring-ring interaction is sufficiently strong than it will synthesize a cholesteric phase (the chain-chain interaction is weak). However, in the case of long and saturated chain, the liquid crystalline phase cannot be formed if the nucleation and crystallization will take place at temperature more than the required temperature for development of the liquid crystals.

The mesophases of cholesteryl ester exist in two forms – stable phase or metastable phase. Enantiotropic phase transition, a solid crystal gets melt, is responsible for formation of stable liquid crystalline phase. In contrast, a metastable mesophase was formed at lower temperature than that for crystal melts called as monotropic phase transition. It results into formation of under cooled isotropic liquid. Stable liquid crystalline phase maybe exists for an indefinite period, in the temperature scale stuck between the melting of crystals and isotropic liquid phase transition. Metastable liquid crystalline phase crystallizes very quickly or may exist for enough period of time but ultimately may be nucleated with crystalline esters to form an exact crystal which is thermodynamically more stable state (Ginsburg et al., 1984).

Assuming that the nucleation and crystallization do not take place earlier to reheating than almost all the transformation of liquid crystals are perfectly reversible. But if crystallization takes place results into formation of crystal with high melting point, then transitions to liquid crystals will not occurred on reheating, and solid crystals would be basically melts into an isotropic liquid. Distinctively, no liquid crystalline phases are scrutinized in saturated esters with more than 20 fatty acyl carbon atoms and metastability possessed by cholesteryl esters comprising a series of length more than C16 carbon atoms.

The liquid part is described by a maximum level of fluidity and moderately squat viscosity. Birefringence was not exhibit under polarized light by fluid materials and therefore is known as isotropic liquid phase. However, two broad maxima were shown by liquid phase of cholesterol and cholesteryl esters in the X-ray scattering studies. Using molybdenum Kα radiation, it was found that the diffraction-intensity curves are practically the same but the intensity is 5 to 15 percent more for the nematic skeleton in comparison to liquid phase. Sharper peaks with steeper inner slopes associate with the nematic structure indicate more promptness of structure in the plane.

Nematic Phase

Most commonly occurring liquid crystalline phase is nematic. The phrase nematic derived from greek word "*nema*" it means "thread". The word initiate from the thread like topological defect examined in nematic phase that is officially known as "disclination". Also it displays "hedgehog" topological defect. The rod shaped or calamitic organic fragments in nematic liquid crystalline phase are self aligned on their long axis which is approximately parallel to possess a long range directional order with no positional order (Figures 5 and 6) (Rego et al., 2010).

Smectic Phase

Smectic phase, usually exist at temperature lower than that for nematic phase, consist of definite layer of liquid crystals which can stack over one another in similar manner just like surface active agent. This word derived from latin term *smecticus* which means cleaning or possessing properties like soap. The organic fragments in a smectic phase have positional order in one dimension. The orientation of fragments in smectic A type is in the line of plane, however in smectic c type it is tilted away from the plane. In the layers this phases are appeared like liquid. On the basis of difference in degree of order of position and orientation, the variety of smectic phases are characterized (Figure 7) (Gennes & Prost, 1993; Chandrasekhar, 1993).

Smectic A: The fragments are properly arranged into layers.
Smectic C: The fragments are tilted within the layers.

Figure 5. Alignment in nematic phase

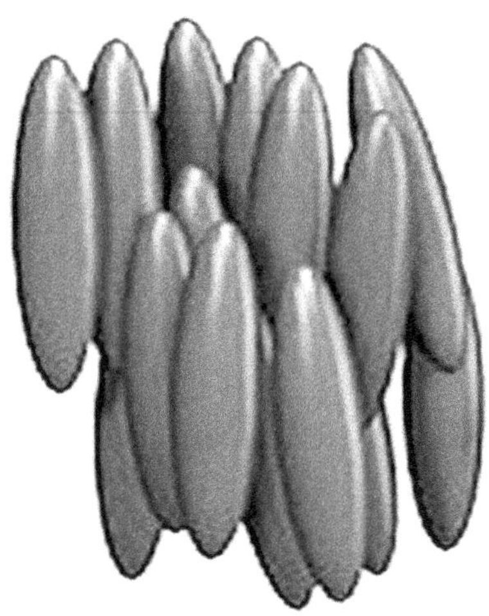

Figure 6. Phase transformation between a nematic (left) and smectic A (right) phases revealed between crossed polarizer and the black colour corresponds to isotropic medium

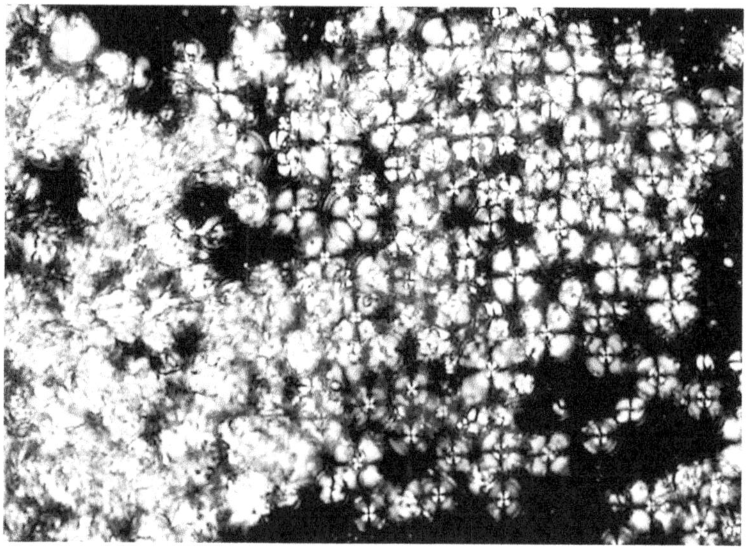

Figure 7. Schematic ordering in smectic phases

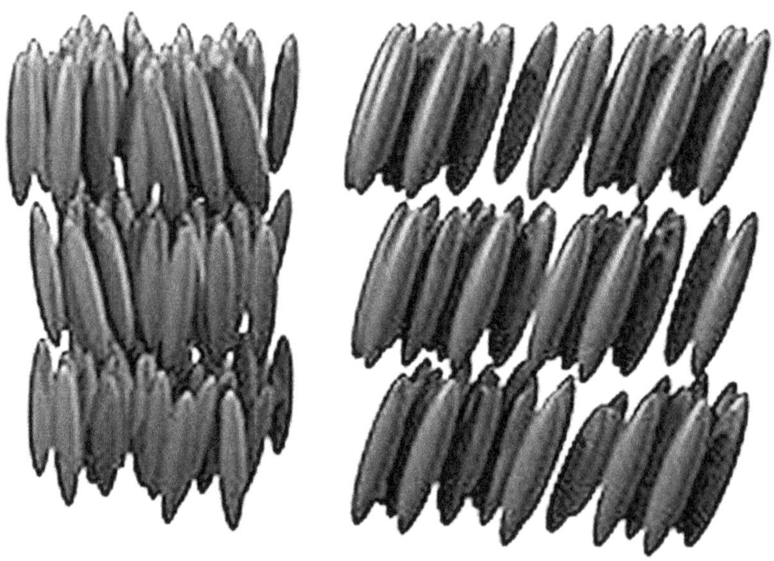

Chiral Phase

As the name indicates the chirality was exhibit by this kind of liquid crystal phase. It is also called as cholesteric phase as this phase was initially examined for derivative of cholesterol. The molecules in which the internal plane of symmetry is lacking will form the chiral phase. This phase was characterized by twisted molecules. The axis of molecule is parallel and its body is perpendicular to the director.

The angle of twisting depends on asymmetric packing of the adjacent molecules that result into longer range of chiral order. In the structure of Smectic C* phase the fragments possess positional ordering and slightly tilted with respect to normal layer by finite angle. An azimuthal twist induced by chirality between layers thereby produced spiral twist of molecular axis (Figure 8) (Gennes & Prost, 1993; Dierking, 2003; Collings & Hird, 1997).

The distance required by molecule of liquid crystalline system to make a complete 360° twist is referred as chiral pitch (p). However, at every half pitch the skeleton of chiral nematic phase repeats with phase director at 0° and ±180° are near about equal (Figure 9).

Blue Phases

This type of liquid crystalline phase exists in the range of temperature betweens the chiral nematic phases and an isotropic liquid phase. In 1981, it was proposed theoretically that an icosahedral arrangement just like quasicrystal can be exhibit by Blue phases. A usual three dimensional cube like framework was displayed by Blue phase having lattice period of several hundred nanometres. Hence a specific Bragg reflection was shown in the light with wavelength fall in the visible range because of cube like external appearance (Kleinert & Maki, 1981; Seideman, 1990).

As a tunable photonic crystal or fast light modulator blue phase is an area of interest to be studied. Blue phase appear in a very short range of temperature, generally not more than few degree celsius. It is confirmed recently that blue phases stabilized at a range of temperature not less than 60 K that includes room temperature (Coles-Harry & Pivenko-Mikhail, 2005; Yamamoto et al., 2005). At room temperature blue phases are remain stable and allowed electro-optical switching in reply to 10^{-4} s order of time (Kikuchi et al., 2002).

Discotic Phase

Disk shaped liquid crystal molecule may familiarize themselves in a layer like design called as discotic phase. Columnar discotic phase consists of disk shaped liquid crystal packed into columns. This column can be organizing them into hexagonal or rectangular array. If liquid crystal molecule in discotic phase shows chirality, then it is known as chiral discotic phase (Figure 10).

Figure 8. Schematic alignment in chiral liquid crystal phases

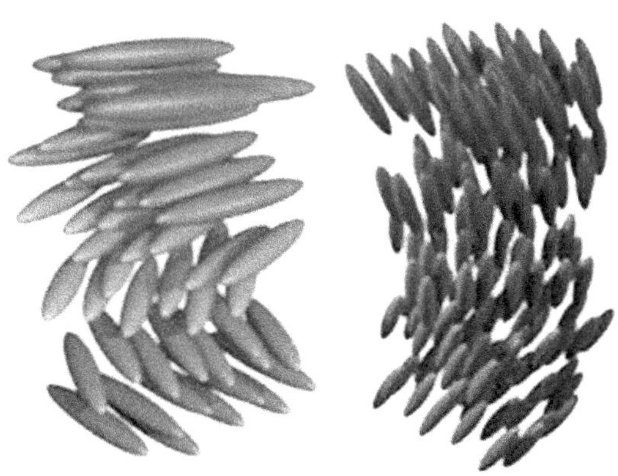

Figure 9. Chiral nematic phase; p refers to the chiral pitch

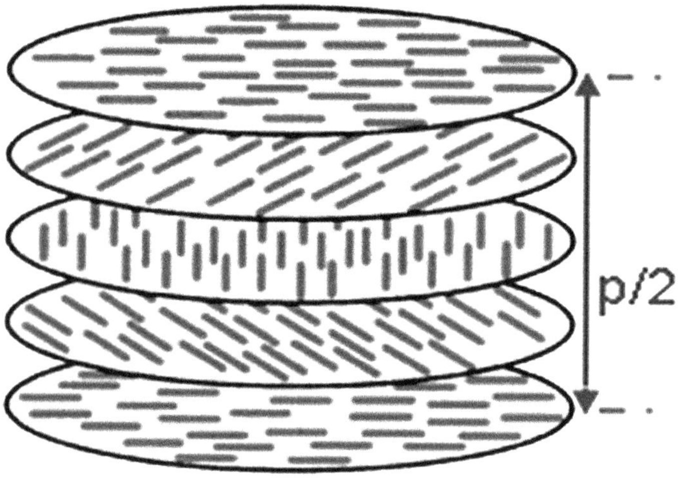

Figure 10. Schematic of columnar phases

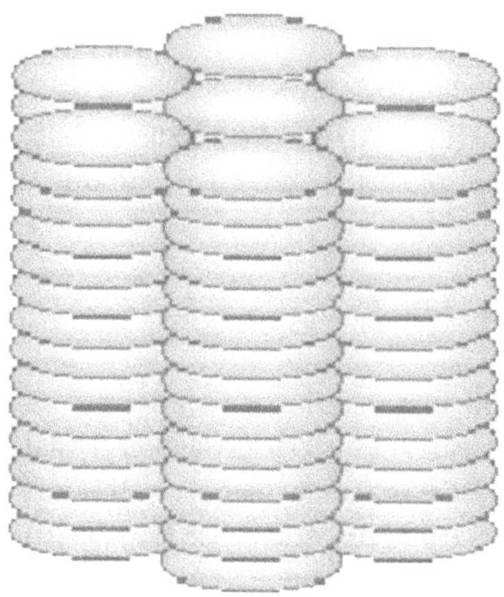

LYOTROPIC LIQUID CRYSTALS

Two or more than two fragments of lyotropic mesophase shows liquid crystalline characteristics in definite range of concentration. The solvent phase of lyotropic liquid crystalline system filled the empty space surrounding the molecule thereby imparts fluidity to the system (Qizhen Liang et al., 2005). An extent of liberty in concentration was enjoyed by lyotropic mesophase which allow them to provoke a range of diverse phases in comparison to thermotropic mesophase.

The amphiphillic moiety consists of two parts - one is hydrophilic and another is hydrophobic in the same skeleton. On the basis of balance between volume of hydrophilic and hydrophobic parts the lyotropic mesophase was exhibited by number of amphiphilic molecules. The structure is form in the course of micro phase separation of two immiscible parts on ananometer magnitude (Figure 11).

Figure 11. Structure of lyotropic liquid crystal, the red heads of surfactant molecules are in contact with water, whereas the tails are immersed in oil (blue): bilayer (left) and micelle (right)

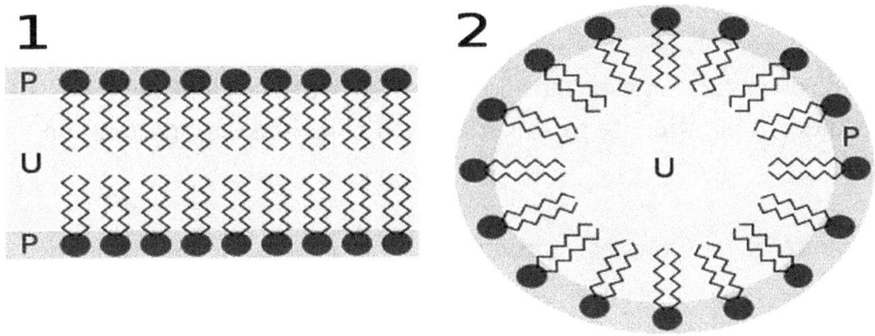

Lyotropic liquid crystal surfactants (surface-active agents) are materials that possess both a glacial moiety (the polar group) and a nonpolar paraffin chain in the same molecule.

Three different type of behavior can take place on addition of water to solid surfactants:

1. Surfactants are virtually insoluble, and remain as solid crystals with an aqueous solution of surfactants monomer.
2. Many surfactants molecule dissolve to forms an aqueous solution consist of micelles.
3. In certain range of concentration, the lyotropic liquid crystal phase is formed.

Surfactant is recommended as non-polar or semi-polar lipid if it is nearly insoluble in water and remains polarised at temperature less than Kraft point. However, at temperature just more than the Kraft point, number of surfactant formed micelle instead of liquid crystal. The lyotropic liquid crystal phase was formed at the temperature region in between the Kraft point and the melting point of surfactant. In the temperature region of 273K to 473K the lyotropic mesogen may be occurred as micellar solution. Some of the surfactant which do not forms micelle will convert into lyotropic LC molecules (Boyd et al., 2006).

In routine life the lyotropic liquid crystal were regularly come across but their existence was not usually familiarized. It also exists through the dissolution of soap and detergent. Even few products of this kind are still sold in the form of liquid crystalline system. The well-known example in industrial zone of lyotropic mesophase is the existence of neat phase in the manufacturing of soap. Analogous phases too exist during the handing of former detergent commodities. In everyday life it also encountered during preparation of cake butters may be composed of stabilized lyotropic liquid crystal emulsion. In the biological science, the lamellar lyotropic mesophase is frequently seen in the form of bilayer arrangement of molecule. Hence these components form the elementary skeleton of number of the biological membrane.

Lamellar liquid crystal phase is one of the most commonly occurring structures amongst lyotropic mesophases, continued by the hexagonal phase and the reverse hexagonal phase. Different types of cubic phases, commonly observe at narrow temperature and concentration ranges, are least common amongst lyotropic liquid crystalline system (Kossena et al., 2004). Two different properties of surfactant are said to be essential for the development of lyotropic liquid crystalline phase are as follows:

1. Degree of repulsive forces stuck between next head group at the interface of surfactant and water. Essential factors contribute to formation of liquid crystal are - power of hydration of head group, steric constraint of alkyl chain and may be the neighboring surfactant molecule have similar, dissimilar or zero charge.
2. The magnitude of contact between the alkyl chain and water, and the degree of alkyl chain conformational disorder. It is influence by the extent and magnitude of unsaturation within alkyl chain (Figure 12).

A general sequence of mesophases, starting from lower concentration to higher concentration of amphiphile are discontinuous cubic phase (micellar cubic phase), hexagonal phase (hexagonal columnar phase) (middle phase), lamellar phase, bicontinuous cubic phase, reverse hexagonal columnar phase and inverse cubic phase (Inverse micellar phase).

Metallotropic Liquid Crystal

Mesophases sometimes may be depends on low melting inorganic compounds like $ZnCl_2$. The accumulation of extended series, just like soap moieties, results into a progression of novel phase which exhibit a range of liquid crystalline behavior. It is a function of both the temperature and content ratio of inorganic phase. Hence such type of phase is called as metallotropic liquid crystal (Martin-James et al., 2006).

Physical Properties of Liquid Crystal

1. **Optical Property:** Optical property (birefringence) of liquid crystalline system can be defined as ability to split the plane polarised light into two different directions of unequal length for example calcite or quartz (Ban et al., 2010).
2. **Dielectric Property:** Dielectric property of liquid crystalline system can be defined as the material that does not conduct electicity readily (Shi et al., 2004)
3. **Diamagnetic Property:** Diamagnetic property of liquid crystalline system can be defined as the characteristics shown by the molecules with a negative magnetic weakness. It means the materials will magnetize in opposite direction to that of an applied magnetic field (Ohki, 2010).

Figure 12. Lyotropic liquid crystals: (a) hexagonal mesophases; (b) cubic mesophases; (c) lamellar mesophase

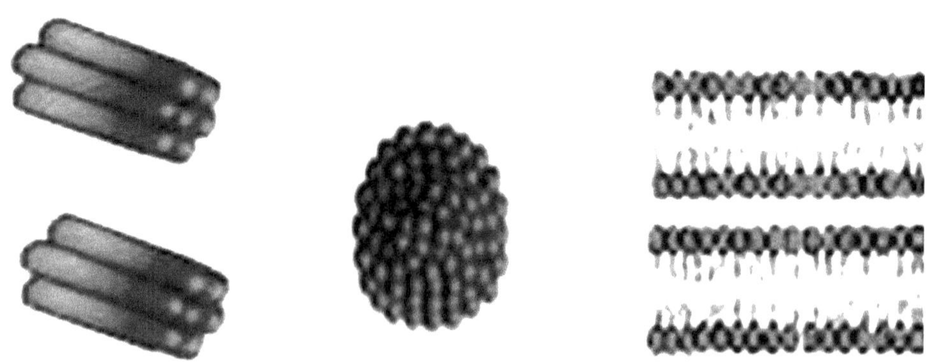

Factors Affecting on Properties of Liquid Crystals:

1. **Effect of Concentration:** The linear relationship exists between concentration of ampiphillic molecules and the properties of mesogen (Winsor, 1968).
2. **Effect of Temperature:** The linear relationship exists between temperature of ampiphillic molecules and the properties of mesogen (Alexandridis et al., 1996).
3. **Effect of Salt Addition:** The boundary of nematic phase was shifted above up to 10^0C due to addition of salts of sodium and potassium. Hence the isotropic phase at room temperature is converted to nematic liquid crystal phase (Kostko et al., 2005).
4. **Effect of pH:** The addition of salt to the solution or lowering of pH of the system will leads to reduction in interaction of hydrophilic head and lowering of interfacial area (Ibrahim et al., 1993).

Chemical Properties of Liquid Crystals

Two different types of liquid crystalline system – thermotropic and lyotropic liquid crystals are differ from each other on the basis of their self-arrangement mechanism. In thermotropic system as the name indicates the transition, responsible for fabrication of liquid crystals, are bring about thermally. It indicates that the liquid crystalline phase can be attained by either increasing the temperature of solid materials or decrease in temperature of liquid medium. In fact, anisotropic distribution forces within the moieties and packing interactions between the molecules are responsible for existence of thermotropic liquid crystal phase (Figure 13).

Two prime parameter rigidity and rod like shape should possess molecules in order to exhibit a liquid crystalline structure. The two cyclic units may be interconnected to attained rigid skeleton. A linear planar conformation was exhibit by the liquid crystalline system due to interconnection of groups. The compounds consist of groups with double bond just like - (HC=N)-, -N=N-, -(HC=CH)-, -HC=N-N=CH- will confine the liberty for rotation. The anisotropic polarizing ability is enhancing by conjugation of liquid crystalline group with phenylene ring. It also attributes the rigidity to the skeleton and enlarges the length of molecular system

Liquid Crystal Stabilization

The primary action in stabilization of liquid crystals is its isolation from the environment by a defensive barrier and converting it into a simply easy to use form. If outer packaging provides principal protec-

Figure 13. 5CB P-N pentyl-p-cyanobiphenyl (PCB)

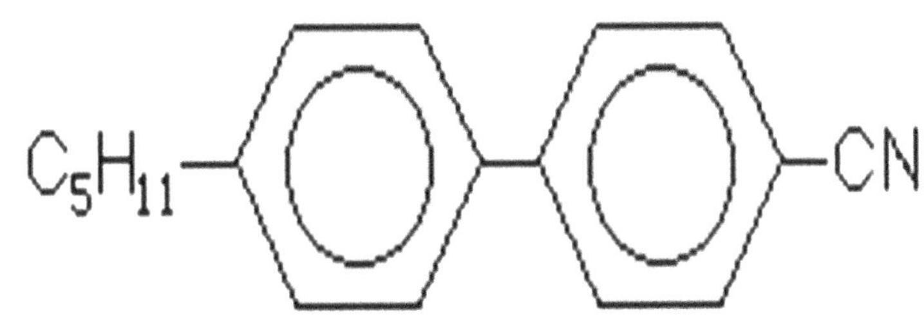

tion of liquid crystalline system against deprivation, then by incorporation of UV absorbing (stabilizing) property in the material, the secondary protection is provided, used in combination with the liquid crystal phase for making devices.

Recently, the most extensively used multipurpose and successful technique of stabilizing, packing and protecting mesophase mixtures is microencapsulation method. In easy words, a microsphere is tiny balls with an even wall surrounded it and in microencapsulation method small droplets of mesophase are coated with an unbroken polymer film to create distinct microsphere. The diameter of microcapsule usually measures in the size range of micron to millimetre.

POLYMERS USED IN LIQUID CRYSTALLINE SYSTEM

The rigid components when fused with the backbone of elastic polymer will form core polymeric chain of liquid crystalline system. The rigid region beside the chain permits the polymer to arrange them in a way like a regular mesophase and hence shows liquid crystalline characteristics. The behavior in which rigid region are formed, the liquid crystals are distinguished into two different groups of polymeric liquid crystals (PLC).

A rigid, rod shaped characteristic was processed by first monomeric group on the core chain of liquid crystal made up of polymer. Numerous aromatic rings are responsible for making up such monomers and providing them essential size. The following figure exhibit a pattern of such kind of PLC.

In polymer liquid crystal system, the more dominant and second group of core chain is distinguished because in this a mesogen is directly incorporated into the chain. Similar to the rigid areas in the first group the mesogen acts. Usually, two or more aromatic rings are required for making up the mesogenic units and also to exhibit liquid crystal property as well as to obtain essential control on movement of polymeric units. The limitations on rotation produced by the steric hindrance and resonance results into stiffness essential for liquid crystallinity of mesogenic units. Axial ratio is additional feature of mesogen defined as ratio of "length of molecule to the diameter"r ($x = L/d$). Investigational result shows that the molecules must be minimally three times longer as their width. If it is not obeyed, then the molecules are not rod shaped enough to show mesophasic characters.

This fraction is distinguished from the initial one either in manner that liquid crystals are segregated or decoupled by an elastic link known as spacer. Decoupling offers free movement of the fragments which enables suitable orientation within the system. The diagram of such type of core chain polymer liquid crystals is as follows.

Note the flexible spacer is the methylene group and the rigid mesogen is represented by aromatic rings and double bond (Figure 14).

ADVANTAGES

- Direct inner contact with the crystal healing energies and geometric structure permit the major benefit for a lot of peoples relating the liquid crystals.
- Through the liquid crystal, one can reach to the uppermost aspect of the mineral kingdom.

Figure 14. Structure of Ply (p-phenyleneterephthalate)

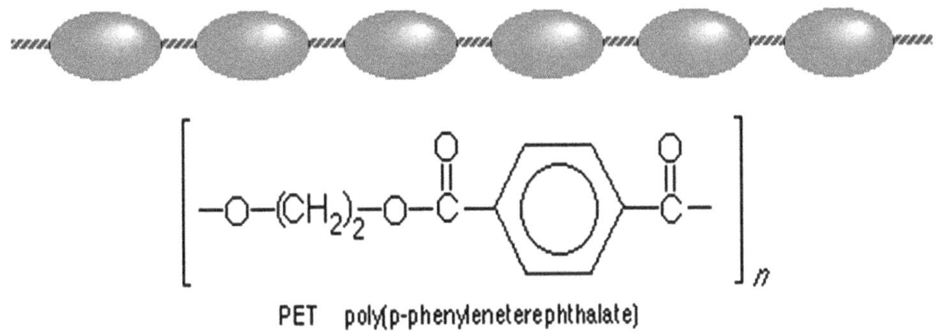

- The liquid crystals, even in a liquid form also preserve its programmability and permitting us to work on them how and where it is needed still inside the body also.
- When crystals from each part of the world are reunited and brought into singleness, the mesophase is the most complete illustration of the mineral kingdom and is the most powerful form of crystalline energy on the globe.
- Mesogen uses the curative energy and conducting capacity of water that enhances the outcomes of the therapy.

GENERAL METHOD FOR THE PREPRATION OF LIQUID CRYSTALLINE SYSTEM

The liquisolid system can be form from a liquid devoid of any modification. Alternatively, if a formulation of the water-insoluble drugs like hydrochlorthiazide, prednisone etc is done then initially it should be dissolved or suspended in a suitable non-volatile solvent system to [repare a solution or suspension of drug having required concentration. After that, the calculated amount of the ready drug solution or suspension or if the drug is in liquid form then the liquid drug is taken as it is and it is combined with a certain specified quantity of carrier which is porous in nature and which possess good absorbing properties like the granular and powder grade micro crystalline cellulose and amorphous cellulose are mostly preferred as carriers. The resultant damp mixture is then converted into a dry, having no adherence property, with free flow and readily compressible powder with addition of premeditated amount of coating material (Figure 15) (Sunit et al., 2012).

EVALUATION PARAMETERS OF LIQUID CRYSTALLINE SYSTEM

Macroscopy Study

Liquid crystals and its transition is identified by trained scientist who have long experience in the field of a new tool optical polarizing microscopy to check various non familiar materials.

Figure 15. General method of preparation of the liquisolid compact

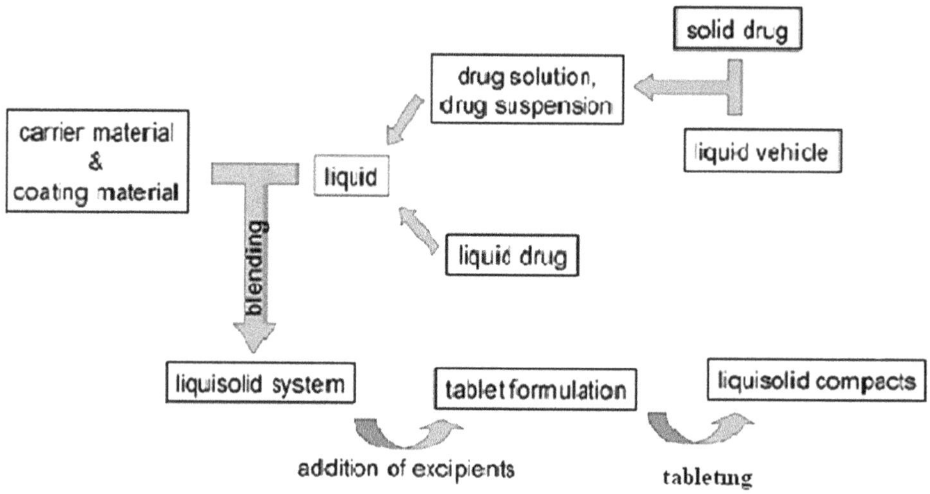

X-Ray Diffraction

X-Ray diffraction is very useful tool in recognition of various liquid crystalline systems and phases and their transitions. It is useful in determining surface texture of liquid crystal during phase transition process (Nounesis & Shivkumar, 1995).

Bragg's experiment cleared the basic and hurdle in understanding of x-ray diffraction principle. In this experiment the reflected light is linked with evenly spaced sheets passing through the centers of the atoms of the crystal lattice. Three Miller indices (h, k, l) are used to identify the direction of a particular set of sheets and the results are noted as *d*. All the scattered rays from neighboring planes will merge constructively (constructive interference). The angle in degrees (θ) *in* between the any plane and reflected x-rays results into difference in a path-length, which is an integer number in multiples *n* of the x-ray wavelength λ (Woolfson, 1997).

The different interfererence pattern occurs because of the distance between internal layer of crystal "d".

Bragg's equation, $d= n (\lambda /2) \sin \theta$

where

d = wavelength of X ray.
n= integer.
Θ= angel at which occurrence of interferences.

The above equation given by Bragg concludes that *d* (interlayer spacing) is inversely proportional to θ (angle of reflected light). X- ray diffraction of greater *d* in the area of longer order range can be estimated by SAXD (small-angle x-ray diffraction) while in case of small *d* values in the area of short-range order can be checked by WAXD (wide-angle x-ray diffraction).

Rheological Study

Rheometer is used for the rheological study of LCs. Different LCs shows different rheological behavior, rise in microstructure of LCs result into increase in consistency with increased viscosity. Lyotropic crystals like cubic and hexagonal crystals have low flow ability due to its 3 & 2 dimensional order. Mesophases from lamellar class are one dimensional in nature and have long range thus possess high flow ability due to gel character, while in case of cubic & hexagonal mesophases show stress still system is not able to flow.

Vesicle Size

Vesicle size of systems is measured by laser light scattering technique; it is quick method which is for applied for particles >1nm.

Differential Scanning Calorimetry

Differential scanning calorimetry is useful for technique in the study of transitions of liquid crystal phases. Heat supplied or extracted during phase transition in LCs can be noted (Nounesis & Shivkumar., 1995).

Transitions in phases are come with changes in the free energy which is due to change in enthalpy (ΔH) or entropy (ΔS) of the LCs. Thus endothermic or exothermic peaks are obtained in DSC thermograms. Phase transitions occurred due to change in entropy, recognized by an alteration in baseline slope of thermogram, which is because of alteration of specific heat capacity. LC polymer phase transitions are occurring due to change in entropy and considered as second order transitions e.g. rubber or glass, called as glass transitions (Miller-Goymann, 2004).

Crystalline phase to amorphous phase such type of transition requires a high energy while in contrast for crystalline transitions to liquid crystalline and liquid crystalline to amorphous transitions requires less quantity of energy, thus device has capability to detect lower values.

Estimation Solubility of Drugs in Semisolids

It's very difficult to determine solubility of drug present in semi-solids so, additional amount of drug is required to prepare saturated system, it's lavish and formulation is not cost effective. Number of techniques are available to assess solubility of drugs in semi-solids such as microscopic study (Gopferich & Lee, 1992); differential scanning calorimetry (DSC) (Jenquin & Mcginity, 1994; Theeuwes et al.,1974); x-ray powder diffraction (Suryanarayanan et al., 1992) HyperDS (Gramaglia et al., 2005); Higuchi release data (Chowhan & Pritchard., 1975) and infra-red ATR spectroscopy (Cantor, 1999). While DSC, XRPD and release data additionally provides release kinetics and drug evaluation.

- **Content Uniformity:** Sample is dissolve in appropriate solvent to determine uniformity of content. Whatman filter paper is used to filter the solution. Lastly the content of drug was estimated using UV-VIS spectrophotometer at specified wavelength (Lee & Kellaway, 2000).
- **Flow Property:** Flow properties of the LCs are calculated by evaluating Carr's index, angle of repose and Hausner's ratio. Fixed funnel method is used for evaluation of angle of repose. The

both densities bulk and tapped required for the calculation of Carr's index and Hausner's ratio (Ansel et al., 1999).

- **Fourier Transform Infra-Red Study:** IR spectrum of optimized formulation was determined by KBr plate method using Fourier FTIR. Dried potassium bromide is used for the baseline correction and then the FTIR spectrum of sample with potassium bromide was recorded. The LCs sample was scanned in IR region ranges from 4000 to 400 cm^{-1}. The compatibility of drug and other excipients in formulation was confirmed by comparing drug and formulation spectra.
- **TEM Study (Transmission Electron Microscopy):** TEM have high magnification power thus the microscopic view of liquid crystals is easy visualize. Sample must be free from water as water will not exist at high vacuum of electron microscope. Thus freeze fracture a special technique is used for the preparation of sample (Ahmed et al., 2004).

APPLICATIONS

Liquid crystal concept has many applications in the different areas such as pharmacy, science, engineering etc. These liquid crystalline systems are still in need of new inventions to show its miracle powers for the society to overcome number of problems.

Pharmaceutical Application

- **Enhancement of Solubility in Case of Poorly Soluble Drugs:** In lyotropic liquid crystals more number of substances is soluble (e.g. hydrocortisone) due to its solubilising nature. Most of times, systems which are applied through dermal route LCs can be used but it have limited applications. As in case of hydrocortisone when used upto 4%, then use specified concentration range of LCs upto 1% only(Makai et al., 2003).

Examples of applications of liquid crystal formulations in drug delivery are shown in Table 3 (Lee et al., 2009; Lara et al., 2005; Esposito et al., 1996).

- **Controlled/Sustained Release of Drug:** All of the applications of mesophases (liquid crystal) in pharmaceutical field depend on their characteristics. Polar lipids when in contact with aqueous atmosphere liquid crystalline materials of lipid-based are formed by mechanism of swelling. Thus they are able to release the drug in sustained manner (Drummond & Fong, 1999; Kraineva et al., 2006).
    - E.g. In treatment of periodontal diseases lyotropic liquid crystal can be used.

This study was done for development of unaqueous lyotropic liquid crystalline systems, which is composed of oils (Miglyol 801) and surface active agents (Cremophor EL, Cremophor RH40), as they easily form lyotropic liquid crystalline phase in aqueous surroundings. Low viscosity systems can be injected into the periodontal pocket very easily and release of drug is in controlled manner, when they are changed into liquid crystalline phase of highly viscous nature (Feher et al., 2008).

Table 3. Examples of applications of liquid crystal formulations in drug delivery

Formulation Components	Phases	Drug	Delivery Route	Release Kinetics
Brij 96/Water/liquid petrolatum/glycerol Gel	Lamellar	Ephedrine hydrochloride	*In vitro*	First order and zero order
Glyceryl monooleate	Lamellar, Cubic	Dadle	*In vitro*	Not tested
Oleylglycerate, Phytanylglycerate	Reverse hexagonal	Paclitaxel, Glucose, Histidine	*In vitro*	Higuchi kinetics
Phytantriol	Reverse hexagonal	Glucose, Allura red	Oral	Diffusion controlled
Glyceryl monooleate	Cubic	Salicylic acid	*In vitro*	Second order swelling kinetics, Fickian diffusion
Monoolein	Cubic	α- chymotrypsin, cytochrome C	*In vitro*	Not tested
Lauric acid	Cubic	Cinnarizine	Duodenal	Not tested
Monoolein	Cubic	Atenolol, Pindolol, Propranolol, Pyrimethamine	*In vitro*	First order and zero order
Glyceryl monooleate	Cubic	Insulin	*In vitro*	Not tested
Poloxamer, Monoglyceride	Cubic	Tetracycline	Periodontal	Fickian diffusion
4-pentyl-4-cyanobiphenyl (k15) 4-heptyl-4-cyanobiphenyl (k21) membrane	Thermotropic	Paracetamol, Methimazole	*In vitro*	Not tested
Cholesteryloleyl carbonate	Thermotropic	Salbutamol sulphate	*In vitro*	Not tested

*NT: not tested.

- **Example of Lamellar Liquid Crystals Containing Glycerol:** Lamellar lyotropic liquid crystal was formed by using poly-oxyethylene-10-oleyl ether (Brij 96) water, liquid petroleum (LP) and glycerol.
- **Stability of Drug:** In the manufacturing of stable hydrocarbon foam the lyotropic liquid crystals are used. In past it's a challenge and very difficult to prepare hydrocarbon foams but now lyotropic liquid crystal molecules change from inverse micelles to easily prepare foams. Hydrocarbon compounds and the surface active agents are miscible with each other while surfactants are not soluble in water, even though water is able to solubilise in the surfactant and lastly mix to prepare the liquid crystal (Paavola et al., 2005).
- **Effect of Liquid Crystalline Systems on Drug Release Profile:** The release of systems is modified after the effect of chlorhexidine species, chlorhexidine base and their salts on the physicochemical characteristics of LCs and also on drug transport through lipoid barriers. It can be possible by use of non-ionic surfactant such as Synperonic A7(PEG7-C13-15) during formulation of liquid crystal (Farkase et al., 2007).
- **For the Formulation of Nanostructure Compounds by Photo-Polymerization of Lyotropic Liquid Crystalline Systems:** A novel route to fabricating such materials is through the use of LLCs that have nanostructures of high order. However, lyotropic liquid crystals being short of required strength. So, templating lyotropic liquid crystals morphology on different compounds (organic polymer) would give a nanostructure retained as part of a robust polymeric matrix. This study focuses on photo polymerization behavior and structure reteintion of hydroxyethyl

acrylate(HEA)/dodecyltrimethyl ammonium bromide(DTAB)/water system in a select liquid crystal phase (Lee et al.,2003).

- **Nanostructure Hexosome for Injectable Drug Delivery:** The formation of reverse hexagonal phase in excess of water by addition of amphiphiles of glycerate head groups, to form hexosome dispersion contain particles of size 200 nm able to retain nanostructure of hexosome phase internally. In the formulation of new parenteral systems of irinotecan was explored (Boyd et al., 2006).
- **Temperature Adjusted Permeation of Drug Throughout Liquid Crystal Surrounded Cellulose Membrane:** The membranes which are stimuli-sensitive work as "permeability valves" or "on-off switches", able to release the drug in pulsatile manner, where transfer rate of mass and time required for it can be guarded by external or environmental conditions. For drug permeation the thermoresponsive barriers are needed which are developed by thermotropic liquid crystals present in between cellulose nitrate (CN) and cellulose acetate (CA). The nematic to isotropic phase transition temperature 41.5^0C in case of transitions of low molecular weight thermotropic liquid crystal of n-heptyl-cyanobiphenyl can be used to adjust permeation of drug. It was found that upon changing temperature, both cellulose membrane without liquid crystal illustrate no temperature sensitivity for the permeation of drug, whereas the marks for liquid crystal captured membranes show a split jumps in permeability when there is rise in temperature more than its transition temperature of drug liquid crystal (Lin et al.,2001; Dinarvand et al., 2006; Atyabi et al., 2007).
- **Liquid Crystal for Treatment of Cancer and Other Disease:** Recently the LCs can be used in the treatment of cancer as new drug is developed name das Tolecine developed by Tsai, compound that also have antiviral and antibacterial activity, this technology can be used in treatment of certain diseases.

The combination of Tolecine and Aoatone® patented, which is specifically for treatment of cancer through different pathways with better efficacy as well as FDA permitted Apatone® as orphan drug for the treatment of metastatic bladder cancer in August 2007 (Tsai et al., 2007).

Technological Field

In Displays of LC's

Recent application of LC's is the LCD (liquid crystal displays) most prominently in technical field, which provide billions of rupees of trade in the market. The LC's act as a primary invention for number of discoveries concerned with science and engineering field.

If transitions occur in the certain type of liquid crystals (i.e. smectic and nematic) due to change in temperature, result into change in their optical form and their property of light transmission. They are able to show double refraction by splitting ordinary light beam into two polarized components. This phenomenon has great applications in the egg timers, thermometers, and heat sensors. LC's structure can also be changed in the presence of magnetic field, so can be used in calculators as well as in LCD displays.

Temperature Measuring Device Such as Thermometer

The principle of LC's can be used in the thermometers as we discussed previously in this chapter, the liquid crystals of chiral nematic type able to reflect light of a wavelength which is equal to the pitch as it depend on upon temperature so, the colour which reflected from chiral nematic crystal depend upon temperature. LC's have ability to measure the temperature accurately by looking at thermometer colour. It is more advantages by mixing different types of LC's in one thermometer to measure temperature in between wide range.

Chiral nematic LC's also used in the most popular "mood ring", as it took benefit of the exclusive property of it. LC's have number of applications in the field of medicine and electronic science. Recently it's easy to map the body temperature by adhering modified liquid crystal devices to the skin as tumors have different temperature than that of surrounding tissue. Identification of bad circuit connections can be possible by using liquid crystal temperature sensors, as they have ability to check the distinguishing higher temperature.

In clinical field the LC's thermometers can be used, the technique is called as liquid crystal thermography. It identifies the illness of human being by sticking the tape of LC's thermometer to skin of patient to map body temperature, as it is based on the principle of reflection.

Optical Imaging

The most recent application of liquid crystal is optical imaging technology and recording. A liquid crystal cell is sandwiched in between two photoconductors and light is ready to fall on photoconductor; it is observed that conductivity of material is increased, result into development of electric field which is influenced by change in applied light intensity. The electrode transmits the different electric pattern for different samples and the optical image for the changes can be recorded.

Other Liquid Crystal Applications

In different fields LC's have wide variety of applications few are as follows;

- For nondestructive mechanical testing of materials under stress.
- For the visualization of RF (radio frequency) waves in waveguides.
- Used in medical applications where, for example, transient pressure transmitted by a walking foot on the ground is measured.
- Low molar mass (LMM) liquid crystals have applications including erasable optical disks,
- Full color "electronic slides" for computer-aided drawing (CAD),
- Light modulators for color electronic imaging.

The new properties and types of LC's still investigated, its sure that, these types definitely have great importance in pharmaceutical and other fields.

REFERENCES

Ahmed, A., Barry, B. W., Williams, A. C., & Davis, A. F. (2004). Pencyclovir solubility in Eudragit films: A comparison of x-ray, thermal, microscopic and release rate techniques. *Journal of Pharmaceutical and Biomedical Analysis*, *34*(5), 945–956. doi:10.1016/j.jpba.2003.11.018 PMID:15019028

Alexandridis, P., Zhou, D., & Khan, A. (1996). *Lyotropic liquid crystallinity in amphiphilic block copolymers: temperature effect on phase behavior and structure copolymers of different composition.* Academic Press.

Ansel, H. C., Allen, L. V., & Popovich, N. G. (1999). Pharmaceutical dosage forms and drug delivery systems. Philadelphia: Lippincott Williams and Wilkins.

Atyabi, F., Khodaverdi, E., & Dinarvand, R. (2007). Temeperature modulated drug permeation through liquid crystal embedded cellulose membranes. *International Journal of Pharmaceutics*, *339*(1-2), 213–221. doi:10.1016/j.ijpharm.2007.03.004 PMID:17448615

Ban, J. F., Lu, S. R., & Zhang, C. X. (2010). Synthesis and characterization of biphenylnate liquid crystalline polyurethanes. *Key Engineering Materials*, *428-429*, 158–161. doi:10.4028/www.scientific.net/KEM.428-429.158

Boyd, B. J., Khoob, S., Whittaker, D. V., & Davey, S. M. (2006). Lyotropic liquid crystalline phases formed from glycerate surfactants as sustained release drug delivery systems. *International Journal of Pharmaceutics*, *309*(1-2), 218–226. doi:10.1016/j.ijpharm.2005.11.033 PMID:16413980

Boyd, B. J., Whittaker, D. V., Khoob, S., & Davey, S. M. (2006). Hexosome formed from glycerate surfactants-Formulation as a colloidal carrier for irinotecan. *International Journal of Pharmaceutics*, *318*(1-2), 154–162. doi:10.1016/j.ijpharm.2006.03.010 PMID:16621358

Brown, G. H., & Shaw, W. G. (1957). The mesomorphic state: Liquid crystals. *Chemical Reviews*, *57*(6), 1049–1157. doi:10.1021/cr50018a002

Cantor, A. S. (1999). Drug and excipient diffusion and solubility in acrylate adhesives measured by infrared-attenuated total reflectance (IR-ATR) spectroscopy. *Journal of Controlled Release*, *61*(1-2), 219–231. doi:10.1016/S0168-3659(99)00119-4 PMID:10469917

Chandrasekhar, S. (1993). *Liquid Crystals* (2nd ed.). Cambridge Univ Pr Published.

Chowhan, Z. T., & Pritchard, R. (1975). Release of corticoids from oleaginous ointment bases containing drug in suspension. *Journal of Pharmaceutical Sciences*, *64*(5), 754–759. doi:10.1002/jps.2600640505 PMID:1151642

Coles-Harry, J., & Mikhail, N. (2005). Liquid crystal 'blue phases' with a wide temperature range. *Nature Materials*, *436*(7053), 997–1000. doi:10.1038/nature03932

Collings, P. J., & Hird, M. (1997). *Introduction to Liquid Crystals.* Bristol, PA: Taylor & Francis. doi:10.4324/9780203211199

Dierking, I. (2003). *Textures of Liquid Crystals.* Weinheim: Wiley-VCH. doi:10.1002/3527602054

Dinarvand, R., Khodaverdi, E., Atyabi, F., & Erfan, M. (2006). Thermoresponsive drug delivery using liquid crystal-embedded cellulose nitrate membranes. *Drug Delivery*, *13*(5), 345–350. doi:10.1080/10717540500394729 PMID:16877309

Drummond, C. J., & Fong, C. (1999). Surfactant self-assembly objects as novel drug delivery vehicles. *Current Opinion in Colloid & Interface Science*, *4*(6), 449–456. doi:10.1016/S1359-0294(00)00020-0

Esposito, E., Carotta, V., Scabbia, A., Trombelli, L., D'Antona, P., Menegatti, E., & Nastruzzi, C. (1996). Comparative analysis of tetracycline-containing dental gels: Poloxamer- and monoglyceride-based formulations. *International Journal of Pharmaceutics*, *142*(1), 9–23. doi:10.1016/0378-5173(96)04649-2

Farkas, E., Kiss, D., & Zelk, O. R. (2007). Study on the release of chlorhexidine base and salts from different liquid crystalline structures. *International Journal of Pharmaceutics*, *340*(1-2), 71–75. doi:10.1016/j.ijpharm.2007.03.038 PMID:17467206

Farkas, E., Kiss, D., & Zelkó, R. (2007). Study on the release of chlorhexidine base and salts from different liquid crystalline structures. *International Journal of Pharmaceutics*, *340*(1-2), 71–75. doi:10.1016/j.ijpharm.2007.03.038 PMID:17467206

Feher, A., Urban, E., Eros, I., Szabove, P., & Csanyi, E. (2008). Lyotropic liquid crystal perconcentrates for the treatment of periodontal disease. *International Journal of Pharmaceutics*, *358*(1-2), 23–26. doi:10.1016/j.ijpharm.2008.02.025 PMID:18403142

Gennes, P. G., & Prost, J. (1993). *The Physics of Liquid Crystals*. Oxford, UK: Clarendon Press.

Ginsburg, G. S., Atkinson, D., & Small, D. M. (1984). Physical properties of cholesteric esters. *Progress in Lipid Research*, *23*(3), 135–167. doi:10.1016/0163-7827(84)90002-X PMID:6399750

Gopferich, A., & Lee, G. (1992). Determining the solubility and crystal form of clenbuterol in thin films of Eudragit NE30D. *Drug Development and Industrial Pharmacy*, *18*(3), 319–331. doi:10.3109/03639049209043702

Gramaglia, D., Conway, B. R., Kett, V. L., Malcolm, R. K., & Batchelor, H. K. (2005). High speed DSC (HyperDSC) as a tool to measure the solubility of a drug within a solid or semi-solid matrix. *International Journal of Pharmaceutics*, *301*(1-2), 1–5. doi:10.1016/j.ijpharm.2005.04.038 PMID:16061335

Ibrahim, H. G., Sallam, E., Takieddin, M., & Habboub, M. (1993). Effects of solute characteristics and concentration on a lyotropic liquid crystal: Solute induced phase change. *Pharmaceutical Research*, *10*(5), 5–12. doi:10.1023/A:1018920118631 PMID:8321840

Jenquin, M. R., & McGinity, J. W. (1994). Characterization of acrylic resin matrix films and mechanisms of drug-polymer interactions. *International Journal of Pharmaceutics*, *101*(1-2), 23–34. doi:10.1016/0378-5173(94)90072-8

Kikuchi, H., Yokota, M., Hisakado, Y., Yang, H., & Kajiyama, T. (2002). Polymer-stabilized liquid crystal blue phases. *Nature Materials*, *1*(1), 64–68. doi:10.1038/nmat712 PMID:12618852

Kleinert, H., & Maki, K. (1981). Lattice Textures in Cholesteric Liquid Crystals. *Fortschritte der Physik*, *29*(5), 219–259. doi:10.1002/prop.19810290503

Kossena, G. A., Charman, W. N., Boyd, B. J., & Porter, C. J. (2004). A novel cubic phase of medium chain lipid origin for the delivery of poorly water soluble drugs. *Journal of Controlled Release*, *99*(2), 217–229. doi:10.1016/j.jconrel.2004.06.013 PMID:15380632

Kostko, A. F., Cipriano, B. H., Pinchuk, O. A., Ziserman, L., Anisimov, M. A., Danino, D., & Raghavan, S. R. (2005). Salt effects on the phases behavior,structure and rheology of chromonic liquid crystals. *The Journal of Physical Chemistry B*, *109*(41), 19126–19133. doi:10.1021/jp052575u PMID:16853466

Kraineva, J., Nicolini, C., Thiyagarajan, P., Kondrashkina, E., & Winter, R. (2006). Incorporation of α-chymotrypsin into the 3D channels of bicontinuous cubic lipid mesophases. *Biochimica et Biophysica Acta*, *1764*(3), 424–433. doi:10.1016/j.bbapap.2005.11.004 PMID:16330264

Kulkarni, S. D., Bakliwal, S. R., Rane, B. R., Pawar, S. P., & Gujarathi, N. A. (2012). Evaluation of Liquisolid Compacts Using Response Surface Methodology. *International Journal of Drug Delivery.*, *4*, 427–433.

Lara, M. G., Bentley, M. V., & Collett, J. H. (2005). *In vitro* drug release mechanism and drug loading studies of cubic phase gels. *International Journal of Pharmaceutics*, *293*(1-2), 241–250. doi:10.1016/j.ijpharm.2005.01.008 PMID:15778062

Lee, J., & Kellaway, I. W. (2000). *In vitro* peptide release from liquid crystalline buccal delivery systems. *International Journal of Pharmaceutics*, *195*(1-2), 29–33. doi:10.1016/S0378-5173(99)00356-7 PMID:10675679

Lee, W. Y., Nguyen, T. H., Hanley, T., & Boyd, B. J. (2009). Nanostructure of liquid crystalline matrix determines *in vitro* sustained release and in vivo oral absorption kinetics for hydrophilic model drugs. *International Journal of Pharmaceutics*, *365*(1-2), 190–199. doi:10.1016/j.ijpharm.2008.08.022 PMID:18790030

Lehmann, O. (1889). ÜberfliessendeKrystalle. *Zeitschrift für Physikalische Chemie*, *4*, 462–472.

Lin, S. Y., Ho, C. J., & Li, M. J. (2001). Precision and reproducibility of temperature response of a thermo-responsive membrane embedded by binary liquid crystals for drug delivery. *J. Contrl. Rel*, *73*(2-3), 293–301. doi:10.1016/S0168-3659(01)00300-5 PMID:11516506

Makai, M., Csányi, E., Németh, Z., Pálinkás, J., & Erős, I. (2003). Structure and drug release of lamellar liquid crystals containing glycerol. *International Journal of Pharmaceutics*, *256*(1-2), 95–107. doi:10.1016/S0378-5173(03)00066-8 PMID:12695015

Martin-James, D., Keary-Cristin, L., Thornton-Todd, A., & Novotnak-Mark, P. (2006). Metallotropic liquid crystals formed by surfactant templating of molten metal halides. *Nature Materials*, *5*(4), 271–275. doi:10.1038/nmat1610 PMID:16547520

Müller-Goymann, C. C. (2004). Physicochemical characterization of colloidal drug delivery systems such as reverse micelles, vesicles, liquid crystals and nanoparticles for topical administration. *European Journal of Pharmaceutics and Biopharmaceutics*, *58*(2), 343–356. doi:10.1016/j.ejpb.2004.03.028 PMID:15296960

Nounesis, G., Shi, Y., & Kumars, S. (1995). *X-ray Diffraction and Calorimetric Studies of Nematic – Nematic and Smectic – Sematic phase Transitions.* ACS Meeting, Anaheim, CA.

Ohki, Y. (2010). Development of epoxy resin composites with high thermal conductivity. *IEEE Electrical Insulation Magazine*, *26*(1), 1–49. doi:10.1109/MEI.2010.5383936

Paavola, A., Kilpelaine, I., Yliruusi, J., & Rosenberg, P. (2005). Controlled release of vancomycine from poloxamer 407 gels. *International Journal of Pharmaceutics*, *288*(2), 235–244. doi:10.1016/j.ijpharm.2004.09.028 PMID:15620863

Qizhen, L., Pengtao, L., Cheng, L., Xigao, J., Dingyi, H., & Yang, L. (2005). Synthesis and Properties of Lyotropic Liquid Crystalline Copolyamides Containing Phthalazinone Moieties and Ether Linkages. *Polymer*, *46*(16), 6258–6265. doi:10.1016/j.polymer.2005.05.059

Rego, J. A., Harvey, J. A. A., MacKinnon, A. L., & Gatdula, E. (2010). Asymmetric synthesis of a highly soluble 'trimeric' analogue of the chiral nematic liquid crystal twist agent Merck S1011. *Liquid Crystals.*, *37*(1), 37–43. doi:10.1080/02678290903359291

Reinitzer, F. (1888). BeiträgezurKenntniss des Cholesterins. *MonatsheftefürChemie (Wien)*, *9*(1), 421–441.

Seideman, T. (1990). The liquid-crystalline blue phases. *Reports on Progress in Physics*, *53*(6), 659–705. doi:10.1088/0034-4885/53/6/001

Shao, Y., & Zerda, T. W. (1998). Phase Transitions of Liquid Crystal PAA in Confined Geometries. *The Journal of Physical Chemistry B*, *102*(18), 3387–3394. doi:10.1021/jp9734437

Shi, M. Q., Zhang, M. Z., Rong, B., Wetzel, K., & Friedrich, K. (2004). Sliding wear behavior of epoxy containing nano-Al_2O_3 particles with different pretreatments. *Wear*, *256*(11-12), 1072–1081. doi:10.1016/S0043-1648(03)00533-7

Sluckin, T. J., Dunmur, D. A., & Stegemeyer, H. (2004). *Crystals That Flow – classic papers from the history of liquid crystals*. London: Taylor & Francis.

Suryanarayanan, R., Venkatesh, S., Hodgin, L. P., & Hanson, P. (1992). Hanson. Determination of the physical state of salicylic acid in hydrogel formulations by x-ray diffractometry. *International Journal of Pharmaceutics*, *78*(1-3), 77–83. doi:10.1016/0378-5173(92)90357-8

Tai, H. S., & Lee, J. Y. (1990). Phase transition behaviors and selective optical properties of a binary cholesteric liquid crystals system: Mixtures of cholesteryloleyl carbonate and cholesteryl nonanoate. *Journal of Applied Physics*, *67*(2), 1001–1006. doi:10.1063/1.345807

Theeuwes, F., Hussain, A., & Higuchi, T. (1974). Quantitative analytical method for determination of drugs dispersed in polymers using differential scanning calorimetry. *Journal of Pharmaceutical Sciences*, *63*(3), 427–429. doi:10.1002/jps.2600630325 PMID:4820377

Tsai, C., Jamison, J., & Miller, T. (2007). New liquid crystal technology hope for treatment of cancer and other diseases. Kent State University.

Winsor, P. A. (1968). Binary and multicomponent solution of amphiphilic compounds solubilization and the formation structure and theoretical significance of liquid crystalline solutions. *Chemical Reviews*, *68*(1), 1–40. doi:10.1021/cr60251a001

Yamamoto, J., Nishiyama, I., Inoue, M., & Yokoyama, H. (2005). Optical isotropy and iridescence in a smectic blue phase. *Nature Materials*, *437*(7058), 525–528. doi:10.1038/nature04034 PMID:16177785

Chapter 9
Liquid Crystal Systems in Drug Delivery

Kamal Kumar Chaudhary
IIIT Allahabad, India

Pooja Kannojia
HNB Garhwal University, India

Nidhi Mishra
IIIT Allahabad, India

ABSTRACT

Liquid crystals have been recently studied as novel drug delivery system. The reason behind this is their similarity to colloidal systems in living organisms. They have proven to be advantageous over Traditional, Dermal, Parentral and Oral Dosage forms. Liquid crystals are thermodynamically stable and possess long shelf life. Liquid crystals show bio adhesive properties and sustained release effects. Objective of this book chapter is to provide in-depth information of Pharmaceutical crystal technology. It shall deal with cubic and hexagonal liquid crystal and their applications in Drug delivery system.

INTRODUCTION

Liquid Crystals (LCs) are determined as one of the most important state of matter subsisting amongst the crystalline solid and the liquid, qualified by the fond or consummate loss of perspective order in crystalline solids, although holding the orientational order of the constituent molecules. This orientational order can remain in the solid state and therefore LCs might demonstrate mechanical stableness like solids as well as flow like liquids. LCs demonstrates universal attributes like double refraction, reaction to magnetized and electrical areas, optical activity in twisted nematic phases and sensitiveness to temperature leading in color changes. Molecular orientation in LCs is the origin of the double refraction that is not exhibit in the glassy state, as it does not have the molecular orientational order. All LCs are condensed state of matter organized by anisotropic organic molecules but all the anisotropic molecules cannot form LCs. These molecules are named mesogens and are either of rod shape or less normally disc shape.

DOI: 10.4018/978-1-5225-0751-2.ch009

Summary of several classes of drugs examined for liquid crystals as drug delivery system given in Table 1. Crystalline solids are characterized by long-range positional and orientational order in three dimensions. Whereas amorphous liquids lack long-range order in any dimensions. LCs (mesophases) depict structural, mechanical and optical attributes intermediate to those of crystalline solids, amorphous and liquid state of matter as shown in Figure 1. LCs, nevertheless, are not a mixture of solids and liquids, but surely a separate state of matter (Lara, 2005). Liquid crystalline systems (mesophases) have been looked into as modern formulations by many authors (Lasson, 2009; Libster, 2007; Liu & Guo, 2007; Bunjes & Rades, 2005; Cervin et al., 2009).

A liquid crystalline material is called lyotropic if phases having long-ranged orientational order are induced by the addition of a solvent. Lipid-based lyotropic liquid crystals can be mainly classified into lamellar phase (L_{α}), cubic phase (V2), and hexagonal phase (H2) according to their different internal structures. Among them, V2 and H2 are the most important and recently have received much attention because of their extremely ordered internal structures, which offers the potential as a slow release matrix for active pharmaceutical ingredients with various sizes and polarities (Drummond& Fong, 1999; Shah et al., 2001). Cubic and hexagonal liquid crystals are often spontaneously formed by the addition of certain amphiphilic lipids in an aqueous environment (Kaasgaard & Drummond, 2006). When cubic and hexagonal liquid crystals are dispersed into nanoparticles with excess water with the addition of stabilizers such as Pluronic copolymers (Chong et al., 2011) and Myrj series (Chong et al., 2012), they form stable colloidal dispersions which are termed cubosomes and hexosomes, respectively (Spicer, 2005; Yaghmur & Glatter, 2009; Lancelot et al., 2014; Hirlekar et al., 2010). In general, the preparation methods of cubic and hexagonal liquid crystals are easier than their dispersions. For example, cubic and hexagonal liquid crystals can be formulated by simply blending lipid and aqueous phases by vortex

Table 1. Drugs in form of liquid crystals as drug delivery system

Drug Substances Forming LCs	Category	Type of Liquid Crystals	References
Arsphenamine	Antimicrobial agents	Nematic thermotropic LCs	(Mueller, 2002)
Nafcillin	Antimicrobial agents	Lamellar, lyotropic LCs	(Bogardus, 1982; Milton, 1996)
Tobramycin	Antimicrobial agents	Nematic thermotropic LCs	(Stevenson, 2005)
Itraconazol	Antimicrobial agents	Nematic thermotropic LCs	(Six et al., 2001; Six et al., 2003; Nesseem, 2001)
Methotrexate	Anticancer	Nematic thermotropic LCs	(Lechuga et al., 2003; 15.Chan & Gonda, 1991; Abdul, 2003)
Leuprolide	Anticancer	Smectic thermotropic LCs	(Powell et al., 1991; Powell et al., 1994; Tan et al., 1998)
Nafarelin	Anticancer	Smectic thermotropic LCs	(Powell et al., 1991; Powell et al., 1994; Tan et al., 1998)
Detirelix	Anticancer	Smectic thermotropic LCs	(Powell et al., 1991; Powell et al., 1994; Tan et al., 1998)
Fenoprofen and its salts	NSAID	Lamellar, lyotropic LCs or smectic thermotropic LCs	(Zhu et al., 2001; Rades & Muller, 1992; Rades & Muller, 1997)
Ibuprofen	NSAID	Lamellar lyotropic LCs	(Muller, 2002)
Diclofenac	NSAID	Lamellar, lyotropic LCs	(Muller, 2002)
Leukotriene	Anti-inflammatory	Thermotropic LCs	(Vadas et al., 1991)
Cromolyn	Antiasthmatic	Cholesteric lyotropic LCs or smectic thermotropic LCs	(Cox et al., 1971; 25. Hartshorne & Woodard, 1973; 26. Stephenson & Diseroad, 2000)
Cyclosporine	Immunosuppresive	Smectic thermotropic LCs	(Liu & Guo, 2007; Lechuga et al., 2003; Loosli et al., 1985; Bennett et al., 1999)

Figure 1. The schematic structures of (a) cubic phase (Pn3m) and (b) hexagonal phase; possible localizations of drugs in the liquid crystals are pointed out
Adapted from Guo et al., 2010 and Yulin et al. (2014).

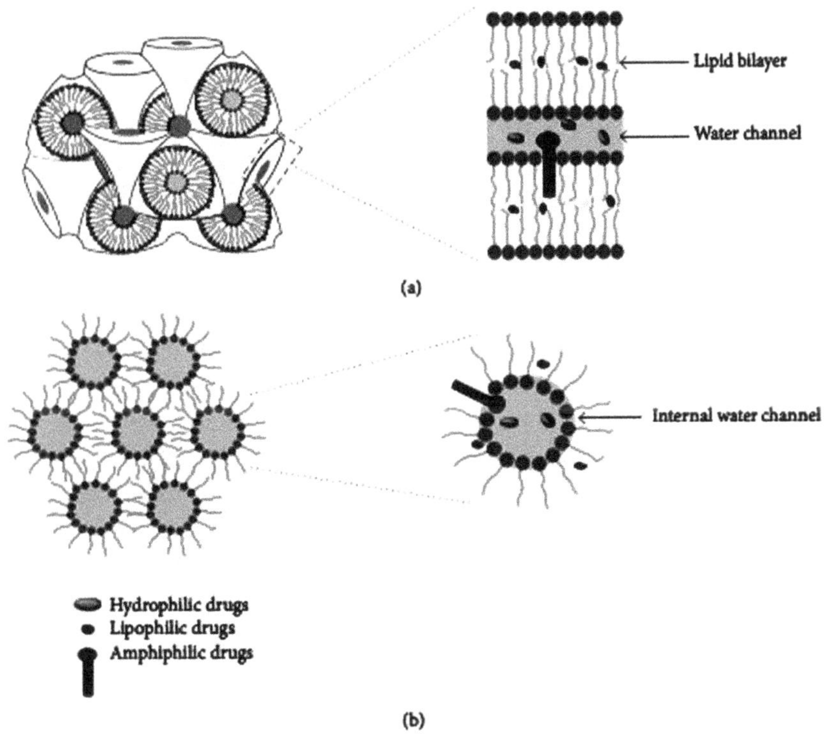

(Boyd et al., 2006). In contrast, the formulation of cubosomes or hexosomes is complicated to a greater extent. There are two commonly used techniques to prepare cubosomes or hexosomes. The first one is called the top-down approach. In this method, a mixture of the structure-forming lipid and stabilizers is first hydrated to allow them to self-assemble in a viscous bulk. The bulk is then disseminated into an aqueous solution through the input of high level energy (such as high-pressure homogenization (Orle et al., 2007) and ultrasonication (Gustafsson et al., 1997)) to form cubosomes or hexosomes. The second preparation technique is called the bottom-up approach. In this approach, the key factor is the presence of hydrotropes, which can dissolve water-insoluble lipid to create liquid precursor and prevent the formation of liquid crystal at high concentration (Mezzenga et al., 2005; Swarnakar et al., 2007). Controlled addition of aqueous medium into the above mixed solution rapidly reduces the lipid solubility and thus results in the formation of cubosomes or hexosomes. This approach needs less energy input and has the advantage to produce nanoparticles with improved stability (Spicer et al., 2001).

The structure of cubic phase is unique and comprises of two uninterrupted but nonintersecting water channels distinguished by a lipid bilayer (Drummond & Fong, 1999; Yaghmur & Glatter, 2009). Established on X-ray crystallographic analysis, cubic phase is divided into three types: the double diamond lattice cubic phase (Pn3m), the body-centered cubic lattice cubic phase (Im3m), and the gyroid lattice cubic phase (Ia3d) (Larsson, 2009; Larsson, 2000). The schematic structure of the double-diamond lattice cubic phase (Pn3m) is shown in Figure 1a. The cubic phases are used as the carriers for hydrophilic, lipophilic, or amphiphilic drugs. Hydrophilic drugs will be settled close to the polar head of lipid or in the water channels, whereas lipophilic drugs will be loaded in the lipid bilayer and amphiphilic drugs in the interface (Figure 1a) (Sagalowicz et al., 2006). The hexagonal phase is compiled of cylindrical micelles compacted in a hexagonal pattern (Figure 1b). In counterpoint to the cubic phase, the water channels in the hexagonal phase are unopened (Libster et al., 2007; Sagalowicz et al., 2006). The distribution of drugs in hexagonal phase is similar to that in cubic phase (Figure 1b).

In recent years, cubic and hexagonal phases have experienced significant attention due to their potential as drug delivery systems. Cubic and hexagonal phases provide a slow drug release matrix and protect peptides, proteins, and nucleic acids from chemical and physical degradation (Clogston & Caffrey, 2005; Mezzenga et al., 2005; Ubbink et al., 2008; Mohammady et al., 2009). The liquid crystal-forming lipids are nontoxic and biodegradable (Ganem et al., 2000) and can be used for various routes of administration. In this chapter, we briefly introduce the lipids utilized to prepare cubic phase and hexagonal phase at physiologic temperature, as well as the determining components on the phase conversion of liquid crystals. Particularly, the investigation of present status of cubic and hexagonal liquid crystals, along with their dispersions as drug delivery systems, will be discussed. This chapter is not intended to provide a comprehensive overview but focuses on lipid-based cubic and hexagonal liquid crystals and their practical applications in drug delivery systems.

CLASSIFICATION

LCs are classified on the substructure of positional order (i.e. Subatomic particles are ordered in arbitrarily structured lattice) and orientational order (i.e. Subatomic particles are predominately directing in the same way). Furthermore, order can be either short-range (merely amongst particles near to one another) or long-range (covering to more prominent, sometimes macroscopical). LCs are classified by their methodology of formulation into the lyotropic and thermotropic LCs (Kawamoto, 2002; Mueller & Hamann, 1993; Mueller & Frank, 1986; Omray, 2013).

Lyotropic Liquid Crystals

A lyotropic liquid crystal comprises of two or more constituents that demonstrate liquid-crystalline attributes in certain concentration ranges. In the lyotropic phases, solvent molecules fill the space around the compounds to furnish fluidness to the arrangement. In contrast to thermotropic liquid crystals, these lyotropics have another degree of freedom of concentration that changes them to induce a variety of different phases. A compound which has two immiscible hydrophilic and hydrophobic parts within the same molecule is called an amphiphilic molecule. Many amphiphilic molecules show lyotropic liquid-crystalline phase sequences depending on the volume balances between the hydrophilic part and hydrophobic part. These structures are formed through the micro-phase segregation of two incompatible components on a nanometer scale. Soap is an everyday example of a lyotropic liquid crystal. The content of water or other solvent molecules changes the self-assembled structures. At very low amphiphile concentration, the molecules will be dispersed randomly without any ordering. At slightly higher (but still low) concentration, amphiphilic molecules will spontaneously assemble into micelles or vesicles. This is done so as to 'hide' the hydrophobic tail of the amphiphile inside the micelle core, exposing a hydrophilic (water-soluble) surface to aqueous solution. These spherical objects do not order themselves in solution, however. At higher concentration, the assemblies will become ordered. A typical phase is a hexagonal columnar phase, where the amphiphiles form long cylinders (again with a hydrophilic surface) that arrange themselves into a roughly hexagonal lattice. This is called the middle soap phase. At still higher concentration, a lamellar phase (neat soap phase) may form, wherein extended sheets of amphiphiles are separated by thin layers of water. For some systems, a cubic (also called viscous isotropic) phase may exist between the hexagonal and lamellar phases, wherein spheres are formed that create a dense cubic lattice. These spheres may also be connected to one another, forming a bicontinuous cubic phase. The objects created by amphiphiles are usually spherical (as in the case of micelles), but may also be disc-like (bicelles), rod-like, or biaxial (all three micelle axes are distinct). These anisotropic self-assembled nano-structures can then order themselves in much the same way as liquid crystals do, forming large-scale versions of all the thermotropic phases (such as a nematic phase of rod-shaped micelles) (Box 1).

Thermotropic Liquid Crystals

Thermotropic phases are those that occur in a certain temperature range. If the temperature is raised too high, thermal motion will destroy the delicate cooperative ordering of the LC phase, pushing the material into a conventional isotropic liquid phase. At too low a temperature, most LC materials will form a conventional (though anisotropic) crystal. Many thermotropic LCs exhibit a variety of phases as temperature is changed. For instance, a particular mesogen may exhibit various smectic and nematic (and finally isotropic) phases as temperature is increased (Box 2).

Box 1. Lyotropic liquid crystals

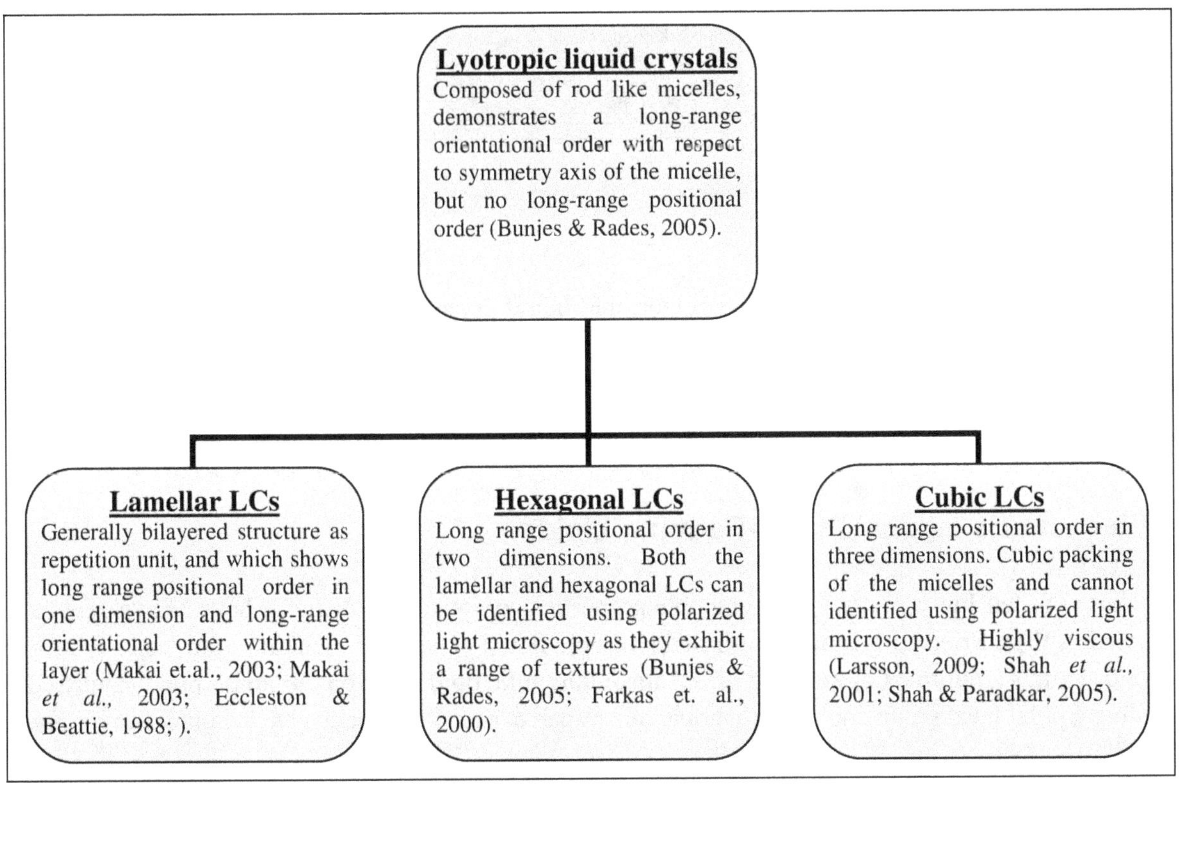

Box 2. Thermotropic liquid crystals

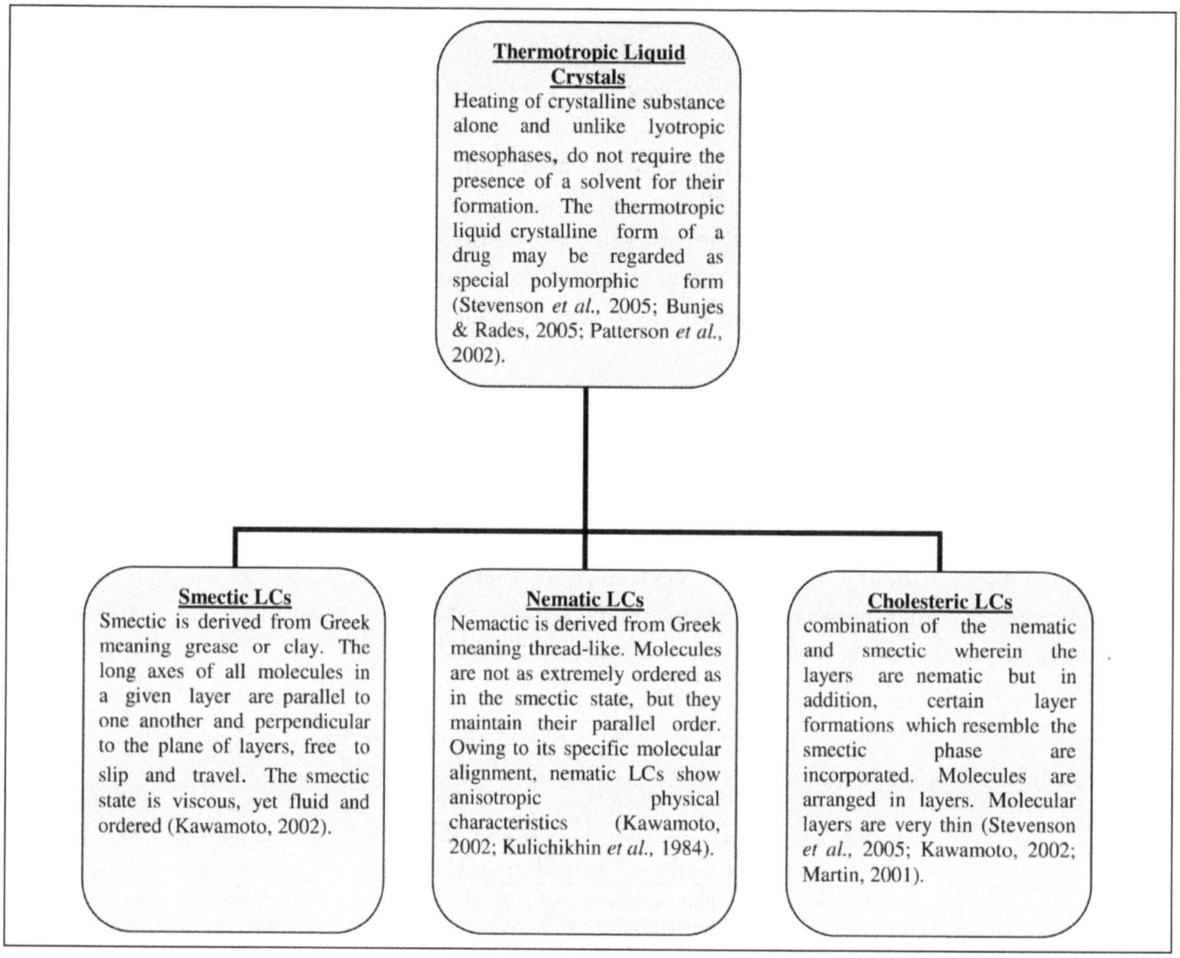

CHARACTERIZATION

Various methods are used to characterize lyotropic liquid crystals which are often employed in drug development and might be utilized in pharmaceutical laboratories. This type of methods is established on some microscopic and macroscopic findings i.e. polarized light microscopy, electron microscopy, x-ray scattering pattern, differential scanning calorimetry, rheological measurements, determination of vesicle size and their distributions (Omray, 2013).

Cubic and Hexagonal Phase-Forming Lipids

Because of their low toxic and biodegradable properties, various types of lipids have been extensively studied as the carriers to prepare lipid-based lyotropic liquid crystals. In general, lipid-based lyotropic liquid crystals are formed by swelling of certain amphiphilic lipids due to their amphiphilic nature containing a polar head group and a hydrophobic tail. When exposed to aqueous environment, amphiphilic lipids spontaneously form thermodynamically stable self assembled structures and eventually develop into cubic and/or hexagonal liquid crystals depending on temperature and water content. Up until now, there have been few materials known to exhibit this kind of phase behavior. In this part, we mainly introduce the lipids which are commonly used to form cubic and/or hexagonal liquid crystals at physiological temperature.

Cubic Phase-Forming Lipids

Glyceryl monooleate (GMO, 2,3-dihydroxypropyl oleate) (Shah et al., 2001; Peng et al., 2010), phytantriol (PT, 3,7,11,15-tetramethyl-1,2,3-hexadecanetriol) (Barauskas & Landh, 2003; Han et al., 2010) and other lipids such as mono linolein (Negrini & Mezzenga, 2011; Yaghmur et al., 2005; Tang et al., 2012), monoelaidin (Chung & Caffrey, 1995; Czeslik et al., 1995; Kulkarni, 2011), phosphatidylethanolamine (Boni & Hui, 1983; Tenchov et al., 1996; Tenchov et al., 1998), oleoylethanolamide (Mohammady et al., 2009), phospholipids (Sjolund et al., 1987; Marsh, 1990; Eriksson & Lindblom, 1993; Takahashi et al. 1996), PEGylated phospholipids (Koynova et al., 1997), alkyl glycerates (Boyd et al., 2006, Fong et al., 2007), and glycolipids (Hato & Minamikawa, 1996) have been reported to form cubic phase. Among them GMO and PT are the most commonly studied to form cubic phase liquid crystals as drug delivery systems. GMO, or monoolein, is a polar unsaturated monoglyceride. The chemical structure of GMO is shown in Figure 2a. GMO is a nontoxic, biodegradable, and biocompatible material and is listed in the FDA's Inactive Ingredients Guide. Although GMO is a well-known emulsifying agent and food additive

Figure 2. Molecular structures of (a) GMO and (b) PT. Phase behaviors of (c) GMO-water and (d) PT-water system. Phase notations: L_C: liquid crystal; L_2: fluid isotropic solution; L_α: lamellar phase; H2: reversed hexagonal phase; VG: gyroid lattice cubic phase (Ia3d); VD: double diamond lattice cubic phase (Pn3m).
Adapted with modifications from Wadsten et al. (2007) and Yulin et al. (2014).

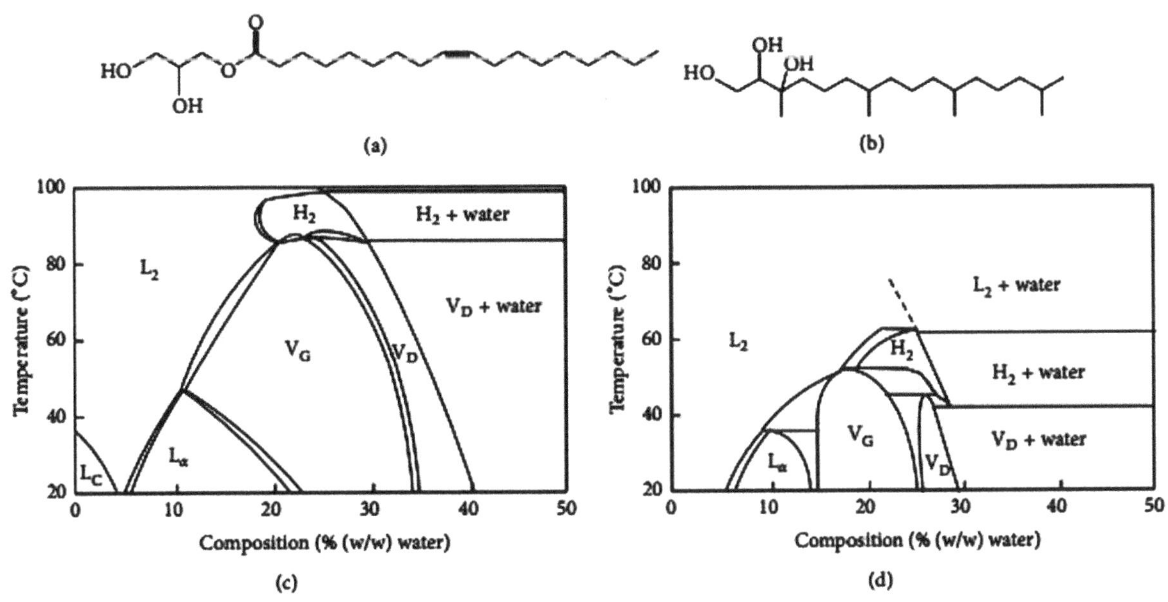

since the 1950s, its potential application in drug delivery has not been discovered until in 1984 when GMO was first proposed as a biocompatible material (Engstrom et al., 1984). The phase diagram of GMO and water is shown in Figure 2c. It is clearly demonstrated that GMO forms cubic phase with water in a broad area at physiological temperature. Due to its excellent phase behavior, GMO is widely used for the preparation of cubic liquid crystals at ambient temperatures. Because of the similar phase behavior to GMO, PT also has been widely used as a cubic phase-forming material in the past decade (Barauskas & Landh, 2003; Dong et al., 2006; Barauskas et al., 2005). The chemical structure and phase behavior of PT are illustrated in Figure 2. PT is a well-known active ingredient used in cosmetic industry, such as hair and skin care products (Wagner, 1994). Recently, PT has been receiving more attention since it has a phytanyl backbone but does not possess an ester bond, which provides an improved chemical stability compared to other fatty acid-based materials, such as GMO, in aqueous and model gastrointestinal conditions (Rizwan et al., 2009, Boyd et al., 2006; Nguyen et al., 2011).

Hexagonal Phase-Forming Lipids

Oleyl glycerate (OG, 2,3-dihydroxypropionic acid octadec-9-enyl ester) and phytanyl glycerate (PG, 2,3-dihydroxypropionic acid 3,7,11,15-tetramethyl-hexadecyl ester) are found to form hexagonal phase at physiological temperature when exposed to excess water, which further expands the lipid domain to form hexagonal phases (Boyd et al., 2004; Boyd et al., 2005; Martin et al., 2013). The molecular structures and phase behaviors of OG and PG are presented in Figure 3. (Boyd et al., 2006) reported that a series of model hydrophobic and hydrophilic drugs, such as paclitaxel, irinotecan, glucose, histidine, and octreotide, can be incorporated into OG- and PG-based hexagonal phases and in vitro drug release was shown to follow the Higuchi diffusion controlled release kinetics. Although the understanding of these new glycerate esters is limited, for example, their long-term safety, tolerability, the susceptibility to esterases, and local toxicity of their degradation products, they are promising materials due to their lower melting point and improved thermal stability compared to GMO (Boyd et al., 2006).

Figure 3. Chemical structures of (a) OG and (b) PG and one-dimensional phase diagrams for (c) OG and (d) PG at 37 °C showing water content at phase boundaries for reverse micellar (L_2) and reverse hexagonal phase (H_2)

Adapted from Boyd et al. (2006); Boyd et al. (2006) and Yulin et al. (2014).

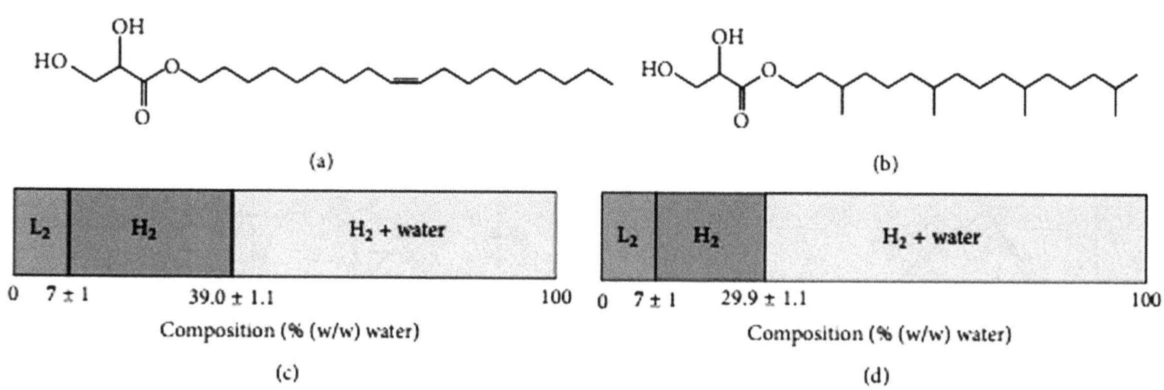

The Influencing Factors for the Phase Transition of Cubic and Hexagonal Liquid Crystals

Many factors influence the phase behaviors of cubic and hexagonal liquid crystals, such as the molecular structures of lipids, pressure, temperature, salt concentration, pH, and addition of a third substance. Full understanding of these influencing factors on the phase transition will provide better quality control as well as expanding the lipid applications in drug development.

The molecular structures of lipids play an important role in the determination of phase behavior. The critical packing parameter (P) is used to predict the nanostructure of formed liquid crystal with the formula $P=V/al$, where P is critical packing parameter, V is the hydrophobic chain volume, a is the cross-sectional area of the polar head group, and l is the hydrophobic chain length (Israelachvili, 1994). It is important to note that the P value (and therefore the self-assembled nanostructure) will change along with other parameters such as temperature and solvent conditions. Depending on P, different self-assembled liquid crystalline structures will be formed (Sagalowicz et al., 2006). When $P=1$, lamellar liquid crystalline structure forms. When $P<1$, oil-in-water self-assembled structures form, such as normal micelles (L1), normal cubic structure (V1), and normal hexagonal phases (H1). When $P>1$, water-in-oil self-assembled structures form, such as reversed micelles (L2), reversed cubic structure (V2), and reversed hexagonal structure (H2). Yaghmur et al., investigated the impact of pressure and temperature on the stability of the inverted type discontinuous cubic phase (Fd3m) versus the inverted type hexagonal phase (H2) (Yaghmur et al., 2010). The results showed that compressing the Fd3m phase under ambient temperature induced the transition of Fd3m to H2. Interestingly, the temperature dependent structural transition demonstrated the opposite trend where an increase of temperature induced the structural transition from H2 to Fd3m at isobaric condition. Salt concentration (Awad et al., 2005; Yaghmur et al., 2008; Yaghmur et al., 2011) and pH value (Okamoto et al., 2008; Alam et al., 2011; Muller et al., 2010) also have an impact on the phase behavior of liquid crystals to a certain extent. For example, Awad et al. found out that low concentrations of $Ca2+$induced the $L\alpha$ phase to the cubic phase transition in the suspensions of monoolein and dioleoylphosphatidylglycerol mixtures (Awad et al., 2005). Sallam et al., observed that the reversed hexagonal phase occurred at a lower temperature in simulated gastric fluid than that in simulated intestinal fluid or water, which indicated that the formation of hexagonal phase was favored in an acidic environment (Sallam et al., 2002). In addition, Negrini and Mezzenga suggested that a system composed of monolinolein and linoleic acids (97/3, w/w) was able to reversibly change from a reverse bicontinuous cubic phase to a reverse hexagonal phase, when the pH was dropped from 7 to 2 (Negrini & Mezzenga, 2011). Yaghmur et al. investigated the pH effect on the phase structures of 6% bupivacaine-loaded GMO-based liquid crystals, and it was found out that the different self-assembled structures were formed by increasing the pH from 6.0 to 7.4, which induced the structural transition of Pn3m + H2 →H2 (Yaghmur et al., 2011; Yaghmur et al., 2012). In addition, additives will modulate the textures of liquid crystals which result in phase transition. Yaghmur et al. introduced tetradecane (TC) to the monolinolein-(MLO-) water-poloxamer 407 (F127) system and found out that, when mass of TC/mass of MLO = 19, the system transformed from cubosomes to hexosomes and, when mass of TC/mass of MLO = 75, the system transformed from hexosomes to a concentrated microemulsion (Yaghmur et al., 2005). Later on they (Yaghmur et al., 2006) found out that diglycerol monooleate or soybean phosphatidylcholine had a countereffect on that of tetradecane which turned back the self-assembled nanostructures in the TC-loaded dispersions from hexosomes to cubosomes. Shah and Paradkar (Shah & Paradkar, 2007) studied the effect of the additives with different hydrophilic-lipophilic balances (HLBs of 1.5, 3, 4, 5, 7, 10, and 11) in

GMO matrices on their phase transformation. The results showed that the GMO matrices incorporated with lower HLB additives (HLBs of 1.5, 3, 4, and 5) formed hexagonal phase after 12 h of hydration. This may be because the incorporated hydrophobic additives were dissolved in lipophilic domain of GMO, thus increasing the apparent hydrophobic chain volume of the lipid. Therefore, it might increase the *P* value of GMO and transform mesophase from cubic phase to hexagonal phase. Interestingly, the GMO matrices incorporated with higher HLB additives (HLBs of 7, 10, and 11) formed lamellar phase after 12 h of hydration. The authors proposed that these hydrophilic additives with higher HLB reduced the access of water to GMO and thus caused such transformation. Amar-Yuli and Garti (Amar & Garti, 2005) investigated the impact of incorporation of triglycerides (TAGs) with various chain lengths into the binary GMO/water system, and the results suggested that the solubilization of TAG in the system facilitates transition from lamellar or cubic phases to hexagonal structure at room temperature. Among all the tested TAGs, tricaprylin in the binary GMO/water system provided direct transformation of the lamellar phase to the hexagonal phase, but without the formation of a Cubic structure. They suggested that TAG between GMO tails would change the geometry of monoolein molecules from cylindrical to wedge shape and thereby caused the phase transition. Dong el al. found out that the presence of 5% w/w vitamin E acetate in the PT-water system suppressed the transition temperature of the cubic phase to hexagonal phase from 60 ∘C to below 25 ∘C (Dong el al·, 2006). This indicated that lipophilic components in liquid crystalline formulations, although they account to relatively small amount, may have a significant impact on the phase behavior.

APPLICATIONS AS DRUG DELIVERY SYSTEMS

LCs have given significant sharp-sightedness over the years as a possible drug delivery vehicle. therapeutical chemical compound of various physicochemical attributes such as analgesics, antibiotics, antifungal, anticancer, vitamins, antiasthmatic, immunosuppressive etc. have been either comprised or itself used for the establishment of the LCs with approximately identical promoting results (Stevenson, 2005; Nilsson et al., 2013).

Since the advent of the first patent in1984 (Engstrom et al., 1984) when the highly ordered cubic phase was proposed as an interesting matrix in controlled release preparations, lipid-based liquid crystal systems have been extensively investigated in drug delivery, as well as the potential application in the ranostic nanomedicines (Murgia et al., 2013; Nilsson et al., 2013; Gupta et al., 2014). In this section, some applications of cubic and hexagonal liquid crystals as drug carriers are reviewed. Tables 2 and 3 list some such drug delivery systems in recent years (2007–2014).

CUBIC LIQUID CRYSTALS AS DRUG DELIVERY SYSTEM

Ability to Sustain or Control Drug Release

As drug carriers, cubic phase liquid crystals have the ability to provide sustained drug release. Drugs with a wide range of molecular weights and water solubilities have demonstrated sustained release in a cubic phase, such as aspirin and vitamin E (Wyatt & Dorschel, 1992), propantheline bromide and oxybutynin

Table 2. Cubic phases as drug carriers in recent years (2007–2014)

Type of Cubic Phases	Composition	Bioactive Molecules	Administration Route	Reference
Cubic phase gel	GMO/water and PT/water	14C-glucose, Allura Red, and fluorescein isothiocyanate dextran	Oral	(Lee et al., 2009)
Cubosomes	GMO/F127/water and PT/F127/water	Cinnarizine	Oral	(Nguyen et al., 2011)
Cubosomes	PT/F127/water	Amphotericin B	Oral	(Yang et al., 2013)
Cubic phase gel	GMO/propylene glycol/water	Capsaicin	Transdermal	(Peng et al., 2010)
Cubic phase gel	GMO/water	Paeonol	Transdermal	(Luo et al., 2011)
Cubic phase gel	GMO/water and PT/water	Sulphorhodamine B	Transdermal	(Bender, 2008)
Cubosomes	GMO/F127/water	Cyclosporine A	Ocular	(Chen, 2012)

Table 3. Hexagonal phases as drug carriers in recent years (2007–2014)

Type of Cubic Phases	Composition	Bioactive Molecules	Administration Route	Reference
Hexagonal phase gel	OG/water	Cinnarizine	Oral	(Boyd et al., 2007)
Hexagonal phase gel	GMO/vitamin K/water	Vitamin K	Transdermal	(Lopes et al., 2007)
Hexosomes	GMO/vitamin K/F127/water	Vitamin K	Transdermal	(Lopes et al., 2007)
Hexagonal phase gel	GMO/TAG/water	Sodium diclofenac	Transdermal	(Cohen et al., 2010; Cohen et al., 2012)
Hexosomes	GMO/oleic acid/F68(Pluronic)/ water	Progesterone	Oromucosal	(Swarnakar et al., 2007)

hydrochloride (Geraghty et al., 1996), metronidazole (Norling et al., 1992), tetracycline (Esposito et al., 1996), timolol maleate (Lindell et al., 1998), chlorpheniramine maleate (Chang & Bodmeier, 1997), propranolol hydrochloride (Costa et al., 2010), melatonin, pindolol, propranolol and pyrimethamine (Burrows et al., 1994), hemoglobin (Leslie et al., 1996), cefazolin (Sadhale & Shah, 1998), insulin (Sadhale & Shah, 1999; Sadhale & Shah, 1999), capsaicin (Peng et al., 2010), cinnarizine (Nguyen et al., 2011; Nguyen et al., 2010), and diclofenac salts (Yariv et al., 2010). Lee et al. studied the in vitro sustained release behavior of a number of model hydrophilic drugs with various molecular weights (14 C-glucose, Allura Red, and fluorescein isothiocyanate dextrans FD-4, FD-20, and FD-70) in two types of liquid crystalline matrixes, namely, V2GMO (a cubic phase prepared from GMO) and V2PT (a cubic phase prepared from PT) (Lee et al., 2009). The release samples were constrained in micro beakers with a fixed surface area to ensure a constant release area between the liquid crystals and the release media. The results showed that in all cases the cumulative amount of drug release through the matrix followed a linear relationship with the square root of time, which represented a Higuchi diffusion controlled release profile. The influence of phase structure and molecular weight on drug release was also investigated. It was discovered that the release rate of each drug decreased as the matrix was changed from V2GMO to V2PT and the diffusion coefficient of the model drugs was reduced as the molecular weight increased. The results indicated that phase type and molecular weight of drugs had an influence on their release behavior. In order to confirm whether the in vitro release data were able to translate into in vivo oral absorption dates, the oral absorption kinetics of 14C-glucose formulations were further studied in rats.

In this study, 14C-gl^{uc}ose was chosen as the model drug due to its fast absorption rate; therefore, the kinetics of 14C-gl^{uc}ose in plasma would only be determined by its release rate from the matrix. The pharmacokinetic results showed that the meant Tmax (t_{ime} to peak) of 14C-gl^{uc}ose absorption in solution formulations (1.00 h) was the shortest, followed by V2GMO ($_{1.13}$ h) and V2PT (1 $_{.88}$ h). It was found out that the oral absorption rate of 14C-gl^{uc}ose followed the order observed in the vitro drug release studies, which indicated that the nanostructure of these lipid based liquid crystalline systems had a significant impact on oral absorption of hydrophilic drugs. Recently, Nguyen et al., (2011) firstly demonstrated the sustained absorption of a poorly water-soluble drug (cinnarizine) when incorporated into PT-based cubosomes after oral administration. The plasma profiles showed that the plasma concentration of PT-based cubosomes was maintained at 21.5±1.5 ng/mL within 12 and 48 h, while the plasma concentrations dropped to below quantification limit after 24 h when treated with suspensions or GMO-based cubosomes. They further investigated the mechanism of PT- and GMO-based cubosomes upon oral administration. The small-angle X-ray scattering results showed that the nanostructure of PT-based cubosomes was well maintained over 18 h in both simulated gastric and intestinal fluids. In contrast, the cubic phase structure of GMO-based cubosomes was collapsed within 2 h in simulated intestinal fluid or 18 h in simulated gastric fluid. This suggested that degradation of the nanostructure lead to fast drug release. In addition, in gastrointestinal retention studies, it was found out that over 10% of given PT and cinnarizine remained in stomach at 24 h after oral administration. In sharp contrast, GMO and cinnarizine were below quantification levels after 4 h. Therefore, the nondigestible nature of PT and the maintenance of the cubosome structure contributed to the sustained release and absorption of cinnarizine in stomach. Esposito et al. studied the performance of cubosomes as sustained percutaneous delivery systems with the model drug molecule of indomethacin (Esposito et al., 2005). The in vitro diffusion study showed that the flux of indomethacin from carbomer-indomethacin loaded cubosomes (A) was significantly lower than carbomer-blank cubosomes spiked with free indomethacin (B) and carbomer with an indomethacin water suspension (C). Furthermore, in vivo results indicated that formulation A significantly prolonged the release of indomethacin thus exhibiting a significant long-lasting antiinflammatory activity when exposed to UVB (ultravioletB) irradiation for 6 h, whereas the anti-inflammatory effect of the other two formulations was time-limited. The results confirmed that the main factor controlling drug diffusion is the nanostructure of cubosomes rather than the viscosity of the carbomer gel. In addition, tape-stripping experiment was conducted to understand the drug release mechanism, and it was found out that the amount of indomethacin recovered in the stratum corneum after the removal of formulation A was remarkably higher than that in the other two formulations. Notably, the amount of indomethacin recovered from the removal of formulations B and C was not significantly different. The authors proposed that the cubosomal GMO interacted with the stratum corneum lipids and it might lead to the formation of a cubosomes depot in stratum corneum from which indomethacin was released in a controlled fashion.

Ability to Improve Drug Bioavailability and Reduce Drug Toxicity

Cubic phases are used to improve the drug bioavailability and reduce drug toxicity. Yang et al. prepared PT-based cubosomes containing amphotericin B (AmB) to improve its bioavailability and reduce nephrotoxicity (Yang et al., 2013). After oral administration of an AmB-loaded cubosomal formulation in rats, nephrotoxicity was not observed and the relative bioavailability of AmB was approximately 285% compared to the control group. Chen et al. developed acyclosporine A-loaded GMO/F127 cubosome system to reduce ocular irritancy (Chen et al., 2012). The results showed that cubosomes almost had no irritation, and only transient corneal hyperemia was observed in one rabbit but recovered within 1 h. In addition, no ocular damage or clinically abnormal signs were noticed in cornea, conjunctiva, or iris.

Ability to Enhance the Stability of Drugs

The unique structure of the cubic phase is used to incorporate unstable drug substances and protect them from physical and chemical degradation. Sadhale and Shah studied the ability of cubic phase gel to protect insulin from agitation induced aggregation (Sadhale & Shah, 1999a; Sadhale & Shah, 1999b). The results showed that the native conformation of agitated insulin in cubic phase gels was almost unaffected for 2 months at 37 ∘C, while the majority of Insulin in solution appeared to aggregate and precipitate only after 8 days. Therefore, the cubic phase gel was able to protect insulin from agitation-induced aggregation and subsequent precipitation. Furthermore, they (Sadhale & Shah, 1999a) investigated the effect of agitation on biological activity of insulin in cubic phase gel by subcutaneous injections of the agitated cubic phase gel, nonagitated cubic phase gel, agitated insulin solution, and normal saline to fasted rats and their blood glucose levels were measured. The blood glucose levels given the non-agitated cubic phase gel and the agitated cubic phase gel were significantly lower ($P < 0.05$) than those in the agitated insulin solution or saline from 40 min to 4 h. The results suggested that insulin was biologically active in both agitated and nonagitated cubic phase gels. However, upon agitation, insulin in solution totally lost its hypoglycemic activity. In summary, GMO-based cubic phase gel can protect insulin from agitation-induced aggregation. Sadhale and Shah also evaluated the stability of two model drugs, cefazolin and cefuroxime, in a GMO cubic phase gel (Sadhale & Shah, 1998). The stability of cefazolin was assessed at two different concentrations (200 and 50μg/g), at 22 and 37 ∘C. The results showed that the degradation of cefazolin at lower concentration was 3- and 18 folds lower in cubic phase gel than that in solutions at 22 and 37 ∘C, respectively. At 22 and 37 ∘C, the kinetics of degradation at higher concentration of cefazolin was not first order but a lag phase followed by an exponential loss of cefazolin, which may be due to its oxidation. Later on, the oxidation of cefazolin was confirmed by its 18-fold higher stability in the presence of EDTA and nitrogen in solution. In addition, the degradation rate of cefuroxime was 2 times slower in cubic phase gel than that in solution. In summary, this study clearly demonstrated that cubic phase gel enhanced the chemical stability of cefazolin and cefuroxime.

Ability to Increase the Penetration of Drugs

Cubic phases and cubosomes also have the ability to improve the transdermal/topical delivery of small molecules such as acyclovir (Helledi & Schubert, 2001), paeonol (Luo et al., 2011), δ-aminolevulinic acid (Bender et al., 2005), sulphorhodamine B (Bender et al., 2008), calcein (Yamada et al., 2011), and diclofenac salts (Yariv et al., 2010), as well as macromolecules such as cyclosporin A (Chen et al., 2012; Lopes et al., 2006). Helledi and Schubert reported that the cubic phase enhanced the penetration of acyclovir by 6 times compared to its commercial product (Helledi & Schubert, 2001). Luo et al. prepared a cubic gel containing 3% paeonol, 30% water, and 67% GMO, and the in vitro skin permeability test showed that the permeability coefficient of cubic gel was 8.34 ±0.49×10 −3 cm/hour, which was significantly higher ($P < 0.05$) compared to the micro emulsion gel (5.88±0.28×10 −3 cm/hour) and the control solution (3.06±0.10×10 −3 cm/hour) (Luo et al., 2011). The results indicated that paeonol in cubic gel had higher permeability than that of paeonol in microemulsion gel and the control solution;

therefore, cubic gel would be a better carrier for paeonol in transdermal delivery. Lopes et al. reported that the cubic phase increased the penetration of cyclosporine A in stratum corneum and epidermis plus dermis ([E + D]) at 12 h post application in vitro (Lopes et al., 2006). The in vivo penetration study showed that the cubic phase increased the concentration of cyclosporin A in the stratum corneum and [E + D] by 2.5 and 2 times, respectively, when compared to the control formulation. Chen et al. prepared a cyclosporine A loaded cubosome system for ocular drug delivery to improve corneal penetration (Chen et al., 2012). The in vitro corneal penetration study showed that the steady-state permeation rate of cyclosporine A was 1.52-fold compared to that of the oil solution. In addition, cyclosporine A-loaded cubosomes demonstrated a significantly enhanced initial penetration rate, where the cumulative amount of cyclosporine A in the first 0.5 h was about2-fold compared to that of the oil solution. The authors concluded that the main mechanism of the enhanced corneal permeation might be the absorption and/or surface lipid exchange between the liquid crystalline nanoparticles and corneal epithelial cells. In addition, the close adhesion of the small lipid colloidal carriers with a large surface area to the lipophilic epithelium surface could promote a quick initial permeation rate. It was also reported that the periodically curved lipid bilayer of liquid crystalline nanoparticles was very similar to the microstructure of the cell membrane (Larsson, 1989; Giorgione et al., 1998) and the cubic architecture in stratum corneum was quite similar to the structure of cubic phases (Norlen & Al-Amoudi, 2004). Furthermore, the interaction between biological tissues and cubic phases may contribute fast permeation rate as well, and this property makes the development of cubosome-based products more promising. Recently, some advanced optical technologies have been used to investigate the penetration mechanism of fluorescent materials. The method of fluorescent quantification at the skin surface was used to quantify the penetration of δ-aminolevulinic acid (ALA) and its methyl ester into the tissue (Bender et al., 2005). ALA is a precursor of heme which can induce the production of the photosensitizer protoporphyrin IX (PpIX) in living tissues. A fiber-optic probe coupled to a spectrophotometer was used to measure the PpIX fluorescence at the skin surface after topical administration of cubic phases. The results showed that, after 1 h application, GMObased cubic systems and PT/propylene glycol/water cubic systems showed significantly higher fluorescence than the standard ointment over 10 h ($P < 0.05$), and this was probably due to the enhanced drug penetration. The authors also analyzed the difference between GMO and PT cubic systems in terms of enhanced drug permeation and concluded that the difference mainly relied on the swelling extent and the rheological property of the systems. Notably, the maximum amount of water in the PT-based cubic phase (about 28%) was less than that in GMO-based cubic phase (about 40%), which implied that PT-based cubic phase had more narrow water channels thus resulting in a slower release. In terms of rheological property, PT-based cubic phase had higher viscosity which made it quite difficult to handle and contact with skin thereby led to a lower PpIX level. In addition, propylene glycol was introduced into PT-based cubic phase to make the system softer, and this may be a partial explanation for the higher PpIX level in the PT-based cubic phase with propylene glycol. In another study, two-photon microscopy (Bender et al., 2008) was used to visualize the uptake of sulphorhodamine B (incorporated into GMO-/PT-based cubic phases) in full thickness human skin. This technology is able to take images of fluorophores of sulphorhodamine B much deeper into highly light-scattering and light-absorbing tissues compared to confocal laser scanning microscopy, but with minimal photobleaching and phototoxic effects. The results suggested that the dominating delivery route of the cubic phases is via micro fissures caused by microscopic clustering of the keratinocytes in the skin. Therefore, sulphorhodamine B delivered by cubic phases diffused into the surrounding intercellular lipid matrix through these microfissures and acted like a source for its sustained release.

HEXAGONAL LIQUID CRYSTALS AS DRUG DELIVERY SYSTEM

Application of OG-Based and PG-Based Hexagonal Phase

Due to the limit of materials and preparation conditions, hexagonal liquid crystals as drug carriers are less reported than those of cubic liquid crystals. Fortunately, in recent years, Boyd et al. synthesized a new class of materials with glycerate headgroups to form lyotropic liquid crystal (Boyd et al., 2006). Among these materials, OG and PG were found to form hexagonal phase in excess water at physiological temperature. Thereafter, the OG- and PG-based hexagonal phase matrices were applied as the carriers for a series of model hydrophobic and hydrophilic drugs, such as paclitaxel, irinotecan, glucose, histidine, and octreotide, and the in vitro release studies showed that in all cases their release behavior obeyed Higuchi kinetics. This suggested that OG- and PG based hexagonal phases have the ability to provide sustained drug release.

In another study, Boyd et al. reported that the OG based hexagonal phase improved the oral bioavailability of cinnarizine up to 3.5 and 3 times than that of the control suspension and GMO-based cubic phase, respectively (Boyd et al., 2007). The in vitro lipolysis experiments showed that all of the GMO had been digested within the first 5 min. In contrast, although the hydrolysis of OG was also fast in the first 5 min, it kept steady in the following 55 min. It suggested that OG was less susceptible to hydrolysis by pancreatic lipase than GMO and this might be responsible for increased oral bioavailability of cinnarizine when incorporated into OG formulations. OG-based hexosomes were also used to improve the stability of irinotecan (Boyd et al., 2006). Irinotecan is a highly effective anticancer drug which displays a pH dependent equilibrium between its active lactone and inactive carboxylate forms, with rapid conversion to the carboxylate form occurring at a neutral pH. The stability studies showed that over 53-day storage of irinotecan-loaded hexosomes at 40∘C, the lactone: carboxylate ratio increased from the initial value of 94: 6 to 100: 0, and 4% of the OG was hydrolysed to glyceric acid which led to the reduction of pH of the system from 6.6 to 3.5. The decreased pH may favor the equilibrium towards the lactone form of irinotecan. The results suggested that OG based hexosomes improved the retention of irinotecan as the lactone form and might be a promising alternative to current irinotecan formulations.

Ability to Increase the Penetration of Drugs

Hexagonal phases and hexosomes also have the ability to enhance the penetration of incorporated drugs. Lopes et al. reported that, when incorporated into GMO-based hexagonal phase gel (GMO/vitamin K/water at 77.5/2.5/20, w/w/w) or GMO-based hexosomes (GMO/vitamin K/F127/water at 15/2.5/0.9/81.6, w/w/w/w), vitamin K was delivered to stratum corneum and [E + D] was increased to 2–3.7 times than that in a vaseline control solution (Lopes et al., 2007). In another article, Lopes et al. evaluated the ability of GMO-based hexosomes (GMO/oleic acid/F127/water at 8/2/0.9/89.1, w/w/w/w) to improve the skin penetration of a model peptide (cyclosporine A) both in vitro and in vivo (Lopes et al., 2006). An in vitro skin penetration study showed that the maximal concentrations of cyclosporine A in the stratum corneum and in the [E + D] were 2-fold higher when incorporated into hexosomes than the control formulation (olive oil). Similarly, in vivo, the concentration of cyclosporin A-loaded hexosomes was 1.5 and 2.8 times higher than that in the stratum corneum and [E + D], respectively. The results suggested that hexagonal phase enhanced the cutaneous penetration of both vitamin K and cyclosporin A. Recently, penetratin, a cell penetrating peptide which was embedded within the hexagonal phase liquid crystal, was used to improve the transdermal delivery of incorporated sodium diclofenac (Cohen et al.,

2010; Cohen et al., 2012). An in vitro skin penetration study revealed that the permeability coefficient of sodium diclofenac enhanced 2.2 times in the presence of 1.4 wt% penetratin. The mechanism of penetratin-enhanced sodium diclofenac permeation through porcine skin in vitro was studied with an attenuated total reflectance Fourier transform infrared (ATR FTIR) technique. ATR-FTIR skin studies implied that penetratin accelerated the structural transition of skin lipids from a hexagonal symmetry to a liquid-disordered state. This structural change resulted in faster diffusion of sodium diclofenac through the stratum corneum. Swarnakar et al., (2007) prepared a progesterone loaded hexosome system for mucosal delivery and investigated the possible penetration mechanisms of the carriers. After the application of progesterone-loaded hexosomes to the excised rabbit buccal mucosa for 12 h, the observed flux was 5 times higher than that of a progesterone-loaded gel and nearly 4times higher than a plain progesterone suspension. Fourier transform infrared spectrum and confocal laser scanning microscopy of treated mucosa showed lipid extraction phenomena as well as evident pores, indicating a probable intercellular "virtual channel" available to facilitate the penetration of hexosomes.

Application in Stimuli Responsive Drug Delivery System

Because of the possibility to switch between the cubic phase (fast release) and hexagonal phase (slow release) by adjusting temperature and/or pH, researchers have designed a series of stimuli responsive drug delivery systems. Fong et al. developed an externally regulated thermo responsive liquid crystalline system for subcutaneous injection of hydrophilic drugs (glucose) (Fong et al., 2009). In in vivo absorption studies, the drug was released slowly from hexagonal phase when subcutaneously injected at physiological temperature. After application of a cool pack at the injection site, the plasma concentration was significantly increased due to the structure transformed into cubic phase. The authors suggested that this system would be a suitable carrier for the delivery of short acting hormones. Negrini and Mezzenga developed a food-grade lyotropic liquid crystal system, which was composed of monolinolein and linoleic acids (97/3, w/w) in the presence of excess water (Negrini & Mezzenga, 2011). The system was able to reversibly convert from cubic phase to hexagonal phase, when changing the pH from neutral (pH 7) to acidic (pH 2) conditions. In vitro drug release and diffusion experiments showed that drug release rate was 4 times faster in cubic phase at pH 7 (intestine) than the hexagonal phase at pH 2 (stomach), which suggested that this system may be an ideal candidate for intestine- or colon-targeted delivery.

CONCLUSION

Liquid crystalline structures furnish a broad range of structural and functional characteristics. They hold power to vehicle hydrophobic and hydrophilic drug(s). It seems that these assigns can be well employed in drug delivery gainsays, constructing surfactant established drug delivery system a productive approach. This book chapter mainly discusses the investigation of current status of lipid-based liquid crystalline phases as drug delivery systems. Although the cubic and hexagonal phases have been extensively investigated as potential sustained release systems for nearly 30 years, more work needs to be done to further evaluate them in drug delivery systems. Studies with respect to the interactions between the drug and the liquid crystalline phases in vivo are very limited, and the impact of the biological environment on drug release kinetics and biodegradation is also not well understood. The commercialization of these systems in clinical application is challenging, primarily due to the lack of a suitable, scalable manufacturing method. In addition, the choice of commercially available lipids with a desired phase behavior is limited. Nevertheless, the future of lipid-based liquid crystalline delivery systems remains exciting in both academic and industrial sectors.

REFERENCES

Abdul-Fatta, A., Zhang, J., Bennett, D. B., & Ballesteros Lechuga, D. (2003). Characterization of spray-dried powders in the liquid crystalline state. *Journal of Pharmaceutical Sciences*, *4*, 1286–1289.

Alam, M. M., Oka, T., Ohta, N., & Yamazaki, M. (2011). Kinetics of low pH-induced lamellar to bicontinuous cubic phase transition in dioleoyl phosphatidyl serine/monoolein. *The Journal of Chemical Physics*, *134*(14), 145102. doi:10.1063/1.3575240 PMID:21495771

Amar Yuli, I., & Garti, N. (2005). Transitions induced by solubilized fat into reverse hexagonal mesophases. *Colloids and Surfaces. B, Biointerfaces*, *43*(2), 72–82. doi:10.1016/j.colsurfb.2005.03.011 PMID:15921902

Awad, T. S., Okamoto, Y., Masum, S. M., & Yamazaki, M. (2005). Formation of cubic phases from large unilamellar vesicles of dioleoylphosphatidylglycerol/monoolein membranes induced by low concentrations of Ca^{2+}. *Langmuir*, *21*(25), 11556–11561. doi:10.1021/la051782i PMID:16316079

Barauskas, J., Johnsson, M., & Tiberg, F. (2005). Self-assembled lipid superstructures: Beyond vesicles and liposome. *Nano Letters*, *5*(8), 1615–1619. doi:10.1021/nl050678i PMID:16089498

Barauskas, J., & Landh, T. (2003). Phase behavior of the phytantriol/water system. *Langmuir*, *19*(23), 9562–9565. doi:10.1021/la0350812

Bender, J., Ericson, M. B., Merclin, N., Iani, V., Rosén, A., Engström, S., & Moan, J. (2005). Lipid cubic phases for improved topical drug delivery in photodynamic therapy. *Journal of Controlled Release*, *106*(3), 350–360. doi:10.1016/j.jconrel.2005.05.010 PMID:15967535

Bender, J., Simonsson, C., Smedh, M., Engstrom, S., & Ericson, M. B. (2008). Lipid cubic phases in topical drug delivery: Visualization of skin distribution using two-photon microscopy. *Journal of Controlled Release*, *129*(3), 163–169. doi:10.1016/j.jconrel.2008.04.020 PMID:18538886

Bennett, D., Cabot, K., Foster, L., Lechuga-Ballesteros, D., & Tan, T. (1999). *Liquid crystal forms of cyclosporin.* US Patent Application 990352, WO 99/42124.

Bogardus, J. B. (1982). Phase equilibria of nafcillin sodium–water. *Journal of Pharmaceutical Sciences*, *71*(1), 105–109. doi:10.1002/jps.2600710125 PMID:7057360

Boni, L. T., & Hui, S. W. (1983). Polymorphic phase behaviour of dilinoleoyl phosphatidyl ethanolamine and palmitoyl oleoyl phosphatidyl choline mixtures. Structural changes between hexagonal, cubic and bilayer phases. *Biochimica et Biophysical Acta Biomembranes*, *731*(2), 177–185. doi:10.1016/0005-2736(83)90007-X PMID:6849915

Boyd, B. J., Davey, G., & Drummond, C. J. (2004). *Surfactants and lyotropic phases formed there from.* International patent WO, 2004/022530.

Boyd, B. J., Davey, G., Khoo, S. M., & Whittaker, D. V. (2005). *Compositions and methods of delivery of biologically active agents.* International patent WO2005021046.

Boyd, B. J., Khoo, S. M., Whittaker, D. V., Davey, G., & Porter, C. J. H. (2007). A lipid-based liquid crystalline matrix that provides sustained release and enhanced oral bioavailability for a model poorly water soluble drug in rats. *International Journal of Pharmaceutics, 340*(1), 52–60. doi:10.1016/j.ijpharm.2007.03.020 PMID:17467935

Boyd, B. J., Whittaker, D. V., Khoo, S. M., & Davey, G. (2006). Lyotropic liquid crystalline phases formed from glycerate surfactants as sustained release drug delivery systems. *International Journal of Pharmaceutics, 309*(1-2), 218–226. doi:10.1016/j.ijpharm.2005.11.033 PMID:16413980

Boyd, B. J., Whittaker, D. V., Khoo, S. M., & Davey, G. (2006). Hexosomes formed from glycerate surfactants-formulation as a colloidal carrier for irinotecan. *International Journal of Pharmaceutics, 318*(1-2), 154–162. doi:10.1016/j.ijpharm.2006.03.010 PMID:16621358

Bunjes, H., & Rades, T. (2005). Thermotropic liquid crystalline drugs. *The Journal of Pharmacy and Pharmacology, 57*(7), 807–816. doi:10.1211/0022357056208 PMID:15969938

Burrows, R., Collett, J. H., & Attwood, D. (1994). The release of drugs from monoglyceride-water liquid crystalline phases. *International Journal of Pharmaceutics, 111*(3), 283–293. doi:10.1016/0378-5173(94)90351-4

Cervin, C., Vandoolaeghe, P., Nistor, C., Tiberg, F., & Johnssona, M. (2009). A combined in vitro and in vivo study on the interactions between somatostatin and lipid-based liquid crystalline drug carriers and bilayers. *European Journal of Pharmaceutical Sciences, 36*(4-5), 377–385. doi:10.1016/j.ejps.2008.11.001 PMID:19041716

Chan, H. K., & Gonda, I. (1991). Methotrexate: Existence of different types of solid. *International Journal of Pharmaceutics, 68*(1-3), 179–190. doi:10.1016/0378-5173(91)90140-J

Chang, C. M., & Bodmeier, R. (1997). Swelling of and drug release from monoglyceride-based drug delivery systems. *Journal of Pharmaceutical Sciences, 86*(6), 747–752. doi:10.1021/js960256w PMID:9188059

Chen, Y., Lu, Y., Zhong, Y., Wang, Q., Wu, W., & Gao, S. (2012). Ocular delivery of cyclosporine A based on glyceryl monooleate/poloxamer 407 liquid crystalline nanoparticles: Preparation, characterization, in vitro corneal penetration and ocular irritation. *Journal of Drug Targeting, 20*(10), 856–863. doi:10.3109/1061186X.2012.723214 PMID:23050903

Chong, J. Y. T., Mulet, X., Waddington, L. J., Boyd, B. J., & Drummond, C. J. (2011). Steric stabilisation of self-assembled cubic lyotropic liquid crystalline nanoparticles: High throughput evaluation of triblock polyethylene oxide-polypropylene oxidepolyethylene oxide copolymers. *Soft Matter, 7*(10), 4768–4777. doi:10.1039/c1sm05181d

Chong, J. Y. T., Mulet, X., Waddington, L. J., Boyd, B. J., & Drummond, C. J. (2012). High-throughput discovery of novel steric stabilizers for cubic lyotropic liquid crystal nanoparticle dispersions. *Langmuir, 28*(25), 9223–9232. doi:10.1021/la301874v PMID:22630595

Chung, H., & Caffrey, M. (1995). Polymorphism, mesomorphism, and metastability of monoelaidin in excess water. *Biophysical Journal, 69*(5), 1951–1963. doi:10.1016/S0006-3495(95)80065-2 PMID:8580338

Clogston, J., & Caffrey, M. (2005). Controlling release from the lipidic cubic phase. Amino acids, peptides, proteins and nucleic acids. *Journal of Controlled Release*, *107*(1), 97–111. doi:10.1016/j.jconrel.2005.05.015 PMID:15990192

Cohen Avrahami, M., Aserin, A., & Garti, N. (2010). HII mesophase and peptide cell-penetrating enhancers for improved transdermal delivery of sodium diclofenac. *Colloids and Surfaces. B, Biointerfaces*, *77*(2), 131–138. doi:10.1016/j.colsurfb.2010.01.013 PMID:20189781

Cohen-Avrahami, M., Libster, D., Aserin, A., & Garti, N. (2012). Penetratin-induced transdermal delivery from H *II* mesophases of sodium diclofenac. J*ournal of Controlled Release,* 159*(3)*, 419–428. doi:10.1016/j.jconrel.2012.01.025 PMID:22306174

Costa Balogh, F. O., Sparr, E., Sousa, J. J. S., & Pais, A. C. (2010). Drug release from lipid liquid crystalline phases: Relation with phase behavior. *Drug Development and Industrial Pharmacy*, *36*(4), 470–481. doi:10.3109/03639040903261997 PMID:19848561

Cox, J. S. G., Woodard, G. D., & McCrone, W. C. (1971). Solid state chemistry of cromolyn sodium (disodium cromoglycate). *Journal of Pharmaceutical Sciences*, *60*(10), 1453–1465. doi:10.1002/jps.2600601003 PMID:5001963

Czeslik, C., Winter, R., Rapp, G., & Bartels, K. (1995). Temperature and pressure-dependent phase behavior of monoacylglycerides monoolein and monoelaidin. *Biophysical Journal*, *68*(4), 1423–1429. doi:10.1016/S0006-3495(95)80315-2 PMID:7787028

Dong, Y. D., Larson, I., Hanley, T., & Boyd, B. J. (2006). Bulk and dispersed aqueous phase behavior of phytantriol: Effect of vitamin E acetate and F127 polymer on liquid crystal nanostructure. *Langmuir*, *22*(23), 9512–9518. doi:10.1021/la061706v PMID:17073473

Drummond, C. J., & Fong, C. (1999). Surfactant self-assembly objects as novel drug delivery vehicles. *Current Opinion in Colloid & Interface Science*, *4*(6), 449–456. doi:10.1016/S1359-0294(00)00020-0

Eccleston, G. M., & Beattie, L. (1988). Micro structural changes during the storage of system containing cetostearyl alcohol/polyxyethylene alkyl ether surfactant. *Drug Development and Industrial Pharmacy*, *14*(15-17), 2499–2518. doi:10.3109/03639048809152029

Engstrom, S., Larsson, K., & Lindman, B. (1984). *Method of preparing controlled-release preparations for biologically active materials.* European Patent EP0126751 A1.

Eriksson, P. O., & Lindblom, G. (1993). Lipid and water diffusion in bicontinuous cubic phases measured by NMR. *Biophysical Journal*, *64*(1), 129–136. doi:10.1016/S0006-3495(93)81347-X PMID:8431537

Esposito, E., Carotta, V., Scabbia, A., Trombellib, L., D'Antonac, P., Menegattia, E., & Nastruzzi, C. (1996). Comparative analysis of tetracycline-containing dental gels: Poloxamer- and monoglyceride-based formulations. *International Journal of Pharmaceutics*, *142*(1), 9–23. doi:10.1016/0378-5173(96)04649-2

Esposito, E., Cortesi, R., Drechsler, M., Paccamiccio, L., Mariani, P., Contado, C., & Puglia, C. et al. (2005). Cubosome dispersions as delivery systems for percutaneous administration of indomethacin. *Pharmaceutical Research*, *22*(12), 2163–2173. doi:10.1007/s11095-005-8176-x PMID:16267633

Farkas, E., Zelko, R., Nemeth, Z., Palinkas, J., Marton, S., & Racz, I. (2000). The effect of liquid crystalline structure on chlorhexidine diacetate release. *International Journal of Pharmaceutics*, *193*(2), 239–245. doi:10.1016/S0378-5173(99)00346-4 PMID:10606788

Fong, C., Wells, D., Krodkiewska, I., Booth, J., & Hartley, P. G. (2007). Synthesis and mesophases of glycerate surfactants. *The Journal of Physical Chemistry B, 111*(6), 1384–1392. doi:10.1021/jp0659655 PMID:17286353

Fong, W. K., Hanley, T., & Boyd, B. J. (2009). Stimuli responsive liquid crystals provide 'on-demand' drug delivery *in vitro* and *in vivo. Journal of Controlled Release, 135*(3), 218–226. doi:10.1016/j.jconrel.2009.01.009 PMID:19331865

Ganem-Quintanar, A., Quintanar-Guerrero, D., & Buri, P. (2000). Monoolein: A review of the pharmaceutical applications. *Drug Development and Industrial Pharmacy, 26*(8), 809–820. doi:10.1081/DDC-100101304 PMID:10900537

Geraghty, P. B., Attwood, D., Collett, J. H., & Dandiker, Y. (1996). The in vitro release of some antimuscarinic drugs from monoolein/water lyotropic liquid crystalline gels. *Pharmaceutical Research, 13*(8), 1265–1271. doi:10.1023/A:1016036908947 PMID:8865324

Giorgione, J. R., Huang, Z., & Epand, R. M. (1998). Increased activation of protein kinase C with cubic phase lipid compared with liposomes. *Biochemistry, 37*(8), 2384–2392. doi:10.1021/bi970873e PMID:9485386

Guo, C., Wang, J., Cao, F., Lee, R. J., & Zhai, G. (2010). Lyotropic liquid crystal systems in drug delivery. *Drug Discovery Today, 15*(23-24), 1032–1040. doi:10.1016/j.drudis.2010.09.006 PMID:20934534

Gupta, A., Stait-Gardner, T., de Campo, L., Waddington, L. J., Kirby, N., Price, W. S., & Moghaddam, M. J. (2014). Nano assemblies of Gd-DTPA-monooleyl and glycerol monooleate amphiphiles as potential MRI contrast agents. *Journal of Materials Chemistry B, 2*(9), 1225–1233. doi:10.1039/c3tb21069c

Gustafsson, J., Ljusberg Wahren, H., Almgren, M., & Larsson, K. (1997). Submicron particles of reversed lipid phases in water stabilized by a nonionic amphiphilic polymer. *Langmuir, 13*(26), 6964–6971. doi:10.1021/la970566+

Han, K., Pan, X., Chen, M., Wang, R., Xu, Y., Feng, M., & Wu, C. (2010). Phytantriol-based inverted type bicontinuous cubic phase for vascular embolization and drug sustained release. *European Journal of Pharmaceutical Sciences, 41*(5), 692–699. doi:10.1016/j.ejps.2010.09.012 PMID:20883779

Hartshorne, N. H., & Woodard, G. D. (1973). Mesomorphism in the system disodium chromoglycate-water. *Molecular Crystals & Liquid Crystals, 23*(3-4), 343–368. doi:10.1080/15421407308083381

Hato, M., & Minamikawa, H. (1996). The effects of oligosaccharide stereochemistry on the physical properties of aqueous synthetic glycolipids. *Langmuir, 12*(6), 1658–1665. doi:10.1021/la950326z

Helledi, L. S., & Schubert, L. (2001). Release kinetics of acyclovir from a suspension of acyclovir incorporated in a cubic phase delivery system. *Drug Development and Industrial Pharmacy, 27*(10), 1073–1081. doi:10.1081/DDC-100108370 PMID:11794810

Hirlekar, R., Jain, S., Patel, M., Garse, H., & Kadam, V. (2010). Hexosomes: A novel drug delivery system. *Current Drug Delivery, 7*(1), 28–35. doi:10.2174/156720110790396526 PMID:20044910

Israelachvili, J. (1994). The science and applications of emulsions- an overview. *Colloids and Surfaces. A, Physicochemical and Engineering Aspects, 91*, 1–8. doi:10.1016/0927-7757(94)02743-9

Kaasgaard, T., & Drummond, C. J. (2006). Ordered 2-D and 3-D nanostructured amphiphile self-assembly materials stable in excess solvent. *Physical Chemistry Chemical Physics*, *8*(43), 4957–4975. doi:10.1039/b609510k PMID:17091149

Kawamoto, H. (2002). The history of liquid crystal display.*Proceedings of the IEEE*, 460-499.

Koynova, R., Tenchov, B., & Rapp, G. (1997). Low amounts of PEG-lipid induce cubic phase in phosphatidyl ethanolamide dispersions. *Biochimica et Biophysica Acta*, *1326*(2), 167–170. doi:10.1016/S0005-2736(97)00067-9 PMID:9218547

Kulichikhin, V. G., Malkin, A. Y., & Papkov, S. P. (1984). Rheological properties of liquid crystalline polymer systems Review. *Polymer Science USSR*, *26*(3), 499–524. doi:10.1016/0032-3950(84)90384-8

Kulkarni, C. V. (2011). Nanostructural studies on monoelaidin-water systems at low temperatures. *Langmuir*, *27*(19), 11790–11800. doi:10.1021/la201235h PMID:21846133

Lancelot, A., Sierra, T., & Serrano, J. L. (2014). Nanostructured liquid crystalline particles for drug delivery. *Expert Opinion on Drug Delivery*, *11*(4), 1–18. doi:10.1517/17425247.2014.884556 PMID:24490701

Lara, M. G., Bentley, M. V. L. B., & Collett, J. H. (2005). In vitro drug release mechanism and drug loading studies of cubic phase gels. *International Journal of Pharmaceutics*, *293*(1-2), 241–250. doi:10.1016/j.ijpharm.2005.01.008 PMID:15778062

Larsson, K. (1989). Cubic lipid-water phases: Structures and biomembrane aspects. *Journal of Physical Chemistry*, *93*(21), 7304–7314. doi:10.1021/j100358a010

Larsson, K. (2000). Aqueous dispersions of cubic lipid-water phases. *Current Opinion in Colloid & Interface Science*, *5*(1-2), 64–69. doi:10.1016/S1359-0294(00)00040-6

Larsson, K. (2009). Lyotropic liquid crystals and their dispersions relevant in foods. *Current Opinion in Colloid & Interface Science*, *14*(1), 16–20. doi:10.1016/j.cocis.2008.01.006

Lechuga-Ballesteros, D., Abdul-Fattah, A., Stevenson, C. L., & Bennett, D. (2003). Properties and stability of a liquid crystal form of cyclosporine-the first reported naturally occurring peptide that exists as a thermotropic liquid crystal. *Journal of Pharmaceutical Sciences*, *92*(9), 1821–1831. doi:10.1002/jps.10444 PMID:12950000

Lee, K. W. Y., Nguyen, T. H., Hanley, T., & Boyd, B. J. (2009). Nanostructure of liquid crystalline matrix determines in vitro sustained release and in vivo oral absorption kinetics for hydrophilic model drugs. *International Journal of Pharmaceutics*, *365*(1-2), 190–199. doi:10.1016/j.ijpharm.2008.08.022 PMID:18790030

Leslie, S. B., Puvvada, S., Ratna, B. R., & Rudolph, A. S. (1996). Encapsulation of hemoglobin in a bicontinuous cubic phase lipid. *Biochimica et Biophysica Acta*, *1285*(2), 246–254. doi:10.1016/S0005-2736(96)00169-1 PMID:8972709

Libster, D., Aserin, A., Wachtel, E., Shoham, G., & Garti, N. (2007). An HII liquid crystal-based delivery system for cyclosporin A: Physical characterization. *Journal of Colloid and Interface Science*, *308*(2), 514–524. doi:10.1016/j.jcis.2006.12.084 PMID:17276444

Lindell, K., Engblom, J., Jonstromer, M., Carlsson, A., & Engstrom, S. (1998). Influence of a charged phospholipid on the release pattern of timolol maleate from cubic liquid crystalline phases. *Progress in Colloid & Polymer Science*, *108*, 111–118.

Liu, T., & Guo, R. (2007). Structure and transformation of the niosome prepared from PEG 6000/Tween80/Span80/H2O lamellar liquid crystal. *Colloids and Surfaces. A, Physicochemical and Engineering Aspects*, *295*(1-3), 130–134. doi:10.1016/j.colsurfa.2006.08.041

Loosli, H. R., Kessler, H., Oschkinat, H., Weber, H. P., Petcher, T., & Wider, A. (1985). The conformation of cyclosporin A in the crystal and in solution. *Helvetica Chimica Acta*, *68*, 682–703. doi:10.1002/hlca.19850680319

Lopes, L. B., Ferreira, D. A., De Paula, D., Garcia, M. T. J., Thomazini, J. A., Fantini, M. C. A., & Bentley, M. V. L. B. (2006). Reverse hexagonal phase nano dispersion of monoolein and oleic acid for topical delivery of peptides:in vitro andin vivo skin penetration of cyclosporin A. *Pharmaceutical Research*, *23*(6), 1332–1342. doi:10.1007/s11095-006-0143-7 PMID:16715364

Lopes, L. B., Lopes, J. L. C., Oliveira, D. C. R., Thomazini, J. A., Garcia, M. T. J., Fantini, M. C. A., & Bentley, M. V. L. B. et al. (2006). Liquid crystalline phases of mono olein and water for topical delivery of cyclosporin A: Characterization and study of *in vitro* and *in vivo* delivery. *European Journal of Pharmaceutics and Biopharmaceutics*, *63*(2), 146–155. doi:10.1016/j.ejpb.2006.02.003 PMID:16621488

Lopes, L. B., Speretta, F. F. F., & Bentley, M. V. L. B. (2007). Enhancement of skin penetration of vitamin K using monoolein-based liquid crystalline systems. *European Journal of Pharmaceutical Sciences*, *32*(3), 209–215. doi:10.1016/j.ejps.2007.07.006 PMID:17900879

Luo, M., Shen, Q., & Chen, J. (2011). Transdermal delivery of paeonol using cubic gel and microemulsion gel. *International Journal of Nanomedicine*, *6*, 1603–1610. PMID:21904450

Makai, M., Csanyi, E., Dekany, I., Nemeth, Z., & Eros, I. (2003). Structural properties of non-ionic surfactant/glycerol/paraffin lyotropic crystals. *Colloid & Polymer Science*, *281*, 839–844. doi:10.1007/s00396-002-0851-4

Makai, M., Csanyi, E., Nemeth, Z. S., Palinkas, J., & Eros, I. (2003). Structure and drug release of lamellar liquid crystals containing glycerol. *International Journal of Pharmaceutics*, *256*(1-2), 95–107. doi:10.1016/S0378-5173(03)00066-8 PMID:12695015

Marsh, D. (1990). Spin label ESR and 31P-NMR studies of the cubic and inverted hexagonal phases of dimyristoyl phosphatidyl choline/myristic acid (1:2, mol/mol) mixtures. *Biochimica et Biophysica Acta*, *1024*(1), 89–94. doi:10.1016/0005-2736(90)90211-6 PMID:2159807

Martin, A. (2001). *Physical pharmacy* (4th ed.). Lippincott Williams and Wilkins. Printed in India at Gopsons Papers Ltd, Noida.

Martin-Bertelsen, B., Korsholm, K. S., Rose, F., Nordly, P., Franzyk, H., Andersen, P., & Foged, C. (2013). The supra molecular structure is decisive for the immune stimulatory properties of synthetic analogues of a mycobacterial lipid in vitro. *RSC Advances*, *3*(43), 20673–20683. doi:10.1039/C3RA42737D

Mezzenga, R., Meyer, C., Servais, C., Romoscanu, A. I., Sagalowicz, L., & Hayward, R. C. (2005). Shear rheology of lyotropic liquid crystals: A case study. *Langmuir*, *21*(8), 3322–3333. doi:10.1021/la046964b PMID:15807570

Mezzenga, R., Schurtenberger, P., Burbidge, A., & Michel, M. (2005). Understanding foods as soft materials. *Nature Materials*, *4*(10), 729–740. doi:10.1038/nmat1496 PMID:16195765

Milton, N., & Nail, S. L. (1996). The physical state of nafcillin sodium in frozen aqueous solutions and freezedried powders. *Pharmaceutical Development and Technology*, *1*(3), 269–277. doi:10.3109/10837459609022595 PMID:9552309

Mohammady, S. Z., Pouzot, M., & Mezzenga, R. (2009). Oleoylethanolamide-based lyotropic liquid crystals as vehicles for delivery of amino acids in aqueous environment. *Biophysical Journal*, *96*(4), 1537–1546. doi:10.1016/j.bpj.2008.10.057 PMID:19217870

Mueller-Goymann, C. C. (2002). Liquid crystals in drug delivery. In J. Swarbrick & J. C. Boylan (Eds.), *Encyclopedia of Pharmaceutical Technology* (pp. 834–853). New York, Basel: Marcel Dekker.

Mueller-Goymann, C. C., & Frank, S. G. (1986). Interaction of lidocaine and lidocaine hydrochloride with liquid crystal structure of topical preparation. *International Journal of Pharmaceutics*, *29*(2-3), 147–159. doi:10.1016/0378-5173(86)90112-2

Mueller-Goymann, C. C., & Hamann, H. J. (1993). Sustained release from reverse micellar solutions by phase transformation into lamellar liquid crystals. *Journal of Controlled Release*, *23*(2), 165–174. doi:10.1016/0168-3659(93)90042-4

Muller, F., Salonen, A., & Glatter, O. (2010). Monoglyceride-based cubosomes stabilized by Laponite: Separating the effects of stabilizer, pH and temperature. *Colloids and Surfaces. A, Physicochemical and Engineering Aspects*, *358*(1–3), 50–56. doi:10.1016/j.colsurfa.2010.01.021

Murgia, S., Bonacchi, S., Falchi, A. M., Lampis, S., Lippolis, V., Meli, V., & Caltagirone, C. (2013). Drug-loaded fluorescent cubosomes: Versatile nanoparticles for potential the ranostic applications. *Langmuir*, *29*(22), 6673–6679. doi:10.1021/la401047a PMID:23642193

Negrini, R., & Mezzenga, R. (2011). PH-responsive lyotropic liquid crystals for controlled drug delivery. *Langmuir*, *27*(9), 5296–5303. doi:10.1021/la200591u PMID:21452814

Nesseem, D. I. (2001). Formulation and evaluation of itraconazole via liquid crystal for topical delivery system. *Journal of Pharmaceutical and Biomedical Analysis*, *26*(3), 387–399. doi:10.1016/S0731-7085(01)00414-9 PMID:11489384

Nguyen, T. H., Hanley, T., Porter, C. J. H., & Boyd, B. J. (2011). Nanostructured liquid crystalline particles provide long duration sustained-release effect for a poorly water soluble drug after oral administration. *Journal of Controlled Release*, *153*(2), 180–186. doi:10.1016/j.jconrel.2011.03.033 PMID:21497623

Nguyen, T. H., Hanley, T., Porter, C. J. H., Larson, I., & Boyd, B. J. (2010). Phytantriol and glyceryl monooleate cubic liquid crystalline phases as sustained-release oral drug delivery systems for poorly water-soluble drugs II. In-vivo evaluation. *The Journal of Pharmacy and Pharmacology*, *62*(7), 856–865. doi:10.1211/jpp.62.07.0006 PMID:20636873

Nilsson, C., Barrios-Lopez, B., Kallinen, A., Laurinmäki, P., Butcher, S. J., Raki, M., & Yaghmur, A. (2013). SPECT/CT imaging of radiolabeled cubosomes and hexosomes forpotential theranostic applications. *Biomaterials*, *34*(33), 8491–8503. doi:10.1016/j.biomaterials.2013.07.055 PMID:23932247

Norlen, L., & Al-Amoudi, A. (2004). Stratum corneum keratin structure, function, and formation: The cubic rod-packing and membrane templating model. *The Journal of Investigative Dermatology*, *123*(4), 715–732. doi:10.1111/j.0022-202X.2004.23213.x PMID:15373777

Norling, T., Lading, P., Engstrom, S., Larsson, K., Krog, N., & Nissen, S. S. (1992). Formulation of a drug delivery system based on a mixture of monoglycerides and triglycerides for use in the treatment of periodontal disease. *Journal of Clinical Periodontology*, *19*(9), 687–692. doi:10.1111/j.1600-051X.1992.tb02529.x PMID:1447387

Okamoto, Y., Masum, S. M., Miyazawa, H., & Yamazaki, M. (2008). Low-pH-induced transformation of bilayer membrane into bicontinuous cubic phase in dioleoyl phosphatidyl serine/monoolein membranes. *Langmuir*, *24*(7), 3400–3406. doi:10.1021/la7036795 PMID:18302439

Omray, L. K. (2013). Liquid crystals as novel vesicular delivery system: A review. *Current Trends in Technology and Science*, *II*(VI), 347–353.

Orle, G. W., Drechsler, M., Koch, M. H. J., Siekmann, B., Westesen, K., & Bunjes, H. (2007). Influence of composition and preparation parameters on the properties of aqueous monoolein dispersions. *International Journal of Pharmaceutics*, *329*(1-2), 150–157. doi:10.1016/j.ijpharm.2006.08.023 PMID:16987623

Patterson, J., Bary, A., & Rades, T. (2002). Physical stability and solubility of the thermotropic mesophases of fenoprofen calcium as pure drug and in a tablet formulation. *International Journal of Pharmacy and Pharmaceutical Sciences*, *247*, 147–157. PMID:12429493

Peng, X., Wen, X., Pan, X., Wang, R., Chen, B., & Wu, C. (2010). Design and In Vitro evaluation of capsaicin transdermal controlled release cubic phase gels. *AAPS PharmSciTech*, *11*(3), 1405–1410. doi:10.1208/s12249-010-9481-1 PMID:20839080

Powell, M. F., Fleitman, J., Sanders, L. M., & Si, V. C. (1994). Peptide liquid crystals: Inverse correlation of kinetic formation and thermodynamic stability in aqueous solution. *Pharmaceutical Research*, *11*(9), 1352–1354. doi:10.1023/A:1018963016079 PMID:7816768

Powell, M. F., Sanders, L. M., Rogerson, A., & Si, V. (1991). Parenteral Peptide formulations: Chemical and physical properties of native luteinizing hormone releasing hormone and hydrophobic analogues in aqueous solution. *Pharmaceutical Research*, *8*(10), 1258–1263. doi:10.1023/A:1015847628047 PMID:1839059

Rades, T., & Muller-Goymann, C. C. (1992). Structural investigations on the liquid crystalline phases of fenoprofen. *Pharmacol Biochem Prop Drug Sust*, *2*, 131–134.

Rades, T., & Muller-Goymann, C. C. (1997). Electron and light microscopical investigation of defect structures in mesophases of pharmaceutical substances. *Colloid & Polymer Science*, *275*(12), 1169–1178. doi:10.1007/s003960050198

Rizwan, S. B., Hanley, T., Boyd, B. J., Rades, T., & Hook, S. (2009). Liquid crystalline systems of phytantriol and glyceryl mono oleate containing a hydrophilic protein: Characterisation, swelling and release kinetics. *Journal of Pharmaceutical Sciences*, *98*(11), 4191–4204. doi:10.1002/jps.21724 PMID:19340889

Sadhale, Y., & Shah, J. C. (1998). Glyceryl monooleate cubic phase gel as chemical stability enhancer of cefazolin and cefuroxime. *Pharmaceutical Development and Technology*, *3*(4), 549–556. doi:10.3109/10837459809028637 PMID:9834958

Sadhale, Y., & Shah, J. C. (1999a). Biological activity of insulin in GMO gels and the effect of agitation. *International Journal of Pharmaceutics*, *191*(1), 65–74. doi:10.1016/S0378-5173(99)00287-2 PMID:10556741

Sadhale, Y., & Shah, J. C. (1999b). Stabilization of insulin against agitation-induced aggregation by the GMO cubic phase gel. *International Journal of Pharmaceutics*, *191*(1), 51–64. doi:10.1016/S0378-5173(99)00288-4 PMID:10556740

Sagalowicz, L., Leser, M. E., Watzke, H. J., & Michel, M. (2006). Monoglyceride self-assembly structures as delivery vehicles. *Trends in Food Science & Technology*, *17*(5), 204–214. doi:10.1016/j.tifs.2005.12.012

Sagalowicz, L., Mezzenga, R., & Leser, M. E. (2006). Investigating reversed liquid crystalline mesophases. *Current Opinion in Colloid & Interface Science*, *11*(4), 224–229. doi:10.1016/j.cocis.2006.07.002

Sallam, A. S., Khalil, E., Ibrahim, H., & Freij, I. (2002). Formulation of an oral dosage form utilizing the properties of cubic liquid crystalline phases of glyceryl monooleate. *European Journal of Pharmaceutics and Biopharmaceutics*, *53*(3), 343–352. doi:10.1016/S0939-6411(02)00016-4 PMID:11976023

Shah, J. C., Sadhale, Y., & Chilukuri, D. M. (2001). Cubic phase gels as drug delivery systems. *Advanced Drug Delivery Reviews*, *47*(2-3), 229–250. doi:10.1016/S0169-409X(01)00108-9 PMID:11311994

Shah, M. H., & Paradkar, A. (2005). Cubic liquid crystalline glyceryl monooleate matrices for oral delivery of enzyme. *International Journal of Pharmaceutics*, *294*(1-2), 161–171. doi:10.1016/j.ijpharm.2005.01.019 PMID:15814241

Shah, M. H., & Paradkar, A. (2007). Effect of HLB of additives on the properties and drug release from the glyceryl monooleate matrices. *European Journal of Pharmaceutics and Biopharmaceutics*, *67*(1), 166–174. doi:10.1016/j.ejpb.2007.01.001 PMID:17353118

Six, K., Berghmans, H., Leuner, C., Dressman, J., Van Werde, K., Mullens, J., & Van den Mooter, G. et al. (2003). Characterization of solid dispersions of itraconazole and hydroxyl propyl methyl cellulose prepared by melts extrusion, part II. *Pharmaceutical Research*, *20*(7), 1047–1054. doi:10.1023/A:1024414423779 PMID:12880291

Six, K., Verreck, G., Peeters, J., Augustijns, P., Kinget, R., & Van den Mooter, G. (2001). Investigation of thermal properties of glassy itraconazole: Identification of a monotropic mesophase. *Thermochimica Acta*, *376*(2), 175–181. doi:10.1016/S0040-6031(01)00563-9

Sjolund, M., Lindblom, G., Rilfors, L., & Arvidson, G. (1987). Hydrophobic molecules in lecithin-water systems. I. Formation of reversed hexagonal phases at high and low water contents. *Biophysical Journal*, *52*(2), 145–153. doi:10.1016/S0006-3495(87)83202-2 PMID:2822159

Spicer, P. T. (2005). Progress in liquid crystalline dispersions: Cubosomes. *Current Opinion in Colloid & Interface Science*, *10*(5-6), 274–279. doi:10.1016/j.cocis.2005.09.004

Spicer, P. T., Hayden, K. L., Lynch, M. L., Ofori-Boateng, A., & Burns, J. L. (2001). Novel process for producing cubic liquid crystalline nanoparticles (cubosomes). *Langmuir*, *17*(19), 5748–5756. doi:10.1021/la010161w

Stephenson, G. A., & Diseroad, B. A. (2000). Structural relationship and desolvation behavior of cromolyn, cefazolin and fenoprofen sodium hydrates. *International Journal of Pharmaceutics*, *198*(2), 167–177. doi:10.1016/S0378-5173(00)00331-8 PMID:10767566

Stevenson, C. L., Bennett, D. B., & Ballesteros, D. L. (2005). Pharmaceutical liquid crystals: The relevance of partially ordered systems. *Journal of Pharmaceutical Sciences*, *94*(9), 1861–1879. doi:10.1002/jps.20435 PMID:16052511

Swarnakar, N. K., Jain, V., Dubey, V., Mishra, D., & Jain, N. K. (2007). Enhanced oromucosal delivery of progesterone via hexosomes. *Pharmaceutical Research*, *24*(12), 2223–2230. doi:10.1007/s11095-007-9409-y PMID:17828445

Takahashi, H., Hatta, I., & Quinn, P. J. (1996). Cubic phases in hydrated 1:1 and 1:2 dipalmitoyl phosphatidyl choline- dipalmitoyl glycerol mixtures. *Biophysical Journal*, *70*(3), 1407–1411. doi:10.1016/S0006-3495(96)79699-6 PMID:8785296

Tan, M. M., Corley, C. A., & Stevenson, C. L. (1998). Effect of gelation on the chemical stability and conformation of leuprolide. *Pharmaceutical Research*, *15*(9), 1442–1448. doi:10.1023/A:1011914007940 PMID:9755898

Tang, T. Y. D., Brooks, N. J., Jeworrek, C., Ces, O., Terrill, N. J., Winter, R., & Seddon, J. M. (2012). Hydrostatic pressure effects on the lamellar to gyroid cubic phase transition of monolinolein at limited hydration. *Langmuir*, *28*(36), 13018–13024. doi:10.1021/la3025843 PMID:22894718

Tenchov, B., Koynova, R., & Rapp, G. (1998). Accelerated formation of cubic phases in phosphatidyl ethanolamine dispersions. *Biophysical Journal*, *75*(2), 853–866. doi:10.1016/S0006-3495(98)77574-5 PMID:9675186

Tenchov, B., Rappolt, M., Koynova, R., & Rapp, G. (1996). New phases induced by sucrose in saturated phosphatidyl ethanolamines: An expanded lamellar gel phase and a cubic phase. *Biochimica et Biophysica Acta*, *1285*(1), 109–122. doi:10.1016/S0005-2736(96)00156-3 PMID:8948481

Ubbink, J., Burbidge, A., & Mezzenga, R. (2008). Food structure and functionality: A soft matter perspective. *Soft Matter*, *4*(8), 1569–1581. doi:10.1039/b802183j

Vadas, E., Toma, P., & Zografi, G. (1991). Solid state phase transitions initiated by water vapor sorption of crystalline L-660-711, a leukotriene D4 receptor antagonist. *Pharmaceutical Research*, *8*(2), 148–155. doi:10.1023/A:1015871415925 PMID:2023861

Wadsten-Hindrichsen, P., Bender, J., Unga, J., & Engstrom, S. (2007). Aqueous self-assembly of phytantriol in ternary systems: Effect of monoolein, distearoyl phosphatidyl glycerol and three watermiscible solvents. *Journal of Colloid and Interface Science*, *315*(2), 701–713. doi:10.1016/j.jcis.2007.07.011 PMID:17655855

Wagner, E. (1994). Panthenol and phytantriol in cosmetics. *Parfumerie Und Kosmetik*, *75*(4), 260–267.

Wyatt, D., & Dorschel, D. (1992). A cubic-phase delivery system composed of glyceryl monooleate and water for sustained release of water-soluble drugs. *Pharmaceutical Technology*, *16*(10), 116–130.

Yaghmur, A., Campo, L., & De, . (2005). Emulsified microemulsions and oil-containing liquid crystalline phases. *Langmuir*, *21*(2), 569–577. doi:10.1021/la0482711 PMID:15641825

Yaghmur, A., Campo, L., & De, . (2006). Control of the internal structure of MLO-based isasomes by the addition of diglycerol monooleate and soybean Phosphatidyl choline. *Langmuir*, *22*(24), 9919–9927. doi:10.1021/la061303v PMID:17106981

Yaghmur, A., & Glatter, O. (2009). Characterization and potential applications of nanostructured aqueous dispersions. *Advances in Colloid and Interface Science*, *147-148*, 333–342. doi:10.1016/j.cis.2008.07.007 PMID:18804754

Yaghmur, A., Kriechbaum, M., Amenitsch, H., Steinhart, M., Laggner, P., & Rappolt, M. (2010). Effects of pressure and temperature on the self-assembled fully hydrated nanostructures of monoolein-oil systems. *Langmuir*, *26*(2), 1177–1185. doi:10.1021/la9023019 PMID:19681634

Yaghmur, A., Laggner, P., Sartori, B., & Rappolt, M. (2008). Calcium triggered $L\alpha$ -*H*2phase transition monitored by combined rapid mixing and time-resolved synchrotron SAXS. PLo*S ONE, 3*(4*)*, e2072. doi:10.1371/journal.pone.0002072 PMID:18446202

Yaghmur, A., Larsen, W., Schmitt, M., Ostergaard, J., Larsen, C., Jensen, H., & Rappolt, M. (2011). In situ characterization of lipidic bupivacaine-loaded formulations. *Soft Matter*, *7*(18), 8291–8295. doi:10.1039/c1sm05854a

Yaghmur, A., Rappolt, M., Ostergaard, J., Larsen, C., & Larsen, S. W. (2012). Characterization of bupivacaine-loaded formulations based on liquid crystalline phases and microemulsions: The effect of lipid composition. *Langmuir*, *28*(5), 2881–2889. doi:10.1021/la203577v PMID:22247936

Yaghmur, A., Sartori, B., & Rappolt, M. (2011). The role of calcium in membrane condensation and spontaneous curvature variations in model lipidic systems. *Physical Chemistry Chemical Physics*, *13*(8), 3115–3125. doi:10.1039/C0CP01036G PMID:21049109

Yamada, K., Yamashita, J., Todo, H., Miyamoto, K., Hashimoto, S., Tokudome, Y., & Sugibayashi, K. (2011). Preparation and evaluation of liquid-crystal formulations with skin-permeation enhancing abilities for entrapped drug. *Journal of Oleo Science*, *60*(1), 31–40. doi:10.5650/jos.60.31 PMID:21178315

Yang, Z., Tan, Y., Chen, M., Dian, L., Shan, Z., Peng, X., & Wu, C. (2013). Development of amphotericin B-loaded cubosomes through the Sol Emuls technology for enhancing the oral bioavailability. *AAPS PharmSciTech*, *13*(4), 1483–1491. doi:10.1208/s12249-012-9876-2 PMID:23090113

Yariv, D., Efrat, R., Libster, D., Aserin, A., & Garti, N. (2010). In vitro permeation of diclofenac salts from lyotropic liquid crystalline systems. *Colloids and Surfaces. B, Biointerfaces*, *78*(2), 185–192. doi:10.1016/j.colsurfb.2010.02.029 PMID:20363601

Yulin, C., Ping, M., & Shuangying, G. (2014). Cubic and Hexagonal Liquid Crystals as Drug Delivery Systems. *BioMed Research International*, *2014*, 815981. PMID:24995330

Zhu, H., Xu, J., Varlashkin, P., Long, S., & Kidd, C. (2001). Dehydration, hydration behavior and structural analysis of fenoprofen calcium. *Journal of Pharmaceutical Sciences*, *90*(7), 845–859. doi:10.1002/jps.1038 PMID:11458334

Section 8
Dendrimers

Chapter 10
Multifunctional Dendrimers for Drug Nanocarriers

Tingbin Zhang
National Center for Nanoscience and Technology, China & Tianjin University, China

Jing Xu
National Center for Nanoscience and Technology, China

Chunqiu Zhang
National Center for Nanoscience and Technology, China

Chan Li
National Center for Nanoscience and Technology, China

Jinfeng Xing
Tianjin University, China

Paul C. Wang
Howard University, USA

Xing-Jie Liang
National Center for Nanoscience and Technology, China

ABSTRACT

Dendrimers are nanosized, monodisperse, highly branched polymers with well-defined topological structure which have attracted much attention for drug delivery recently. To further improve the performance of dendrimers in drug delivery, various functional dendrimers are developed by decorating the dendrimers with targeting agents, imaging agents, or stimuli-sensitive moieties. They show good biocompatibility, visibility, tumor targeting and stimuli-sensitive properties for drug or gene delivery. This chapter will focus on the design of multifunctional nanocarriers based on the dendrimers. Therefore, the chapter will provide the ideas for designing the dendrimers based nanocarriers for controllable drug delivery and let more people know the development of dendrimers for drug delivery in recent years.

INTRODUCTION

In the recent years, significant progress has been achieved in the field of nanotechnology, especially in drug delivery (Shi, Votruba, Farokhzad, & Langer, 2010; Elsabahy & Wooley, 2012; Markman, Rekechenetskiy, Holler, & Ljubimova, 2013). Some traditional drugs have to face the drawbacks, such as poor aqueous solubility, undesired side-effects and low bioavailability (Allen & Cullis, 2013; Patel, Zhou,

DOI: 10.4018/978-1-5225-0751-2.ch010

Piepmeier, & Saltzman, 2012), which dramatically decrease their applications in clinic. With the quick development of nanotechnology, numerous nanocarriers have been employed to solve these problems, because of their outstanding performance with targeting, delayed release, high solubility and dispensability. Most widely used nanocarriers based on polymers such as nanoparticles, micelles and liposomes are efficient, while they are metastable *in vivo* for the self-assembled nanocarriers and it is difficult to precisely control the size, structure and the surface properties of the nanocarriers (Markman et al., 2013; Torchilin, 2014). Furthermore, conventional polymers are typically polydisperse in molecular weight, resulting in poorly controlled the physicochemical properties of nanocarriers, which inevitably cause serious issues in pharmacokinetic study in clinical trials.

Contrast to the conventional polymers, dendrimers are nanosized, monodisperse, highly branched polymers with well-defined topological structure which have attracted much attention for drug delivery applications (Astruc, Boisselier, & Ornelas, 2010; Mintzer & Grinstaff, 2011). Most of them can improve the aqueous solubility and bioavailability of drugs by physically encapsulating in the voids or covalently attaching to the surface groups (D'Emanuele & Attwood, 2005). Dendrimers also have other advantages in drug delivery, such as stable structure, passive tumor targeting by enhanced penetration and retention (EPR) effect, large number of peripheral functional groups, monodisperse size, reproducible synthesis and hydrophobic interiors for drug encapsulation (Cheng, Zhao, Li, & Xu, 2011; Lee, MacKay, Fréchet, & Szoka, 2005; Medina & El-Sayed, 2009). In addition, the dendrimers are feasible modified by functional groups such as active targeting moieties, drugs, imaging agents and stimuli-sensitive elements (Cheng et al., 2011; Singh, Gupta, Asthana, & Jain, 2008). More importantly, the use of dendrimers as drug carriers has reproducible pharmacokinetics which plays a vital role for the drug delivery system in clinical application (Cheng et al., 2011).

The original research of dendrimers started in 1978 by Vögtle and his coworkers, who synthesized the dendritic arms with a central core in a controllable way (Vögtle, Buhleier, &Wehner, 1978). In the early 1980, the dendrimers were boosted by Denkewalter, Tomalia (Tomalia et al., 1985), and Newkome (Newkome, Yao, Baker, & Gupta, 1985). Until now, various dendrimers have been developed, such as polyamidoamine (PAMAM), poly(propyleneimine) (PPI), peptide dendrimers and hybrid dendrimers. The idea of encapsulating guest molecules in dendritic hosts was first proposed by Maciejewski' in 1982. Since then, more and more researchers focused on the development of dendrimers as drug carriers. Jansen et al. (1995) demonstrated that the release of guest molecules entrapped in a "dendritic box" was related to the shapes of the guest molecules, the interior cavities and architecture of the dendrimers. One of the earliest examples that dendrimers served as antitumor drug carriers was achieved by conjugating cisplatin (20–25% by weight) onto the surface groups of a generation (G)-3.5 sodium carboxylate terminated PAMAM dendrimer (Malik, Evagorou, & Duncan, 1999). The solubility of cisplatin was enhanced tenfold and the tumor accumulation levels of platinum (from cisplatin) by EPR effect were fiftyfold greater for the dendrimer-cisplatin than free cisplatin at equivalent doses. In addition, the dendrimer-cisplatin showed better antitumor activity than free cisplatin *in vivo*. In another study, Ihre et al. (2002) reported another polyester dendritic system based on the monomer unit 2,2-bis(hydroxymethyl) propanoic acid for drug delivery. The antitumor drug doxorubicin (DOX) was conjugated on the surface of the dendrimer via a pH-sensitive linkage, demonstrating the feasibility of applying these polyester dendrimers in drug delivery.

While, the conventional dendrimers also face some barriers for more efficient drug delivery as carriers, such as unsatisfied tumor targeting capability, serious side-effects on normal organs, premature release of drugs and fast renal excretion. Therefore, the development of multifunctional nanocarriers based on dendrimers is an active area of current research. The dendrimers can be modified by the active targeting or imaging agents to enhance the accumulation of drugs around the targeted site or monitor the biodistribution and target accumulation of dendrimers. The introduction of stimuli-sensitive moieties (such as hydrozone bond, disulphide bond et al) into the dendrimers is an effective way to achieve the controllable drug release and reduce the side-effects of dendrimers. Additionally, by combination the advantages of liposomes or micelles with dendrimers is also an effective way to enhance the drug loading capacity and prolong the circulation time of nanocarriers. This chapter will focus on the design of multifunctional nanocarriers based on the dendrimers with good biocompatibility, visibility, tumor targeting and stimuli-sensitive properties for drug or gene delivery (Figure 1).

Figure 1. A schematic description of the multifunctional dendrimers based nanocarriers for drug delivery. PEGlyation of the dendrimers can prolong the circulation time and improve the biocompatibility of them. The tumor targeting agents can be attached to the end of polyethylene glycol (PEG) chains to increase the tumor accumulation of dendrimers. The antitumor drugs/imaging agents can be encapsulated in the interiors or conjugated on the peripheral groups of dendrimers. In addition, the conjugated drugs can also be attached via the cleavable units, such as pH, enzyme, redox, temperature or light sensitive moieties to achieve the controllable drug release.

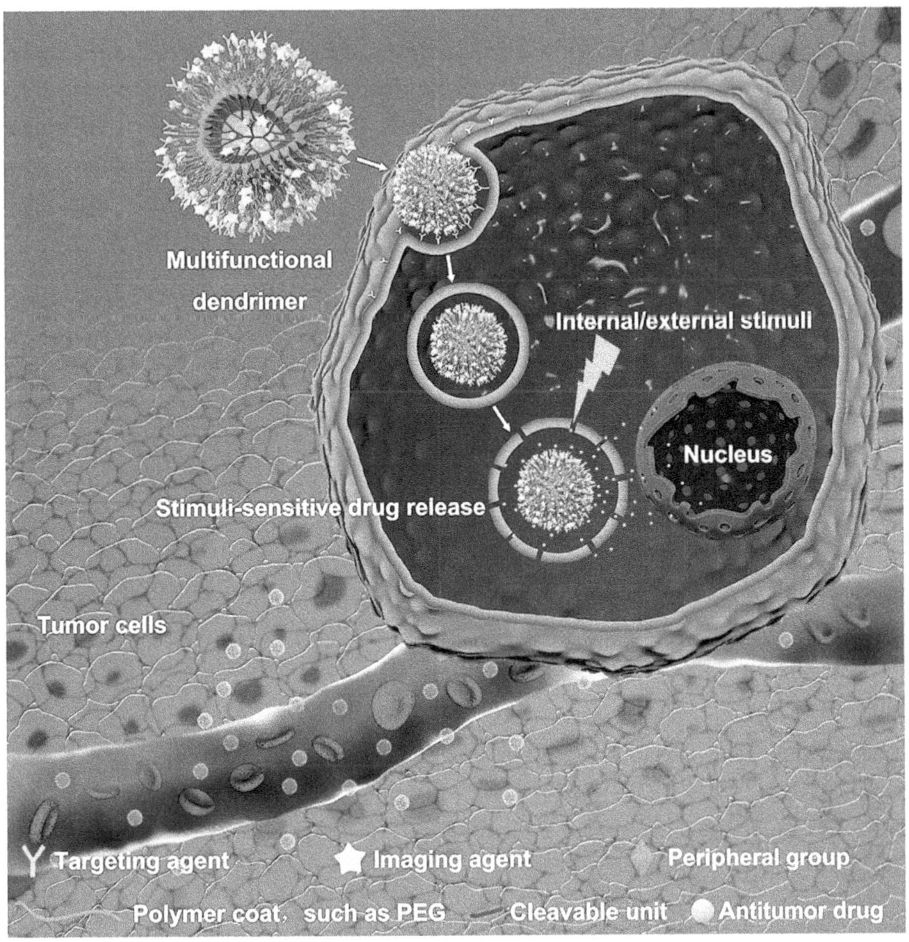

THE APPROACHES TO DENDRIMER SYNTHESIS

Dendrimers have monodisperse molecular weight and well-defined 3D architecture, which can be divided into three parts: core, branches and peripheral groups (Figure 2A). They can be synthesized from the core to periphery or from the periphery to core. Owing to the dendrimer synthesis has been systematically described in recent reviews. In addition, the synthesis of multifunctional dendrimer is based on the conventional dendrimer. In this chapter, brief description of the dendrimer synthesis will be given, including divergent, convergent, orthogonal and 'click' chemistry approaches.

The Original Approaches to Dendrimer Synthesis

Historically, the dendrimers are synthesized by divergent and convergent approaches in a stepwise fashion. As show in Figure 2B, the G2 dendrimer is synthesized with the divergent and convergent approach, respectively. The divergent dendrimer synthesis starts with the functional core molecule and builds up generations to the periphery, which demands large number of reactions to protect and deprotect the reactive groups. So the divergent approach is a slow and costly process and it is difficult to obtain the perfect dendrimers especially for the high generation dendrimer. For example, although the transformation efficiency was 99.5% for each reaction, the yield of monodisperse G5 dendrimer was only 29% (Bosman, Janssen, & Meijer, 1999). Unlike the divergent approach, the convergent dendrimer synthesis is relative more effective and more probable to obtain the perfect dendrimer. The convergent synthesis builds up dendrons firstly from the periphery to core. Then the dendrons are joint together with the functional core to form dendrimer. Compared to divergent approach, the convergent approach demands less reactive sites and the purification is easier with less possible to get the defect dendrimer. Kawaguchi et al. (1995) reported a double exponential growth by combination the divergent and convergent approach to further accelerate the growth rate of dendrimer synthesis. The method is a bi-directional synthesis by

Figure 2. Schematic anatomy of a dendrimer (A) and description of the dendrimer synthesis by divergent and convergent approaches (B)

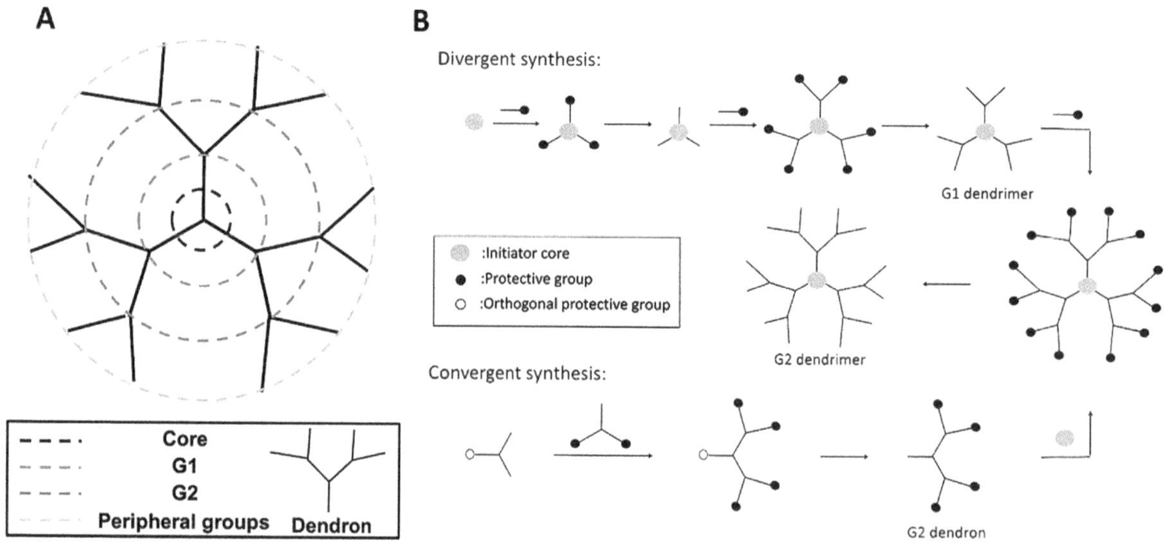

selective protection and deprotection of the reactive groups at the core or periphery. The disadvantages also exist in this method, such as difficult to synthesize the high generation dendrimer because of the steric hindrance and much more complicated protection and deprotection process.

Orthogonal Chemistry and 'Click' Chemistry

The complicated, slow and costly dendrimer synthesis is mainly due to the repeated protection and deprotection process of the reactive groups. So the reduction of the protecting-group amount may be an effective way to improve the rate of the dendrimer synthesis. The orthogonal chemistry is a protecting-group-free approach which has been used in many areas of chemistry, including the synthesis of oligo-saccharides, oligonucleotides and peptides. By combination the divergent or convergent approach with the orthogonal chemistry, the concept of the dendrimer synthesis may be changed thoroughly. The first orthogonal dendrimer synthesis was reported by Zeng and Zimmerman (1996) who synthesized a G4 dendrimer in four steps avoiding the process of protection or deprotection. In order to further improve the efficiency of dendrimer synthesis by this approach, the original monomer was replaced by Fréchet's branched monomer which could grow two generation simultaneously (Wooley, Hawker, & Fréchet, 1994). The G6 dendrimer was obtained in only three steps from the branched monomer which remained the fastest dendrimer synthesis until now.

Although the rate of the dendrimer can be substantially improved, the yield of each reaction remains unsatisfied, resulting in the low efficiency to obtain the perfect dendrimer. It is known that 'click' chemistry is a fast, high yielding and nonreversible reaction with few inoffensive by-products that are easily removed by non-chromatographic methods. Thus, by application the 'click' chemistry in the synthesis of dendrimer, the yield of the perfect dendrimer will be increased substantially. Similarly, by the combination of orthogonal chemistry and 'click' chemistry, the dendrimer synthesis will be fast and high yielding. This approach was verified by Killops et al. (2008). They synthesized a G4 dendrimer by the combination of divergent approach with thiol-ene 'click' chemistry. The reaction can be conducted at room temperature, in the presence of oxygen, without the use of any metal catalysts, by irradiation with 365 nm UV light. The efficiency of G4 dendrimer synthesis was unprecedented under the benign reaction conditions. Recently, Kottari et al. (2014) reported a multifunctional dendrimer utilizing carbohydrate building blocks by the application of orthogonal chemistry, thiol-ene 'click' chemistry and nucleophilic substitution (SN2) reactions. The synthesized process of the dendrimer did not carry out the protection-deprotection steps. In addition, they found that the low generation, globular dendrimer showed higher affinity with the Lec Alectin.

THE DENDRIMERS WITH ACTIVE TUMOR-TARGETING CAPACITY

The tumor usually has increased vascular permeability as well as poor lymphatic drainage, which provides a good opportunity for nanocarriers (in the size range of 20-200 nm) to accumulate inside the interstitial space of tumor and retain in the tumor (Danhier, Feron, & Préat, 2010). This passive targeting phenomenon is called by "EPR effect", discovered by Matsumura and Maeda (Matsumura & Maeda, 1986). Surprisingly, the well-designed nanocarriers can enhance the drug concentration in tumors about 10-30 times compared to the blood due to EPR effect (Maeda, Sawa, & Konno, 2001). Therefore, various nanocarriers such as nanoparticles, micelles, liposomes and dendrimers have been designed to enhance the anticancer effect by EPR effect (Maeda, Bharate, & Daruwalla, 2009; V. Torchilin, 2011). Dendrimers with well-defined architecture and reproducible pharmacokinetics are one of the promising nanocarriers for drug delivery (Caminade & Turrin, 2014).

According to the generation, size and surface charge of dendrimers, the circulation and transportation of them *in vivo* are different. Generally, the cationic dendrimers are inclined to accumulate in each organ owing to their favorable electrostatic interaction with the negatively charged cell membranes of epithelial and endothelial cells. The low generation dendrimers with small size (always smaller than 10 nm) are easily cleared through renal filtration. Therefore, the negative charged or uncharged, high generation dendrimers always show a relative long-circulation time and improve their accumulation in tumor tissues by EPR effect (Okuda et al., 2006). PEGlyation (water soluble polymers) of dendrimers is also an effective approach to prolong the circulation time and improve the biocompatibility of dendrimers, which can increase the size, molecular weight of dendrimers and reduce the interaction with proteins *in vivo* (Kaminskas et al., 2008; Lim et al., 2008).

Unlike the passive targeting, Saad et al. (2008) found that the influence of polymer structure, composition, size and molecular weight on the distribution and the anticancer efficacy of the active targeting nanoparticles was minimized by comparing the properties of three widely used nanocarriers: linear polymer, dendrimer and liposome in drug delivery. After the introduction of the active targeting agents, the cellular internalization and intra tumoral accumulation of nanocarriers were significantly enhanced and the adverse side-effects on healthy organs were minimized. However, the active targeting process cannot be separated from the passive targeting since it occurs only after passive accumulation around the tumors (Danhier et al., 2010). In order to facilitate the dendrimers based nanocarriers with good tumor-targeting capability, researchers synthesized a series of modified dendrimers by conjugation the hydrophilic molecules and active targeting agents such as peptides (Shukla et al., 2005), antibodies (Shukla et al., 2006), vitamins (Kukowska-Latallo et al., 2005) or carbohydrate residues (Barata, Shaunak, Teo, Zloh, & Brocchini, 2011) on the surface of dendrimers.

With the purpose of improving the tumor-targeting, Singh et al. (2008) synthesized the fourth generation (G4) folate-PAMAM dendrimer and folate-PEG-PAMAM dendrimer. The folate molecules can specifically target to the folate receptor which is overexpressed on many human tumors cells including kidney, breast, myeloid cells, ovary, brain and lung (Lu & Low, 2012). They found that the folate-PEG-PAMAM dendrimer was non-cytotoxic and effective to deliver the anticancer drug 5-fluorouracil to solid tumors created by KB cells compared to the non-PEGylated formulation. Based on the similar methods, Zhu et al. (2011) synthesized a tumor neovascular endothelial cells and tumor cells targeted PAMAM dendrimers via the conjugation of cyclized arginine–glycine–aspartic (RGD) peptides and acid-sensitive DOX with PEGlyated PAMAM dendrimers (RGD-PPCD). The RGD can selective target to the integrin $\alpha_v\beta_3$. The PEGlyated PAMAM dendrimers exhibited long circulation time and the DOX showed controllable release profile in weakly acidic lysosomes. Moreover, the constructed RGD-PPCD nanocarriers exhibited significantly improved therapeutic effect against murine B16 melanoma, which might be caused by the higher tumor accumulation of RGD-PPCD and its strong capability to induce apoptosis of tumor neovascular endothelial cells. In another study, Yang et al. (2015) developed an ultra small iron oxide nanoparticles (NPs) functionalized RGD-modified dendrimers (G5.NHAc-RGD-Fe_3O_4 NPs) for targeted magnetic resonance (MR) imaging (Figure 3). The G5.NHAc-RGD-Fe_3O_4 NPs showed high affinity for C6 cells and the C6 tumor in nude mice that overexpress $\alpha_v\beta_3$ receptors. Therefore, the G5.NHAc-RGD-Fe_3O_4 NPs is a promising nanosystem for targeted MR imaging in different types of tumors.

Figure 3. Schematic representation of the G5.NHAc-RGD-Fe_3O_4 NPs and its active targeting of $\alpha_v\beta_3$ receptors (A) and MR images of tumors after intravenous injections of 0.1 mL of PBS solutions containing G5.NHAc-RGD-Fe_3O_4 NPs (600 μg Fe) at different times (B)

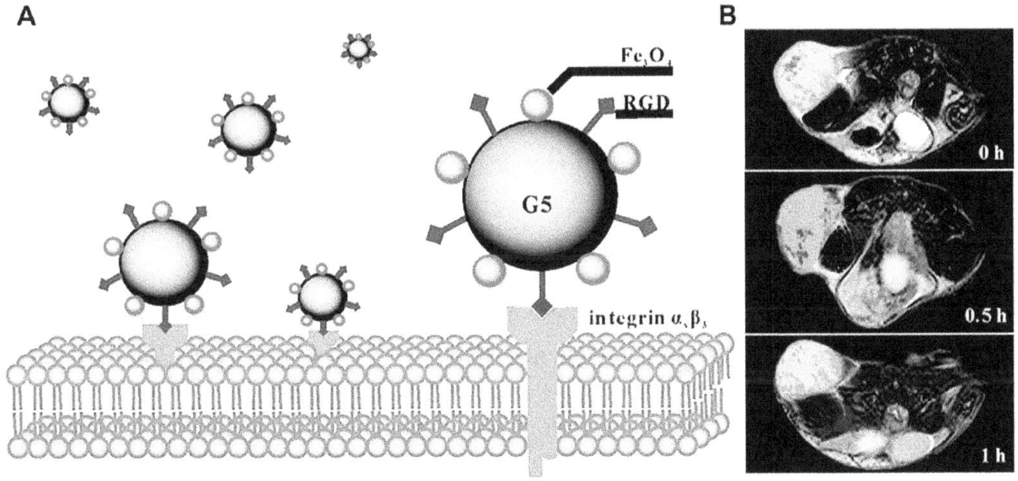

Researchers also attempted to apply the targeted dendrimers in the treatment of brain tumor. Owing to the barrier of blood-brain barrier (BBB) composed by endothelial cells, pericytes, microglial and astrocytes cells, the treatment of brain tumors remains a great challenge (Wohlfart, Gelperina, & Kreuter, 2012). However, the nanotechnology has been proved to be a promising way to deliver drugs across the BBB by adjusting the molecular weight, size, charge and targeted agents of nanocarriers. Y. Li et al. (2012) reported a dual-targeting nanocarrier based on G4 PAMAM dendrimers for treating brain gliomas. The transferrin (Tf) as an active targeting agent was conjugated on the surface of the dendrimers with PEG as spacer to enhance the cellular uptake by brain capillary endothelium and many malignant cells which expressed the Tf receptor (Jefferies et al., 1984; H. Li & Qian, 2002). The tamoxifen (TAM) as an estrogen receptor modulator was physical encapsulated in the interiors of the dendrimers to inhibit multidrug resistance and enhance the BBB transporting (Kayyali, Marriott, & Wiseman, 1994). The DOX was also conjugated on the surface of dendrimers via an acid labile hydrazone bond to facilitate the controllable drug release profile. The dual-targeting nanocarrier showed high BBB transportation capability with the transporting ratio of 6.06% in 3 h and effective inhibition the growth of glioma spheroids.

Although the dendrimers based targeted nanocarriers can deliver the drugs to tumors with strong penetration capability, the circulation time is limited for the nonspecific interaction with the proteins or normal organs and fast clearance through renal filtration. It is known that the nanoparticles with the size of 50-200 nm in diameter always have long circulation time *in vivo* but the tumor penetration capability is limited for the relative large size (Chan et al., 2014; Gref et al., 2012). Thus, Sunoqrot et al. (2014) developed a multi-scale hybrid nanoparticles platform by encapsulating the smaller FA modified PAMAM dendrimers (~5 nm in diameter) into larger poly(ethylene glycol)-b-poly(*D,L*-lactide) (PEG-PLA) NPs (~70 nm) to prolong blood circulation and enhance tumor penetration simultaneously. The PEG-PLA NPs allowed the passive accumulation around the tumor site through the EPR effect for which can reduce the premature renal elimination and enhance the blood circulation time. When the hybrid NPs accumulated at the tumor site, the gradually released dendrimers would target to individual cancer cells, with more efficient tumor distribution and penetration. Therefore, the multi-scale hybrid nanoparticles platform is a promising nanocarrier with long circulation capability and strong penetration capability for tumor-targeted drug delivery.

THE DENDRIMERS WITH IMAGING CAPACITY FOR DRUG DELIVERY

The development of novel nanoplatforms for diagnosis and/or treatment of different diseases, especially the early-stage diseases has been received a great deal of attention in recent years in order to identify the diseases as early as possible and enhance the percent of cure rate. Dendrimers with well-defined 3D spherical shape, large number of surface functional groups and hydrophobic cavities are the perfect carriers for diagnosis and/or treatment of diseases. By decorating the imaging agents at the periphery or in the interiors of the dendrimers, the dendrimers based nanoplatform allow the application of various modern imaging technologies, such as fluorescence imaging (FI) (Talanov et al., 2006), magnetic resonance (MR) imaging (Andolina, Klemm, Floyd III, Fréchet, & Raymond, 2012), computed tomography (CT) (Cao et al., 2015), single-photon emission tomography (SPECT) (Y. Zhang, Sun, Xu, Zhang, et al., 2010), positron emission tomography (PET) (Almutairi et al., 2009) for diagnosis and recognition of disease especially tumors (Chen et al., 2013; Qiao & Shi, 2014). In order to enhance the diagnosis accuracy, dual mode imaging technology has also been equipped in dendrimers based nanoplatforms. Moreover, the theranostic nanoplatforms based on dendrimers are also applied for diagnosis and treatment of tumor simultaneously (Barreto et al., 2011).

Xu et al. (2013) reported a functionalized fluorescent dendrimer with the fluorescent perylene-3,4,9,10-tetracarboxydiimide chromophore (PDI) as core and cationic dendritic polyesters as the outer part for drug delivery. The central PDI chromophore allowed tracing the distribution of the dendrimers. The outer degradable dendritic polyester units provided the hydrophobic cavities for encapsulating the hydrophobic drug and the peripheral primary amines for enhancing the cellular uptake and water solubility of the dendrimers. The dendrimer-based nanocarriers could enhance the water solubility of a hydrophobic pesticide, thiamethoxam, and significantly increase the cytotoxicity of the drug, which were distributed in all tested tissues of Heliothis armigera by detection the fluorescence of PDI (X. Liu et al., 2015). X. Xu et al. (2014) synthesized the bio-inspired supramolecular hybrid dendrimers (SHDs) for gene delivery and biological tracking. The quantum dots (QDs) were used as model templates as the core of the dendrimers for their fluorescent properties. The low generation peptide dendrons with arginine-rich peptide as the surface groups could self-assemble onto surface of QDs via coordination interactions to form multifunctional SHDs, which had well-defined, hierarchical, and stable nanostructure. The multifunctional SHDs could monitor the intracellular traffic, protein expression and imaging *in vivo* to further investigate the gene delivery pathways. In addition, high transfection efficiency, low cytotoxicity and serum resistance were achieved by SHDs both *in vitro* and *in vivo*.

Although gold nanoparticles (AuNPs) have received increasing attention to be used for X-ray CT imaging for its higher X-ray absorption coefficient, non-cytotoxicity and feasible functionalization (Sun et al., 2009), the stability and circulation time of AuNPs *in vivo* are unsatisfied. Qiao and Shi (2014) developed a series of modified dendrimers entrapped AuNPs nanosystems for xenograft tumor model or blood pool CT imaging. Amine terminated G5 PAMAM dendrimers were used originally, followed by acetylation of the residual dendrimer surface amines to neutralize the excess positive charge and improve biocompatibility (H. Wang et al., 2011). Moreover, PEG and active target agents such as lactobionic acid and folic acid (FA) modified dendrimers were also synthesized to facilitate the nanosystems with good stability, significantly enhanced biocompatibility and tumor-targeting capability for CT imaging (Cao et al., 2015; Peng et al., 2013; Peng et al., 2012). The dendrimers can also be applied for T_1 MR imaging by conjugation the small molecular Gd(III)-chelates or T_2 MR imaging by assembly onto iron oxide NPs. Huang et al. (2012) synthesized the G3 biodegradable polydisulfide dendrimer nanoclusters for T_1 MR imaging. The G3 PAMAM dendrimers were connected by the redox-sensitive disulphide bonds firstly to properly prolong the circulation time for high-quality MR images (Figure 4). Additionally, the nanoclusters can also be reduced to small degradation products during circulation and undergo efficient renal excretion to reduce possibility of toxic side effects caused by the accumulation and transmetalation of chelated Gd. Subsequently, the Gd chelates were conjugated on the surface of dendrimers which can be further labeled with Gd for T_1 MR imaging. The nanoclusters showed a circulation half-life of >1.6 h in mice and produced a statistically significant enhancement in the abdominal aorta and kidneys for as long as 4 h. Through the method of layer-by-layer (LbL) self-assembly, Shi et al. (2008) constructed the shell-crosslinked Fe_3O_4 nanoparticles for *in vivo* T_2 MR imaging of tumors. FA functionalized G5 acetylated dendrimers were assembled onto Fe_3O_4 NPs through electrostatic interaction to facilitate the nanoparticles with active targeting capability and stability *in vivo*. From the results of MR imaging, the nanoparticles could specifically target the FA receptors expressing tumor model with good water-solubility, stability, and biocompatibility.

The dendrimers based nanosystems can also achieve dual mode imaging by encapsulating the different imaging agents in the cavities or connecting on the core or periphery of the dendrimers to collect more necessary and reliable information (Jennings & Long, 2009; Talanov et al., 2006). Chen et al. (2013) and S. Wen et al. (2013) developed a G5 dendrimer-based dual mode imaging nanoplatform by entrapping AuNPs within the interiors of dendrimers and loading Gd(III) ions via the conjugation of Gd chelates on the periphery of dendrimers for dual mode CT/T_1 MR imaging of animal organs. The targeting ligands, such as folic acid (FA), were linked onto the periphery of dendrimer with PEG as the spacer (Chen et al., 2015). The remaining terminal amines were acetylated to enhance the biocompatibility of the nanoplatform. The formed dendrimer-based dual mode imaging nanoplatform was water dispersible, colloidally stable and noncytotoxic in the given concentration range. Moreover, the nanoplatform enabled targeted dual modality CT/T_1 MR imaging of the xenograft tumor model which is overexpressing the specific binding receptor *in vivo*. In another study, Talanov et al. (2006) reported a G6 PAMAM dendrimer-based nanoprobe for dual modality T_1 MR and fluorescence imaging. The 1B4M-DTPA, a Gd(III) chelate moiety for MR imaging, and Cy5.5, a NIR fluorescent dye for FI, were conjugated to the surface of the dendrimers via thio urea and amide linkage, respectively. The nanoprobe could be used for efficient visualization of sentinel lymph nodes in mice by dual modality MR and fluorescence imaging.

By incorporating the diagnostic and therapeutic agents into dendrimers simultaneously, theranostic nanoplatforms are achieved, which can concurrently diagnose the diseases and provide the real-time feedback on the pharmacokinetics of the systems (Cheng et al., 2011). Taratula et al. (2015) developed a theranostic nanoplatform by encapsulation the hydrophobic silicon naphthalocyanine (SiNc) into the hydrophobic pockets of the G5 PPI dendrimer following surface PEGlyation for diagnostic and treatment of ovarian cancer. The SiNc-loaded nanoplatform preserved near-infrared (NIR) fluorescence imaging and dual photothermal (PTT) and photodynamic (PDT) properties. Under NIR irradiation (785 nm, 1.3 W/cm^2), strong NIR fluorescence signal was observed in the tumor area and the solid tumors were completely eradicated without tumor recurrence.

Figure 4. (A) Schematic illustrating the synthetic process of gadolinium (Gd)-labeled polydisulfide dendrimer nanoclusters (DNCs). (B) T_1 MR images of nu/nu nude mice at various time points after the tail vein injection of polydisulfide DNCs with gadolinium (Gd)-labeled PAMAM (G3) as control. T_1-weighted images of the kidney were acquired pre-injection and 15 min, 1 h, 2 h, and 4 h post-injection by a 4.7 T small animal horizontal bore Varian INOVA system.

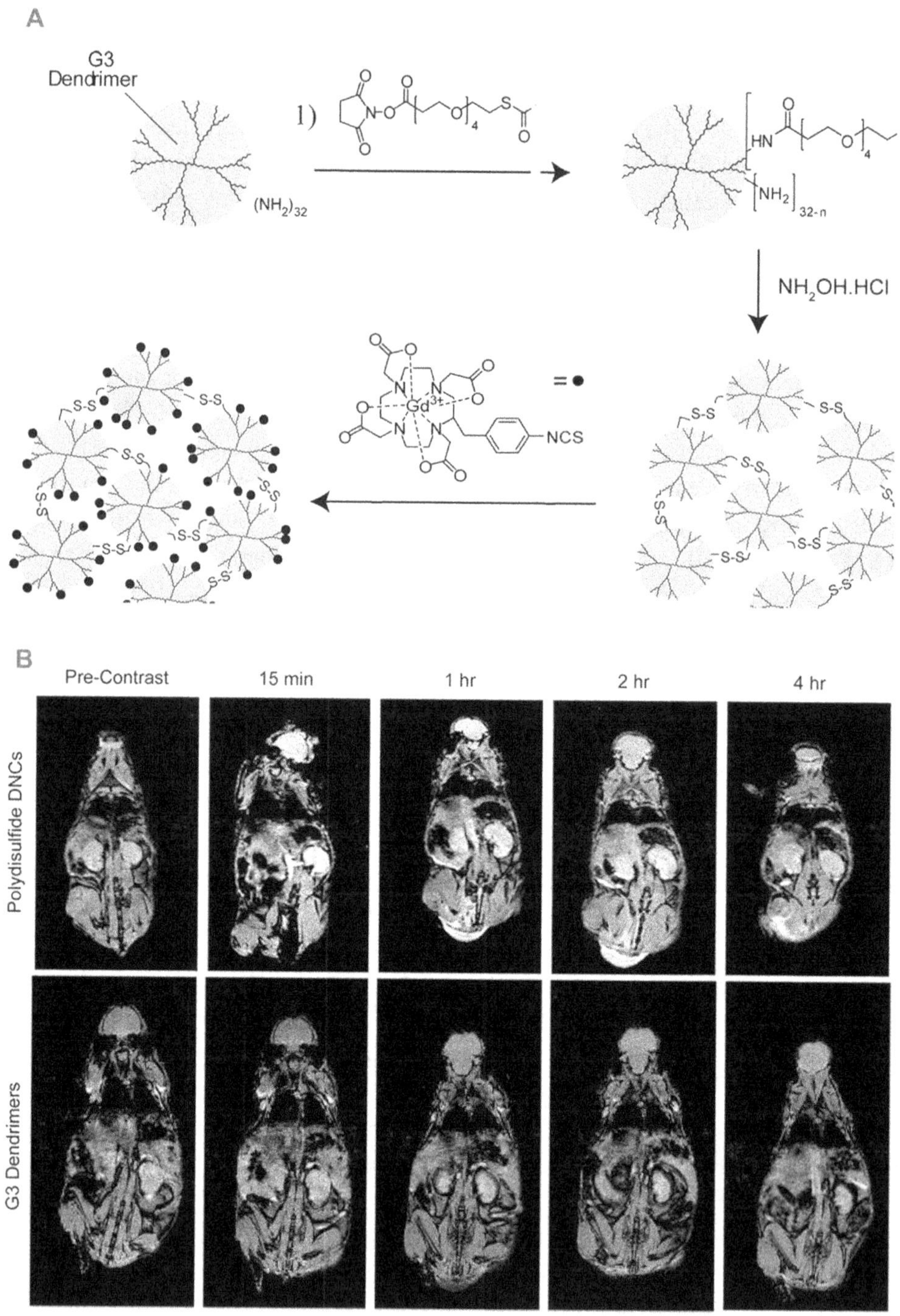

STIMULI-SENSITIVE DENDRIMERS FOR CONTROLLABLE DRUG DELIVERY

Dendrimers with well-defined 3D spherical shape, hydrophobic cavities and large number of functional groups can physically encapsulate or covalently attach the drugs on the surface of dendrimers. However, it is difficult to avoid the premature release of drugs and control the release rate of drugs. The design of stimuli-sensitive dendrimers to facilitate the controllable drug release has received much attention in recent years. The stimuli can be internal in the tumor tissue such as changes in pH, enzyme, redox and temperature, or external such as light.

pH-Sensitive

Owing to the relative more acidic of the tumor extracellular environment (pH 6.5) and endosome or lysosome (pH 5.0-5.5) than the blood or normal tissues (pH 7.4), various pH-sensitive nanocarriers have been developed to control the drug release from nanocarriers at the tumor site (Du, Du, Mao, & Wang, 2011; Mura, Nicolas, & Couvreur, 2013). The pH-sensitive nanocarriers can be obtained by introducing the cleavage covalent bonds, for example hydrozone bond or the zwitterionic polymer such as chitosan and poly(2-(*N*,*N*-diethylamino)ethyl methacrylate) (PDMAEMA) (Jin et al., 2011; Koren, Apte, Jani, & V. P. Torchilin, 2012). Because of the large number peripheral functional groups of the dendrimers, they can be functionalized with drugs, targeting agents, pH-sensitive bonds or hydrophilic groups (Mullen et al., 2011). Additionally, the interiors of dendrimers can physically encapsulate the drugs (He et al., 2015). Therefore, dendrimers are good candidates to serve as the pH-sensitive nanocarriers.

One of the earliest pH-sensitive dendrimers was reported by Kono et al. (1999). They synthesized a G2 polyether dendrimer where the methotrexate was conjugated on the surface of dendrimer via an acid cleavable hydrazide bond for pH-triggered anticancer drug release. Subsequently, Cameron C. Lee et al. (2006) synthesized a novel bow-tie polyester dendrimer by the conjugation of G3 dendron coupled of solubilizing PEG chains and G4 dendron functionalized with drugs via hydrazone bond. The architecture, molecular weight, and drug loading of bow-tie dendrimer could be readily controlled. In addition, the bow-tie dendrimer showed a long circulation time with the half-life of 16±1 h in BALB/c mice bearing C-26 colon carcinomas, while the half-life of the free DOX was less than 10 min. Also, the tumor accumulation of bow-tie dendrimer was ninefold higher than free DOX after 48 h. Interestingly, the bow-tie dendrimer could complete regression the growth of tumor at the highest dose administered with 100% survival of the mice. But no cures were achieved for the free DOX at its maximum tolerated dose (6 mg/kg) or dendrimer-DOX conjugated via a stable carbamate bond.

With the aim of increasing the accumulation of drugs in tumor, Kaminskas et al. (2011) synthesized a pH-sensitive PEGylated polylysine dendrimer for drug delivery. G5 polylysine dendrimer was used where the DOX was conjugated on the surface of dendrimers through an acid labile 4-(hydrazinosulfonyl) benzoic acid (HSBA). When the dendrimers were incubated in pH 7.4 buffer over 3 days, the release of DOX was less than 10%. In contrast, the release of DOX was approximately 100% at pH 5.0. In addition, the distribution of DOX-conjugated, PEGylated polylysine dendrimers in rats bearing Walker 256 tumors revealed higher accumulation in tumor tissue compared with control tissue such as heart (about 3 fold) and muscle (about 8 fold). In another study, Yuan et al. (2010) developed a novel poly(*L*-glutamic acid) dendrimer with both pH-sensitive and active targeting functions for controllable drug delivery (Figure 5). The polyhedral oligomeric silsesquioxane (POSS) was used as the core of the poly(*L*-glutamic acid) dendrimers. The antitumor drug DOX and the active targeting agent (biotin) were conjugated on the

Figure 5. The synthesis of both pH-sensitive and active targeted poly(L-glutamic acid) dendrimers Copyright 2010. Reproduced with permission from the American Chemical Society.

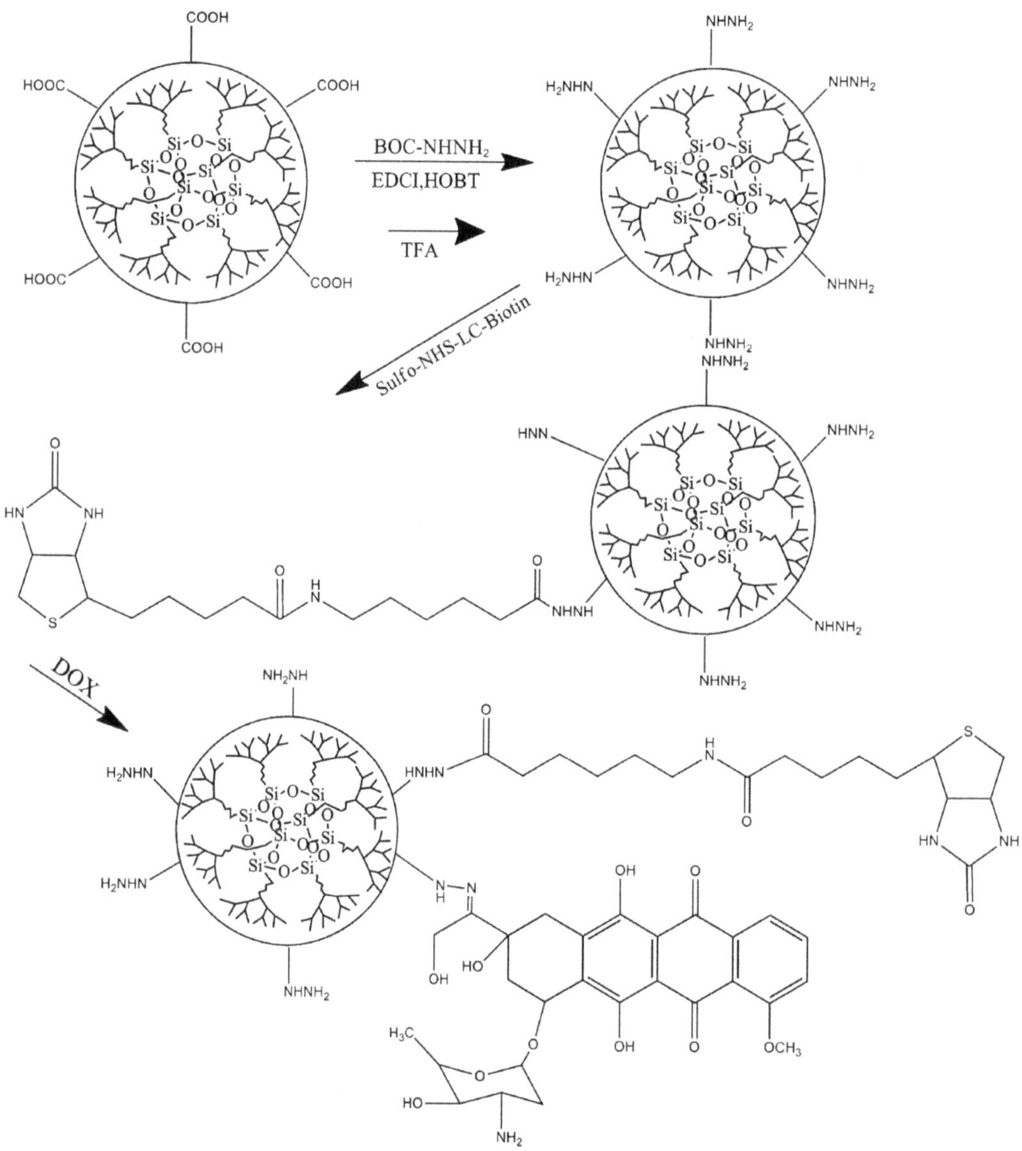

surface of dendrimers via the pH-sensitive hydrazine bonds and amide bonds, respectively. The biotin can specifically target the biotin receptors which are always overexpressed on the surface of tumor cells. The novel dendrimers showed pH-sensitive drug release and much higher cellular uptake through the receptor-mediated endocytosis.

The incorporation of zwitterionic polymer can also facilitate the dendrimer based nanocarriers with pH-sensitive capability. K. C. Liu and Yeo (2013) reported a pH-sensitive drug carrier by coating the zwitterionic chitosan on the surface of amine-terminated PAMAM dendrimer. The chitosan was modified by the succinic anhydride to make it show positive charges at low pH and negative charges at relatively high pH. On one hand, the zwitterionic chitosan could shield the positive charges of dendrimer at pH 7.4

to reduce its cytotoxicity and nonspecific interaction with proteins. On the other hand, positive charges of dendrimer would be exposed because of the charge reverse of chitosan to recover the tumor penetration capability of PAMAM dendrimers. Also, the transition pH of chitosan can be adjusted by changing the ratio of anhydride to amine. In another study, Jin et al. (2011) synthesized a core-shell nanosystem with the G4 PAMAM dendrimer as core and PDMAEMA and PEG chains as shell. The core can physical encapsulate the drugs such as 5-fluorouracil (5-FU). The amphiphilic PDMAEMA can control the release of drugs as they were hydrophobic at pH 7.4 and hydrophilic at pH 6.5. PEG chains could prolong the circulation time of nanosystem in blood vessels. The nanosystem showed high encapsulation efficiency of drugs, high tumor-targeting and controllable release of drugs in low-pH tumor tissues.

Interestingly, Zhou et al. (2012) reported a pH-responsive size-tunable DNA dendrimer with first generation (G1) to fourth generation (G4) by the self-assembly of DNA monomers. Each DNA monomer contained 13-base sticky ends to facilitate the dendrimer with extra stability and easy functionalization. The cytosine-rich strand was incorporated into the dendrimer between the core and first layer to achieve the pH-responsive DNA dendrimer, which would change from the extended duplexunder neutral or basic conditions to the constrained four stranded i-motif structure under slightly acidic conditions because of the non-Watson-Crick base pairing between cytosine residues. The DNA dendrimers showed good biocompatibility and the high generation dendrimers could be facilely obtained in high yield because of the precise recognition of DNA sequences. With the increasing of generation, the size of dendrimer increased from 13.2 to 28.6 nm with narrow size distribution in pH 8.0 buffer. When the dendrimers were incubated in pH 5.0 buffer, the size of different generation dendrimers showed similar decrease around 3 nm. In addition, the shrink of G1 dendrimer was almost 30% upon pH stimulus. Therefore, the pH-responsive DNA dendrimer is a promising candidate to construct functional and smart nanocarriers for drug delivery.

Enzyme-Sensitive

Enzymes play a vital role in cell regulation, which possess outstanding catalytic properties and exceptional biorecognition capabilities. Therefore, the design of enzyme-sensitive nanocarriers is an effective way to specifically target and kill diseased tissue and significantly reduce the side-effects on normal organs (De La Rica, Aili, & Stevens, 2012). Dendrimers with well-defined 3D architecture and large number of functional terminated-groups are promising candidate to construct the enzyme-sensitive nanocarriers for drug delivery. A multifunctional G1 dendrimer was reported by Fuchs et al. (2005) with cathepsin B cleavage site and dansyl for controllable release the drugs and fluorescence imaging, respectively. Cathepsin B as a lysosomal cysteine protease is only found in the intracellular compartment. Thus, the drugs would be released only after the internalization of the dendrimers in the cell by endocytosis, which would avoid the premature release of drugs. The H-Gly-Arg-Phe-Gly-OH sequence equipped with the ligands for Pt^{2+}complexation was chosen as an appropriate substrate of Cathepsin B. The process of internalization of the multifunctional dendrimers in the cell could be visualized by confocal fluorescence microscopy.

Recently, Gu and coworkers also reported several cathepsin B responsive dendrimers based nanoparticles for drug delivery (N. Li et al., 2014; C. Zhang, Pan, Luo, She, et al., 2014). The drug DOX was conjugated on the surface of dendrimer via a cathepsin B sensitive tetra-peptide linker Gly-Phe-Leu-Gly (GFLG) to facilitate the nanoparticles with controllable release profile. The mPEG was conjugated to the periphery of dendrimer via click reaction to prolong the circulation time and reduce the side-effects.

After the conjugation of DOX and mPEG, the dendrimers could assemble into nanoparticles around 100 nm, which would significantly reduce the renal elimination to further improve the accumulation of drugs in tumor by EPR effect. In addition, the incorporation of cathepsin B-sensitive cleavage site can also avoid the premature release of DOX and the DOX would be released only after the internalization of nanoparticles in the tumor cells. Therefore, the dendrimer based nanoparticles showed the high antitumor activity.

Enzyme-responsive micelles based on the amphiphilic dendrimers are also good candidate for controllable drug delivery owing to large voids for drug encapsulation. Generally, the enzyme specific cleavable sequence was located in the hydrophobic side. Once the micelles were encountered with the corresponding enzyme, the hydrophilic–lipophilic balance (HLB) would be changed, leading to the destabilization of the micelles and release of guest molecules. Harnoy et al., (2014) reported an enzyme-responsive micelle with phenyl acetamide as the enzyme penicilin G amidase (PGA)-cleavable hydrophobic end groups and PEG as the hydrophilic part (Figure 6). The amphiphilic PEG-dendron hybrids could self-assemble into micellar nanocarriers that showed the controllable release of encapsulated guest molecules upon enzymatic activation. Comparison of hydrolysis and disassembly rates for the micelles composed by different lengths of the PEG block, they found that the micelle with longer PEG block disassembled faster. Thus, the enzymatic degradation of phenyl acetamide occured at the "monomeric" form of the amphiphilic hybrids, leading to the change in amphiphilicity of micelles and release the guest molecules.

Redox-Sensitive

Disulphide bonds are redox-sensitive which are prone to cleavage by glutathione (GSH). In addition, the degradation rate of nanoparticles stabilized by disulfide groups is different when the concentration

Figure 6. Schematic representation of the enzyme-sensitive nanocarrier for controllable hydrophobic guest delivery and releases the guest molecules when the hydrophobic end groups were cleaved by enzyme
Copyright 2014. Reproduced with permission from the American Chemical Society.

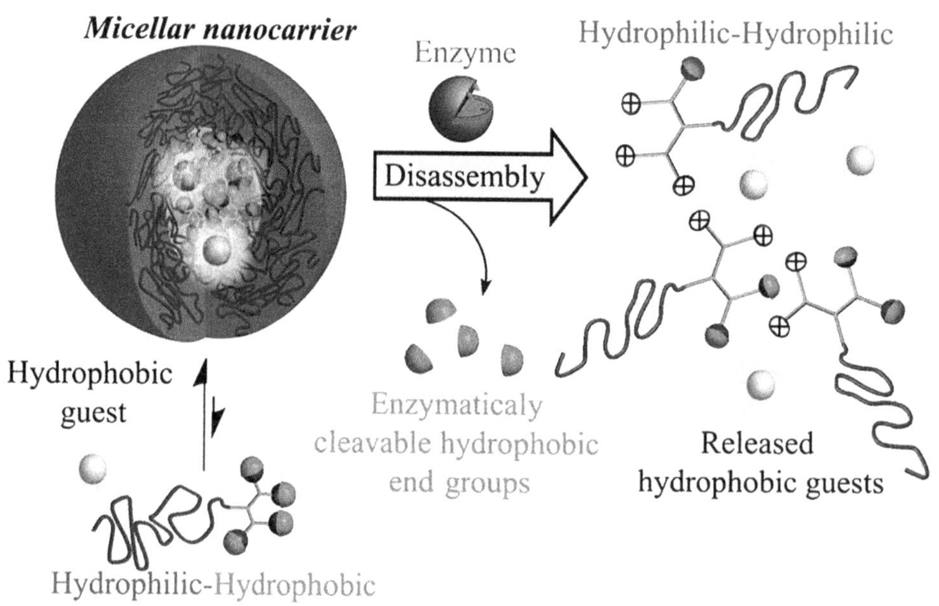

and the amount of available GSH are different (Y. Wen, Zhang, & Li, 2014). It is known that the intracellular concentration of GSH (5-10 mM) is much higher than the extracellular concentration (2-10 μM) (Such, Yan, Johnston, Gunawan, & Caruso, 2015). Moreover, the dendrimer has large number of functional groups which is easy to be functionalized with redox-sensitive groups. The interiors of them can also provide the accommodation for drugs. Therefore, the redox-sensitive dendrimers are promising nanocarriers for controllable drug delivery.

The general method to construct the redox-sensitive dendrimers is to conjugate the redox-sensitive groups with dendrimers. Kurtoglu et al. (2009) reported a dendrimer-drug conjugates via the disulfide linkages for drug delivery. G4 PAMAM dendrimer was chosen as the platform and N-Acetyl cysteine (NAC), an anti-inflammatory agent, was chosen as the model drugs. The PAMAM-S-S-NAC nanosystem showed good stability in the presence of BSA solution, revealing it could protect the conjugated drugs from premature release in blood circulation. However, the percent of drugs released from PAMAM-S-S-NAC nanosystem was about 60% within 1 h at intracellular GSH concentrations, indicating the redox-sensitive of the nanosystem. More importantly, the PAMAM-S-S-NAC nanosystem exhibited an order of magnitude improvement in antioxidant activity of NAC. In order to improve the circulation time and reduce the toxicity of dendrimers, Hu et al. (2014) synthesized a PEGlyated PAMAM dendrimer via the conjugation of cleavable disulfide bonds. The DOX was physically encapsulated in the interiors of dendrimers with the drug loading content of 10%. Interestingly, the dendrimer showed redox and pH dual-responsive DOX release profile. Moreover, the sensitive dendrimer exhibited more significant cytotoxicity to kill B16 and A549 tumor cells compared with its noncleavable counterparts.

In another study, X. Wang et al. (2013) developed a new strategy to synthesize the GSH-triggered drug delivery system based on dendrimer (Figure 7). They chose the biocompatible hydroxyl-terminated

Figure 7. Synthesis route of dendrimer-encapsulated gold nanoparticles and their potential applications as scaffolds for the GSH-responsive drug delivery systems

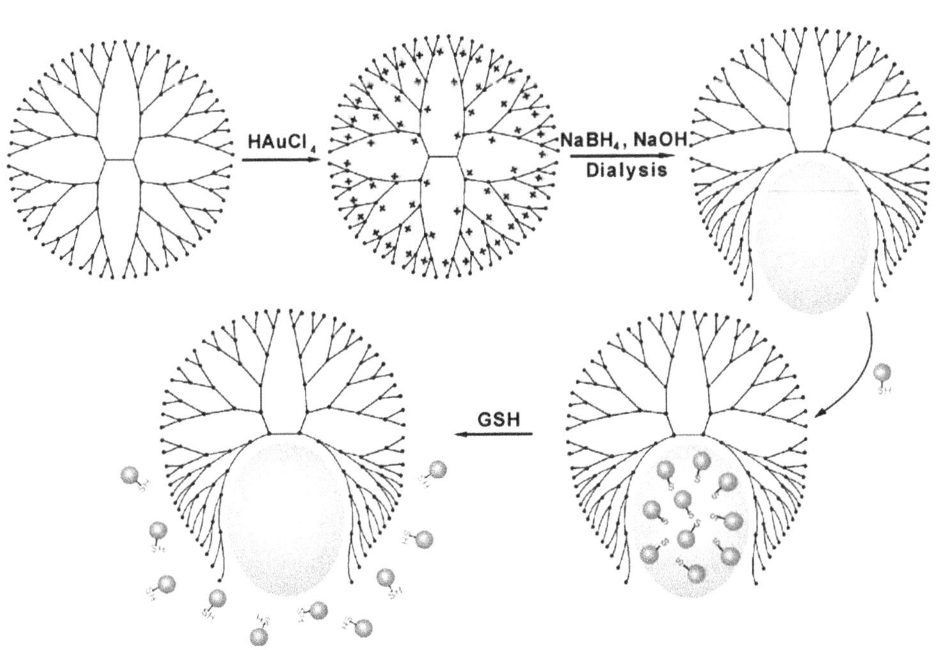

PAMAM dendrimers as templates in which the gold nanoparticles were synthesized in the interiors of dendrimers. Then, the anticancer drugs, such as thiolated DOX and cisplatin (CPT), were conjugated on the surface of AuNPs via the Au-S bond. Although the cytotoxicity of thiolated DOX and CPT loaded within the nanoparticle were much reduced compared with the free anticancer compounds, the cytotoxicity of nanosystem could be enhanced by improving the intracellular GSH. In addition, the nanosystem showed excellent biocompatibility on several cell lines. Therefore, the novel nanosystem can be developed as a stimuli-responsive nanocarrier for anticancer drug delivery.

Thermo-Sensitive

It is known that the dendrimers can physically encapsulate the hydrophobic drugs because of the internal cavities of them. With increasing the generation number of dendrimers, the volume of internal cavities become larger and the drug loading capability is enhanced simultaneously (Morgan et al., 2003). Moreover, by adjusting the net surface charge, internal composition and type and degree of functionalization of surface groups of dendrimers, the drug loading capability can be further enhanced (Bhadra, Bhadra, Jain, & Jain, 2003; Dhanikula, Argaw, Bouchard, & Hildgen, 2008). However, the control of guest drugs release is hard to achieve. Coating the dendrimers with thermo-sensitive polymers, such as PEG and Poly(*N*-isopropylacrylamide) (PNIPAAm) et al, seems an effective way to facilitate the dendrimers with controllable release profile (Z. Wang, Zhou, Liu, & Fan, 2010). When the solution temperature is beyond the lower critical solution temperature (LCST) of polymers, the solubility of polymers will decrease significantly. Thus, the polymers will cover on the surface of dendrimers and the drug will not be released. Once the temperature is lower than the LCST of polymers, the polymers will be hydrophilic and the drug will be released. Therefore, thermo-sensitive polymers functionalized dendrimers are good candidate for controllable drug release.

One of the earliest thermo-sensitive dendrimers was reported by Kimura et al. (2000), which was synthesized by the conjugation the PNIPAAm with the G3 PPI dendrimer. PNIPAAm is one of the most extensively studied thermo-sensitive polymers, exhibiting a LCST at around 33 °C in aqueous solution (H. Wei, Cheng, Zhang, & Zhuo, 2009). The thermo-sensitive PPI dendrimer functionalized with PNIPAAm segments showed the same LCST as PNIPAAm arms. Considering the toxicity issue and short blood circulation time encountered in traditional thermo-sensitive dendrimers, Zhao et al. (2011) developed a PEGlyated thermo-sensitive PAMAM dendrimer for drug delivery. After the PEGlyation of PNIPAAm functionalized PAMAM dendrimers (PAMAM-g-PNIPAAm), the LCST of them was enhanced from 32 °C to 35 °C. In addition, the PEGlyated PAMAM-g-PNIPAAm showed prolonged drug release at the temperature above the LCST of them. With the aim to preserve the molecular uniformity of dendrimers, Kono and coworkers developed a series of thermo-sensitive PAMAM dendrimers by the conjugation of thermo-sensitive groups, such as isobutyramide (IBAM), *n*-butyramide (NBAM), cyclopropane carboxylic acid amide (CPCAM) and Phenylalanine (Phe) with the dendrimers (Haba, Harada, Takagishi, & Kono, 2004; Haba, Kojima, Harada, & Kono, 2006; Tono et al., 2006). The PAMAM dendrimers functionalized with different thermo-sensitive groups showed different LCSTs. In addition, the interiors of thermo-sensitive dendrimers could encapsulate the guest molecules. Thus, the alkylamide-terminated PAMAM dendrimers are good candidate for controllable drug delivery.

A series of PEGlyated thermo-sensitive dendrimers up to the G4 were synthesized by Wu et al. (2014) through CuAAC and amidation reactions (Figure 8). Depending on the generation number of dendrimers, the LCSTs were different. The high generation number of dendrimer showed lower LCST

Figure 8. Synthetic route of the PEGlyated dendrimers. The abbreviation of TEA = triethylamine; DCM = dichloromethane; TFA = trifluoroacetic acid and THF = tetrahydrofuran

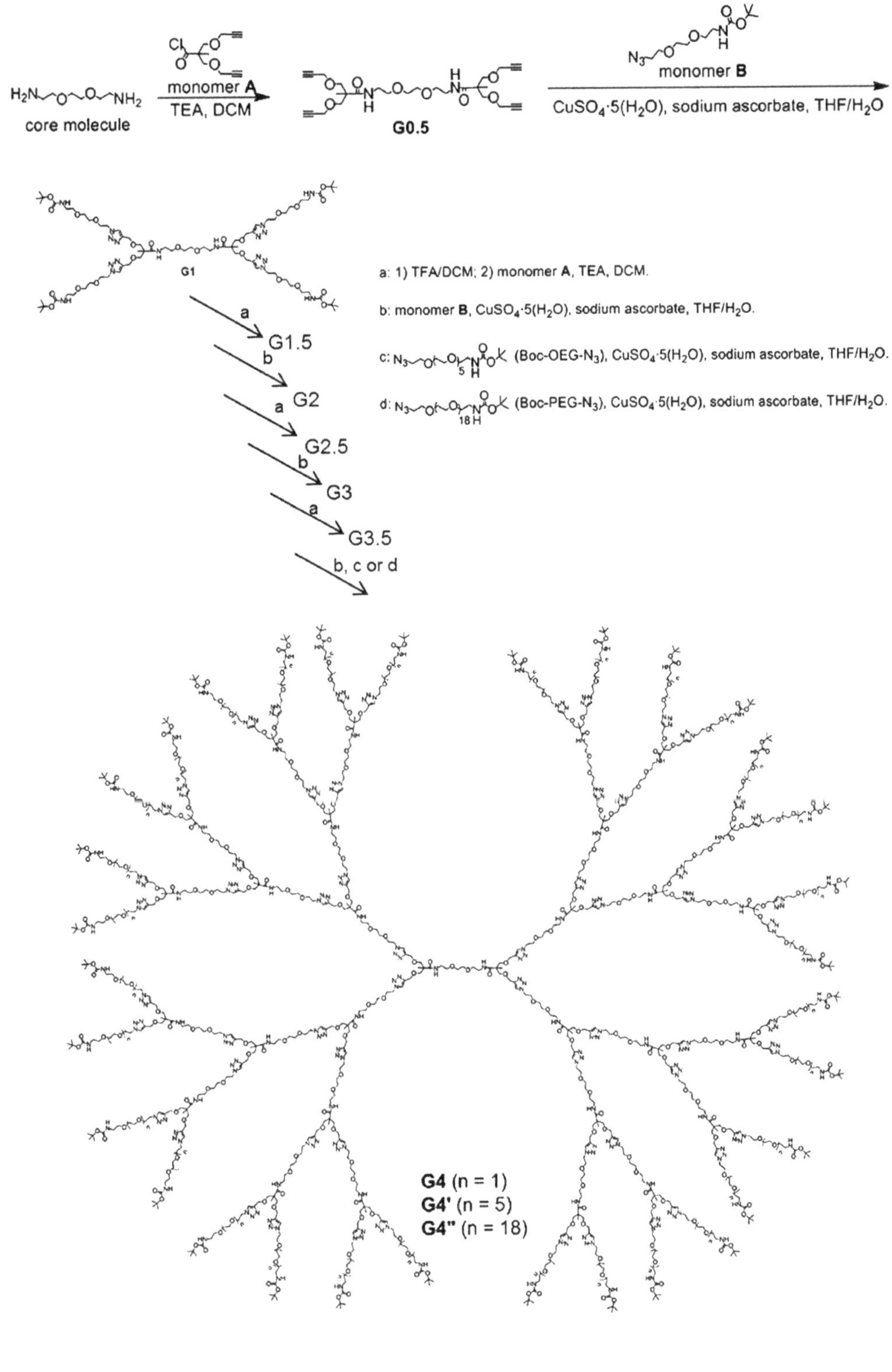

because of its relatively high hydrophobicity. They also investigated the influence of the length of PEG on the tumor accumulation and penetration of G4 dendrimer conjugated with gemcitabine (GEM) with GEM-conjugated G4 PAMAM as control. After the conjugation of GEM with G4 dendrimers, they also showed thermo-sensitivity. Moreover, they also found that the longest peripheral PEG segments showed significantly higher tumor accumulation and penetration compared to the GEM-conjugated PAMAM or GEM-conjugated PAMAM with short PEG segments by the combination of micro positron emission tomography (micro-PET) and multispectral optoacoustic tomography (MSOT) imaging techniques. Thus, the longest PEG functionalized dendrimers exhibited the best antitumor activity.

Light-Sensitive

Owing to their noninvasive and the potential of being site specific, various light-responsive nanocarriers have been developed for controllable drug release. Dendrimers have hydrophobic cavities and numerous functional groups on the surface, which are easy to be functionalized with light-responsive groups. Thus, the photosensitive dendrimers are good candidate for controllable drug delivery. However, the development of photosensitive dendrimers for drug delivery is blocked because of the low penetration depth (~10 mm) of ultraviolet–visible region. Therefore, the present works are mainly involved *in vitro*. A new series of fully photodegradable polyester dendrimers were synthesized by Nazemi et al. (2013). All the backbones of the dendrimers were fully photodegradable by the incorporation of photodegradable o-nitrobenzyl esters. Therefore, the polyester dendrimers could instantaneously release all the encapsulated drugs to kill the tumors once they were irradiated with UV light. In another work, Kostiainen et al. (2007) developed a photo-responsive dendron which could condense DNA in multivalent binding and release the DNA by UV irradiation. The photosensitive o-nitrobenzyl groups were used as the linkers between the dendron and spermine groups which showed multivalent DNA binding. Once the dendrons were irradiated by long-wavelength UV light (λ=350 nm), the leave behind of dendron was negative which will repel the DNA, leading to the release of DNA.

THE NOVEL MICELLE - OR LIPOSOME - LIKE NANOCARRIERS

Micelles and liposomes as two typically nanocarriers have been widely used for drug delivery (Deng, Jiang, Cheng, Meng, & Zhong, 2012; Rösler, Vandermeulen, & Klok, 2012). Micelles are formed by the self-assembly of amphiphilic copolymers beyond the critical micelle concentration (CMC) in aqueous solution (Nicolas, Mura, Brambilla, Mackiewicz, & Couvreur, 2013). The hydrophobic polymers form the core of micelles which can serve as a reservoir for hydrophobic drugs. The hydrophilic polymers form the shell of micelles which can stabilize the micelles. Besides, the size distribution of micelle is fairly narrow with the average diameters of 10-100 nm. Also, the micelles always have long circulation time and passive targeting (EPR) capacity to the tumor. Liposomes are also formed by the self-assembly of amphiphilic copolymers with bilayer phospholipid systems (Allen & Cullis, 2013). Unlike the micelles, liposomes have both the hydrophilic cavities to encapsulate the hydrophilic drugs and hydrophobic part between the lipid bilayers to encapsulate the hydrophobic drugs. Besides, the liposomes showed good biocompatibility, biodegradability and long circulation time (Al-Jamal & Kostarelos, 2011). However, the amphiphilic copolymers of micelles or liposomes are always polydisperse and the structures of them are difficult to precise control. Dendrimers are a class of artificial polymers with homogeneous molecular weight and well-defined hyperbranched structure. Therefore, by combining the properties of dendrimers with micelles or liposomes, the novel nanocarriers may have controllable size, large cavities, long circulation time, good biocompatibility and even reproducible pharmacokinetics. It is no doubt that the novel nanocarriers will be easily modified by functional moieties such as active targeting, imaging and sensitive agents.

In order to enhance anticancer drug efficacy, reduce side-effector overcome the drug resistance of tumor, novel nanocarriers based on dendrimer have been developed by combining the properties of micelle with dendrimers. T. Wei et al. (2015) reported an innovative nanomicellar drug delivery system based on the amphiphilic dendrimer to combat tumor drug resistance both *in vitro* and *in vivo* (Figure 9). The amphiphilic dendrimer composed of a hydrophilic dendritic polymer component and a hydrophobic lipid entity could self-assemble into nanomicelle with large void space in their core. Importantly, the DOX-encapsulated nanomicelle could overcome drug resistance of breast tumor with small size (10 nm), narrow size distribution and high drug-loading capacity (>40%). Moreover, this drug delivery system can abolish significantly the systemic toxicity caused by the free drug.

With the same method to synthesize stimuli-sensitive dendrimers, the nanomicelles composed by amphiphilic dendrons or dendrimers can also be manipulated to show stimuli-sensitive degradation of the dendrimers or disassembly of the micelles to release the drugs. Thayumanavan and coworkers developed a series of biological, physical and chemical stimuli-sensitive micelles or inverse micelles by the supramolecular assembly of amphiphilic dendrons (Molla, Rangadurai, Pavan, & Thayumanavan, 2015; R. Ramireddy, Raghupathi, Torres, & Thayumanavan, 2012; Raghupathi, Guo, Munkhbat, Rangadurai, & Thayumanavan, 2014). Temperature sensitive systems were reported by them to control release the guest molecules. They synthesized three dendrons with different generations with temperature sensitive penta-(ethylene glycol) as the hydrophilic part and decyl groups as hydrophobic part (Aathimanikandan, Savariar, & Thayumanavan, 2005). The three dendrons showed different lower critical solution temperature (LCST) transitions. The higher generation of dendrons, the lower LCST was got. When the temperature was higher than LCST, the solubility of penta-(ethylene glycol) decreased and the guest molecules were released. Interestingly, they found that the G1dendrons had another temperature-sensitive transition named the sub-LCST transition below the LCST where the size of the micelle was decreased sharply and the dendritic host, guest rapidly exchanged (Fuller et al., 2013). With the purpose to construct light-sensitive micelles, the photolabile o-nitrobenzyl ester was introduced as the hydrophobic part of the dendrons (Yesilyurt, Ramireddy, & Thayumanavan, 2011). Thus, the hydrophilic-lipophilic balance (HLB) of the dendrons would be changed when they were exposed by light, resulting in light-triggered disassembly of micelles and release of the drugs. The protein sensitive micelles or inverse micelles were also reported by Azagarsamy et al. (2010) and Yesilyurt et al. (2012). The hydrophilic or hydrophobic of the dendrons was modified by the binding partner of the protein. Thus, when the micelles based on dendrons were exposed by the specific binding protein, the HLB of the dendrons would be significantly changed, due to the attaching of the rather large hydrophilic protein, resulting in protein-triggered release of the drugs. A dual protein-sensitive micelle was also designed by them (Figure 10) (Guo, Zhuang, Wang, Raghupathi, & Thayumanavan, 2014). The enzyme-sensitive coumarin ester was chosen as the hydrophobic moiety and the protein-specific 2,4-dinitrophenyl ligand was chosen as part of the hydrophilic PEG moiety of dendrons. The guest molecules would be released only when the micelles were encountered the two different proteins simultaneously. These multiple stimuli-responsive micelles can further enhance the targeted drug delivery capability of the nanocarriers.

Figure 9. Nanomicelles constructed with amphiphilic dendrimer (AmDM) for tumor therapy. (A) The construction of empty AmDM nanomicelles and DOX-loaded AmDM/DOX nanomicelles. (B) Molecular structure of the AmDM. NOD scid gamma (NSG) mice bearing drug resistant breast cancer MCF-7R tumors were treated with free DOX and AmDM/DOX nanomicelles at doxorubicin dose of 2.5 and 5.0 mg/kg via i.v. administration (twice per week, n = 7) with PBS, AmDM groups as control (n = 7). (C) Tumor volume and (D) mice body weight after injection. (E) Mice survival curves at different conditions. (F) Ki-67 IHC staining of tumor tissues to evaluate tumor proliferation. (G) Histological analysis of heart to assess the toxicity.

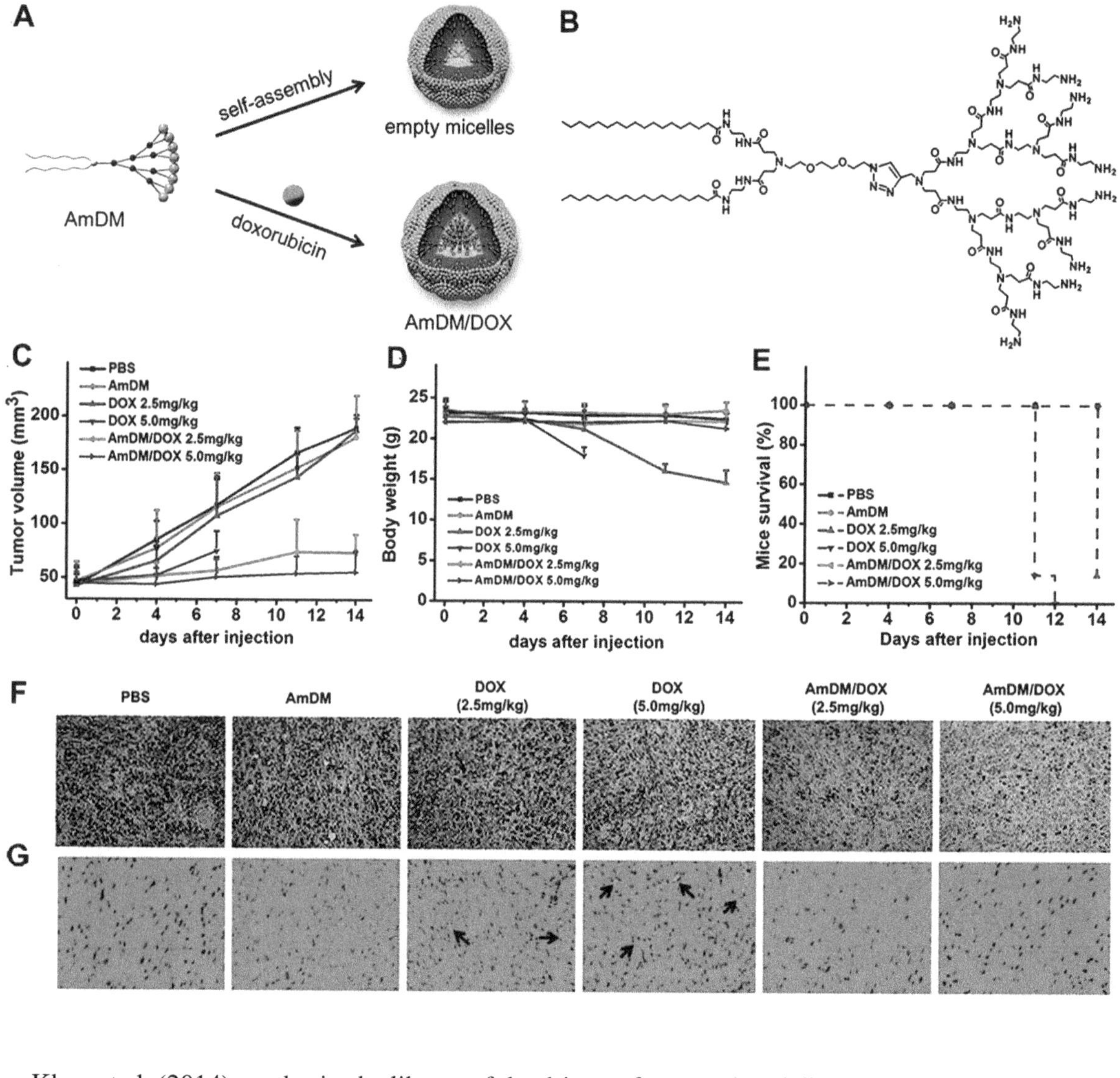

Khan et al. (2014) synthesized a library of dendrimers for targeting delivery small interfering RNA (siRNA) to liver endothelium *in vivo*. They chose the low generation PPI or PAMAM dendrimers modified with epoxide-terminated alkyl chains to formulate the dendrimer-lipid nanocarriers. Cholesterol and 1,2-dimyristoyl-sn-glycero-3-phosphoethanolamine-N-mPEG2000 were used to enhance the stability and efficiency of the nanocarriers. By changing the formulation of dendrimer-lipid nanocarriers, they

Figure 10. Schematic representation of light, protein and enzyme stimuli supramolecular disassembly
Copyright 2014. Reproduced with permission from the American Chemical Society.

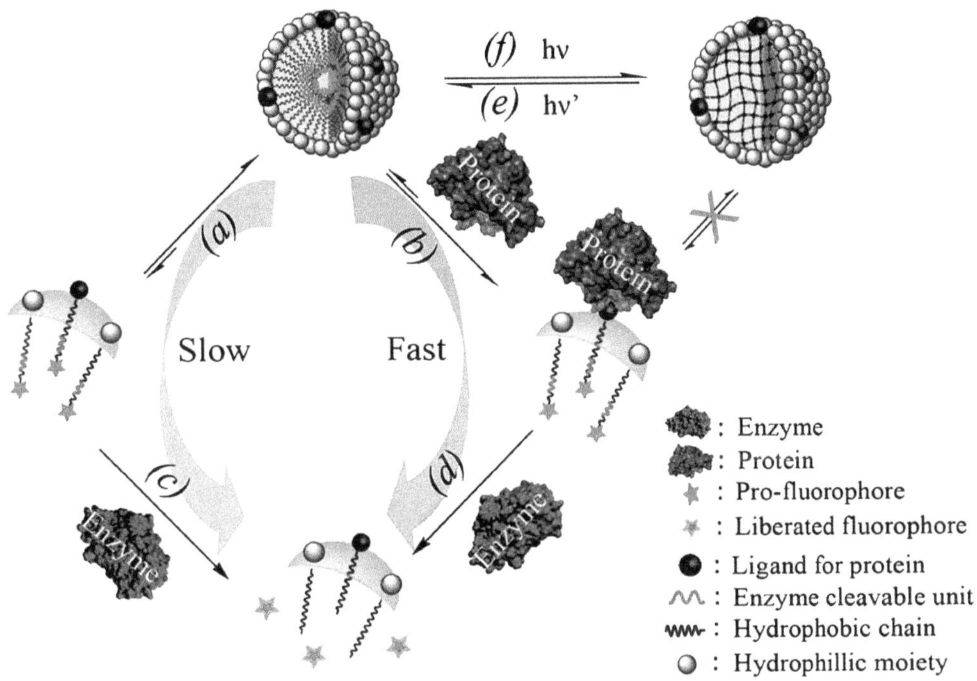

could specifically deliver the siRNA to endothelial cells, hepatocytes and tumor cells *in vivo*. They also found that the dendrimer-lipid nanocarriers can also specifically deliver siRNA to lung endothelial cells by adjusting the formulation (Khan et al., 2015). In addition, dendrimer-lipid nanocarriers did not cause chronic increases inflammation-related cytokines and animals did not suffer body weight reduction due to the toxicity even at high doses.

CONCLUSION AND PERSPECTIVES

The development of multifunctional dendrimers based nanocarriersis receiving much attention in recent years. Compared to conventional dendrimers, they showed improved biocompatibility, high tumor accumulation, real-time imaging, controllable drug release and prolonged circulation times. Thus, the development of multifunctional dendrimers based nanocarriers may accelerate the application of them in clinical trials or application. However, several problems should be taken into account, such as the complicated synthesis of dendrimers especially for high generation, the poor degradation, the fast renal excretion because of the relative small size and the bad balance between passive targeting and active targeting. Moreover, the percent and the location of functional groups should be exactly controlled, which determine the monodispersity and efficiency of the dendrimers as nanocarriers. Finally, the further understanding of the unique physicochemical and biological properties of the tumors will also contribute to the development and improvement of the multifunctional dendrimers based nanocarriers for tumor therapy.

REFERENCES

Aathimanikandan, S. V., Savariar, E. N., & Thayumanavan, S. (2005). Temperature-sensitive dendritic micelles. *Journal of the American Chemical Society*, *127*(42), 14922–14929. doi:10.1021/ja054542y PMID:16231948

Al-Jamal, W. T., & Kostarelos, K. (2011). Liposomes: From a clinically established drug delivery system to a nanoparticle platform for theranostic nanomedicine. *Accounts of Chemical Research*, *44*(10), 1094–1104. doi:10.1021/ar200105p PMID:21812415

Allen, T. M., & Cullis, P. R. (2013). Liposomal drug delivery systems: From concept to clinical applications. *Advanced Drug Delivery Reviews*, *65*(1), 36–48. doi:10.1016/j.addr.2012.09.037 PMID:23036225

Almutairi, A., Rossin, R., Shokeen, M., Hagooly, A., Ananth, A., Capoccia, B., & Fréchet, J. M. J. et al. (2009). Biodegradable dendritic positron-emitting nanoprobes for the noninvasive imaging of angiogenesis. *Proceedings of the National Academy of Sciences of the United States of America*, *106*(3), 685–690. doi:10.1073/pnas.0811757106 PMID:19129498

Andolina, C. M., Klemm, P. J., Floyd, W. C. III, Fréchet, J. M., & Raymond, K. N. (2012). Analysis of lanthanide complex dendrimer conjugates for bimodal NIR and MRI imaging. *Macromolecules*, *45*(22), 8982–8990. doi:10.1021/ma302206g PMID:23226878

Astruc, D., Boisselier, E., & Ornelas, C. (2010). Dendrimers Designed for Functions: From Physical, Photophysical, and Supramolecular Properties to Applications in Sensing, Catalysis, Molecular Electronics, Photonics, and Nanomedicine. *Chemical Reviews*, *110*(4), 1857–1959. doi:10.1021/cr900327d PMID:20356105

Azagarsamy, M. A., Yesilyurt, V., & Thayumanavan, S. (2010). Disassembly of dendritic micellar containers due to protein binding. *Journal of the American Chemical Society*, *132*(13), 4550–4551. doi:10.1021/ja100746d PMID:20232866

Barata, T. S., Shaunak, S., Teo, I., Zloh, M., & Brocchini, S. (2011). Structural studies of biologically active glycosylated polyamidoamine (PAMAM) dendrimers. *Journal of Molecular Modeling*, *17*(8), 2051–2060. doi:10.1007/s00894-010-0907-1 PMID:21161557

Barreto, J. A., O'Malley, W., Kubeil, M., Graham, B., Stephan, H., & Spiccia, L. (2011). Nanomaterials: Applications in cancer imaging and therapy. *Advanced Materials*, *23*(12), H18–H40. doi:10.1002/adma.201100140 PMID:21433100

Bhadra, D., Bhadra, S., Jain, S., & Jain, N. (2003). A PEGylated dendritic nanoparticulate carrier of fluorouracil. *International Journal of Pharmaceutics*, *257*(1), 111–124. doi:10.1016/S0378-5173(03)00132-7 PMID:12711167

Bosman, A. W., Janssen, H. M., & Meijer, E. W. (1999). About Dendrimers: Structure, Physical Properties, and Applications. *Chemical Reviews*, *99*(7), 1665–1688. doi:10.1021/cr970069y PMID:11849007

Caminade, A.-M., & Turrin, C.-O. (2014). Dendrimers for drug delivery. *Journal of Materials Chemistry B*, *2*(26), 4055–4066. doi:10.1039/c4tb00171k

Cao, Y., He, Y., Liu, H., Luo, Y., Shen, M., Xia, J., & Shi, X. (2015). Targeted CT imaging of human hepatocellular carcinoma using low-generation dendrimer-entrapped gold nanoparticles modified with lactobionic acid. *Journal of Materials Chemistry B*, *3*(2), 286–295. doi:10.1039/C4TB01542H

Chan, K. W., Yu, T., Qiao, Y., Liu, Q., Yang, M., Patel, H., & Bulte, J. W. et al. (2014). A diaCEST MRI approach for monitoring liposomal accumulation in tumors. *Journal of Controlled Release*, *180*, 51–59. doi:10.1016/j.jconrel.2014.02.005 PMID:24548481

Chen, Q., Li, K., Wen, S., Liu, H., Peng, C., Cai, H., & Shi, X. et al. (2013). Targeted CT/MR dual mode imaging of tumors using multifunctional dendrimer-entrapped gold nanoparticles. *Biomaterials*, *34*(21), 5200–5209. doi:10.1016/j.biomaterials.2013.03.009 PMID:23583039

Chen, Q., Wang, H., Liu, H., Wen, S., Peng, C., Shen, M., & Shi, X. et al. (2015). Multifunctional Dendrimer-Entrapped Gold Nanoparticles Modified with RGD Peptide for Targeted Computed Tomography/Magnetic Resonance Dual-Modal Imaging of Tumors. *Analytical Chemistry*, *87*(7), 3949–3956. doi:10.1021/acs.analchem.5b00135 PMID:25768040

Cheng, Y., Zhao, L., Li, Y., & Xu, T. (2011). Design of biocompatible dendrimers for cancer diagnosis and therapy: Current status and future perspectives. *Chemical Society Reviews*, *40*(5), 2673–2703. doi:10.1039/c0cs00097c PMID:21286593

D'Emanuele, A., & Attwood, D. (2005). Dendrimer–drug interactions. *Advanced Drug Delivery Reviews*, *57*(15), 2147–2162. doi:10.1016/j.addr.2005.09.012 PMID:16310283

Danhier, F., Feron, O., & Préat, V. (2010). To exploit the tumor microenvironment: Passive and active tumor targeting of nanocarriers for anti-cancer drug delivery. *Journal of Controlled Release*, *148*(2), 135–146. doi:10.1016/j.jconrel.2010.08.027 PMID:20797419

De La Rica, R., Aili, D., & Stevens, M. M. (2012). Enzyme-responsive nanoparticles for drug release and diagnostics. *Advanced Drug Delivery Reviews*, *64*(11), 967–978. doi:10.1016/j.addr.2012.01.002 PMID:22266127

Deng, C., Jiang, Y., Cheng, R., Meng, F., & Zhong, Z. (2012). Biodegradable polymeric micelles for targeted and controlled anticancer drug delivery: Promises, progress and prospects. *Nano Today*, *7*(5), 467–480. doi:10.1016/j.nantod.2012.08.005

Dhanikula, R. S., Argaw, A., Bouchard, J.-F., & Hildgen, P. (2008). Methotrexate loaded polyether-copolyester dendrimers for the treatment of gliomas: Enhanced efficacy and intratumoral transport capability. *Molecular Pharmaceutics*, *5*(1), 105–116. doi:10.1021/mp700086j PMID:18171013

Du, J.-Z., Du, X.-J., Mao, C.-Q., & Wang, J. (2011). Tailor-Made Dual pH-Sensitive Polymer-Doxorubicin Nanoparticles for Efficient Anticancer Drug Delivery. *Journal of the American Chemical Society*, *133*(44), 17560–17563. doi:10.1021/ja207150n PMID:21985458

Elsabahy, M., & Wooley, K. L. (2012). Design of polymeric nanoparticles for biomedical delivery applications. *Chemical Society Reviews*, *41*(7), 2545–2561. doi:10.1039/c2cs15327k PMID:22334259

Fuchs, S., Otto, H., Jehle, S., Henklein, P., & Schlüter, A. D. (2005). Fluorescent dendrimers with a peptide cathepsin B cleavage site for drug delivery applications. *Chemical Communications*, (14): 1830–1832. doi:10.1039/B415651J PMID:15795757

Fuller, J. M., Raghupathi, K. R., Ramireddy, R. R., Subrahmanyam, A. V., Yesilyurt, V., & Thayumanavan, S. (2013). Temperature-Sensitive Transitions below LCST in Amphiphilic Dendritic Assemblies: Host–Guest Implications. *Journal of the American Chemical Society*, *135*(24), 8947–8954. doi:10.1021/ja402019c PMID:23692369

Gref, R., Domb, A., Quellec, P., Blunk, T., Müller, R., Verbavatz, J., & Langer, R. (2012). The controlled intravenous delivery of drugs using PEG-coated sterically stabilized nanospheres. *Advanced Drug Delivery Reviews*, *64*, 316–326. doi:10.1016/j.addr.2012.09.008 PMID:25170183

Guo, J., Zhuang, J., Wang, F., Raghupathi, K. R., & Thayumanavan, S. (2014). Protein AND enzyme gated supramolecular disassembly. *Journal of the American Chemical Society*, *136*(6), 2220–2223. doi:10.1021/ja4108676 PMID:24447098

Haba, Y., Harada, A., Takagishi, T., & Kono, K. (2004). Rendering poly (amidoamine) or poly (propylenimine) dendrimers temperature sensitive. *Journal of the American Chemical Society*, *126*(40), 12760–12761. doi:10.1021/ja047755g PMID:15469255

Haba, Y., Kojima, C., Harada, A., & Kono, K. (2006). Control of temperature-sensitive properties of poly (amidoamine) dendrimers using peripheral modification with various alkylamide groups. *Macromolecules*, *39*(21), 7451–7453. doi:10.1021/ma061019a

Harnoy, A. J., Rosenbaum, I., Tirosh, E., Ebenstein, Y., Shaharabani, R., Beck, R., & Amir, R. J. (2014). Enzyme-Responsive Amphiphilic PEG-Dendron Hybrids and Their Assembly into Smart Micellar Nanocarriers. *Journal of the American Chemical Society*, *136*(21), 7531–7534. doi:10.1021/ja413036q PMID:24568366

He, X., Alves, C. S., Oliveira, N., Rodrigues, J., Zhu, J., Bányai, I., & Shi, X. et al. (2015). RGD peptide-modified multifunctional dendrimer platform for drug encapsulation and targeted inhibition of cancer cells. *Colloids and Surfaces. B, Biointerfaces*, *125*(0), 82–89. doi:10.1016/j.colsurfb.2014.11.004 PMID:25437067

Hu, W., Cheng, L., Cheng, L., Zheng, M., Lei, Q., Hu, Z., & Chen, D. et al. (2014). Redox and pH-responsive poly (amidoamine) dendrimer–poly (ethylene glycol) conjugates with disulfide linkages for efficient intracellular drug release. *Colloids and Surfaces. B, Biointerfaces*, *123*, 254–263. doi:10.1016/j.colsurfb.2014.09.024 PMID:25277289

Huang, C.-H., Nwe, K., Al Zaki, A., Brechbiel, M. W., & Tsourkas, A. (2012). Biodegradable Polydisulfide Dendrimer Nanoclusters as MRI Contrast Agents. *ACS Nano*, *6*(11), 9416–9424. doi:10.1021/nn304160p PMID:23098069

Ihre, H. R., Padilla De Jesús, O. L., Szoka, F. C., & Fréchet, J. M. J. (2002). Polyester Dendritic Systems for Drug Delivery Applications: Design, Synthesis, and Characterization. *Bioconjugate Chemistry*, *13*(3), 443–452. doi:10.1021/bc010102u PMID:12009932

Jansen, J. F. G. A., Meijer, E. W., & de Brabander-van den Berg, E. M. M. (1995). The Dendritic Box: Shape-Selective Liberation of Encapsulated Guests. *Journal of the American Chemical Society*, *117*(15), 4417–4418. doi:10.1021/ja00120a032

Jefferies, W. A., Brandon, M. R., Hunt, S. V., Williams, A. F., Gatter, K. C., & Mason, D. Y. (1984). Transferrin receptor on endothelium of brain capillaries. *Nature*, *312*(5990), 162–163. doi:10.1038/312162a0 PMID:6095085

Jennings, L. E., & Long, N. J. (2009). 'Two is better than one'—probes for dual-modality molecular imaging. *Chemical Communications*, (24): 3511–3524. doi:10.1039/b821903f PMID:19521594

Jin, Y., Ren, X., Wang, W., Ke, L., Ning, E., Du, L., & Bradshaw, J. (2011). A 5-fluorouracil-loaded pH-responsive dendrimer nanocarrier for tumor targeting. *International Journal of Pharmaceutics*, *420*(2), 378–384. doi:10.1016/j.ijpharm.2011.08.053 PMID:21925254

Kaminskas, L. M., Boyd, B. J., Karellas, P., Krippner, G. Y., Lessene, R., Kelly, B., & Porter, C. J. (2008). The impact of molecular weight and PEG chain length on the systemic pharmacokinetics of PEGylated poly l-lysine dendrimers. *Molecular Pharmaceutics*, *5*(3), 449–463. doi:10.1021/mp7001208 PMID:18393438

Kaminskas, L. M., Kelly, B. D., McLeod, V. M., Sberna, G., Owen, D. J., Boyd, B. J., & Porter, C. J. (2011). Characterisation and tumour targeting of PEGylated polylysine dendrimers bearing doxorubicin via a pH labile linker. *Journal of Controlled Release*, *152*(2), 241–248. doi:10.1016/j.jconrel.2011.02.005 PMID:21315119

Kawaguchi, T., Walker, K. L., Wilkins, C. L., & Moore, J. S. (1995). Double Exponential Dendrimer Growth. *Journal of the American Chemical Society*, *117*(8), 2159–2165. doi:10.1021/ja00113a005

Kayyali, R., Marriott, C., & Wiseman, H. (1994). Tamoxifen decreases drug efflux from liposomes: Relevance to its ability to reverse multidrug resistance in cancer cells? *FEBS Letters*, *344*(2), 221–224. doi:10.1016/0014-5793(94)00378-5 PMID:8187888

Khan, O. F., Zaia, E. W., Jhunjhunwala, S., Xue, W., Cai, W., Yun, D. S., & Anderson, D. G. et al. (2015). Dendrimer-inspired nanomaterials for the in vivo delivery of siRNA to lung vasculature. *Nano Letters*, *15*(5), 3008–3016. doi:10.1021/nl5048972 PMID:25789998

Khan, O. F., Zaia, E. W., Yin, H., Bogorad, R. L., Pelet, J. M., Webber, M. J., & Anderson, D. G. et al. (2014). Ionizable Amphiphilic Dendrimer-Based Nanomaterials with Alkyl-Chain-Substituted Amines for Tunable siRNA Delivery to the Liver Endothelium In Vivo. *Angewandte Chemie*, *126*(52), 14625–14629. doi:10.1002/ange.201408221 PMID:25354018

Killops, K. L., Campos, L. M., & Hawker, C. J. (2008). Robust, Efficient, and Orthogonal Synthesis of Dendrimers via Thiol-ene "Click" Chemistry. *Journal of the American Chemical Society*, *130*(15), 5062–5064. doi:10.1021/ja8006325 PMID:18355008

Kimura, M., Kato, M., Muto, T., Hanabusa, K., & Shirai, H. (2000). Temperature-sensitive dendritic hosts: Synthesis, characterization, and control of catalytic activity. *Macromolecules*, *33*(4), 1117–1119. doi:10.1021/ma9914671

Kono, K., Liu, M., & Fréchet, J. M. (1999). Design of dendritic macromolecules containing folate or methotrexate residues. *Bioconjugate Chemistry*, *10*(6), 1115–1121. doi:10.1021/bc990082k PMID:10563782

Koren, E., Apte, A., Jani, A., & Torchilin, V. P. (2012). Multifunctional PEGylated 2C5-immunoliposomes containing pH-sensitive bonds and TAT peptide for enhanced tumor cell internalization and cytotoxicity. *Journal of Controlled Release*, *160*(2), 264–273. doi:10.1016/j.jconrel.2011.12.002 PMID:22182771

Kostiainen, M. A., Smith, D. K., & Ikkala, O. (2007). Optically Triggered Release of DNA from Multivalent Dendrons by Degrading and Charge-Switching Multivalency. *Angewandte Chemie*, *46*(40), 7600–7604. doi:10.1002/anie.200701200 PMID:17729224

Kottari, N., Chabre, Y. M., Shiao, T. C., Rej, R., & Roy, R. (2014). Efficient and accelerated growth of multifunctional dendrimers using orthogonal thiol–ene and SN 2 reactions. *Chemical Communications*, *50*(16), 1983–1985. doi:10.1039/c3cc46633g PMID:24416763

Kukowska-Latallo, J. F., Candido, K. A., Cao, Z., Nigavekar, S. S., Majoros, I. J., Thomas, T. P., & Baker, J. R. et al. (2005). Nanoparticle Targeting of Anticancer Drug Improves Therapeutic Response in Animal Model of Human Epithelial Cancer. *Cancer Research*, *65*(12), 5317–5324. doi:10.1158/0008-5472.CAN-04-3921 PMID:15958579

Kurtoglu, Y. E., Navath, R. S., Wang, B., Kannan, S., Romero, R., & Kannan, R. M. (2009). Poly (amidoamine) dendrimer–drug conjugates with disulfide linkages for intracellular drug delivery. *Biomaterials*, *30*(11), 2112–2121. doi:10.1016/j.biomaterials.2008.12.054 PMID:19171376

Lee, C. C., Gillies, E. R., Fox, M. E., Guillaudeu, S. J., Fréchet, J. M., Dy, E. E., & Szoka, F. C. (2006). A single dose of doxorubicin-functionalized bow-tie dendrimer cures mice bearing C-26 colon carcinomas. *Proceedings of the National Academy of Sciences of the United States of America*, *103*(45), 16649–16654. doi:10.1073/pnas.0607705103 PMID:17075050

Lee, C. C., MacKay, J. A., Fréchet, J. M. J., & Szoka, F. C. (2005). Designing dendrimers for biological applications. *Nature Biotechnology*, *23*(12), 1517–1526. doi:10.1038/nbt1171 PMID:16333296

Li, H., & Qian, Z. M. (2002). Transferrin/transferrin receptor-mediated drug delivery. *Medicinal Research Reviews*, *22*(3), 225–250. doi:10.1002/med.10008 PMID:11933019

Li, N., Li, N., Yi, Q., Luo, K., Guo, C., Pan, D., & Gu, Z. (2014). Amphiphilic peptide dendritic copolymer-doxorubicin nanoscale conjugate self-assembled to enzyme-responsive anti-cancer agent. *Biomaterials*, *35*(35), 9529–9545. doi:10.1016/j.biomaterials.2014.07.059 PMID:25145854

Li, Y., He, H., Jia, X., Lu, W.-L., Lou, J., & Wei, Y. (2012). A dual-targeting nanocarrier based on poly(amidoamine) dendrimers conjugated with transferrin and tamoxifen for treating brain gliomas. *Biomaterials*, *33*(15), 3899–3908. doi:10.1016/j.biomaterials.2012.02.004 PMID:22364698

Lim, J., Guo, Y., Rostollan, C. L., Stanfield, J., Hsieh, J.-T., Sun, X., & Simanek, E. E. (2008). The role of the size and number of polyethylene glycol chains in the biodistribution and tumor localization of triazine dendrimers. *Molecular Pharmaceutics*, *5*(4), 540–547. doi:10.1021/mp8000292 PMID:18672950

Liu, K. C., & Yeo, Y. (2013). Zwitterionic Chitosan–Polyamidoamine Dendrimer Complex Nanoparticles as a pH-Sensitive Drug Carrier. *Molecular Pharmaceutics*, *10*(5), 1695–1704. doi:10.1021/mp300522p PMID:23510114

Liu, X., He, B., Xu, Z., Yin, M., Yang, W., Zhang, H., & Shen, J. et al. (2015). A functionalized fluorescent dendrimer as a pesticide nanocarrier: Application in pest control. *Nanoscale*, *7*(2), 445–449. doi:10.1039/C4NR05733C PMID:25429649

Lu, Y., & Low, P. S. (2012). Folate-mediated delivery of macromolecular anticancer therapeutic agents. *Advanced Drug Delivery Reviews*, *64*, 342–352. doi:10.1016/j.addr.2012.09.020 PMID:12204598

Maeda, H., Bharate, G., & Daruwalla, J. (2009). Polymeric drugs for efficient tumor-targeted drug delivery based on EPR-effect. *European Journal of Pharmaceutics and Biopharmaceutics*, *71*(3), 409–419. doi:10.1016/j.ejpb.2008.11.010 PMID:19070661

Maeda, H., Sawa, T., & Konno, T. (2001). Mechanism of tumor-targeted delivery of macromolecular drugs, including the EPR effect in solid tumor and clinical overview of the prototype polymeric drug SMANCS. *Journal of Controlled Release*, *74*(1), 47–61. doi:10.1016/S0168-3659(01)00309-1 PMID:11489482

Malik, N., Evagorou, E. G., & Duncan, R. (1999). Dendrimer-platinate: A novel approach to cancer chemotherapy. *Anti-Cancer Drugs*, *10*(8), 767–776. doi:10.1097/00001813-199909000-00010 PMID:10573209

Markman, J. L., Rekechenetskiy, A., Holler, E., & Ljubimova, J. Y. (2013). Nanomedicine therapeutic approaches to overcome cancer drug resistance. *Advanced Drug Delivery Reviews*, *65*(13-14), 1866–1879. doi:10.1016/j.addr.2013.09.019 PMID:24120656

Matsumura, Y., & Maeda, H. (1986). A new concept for macromolecular therapeutics in cancer chemotherapy: Mechanism of tumoritropic accumulation of proteins and the antitumor agent smancs. *Cancer Research*, *46*(12 Part 1), 6387–6392. PMID:2946403

Medina, S. H., & El Sayed, M. E. H. (2009). Dendrimers as Carriers for Delivery of Chemotherapeutic Agents. *Chemical Reviews*, *109*(7), 3141–3157. doi:10.1021/cr900174j PMID:19534493

Mintzer, M. A., & Grinstaff, M. W. (2011). Biomedical applications of dendrimers: A tutorial. *Chemical Society Reviews*, *40*(1), 173–190. doi:10.1039/B901839P PMID:20877875

Molla, M. R., Rangadurai, P., Pavan, G. M., & Thayumanavan, S. (2015). Experimental and theoretical investigations in stimuli responsive dendrimer-based assemblies. *Nanoscale*, *7*(9), 3817–3837. doi:10.1039/C4NR04563G PMID:25260107

Morgan, M. T., Carnahan, M. A., Immoos, C. E., Ribeiro, A. A., Finkelstein, S., Lee, S. J., & Grinstaff, M. W. (2003). Dendritic molecular capsules for hydrophobic compounds. *Journal of the American Chemical Society*, *125*(50), 15485–15489. doi:10.1021/ja0347383 PMID:14664594

Mullen, D. G., McNerny, D. Q., Desai, A., Cheng, X.-, DiMaggio, S. C., Kotlyar, A., & Banaszak Holl, M. M. et al. (2011). Design, Synthesis, and Biological Functionality of a Dendrimer-Based Modular Drug Delivery Platform. *Bioconjugate Chemistry*, *22*(4), 679–689. doi:10.1021/bc100360v PMID:21425790

Mura, S., Nicolas, J., & Couvreur, P. (2013). Stimuli-responsive nanocarriers for drug delivery. *Nature Materials*, *12*(11), 991–1003. doi:10.1038/nmat3776 PMID:24150417

Nazemi, A., Schon, T. B., & Gillies, E. R. (2013). Synthesis and degradation of backbone photodegradable polyester dendrimers. *Organic Letters*, *15*(8), 1830–1833. doi:10.1021/ol4004367 PMID:23545015

Newkome, G. R., Yao, Z., Baker, G. R., & Gupta, V. K. (1985). Micelles. Part 1. Cascade molecules: A new approach to micelles. A [27]-arborol. *The Journal of Organic Chemistry*, *50*(11), 2003–2004. doi:10.1021/jo00211a052

Nicolas, J., Mura, S., Brambilla, D., Mackiewicz, N., & Couvreur, P. (2013). Design, functionalization strategies and biomedical applications of targeted biodegradable/biocompatible polymer-based nanocarriers for drug delivery. *Chemical Society Reviews*, *42*(3), 1147–1235. doi:10.1039/C2CS35265F PMID:23238558

Okuda, T., Kawakami, S., Akimoto, N., Niidome, T., Yamashita, F., & Hashida, M. (2006). PEGylated lysine dendrimers for tumor-selective targeting after intravenous injection in tumor-bearing mice. *Journal of Controlled Release*, *116*(3), 330–336. doi:10.1016/j.jconrel.2006.09.012 PMID:17118476

Patel, T., Zhou, J., Piepmeier, J. M., & Saltzman, W. M. (2012). Polymeric nanoparticles for drug delivery to the central nervous system. *Advanced Drug Delivery Reviews*, *64*(7), 701–705. doi:10.1016/j.addr.2011.12.006 PMID:22210134

Peng, C., Qin, J., Zhou, B., Chen, Q., Shen, M., Zhu, M., & Shi, X. et al. (2013). Targeted tumor CT imaging using folic acid-modified PEGylated dendrimer-entrapped gold nanoparticles. *Polymer Chemistry*, *4*(16), 4412–4424. doi:10.1039/c3py00521f

Peng, C., Zheng, L., Chen, Q., Shen, M., Guo, R., Wang, H., & Shi, X. et al. (2012). PEGylated dendrimer-entrapped gold nanoparticles for in vivo blood pool and tumor imaging by computed tomography. *Biomaterials*, *33*(4), 1107–1119. doi:10.1016/j.biomaterials.2011.10.052 PMID:22061490

Qiao, Z., & Shi, X. (2014). Dendrimer-based molecular imaging contrast agents. *Progress in Polymer Science*, *44*, 1–27. doi:10.1016/j.progpolymsci.2014.08.002

Raghupathi, K. R., Guo, J., Munkhbat, O., Rangadurai, P., & Thayumanavan, S. (2014). Supramolecular Disassembly of Facially Amphiphilic Dendrimer Assemblies in Response to Physical, Chemical, and Biological Stimuli. *Accounts of Chemical Research*, *47*(7), 2200–2211. doi:10.1021/ar500143u PMID:24937682

Ramireddy, , R., Raghupathi, K., Torres, D. A., & Thayumanavan, S. (2012). Stimuli sensitive amphiphilic dendrimers. *New Journal of Chemistry*, *36*(2), 340–349. doi:10.1039/c2nj20879b PMID:24039387

Rösler, A., Vandermeulen, G. W. M., & Klok, H.-A. (2012). Advanced drug delivery devices via self-assembly of amphiphilic block copolymers. *Advanced Drug Delivery Reviews, 64,* 270-279.

Saad, M., Garbuzenko, O. B., Ber, E., Chandna, P., Khandare, J. J., Pozharov, V. P., & Minko, T. (2008). Receptor targeted polymers, dendrimers, liposomes: Which nanocarrier is the most efficient for tumor-specific treatment and imaging? *Journal of Controlled Release*, *130*(2), 107–114. doi:10.1016/j.jconrel.2008.05.024 PMID:18582982

Shi, J., Votruba, A. R., Farokhzad, O. C., & Langer, R. (2010). Nanotechnology in Drug Delivery and Tissue Engineering: From Discovery to Applications. *Nano Letters*, *10*(9), 3223–3230. doi:10.1021/nl102184c PMID:20726522

Shi, X., Wang, S. H., Swanson, S. D., Ge, S., Cao, Z., Van Antwerp, M. E., & Baker, J. R. et al. (2008). Dendrimer-Functionalized Shell-crosslinked Iron Oxide Nanoparticles for In-Vivo Magnetic Resonance Imaging of Tumors. *Advanced Materials*, *20*(9), 1671–1678.

Shukla, R., Thomas, T. P., Peters, J., Kotlyar, A., Myc, A., & Baker, J. R. Jr. (2005). Tumor angiogenic vasculature targeting with PAMAM dendrimer–RGD conjugates. *Chemical Communications*, (46): 5739–5741. doi:10.1039/b507350b PMID:16307130

Shukla, R., Thomas, T. P., Peters, J. L., Desai, A. M., Kukowska-Latallo, J., Patri, A. K., & Baker, J. R. et al. (2006). HER2 specific tumor targeting with dendrimer conjugated anti-HER2 mAb. *Bioconjugate Chemistry*, *17*(5), 1109–1115. doi:10.1021/bc050348p PMID:16984117

Singh, P., Gupta, U., Asthana, A., & Jain, N. K. (2008). Folate and Folate–PEG–PAMAM Dendrimers: Synthesis, Characterization, and Targeted Anticancer Drug Delivery Potential in Tumor Bearing Mice. *Bioconjugate Chemistry*, *19*(11), 2239–2252. doi:10.1021/bc800125u PMID:18950215

Such, G. K., Yan, Y., Johnston, A. P. R., Gunawan, S. T., & Caruso, F. (2015). Interfacing Materials Science and Biology for Drug Carrier Design. *Advanced Materials*, *27*(14), 2278–2297. doi:10.1002/adma.201405084 PMID:25728711

Sun, I. C., Eun, D. K., Na, J. H., Lee, S., Kim, I. J., Youn, I. C., & Choi, K. et al. (2009). Heparin-Coated Gold Nanoparticles for Liver-Specific CT Imaging. *Chemistry (Weinheim an der Bergstrasse, Germany)*, *15*(48), 13341–13347. doi:10.1002/chem.200902344 PMID:19902441

Sunoqrot, S., Bugno, J., Lantvit, D., Burdette, J. E., & Hong, S. (2014). Prolonged blood circulation and enhanced tumor accumulation of folate-targeted dendrimer-polymer hybrid nanoparticles. *Journal of Controlled Release*, *191*(0), 115–122. doi:10.1016/j.jconrel.2014.05.006 PMID:24837188

Talanov, V. S., Regino, C. A., Kobayashi, H., Bernardo, M., Choyke, P. L., & Brechbiel, M. W. (2006). Dendrimer-based nanoprobe for dual modality magnetic resonance and fluorescence imaging. *Nano Letters*, *6*(7), 1459–1463. doi:10.1021/nl060765q PMID:16834429

Taratula, O., Schumann, C., Duong, T., Taylor, K. L., & Taratula, O. (2015). Dendrimer-encapsulated naphthalocyanine as a single agent-based theranostic nanoplatform for near-infrared fluorescence imaging and combinatorial anticancer phototherapy. *Nanoscale*, *7*(9), 3888–3902. doi:10.1039/C4NR06050D PMID:25422147

Tomalia, D. A., Baker, H., Dewald, J., Hall, M., Kallos, G., Martin, S., & Smith, P. et al. (1985). A New Class of Polymers: Starburst-Dendritic Macromolecules. *Polymer Journal*, *17*(1), 117–132. doi:10.1295/polymj.17.117

Tono, Y., Kojima, C., Haba, Y., Takahashi, T., Harada, A., Yagi, S., & Kono, K. (2006). Thermosensitive properties of poly (amidoamine) dendrimers with peripheral phenylalanine residues. *Langmuir*, *22*(11), 4920–4922. doi:10.1021/la060066t PMID:16700575

Torchilin, V. (2011). Tumor delivery of macromolecular drugs based on the EPR effect. *Advanced Drug Delivery Reviews*, *63*(3), 131–135. doi:10.1016/j.addr.2010.03.011 PMID:20304019

Torchilin, V. P. (2014). Multifunctional, stimuli-sensitive nanoparticulate systems for drug delivery. *Nature Reviews. Drug Discovery*, *13*(11), 813–827. doi:10.1038/nrd4333 PMID:25287120

Vögtle, F., Buhleier, E., & Wehner, W. (1978). Cascade and Nonskid-Chain-Like Syntheses of Molecular Cavity Topologies. *Synthesis*, *2*, 155–158.

Wang, H., Zheng, L., Peng, C., Guo, R., Shen, M., Shi, X., & Zhang, G. (2011). Computed tomography imaging of cancer cells using acetylated dendrimer-entrapped gold nanoparticles. *Biomaterials*, *32*(11), 2979–2988. doi:10.1016/j.biomaterials.2011.01.001 PMID:21277019

Wang, X., Cai, X., Hu, J., Shao, N., Wang, F., Zhang, Q., & Cheng, Y. et al. (2013). Glutathione-triggered "off–on" release of anticancer drugs from dendrimer-encapsulated gold nanoparticles. *Journal of the American Chemical Society*, *135*(26), 9805–9810. doi:10.1021/ja402903h PMID:23789713

Wang, Z., Zhou, B., Liu, D., & Fan, X. (2010). Thermosensitive Poly (N-isopropylacrylamide)-g-Polyamidoamine Dendrimer Derivatives: Preparation and the Drug Release Behaviors. *Macromolecular Symposia*, *297*(1), 158–166. doi:10.1002/masy.200900055

Wei, H., Cheng, S.-X., Zhang, X.-Z., & Zhuo, R.-X. (2009). Thermo-sensitive polymeric micelles based on poly (N-isopropylacrylamide) as drug carriers. *Progress in Polymer Science*, *34*(9), 893–910. doi:10.1016/j.progpolymsci.2009.05.002

Wei, T., Chen, C., Liu, J., Liu, C., Posocco, P., Liu, X., & Fermeglia, M. et al. (2015). Anticancer drug nanomicelles formed by self-assembling amphiphilic dendrimer to combat cancer drug resistance. *Proceedings of the National Academy of Sciences of the United States of America*, *112*(10), 2978–2983. doi:10.1073/pnas.1418494112 PMID:25713374

Wen, S., Li, K., Cai, H., Chen, Q., Shen, M., Huang, Y., & Zhang, G. et al. (2013). Multifunctional dendrimer-entrapped gold nanoparticles for dual mode CT/MR imaging applications. *Biomaterials*, *34*(5), 1570–1580. doi:10.1016/j.biomaterials.2012.11.010 PMID:23199745

Wen, Y., Zhang, Z., & Li, J. (2014). Highly Efficient Multifunctional Supramolecular Gene Carrier System Self-Assembled from Redox-Sensitive and Zwitterionic Polymer Blocks. *Advanced Functional Materials*, *24*(25), 3874–3884. doi:10.1002/adfm.201303687

Wohlfart, S., Gelperina, S., & Kreuter, J. (2012). Transport of drugs across the blood–brain barrier by nanoparticles. *Journal of Controlled Release*, *161*(2), 264–273. doi:10.1016/j.jconrel.2011.08.017 PMID:21872624

Wooley, K. L., Hawker, C. J., & Fréchet, J. M. (1994). A "Branched-Monomer Approach" for the Rapid Synthesis of Dendimers. *Angewandte Chemie*, *33*(1), 82–85. doi:10.1002/anie.199400821

Wu, W., Driessen, W., & Jiang, X. (2014). Oligo (ethylene glycol)-based thermosensitive dendrimers and their tumor accumulation and penetration. *Journal of the American Chemical Society*, *136*(8), 3145–3155. doi:10.1021/ja411457r PMID:24506735

Xu, X., Jian, Y., Li, Y., Zhang, X., Tu, Z., & Gu, Z. (2014). Bio-Inspired Supramolecular Hybrid Dendrimers Self-Assembled from Low-Generation Peptide Dendrons for Highly Efficient Gene Delivery and Biological Tracking. *ACS Nano*, *8*(9), 9255–9264. doi:10.1021/nn503118f PMID:25184443

Xu, Z., He, B., Shen, J., Yang, W., & Yin, M. (2013). Fluorescent water-soluble perylenediimide-cored cationic dendrimers: Synthesis, optical properties, and cell uptake. *Chemical Communications*, *49*(35), 3646–3648. doi:10.1039/c3cc40330k PMID:23529155

Yang, J., Luo, Y., Xu, Y., Li, J., Zhang, Z., Wang, H., & Zhang, G. et al. (2015). Conjugation of Iron Oxide Nanoparticles with RGD-Modified Dendrimers for Targeted Tumor MR Imaging. *ACS Applied Materials & Interfaces*, *7*(9), 5420–5428. doi:10.1021/am508983n PMID:25695661

Yang, Q., Yang, Y., Li, L., Sun, W., Zhu, X., & Huang, Y. (2015). Polymeric Nanomedicine for Tumor-Targeted Combination Therapy to Elicit Synergistic Genotoxicity against Prostate Cancer. *ACS Applied Materials & Interfaces*, *7*(12), 6661–6673. doi:10.1021/am509204u PMID:25775367

Yesilyurt, V., Ramireddy, R., Azagarsamy, M. A., & Thayumanavan, S. (2012). Accessing Lipophilic Ligands in Dendrimer-Based Amphiphilic Supramolecular Assemblies for Protein-Induced Disassembly. *Chemistry (Weinheim an der Bergstrasse, Germany)*, *18*(1), 223–229. doi:10.1002/chem.201102727 PMID:22127994

Yesilyurt, V., Ramireddy, R., & Thayumanavan, S. (2011). Photoregulated Release of Noncovalent Guests from Dendritic Amphiphilic Nanocontainers. *Angewandte Chemie*, *123*(13), 3094–3098. doi:10.1002/ange.201006193 PMID:21404394

Yuan, H., Luo, K., Lai, Y., Pu, Y., He, B., Wang, G., & Gu, Z. et al. (2010). A novel poly (L-glutamic acid) dendrimer based drug delivery system with both pH-sensitive and targeting functions. *Molecular Pharmaceutics*, *7*(4), 953–962. doi:10.1021/mp1000923 PMID:20481567

Zeng, F., & Zimmerman, S. C. (1996). Rapid synthesis of dendrimers by an orthogonal coupling strategy. *Journal of the American Chemical Society*, *118*(22), 5326–5327. doi:10.1021/ja960317s

Zhang, C., Pan, D., Luo, K., She, W., Guo, C., Yang, Y., & Gu, Z. (2014). Peptide Dendrimer-Doxorubicin Conjugate-Based Nanoparticles as an Enzyme-Responsive Drug Delivery System for Cancer Therapy. *Advanced Healthcare Materials*, *3*(8), 1299–1308. doi:10.1002/adhm.201300601 PMID:24706635

Zhang, Y., Sun, Y., Xu, X., Zhang, X., Zhu, H., Huang, L., & Shen, Y.-M. et al. (2010). Synthesis, Biodistribution, and Microsingle Photon Emission Computed Tomography (SPECT) Imaging Study of Technetium-99m Labeled PEGylated Dendrimer Poly (amidoamine)(PAMAM)-Folic Acid Conjugates. *Journal of Medicinal Chemistry*, *53*(8), 3262–3272. doi:10.1021/jm901910j PMID:20350006

Zhao, Y., Fan, X., Liu, D., & Wang, Z. (2011). PEGylated thermo-sensitive poly(amidoamine) dendritic drug delivery systems. *International Journal of Pharmaceutics*, *409*(1–2), 229–236. doi:10.1016/j.ijpharm.2011.02.005 PMID:21316434

Zhou, T., Chen, P., Niu, L., Jin, J., Liang, D., Li, Z., & Liu, D. et al. (2012). pH-Responsive Size-Tunable Self-Assembled DNA Dendrimers. *Angewandte Chemie*, *124*(45), 11433–11436. doi:10.1002/ange.201205862 PMID:23037637

Zhu, S., Qian, L., Hong, M., Zhang, L., Pei, Y., & Jiang, Y. (2011). RGD-Modified PEG-PAMAM-DOX Conjugate: In Vitro and In Vivo Targeting to Both Tumor Neovascular Endothelial Cells and Tumor Cells. *Advanced Materials*, *23*(12), H84–H89. doi:10.1002/adma.201003944 PMID:21360776

KEY TERMS AND DEFINITIONS

Active Targeting: The drug nanocarriers functionalized with the targeting agents are inclined to accumulate at the target site.

Dendrimer: Dendrimer is a type of synthetic polymer with the nano-sized, well-defined and highly branched achitecture, reminiscent of a tree.

Enhanced Permeability and Retention (EPR) Effect: EPR effect is a phenomenon that the well-defined nanocarriers showed more efficient to accumulate in tumors because of the leaky tumor vessels.

Multifunctional Dendrimers: The multifunctional dendrimer is a new type of nanocarrier for drug delivery, which can have long circulation times, improve the tumor accumulation and penetration, facilitate the controllable the drug release and trace the distribution of the dendrimers.

Nanocarriers: Nanocarrier is a type of drug carrier with the diameter size ranging from 1 to 1000 nm.

Passive Targeting: Owing to the nano-size of the nanocarriers, they tend to accumulate in tumors by EPR effect.

Theranostic Nanoplatform: The nanoplatfom can concurrently diagnose and treat the diseases.

Section 9
Polymetric Systems

Chapter 11
Smart Hydrogels for Pharmaceutical Applications

Snežana S. Ilić-Stojanović
University of Nis, Serbia

Vesna D. Nikolić
University of Nis, Serbia

Ljubiša B. Nikolić
University of Nis, Serbia

Slobodan D. Petrović
University of Belgrade, Serbia

ABSTRACT

The latest development in the field of smart hydrogels application as drugs carriers is shown in this chapter. Hydrogels are three-dimensional polymer network consisting of at least one hydrophilic monomer. They are insoluble in water, but in the excess presence of water or physiological fluids, swell to the equilibrium state. The amount of absorbed water depends on the chemical composition and the crosslinking degree of 3D hydrogel network and reaches over 1000% of the xerogel weight. Stimuli-responsive hydrogels exhibit significant change of their properties (swelling, color, transparency, conductivity, shape) due to small changes in the external environment conditions (pH, ionic strength, temperature, light wavelength, magnetic or electric fields, ultrasound, or a combination thereof). This smart hydrogels, with different physical and chemical properties, chemical structure and technology of obtaining, show great potential for application in the pharmaceutical industry. The application of smart hydrogels is very promising and at the beginning of the development and exploitation.

INTRODUCTION

A short overview of the development and current state-of-art relating to the implementation of "smart" gels as carriers of pharmaceuticals in systems for modified/controlled drug release is presented in this chapter. In today's rapid technology expansion, there is an ever-growing trend for a new generation of "smart" materials. They have the advantage of being less limited by design constraints. One such category of these intelligent materials is "smart" or stimuli-responsive polymers. Researches in this chapter were focused on:

DOI: 10.4018/978-1-5225-0751-2.ch011

- Different ways of synthesis and characterization of stimuli-responsive hydrogels,
- Analysis by the type of stimuli they respond to, and
- Implementation of systems for the controlled delivery of drugs (chemically controlled systems, diffusion controlled systems, systems controlled by the swelling and systems for modulated release) (Milić & Petrović, 2003).

Smart hydrogels with different physical and chemical properties, chemical structure and obtainable technology show great potential for application in the pharmaceutical industry. The aim of this chapter is to provide the latest trend and idea for further research opportunities in the field of smart hydrogels application as drugs carriers. Also, it could be the basis for the synthesis of new smart materials and for their new applications.

Background

Hydrogels are three-dimensional polymer network consisting of at least one hydrophilic monomer. They are insoluble in the water, but in the excess presence of water or physiological fluids, swell to the equilibrium state. Koetting et al. (2015) cited that hydrogels are three dimensional network structures consisting of polymeric chains, joined by tie points or joints and swell in water up to thermodynamic equilibrium. There are some variations of this basic definition. Hydrogel is defined as a solid, crosslinked three-dimensional network which swells in water, and the hydrophilic macromolecules contain 20-95% of water, according to Grant & Hackh's Chemical Dictionary (1987). According to IUPAC recommendations, *hydrogel* is defined as a gel in which the swelling agent is water (Slomkowski et al., 2011). The network component of a hydrogel is usually a polymer network, while a hydrogel in which the network component is a colloidal network may be referred to as an *aquagel*. Polymer network without water is *xerogel*. *Gel* is defined as non-fluid colloidal network or polymer network that is expanded throughout its whole volume by a fluid (Jones et al., 2009). Gels also may be defined as a substantially diluted crosslinked system, which exhibits no flow when in the steady-state (Ferry, 1980). It is consequential to understand difference between the term *gel* and *hydrogel*. Their polymeric network may be similar in chemical composition, but different in physical features. When *gel* is swollen to equilibrium, the further addition of fluid polymer network should be diluted. But, *hydrogel* may absorb large amounts of fluid, increasing the volume to the equilibrium state, while still maintaining a three-dimensional structure and shape (Gupta et al., 2002).

Network structure of the hydrophilic polymer chains absorbs and holds water within the pores. The pores in hydrogels were created during swelling of the polymer network when water molecules penetrate the network and volume of the system increases. The pores are usually not present in the dry network before swelling. The only exception is when the pores are formed intentionally during synthesis of the dry network. The amount of water that the hydrogel may receive depends on the chemical composition and the crosslinking degree of three-dimensional hydrogel network and reaches over 1000% of the weight in the xerogel state (Hoffman, 2002; Pal et al., 2009; Jagur-Grodzinski, 2010). Graham (1861) gave a description of the gel: "while the rigidity of the crystal structure is excluded from the outside looks, the softness of gelatin colloids gives fluidity and allows the colloid to become a medium for the diffusion of liquids, like water itself". He was the first to introduce the term hydrogel in 1864. and described special diffusion properties of the gel (Graham, 1864). Jordan-Lloyd (1926) gave a concise and useful definition for checking: "If it looks like gel, it must be gel", because in colloidal conditions, it is easier to recognize "gel" than to define it. The next work on crosslinked polymers and networks appeared in German literature by the middle 1930s. Meanwhile significant work on the behavior of "natural hydrocolloids" appeared by the late 1930s, but without structural insight (Koetting et al., 2015). The work in that period and in the 1940s concentrated mostly on reaction kinetics and mechanical properties of the ensuing networks. The first report on phase transition of pH-sensitive hydrogels was published in 1950 (The Chemical Industry, 1950) and succeeding studies on the hydrogels biocompatibility were published in 1959. Tanaka and coleague described the phenomenon of swelling and the kinetics of poly(acrylamide) hydrogels (Tanaka & Fillmore, 1979). The tension within the crosslinked polymer network and forces between the polymer network and the solvent are in equilibrium with the polymer chains motion. The characteristic of crosslinked polymers is that they do not dissolve, they only swell in solvents, depending on the crosslinking degree, they are amorphous and insoluble.

HYDROGELS TYPES

There are different ways for hydrogel classification (Ratner & Hoffman, 1976; Peppas, 1986, 1991; Peppas, et al., 2000; Jagur-Grodzinski, 2010).

- According to the origin of monomer, hydrogels may be:
  - Natural hydrogels (obtained by crosslinking of natural polymers, e.g. starch, cellulose, proteins, dextran, chitosan, alginate, fibrin, collagen, gelatin, hyaluronic acid).
  - Synthetic hydrogels (obtained by polymerization reactions and differ in the composition of the monomers and other reactants, as well as in the polymerization reaction, which enables the design for specific applications). The most frequently used monomers are: *N*-isopropylacrylamide, 2-hydroxyethyl methacrylate, 2-hydroxypropyl methacrylate, *N*-vinyl-2-pyrrolidone, vinyl acetate, vinyl benzoate, acrylic acid, methacrylic acid, ethylene oxide, ethylene glycol acrylate, ethylene glycol methacrylate and ethylene glycol dimethacrylate.
  - Combination of natural and synthetic types.
- Hydrogels are divided into physically and chemically crosslinked by the type of chemical bond.
  - Chemicaly crosslinked hydrogels occur through permanent, covalent bonding in the polymerization reaction and crosslinking between mono- and multifunctional components (monomers and crosslinkers). The hydrogels crosslinked by covalent bonds can be obtained by the following reactions:
    - The radical polymerization process of a monomer and crosslinker dissolved in a suitable solvent. The polymerization may be initiated thermally, by radiation (UV, γ, or X-ray) (radiation polymerization), by the microwave field, or using a suitable initiator;
    - Polycondensation crosslinking can be carried out by reaction between functional groups with complementary reactivity such as reactions amine/carboxylic acid, isocyanate/ OH-NH_2 or the formation of Schiff base;
    - Enzymes reactions.
  - Physically crosslinked hydrogels are formed by mutual bonding of polymer chains and establishing physical interactions between different chains.

- In relation to side groups polarity, hydrogels are divided into:
  - Neutral hydrogels have no charged groups in their structure, and their swelling is due to the interaction of water and polymer network to the extent allowed by the network flexibility.
  - Ionic hydrogels contain ionizing lateral functional groups. The main characteristic of ionic hydrogels is that their swelling degree depends on the pH value of the environment. Depending on their lateral functional groups, they may be:
    - Anionic hydrogels, which usually contain a large number of ionizable acidic groups such as carboxylic or sulfonic acid side groups. These pH-sensitive hydrogels are known as polyanions).
    - Cationic hydrogels, that generally have side basic functional groups such as primary, secondary, and tertiary amino groups.
    - Amphiphilic hydrogels contain anionic and cationic side groups.
- According to the nature of the polymer crosslinked network they may include:
  - Homopolymer hydrogels consist of only one type of monomer.
  - Copolymer hydrogels are composed of two or more types of monomers, obtained by polymerization in aqueous solution in the presence of crosslinkers.
  - Interpenetrated network (IPN) is composed of two or more polymers in the network form and when the crosslinked polymer network is in the presence of another
  - Previously crosslinked polymer network (Sperling & Mishra, 1996).
  - Semi-interpenetrated networks (semi-IPN) imply the existence of only one network through which a linear polymer is interwoven in order to provide better mechanical properties. The interactions between the linear polymer and the network may be covalent and non-covalent and, according to the synthesis type, may be sequential, and simultaneous.
- They can be classified based on the physical structure of the networks as:
  - Amorphous,
  - Semi-crystalline,
  - Hydrogen-bonded structures,
  - Super-molecular structures, and
  - Hydro-colloidal aggregates.
- According to the presence and pores size hydrogels were divided into:
  - Superporous (pores size > 100 μm),
  - Macroporous (pores size from 0.1 to 1 μm),
  - Microporous (pores size between 0.1 and 0.01 μm) and
  - Non-porous hydrogels (pores size between 0.001 and 0.01 μm).
- In relation to the behavior in a living organism, hydrogels can be:
  - Non-toxic and
  - Toxic.
- Based on the swelling behavior to variations in the external medium, there are:
  - Conventional hydrogels (weakly crosslinked hydrophilic polymers which are not significantly sensitive to changes in the environment) and
  - Stimuli-responsive hydrogels (which show significant changes in volume, shape and mechanical properties due to changes in the external environment).

Different types of hydrogels, especially physiologically-responsive, have been investigated for pharmaceutical applications. This chapter summarizes the latest research in hydrogels used for pharmaceutical applications, ranging from the type of stimuli (pH, temperature, biomolecules, pressure, ionic strength, electrical impulses, ultrasound, magnetic fields, light). Both natural and synthetic polymers have been applied with different degrees of success in medical applications.

Design and Synthesis of Smart Hydrogels

The integral components for the hydrogels synthesis are monomer, initiator and crosslinker for the hydrogels prepared by radical polymerization. Water or other aqueous solutions can be used as diluents. Polymerization process temperature can be controlled. Some of hydrogels can be prepared by polycondensation (or polyaddition) crosslinking reactions, i.e., without initiator. The chemical nature and number of side-pendant groups can be precisely controlled by the choice of the chemical compounds used in the synthesis. An overview of most commonly used monomers in the hydrogel synthesis in pharmacy (with their acronyms and structures) is given in the Figure 1.

The "smart" hydrogels may be synthesized in the conventional manner to result in hydrogels with small pore sizes or they may be synthesized by various other approaches to result in macroporous hydrogels for different applications. Some of these approaches are by co-polymerization, free radical polymerization, genetic engineering, irradiation, reversible addition-fragmentation chain transfer (RAFT), atom transfer radical polymerization (ATRP) and nitroxide-mediated polymerization (NMP) techniques. The most probable way of monomers bonding during polymerization is formation of mixed structures with random, statistical, unsystematic arrangement. Conformation and flexibility depends on the intermolecular and intramolecular interactions (electrostatic and hydrophobic interactions, dipole-dipole interactions, hydrogen bonds). A possible method of the synthesis and crosslinking of polymer chains of p(NIPAM-HPMet) copolymer network, with the potential formation of intramolecular hydrogen bonds is indicated in Figure 2 (Ilić-Stojanović et al., 2014a; Ilić-Stojanović, 2015).

It is important to remove residual monomers, initiator, crosslinker and impurities from obtained hydrogels as unwanted products produced *via* side reactions during the synthesis. Synthesis of hydrogels with a minimum content of residual reactants is a necessary precondition for application, particularly in the pharmaceutical, dental and hygiene products. The residual monomer content of up to 0.5% and even up to 1.0% or more is often found in polymers produced on an industrial scale. For example, mass of residual reactants NIPAM, HPMet and EGDM in the synthesized copolymer hydrogel p(NIPAM-HPMet) compared to the total weight of the obtained xerogel is shown in Figure 3. The values were 0.12-0.38% for NIPAM, 0.021-0.074% for HPMet and 0.007-0.012% of EGDM, based on the amount of synthesized hydrogels (Ilić-Stojanović et al., 2012a, Ilić-Stojanović, 2015).

The amount of residual monomer in some acrylates and examination of impact of their reduction on the quality of acrylate dental prosthetics by HPLC method were determined (Kostić et al., 2009; 2011). Variations of the properties of hydrogels (e.g., gel content, swelling capacity, the content of residual monomers) in relation to the content and the initiators of the system have been tested in many scientific papers and patent literature (Merrigan et al. 2004; Omidian et al., 2008; Kabiri et al. 2011).

The suitability of a hydrogel as a drug delivery carrier and its performance in a particular application depends to a large extent on its bulk structure (Peppas et al., 2000). The most important parameters used to characterize the network structure of hydrogels are the polymer volume fraction in the swollen state ($\upsilon_{2,s}$), molecular weight of the polymer chain between two neighboring crosslinking points (M_c), and

Figure 1. Monomers for hydrogel synthesis in pharmacy with their abbreviation and structures

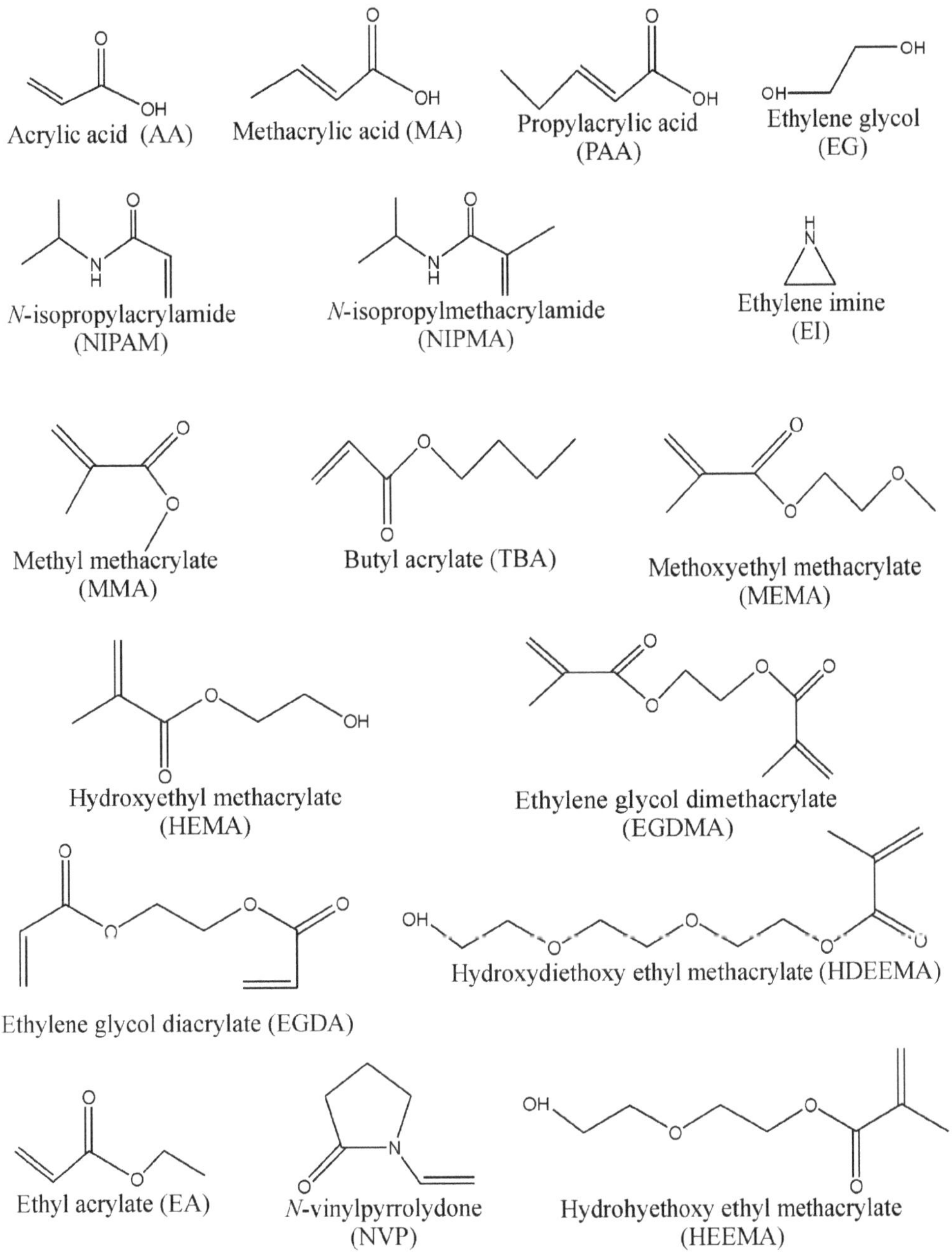

the corresponding mesh size (ξ). Upon a contact of the xerogel with water, water molecules penetrate into the space between the polymer chains, causing an increase in volume and the swelling of the network. *Flory* and *Rehner* (1943) developed a thermodinamical theory of swelling of crosslinked polymer structure that does not contain ionic moieties, which is subject to a statistical distribution. A crosslinked polymer gel, which is immersed in a fluid and allowed to reach equilibrium with its surroundings, is subject only to two opposing forces, the thermodynamic force of mixing and the retractive force of the

Figure 2. A model that shows a possible way of crosslinking p(NIPAM-HPMet) copolymer
Source: Ilić-Stojanović et al. (2014a), © [2013] [John Wiley & Sons, Inc]. Used with permission.

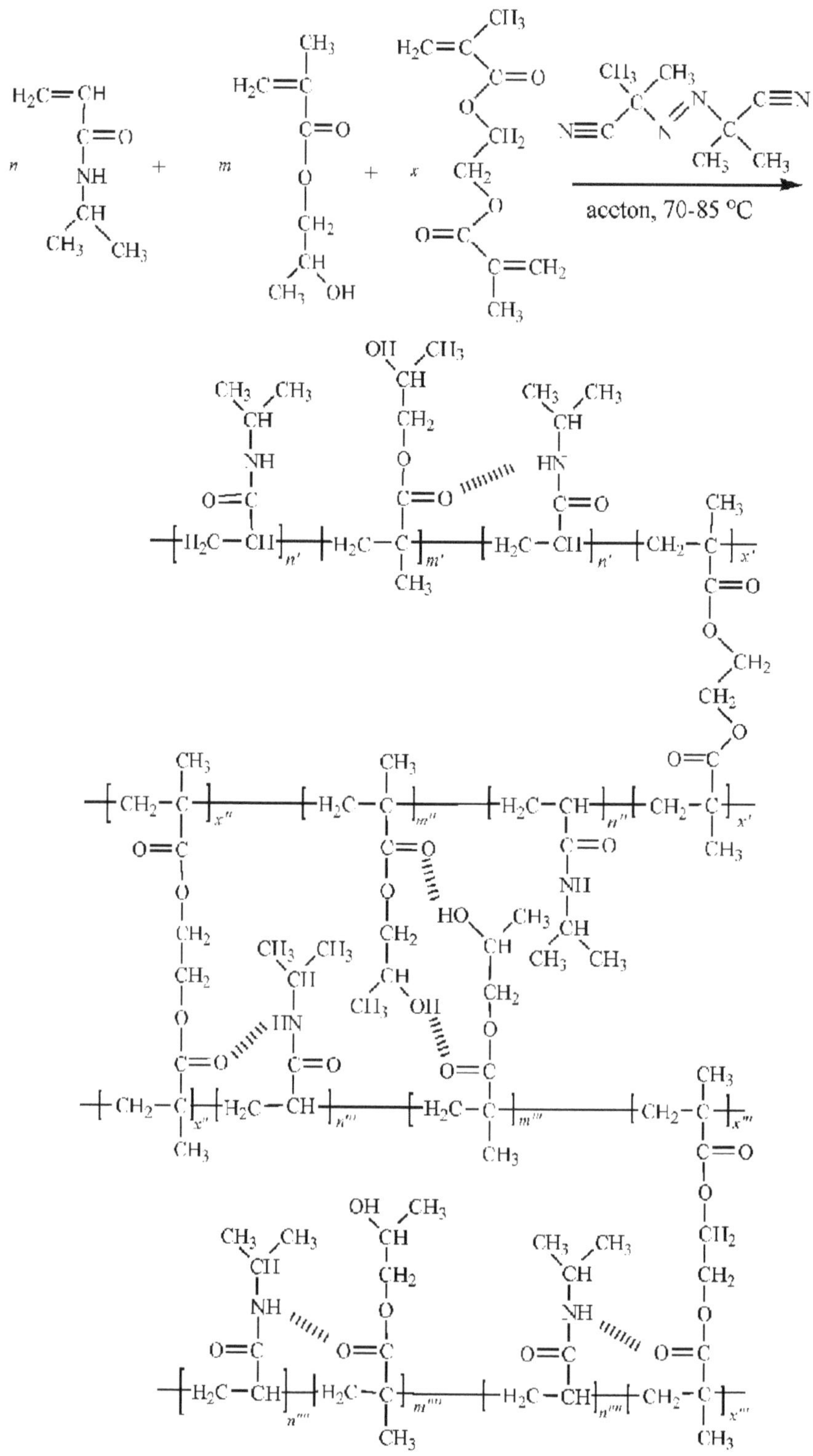

Figure 3. The quantities of residual reactants relative to the total xerogel weight in mg/g for: a) NIPAM, b) HPMet and c) EGDM
Source: Ilić-Stojanović (2015) © [2015] [LAP LAMBERT Academic Publishing]. Used with permission.

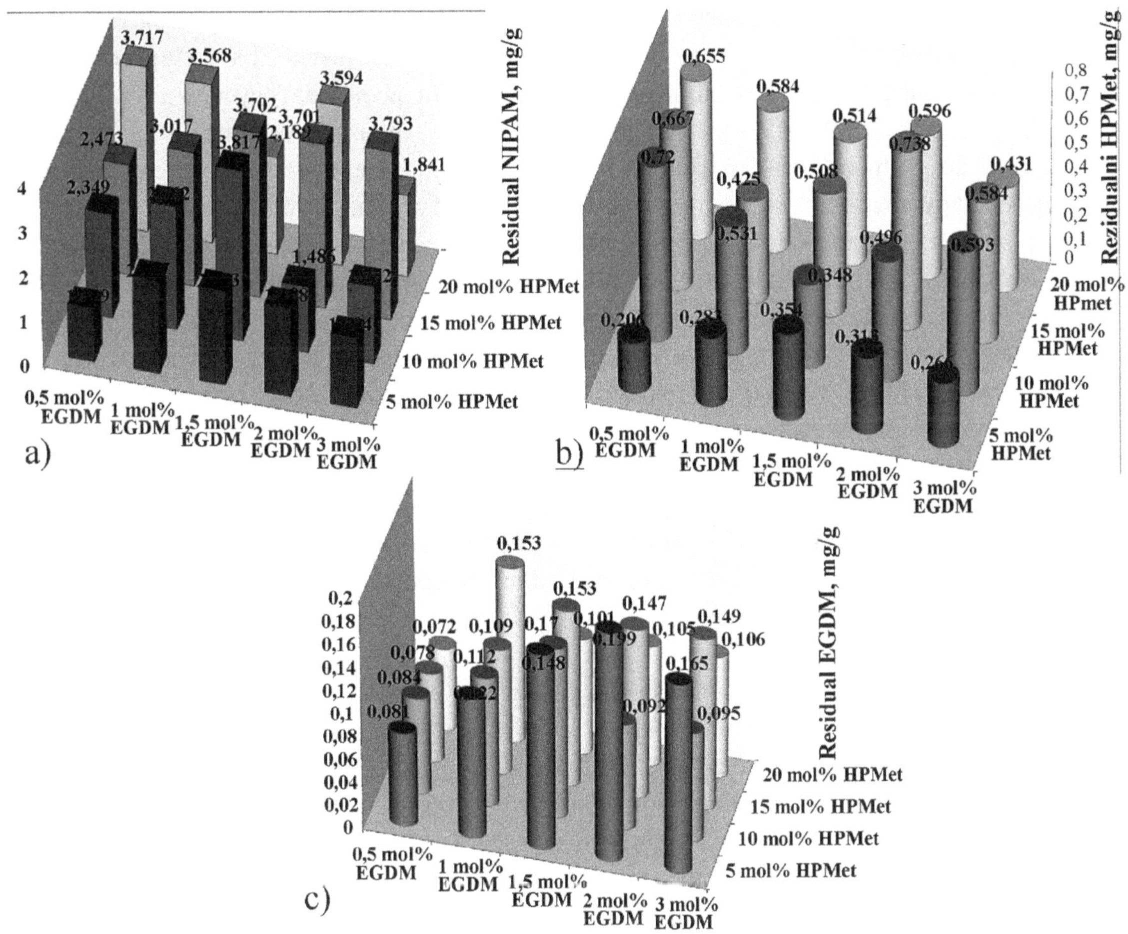

polymer chains. Dušek and Prins (1969) studied the structure and elasticity of non-crystalline polymer networks. They described various kinds of network structures which may exist before or arise during its formation. A number of theories and models have been developed in order to provide a more precise clarification of the swelling process.

HYDROGELS FOR PHARMACEUTICAL APPLICATIONS

The characteristic of marked importance of living systems is their response to external stimuli adapting themselves to changing environmental conditions. There are a lot of scientists in the last fifty years which have been trying to mimic this behaviour designing the stimuli-responsive polymers. Stimuli-responsive hydrogels exhibiting significant change of properties due to small changes in the external environment conditions (pH, ionic strength, temperature, light wavelength, glucose concentration, magnetic or electric fields, ultrasound, or a combination thereof) were developed. Hydrogels respond to external stimuli is manifested as a change of one or more properties, e.g. volume, swelling degree, shape, surface characteristics, network structure, mechanical properties, permeability, phase transitions, degradation. That is why they are called "intelligent" or "smart" gels (Kumar et al., 2007). Hydrogel properties can be controlled and designed by selection of monomers and synthesis parameters, for example delivery systems for drugs, immobilization of enzymes or microorganisms (Chaterji et al., 2007; Gupta et al., 2002).

Hydrogels are materials that can be designed for use in human medicine. They have an important role in controlling the release rate of drugs, they are increasing the solubility and limiting the degradation and toxicity of drugs. Increasing demands for more effective treatment and rapid development in this area, make smart hydrogels one of the „materials for XXI century". They have elastic properties and soft consistency, which is almost similar to the tissue of a living organism (Peppas et al., 2000). They are inert and compatible with the human body tissues, such as skin, eyes and some internal organs. Due to these unique characteristics and possible applications in the pharmacy, e.g., for modified/controlled drug release, different types of stimuli-responsive hydrogels were synthesized and characterized. Traditional pharmaceutical drug forms with targeted release are not suitable for most drugs, because it does not provide satisfactory stability of drug and adequate download in the systemic circulation (Alvarez-Lorenzo et al., 2009). Sustained release formulations provide an extended and not uniform release and reduces the need for anew drug dosage. Systems for controlled drug release which include speed control and the place of release are most preferred. The drug concentration at the site of action must be maintained over a long period of time at a level that ensures maximum therapeutic level and minimal toxicity. Smart hydrogels are used as carriers to achieve:

- A constant concentration of a therapeutically active compound in the blood with minimal oscillations,
- Predictable and reproductive release over an extended period of time,
- Protection of bioactive compounds with regard to their very short half-life,
- Elimination of the side effects and frequent dosing,
- Optimized therapy and an improved safety profile in patients, and
- Solution for the drugs problem stability (Graham, 1992).

Highly porous hydrogel structures allow the absorption of relatively large quantities of drug. When a drug incorporated in the hydrogel comes into a contact with the aqueous medium, water penetrates in the system and dissolves the drug. The drug diffuses out of the delivery system in the surrounding aqueous medium (Bajpai & Saxena, 2004). Swelling kinetic is very important for hydrogels characterization, as well as the drug release kinetics from the hydrogel as a carrier.

Biodegradability of hydrogels is desirable and is achieved by introducing natural polymers or degradable groups (such as ester, anhydride, and amide) into the main chain. The biodegradable block copolymers based on poly(ethylene glycol) and poly(propylene glycol) and copolymers based on p(NIPAM), poly(acrylamide) and poly(dimethylacrylamide) are useful as drug carriers and enzymes (Ashley et al., 2012). Poly(acrylamide) can be synthesized from the monomer acrylamide (a potent neurotoxin and a carcinogen) in the form of linear chains or crosslinked. It is used for the production of soft contact lenses and to correct defects and deformations of soft tissues. During synthesis, there is a small percentage of acrylamide still present (0.01-0.05%). Poly(acrylamide) hydrogels are not considered hazardous, but several of the identified degradation byproducts are (Chalker-Scott, 2013). In dilute aqueous solution, polyacrylamide polymers are susceptible to chemical, thermal and mechanical degradation. However, crosslinked variants of polyacrylamide showed greater resistance to all of these methods of degradation and have proved much more stable (Sojka et al, 2007). By covalently connecting paclitaxel with a structure that is prone to self-assembling, a hydrogel of paclitaxel can be formed without compromising the activity of the paclitaxel (Gao et al., 2014). The other drug delivery system based on a hydrogel and paclitaxel conjugate layer is spread with a thin film of a 2-methacryloyloxyethyl phosphorylcholine layer (Cho & Hong, 2014). They deliver an endodermis growth inhibitory substance to a target lesion to prevent restenosis of a blood vessel. Hauser and Seow (2014) invented the crosslinked hydrogels comprising a plurality of amphiphilic peptides and/or peptoids capable of self-assembling into three-dimensional macromolecular nanofibrous networks, which entrap water and form hydrogels. These hydrogels have various uses, e.g. as cell culture substrates, as wound dressing, as an implant, for drug and gene delivery, in pharmaceutical or cosmetic compositions, in regenerative medicine, in tissue engineering and tissue regeneration. The biodegradable and injectable hydrogel, comprising thiol group, polyethylene glycol and gold chloride prepared in less than 60 seconds, may be administered as blood vessel sealant, a vessel closing device, or a drug delivery carrier (Mellin et al., 2014). Injectable hydrogels crosslinked *in situ* could be implanted simply by the injection of the solution through a catheter to the target site (Loh et al., 2012). The other example of biodegradable *in situ* crosslinking hydrogel was obtained by gamma-polyglutamic acid and applied to sealants of suppressing the leakage of blood or air during surgical operation, tissue adhesives, anti-adhesive agents and drug delivery carriers (Koh et al., 2012). In addition to these examples of biodegradable hydrogels, there are numerous examples of synthetic non-biodegradable hydrogels, which have important medical applications. In example, the non-degradable drug-eluting optically transparent contact lens was obtained using poly(hydroxyethyl methacrylate), p(HEMA), silicone, agarose, alginate, chitosan and hyaluronic acid and applied as anti-bacterial prototype contact lenses by encapsulating ciprofloxacin-PLGA 65:35 films in p(HEMA) (Ciolino et al., 2014).

Drug Delivery Profiles and Systems

The mode of hydrogel delivery to the human body is significant for implementation. The administration routes of hydrogel-based formulations include transdermal, oral, nasal or parenteral. Drug delivery systems can be classified according to the mechanism controlling the drug release, but most drug delivery devices act by combination mechanisms (Peppas & Khare, 1993; Langer & Peppas, 1983):

- **Diffusion-Controlled Systems:** Where drug diffuses through the polymer, the polymer may undergo subsequent biodegradation on exhaustion of the drug. There are two types:
  - **Reservoir (Membrane Systems, or Laminated Matrix Devices):** Are hollow devices in which an inner core of dissolved, suspended or neat drug is surrounded by a polymer membrane. Drug diffusion through the membrane is rate limiting and controls the overall drug release rate.
  - **Matrix (Monolithic Systems):** Contains drug solution uniformly dissolved or dispersed within the polymer matrix.
- **Chemically Controlled Systems:** Where the release of a pharmacologically active agent usually takes place in the aqueous environment using following systems:
  - **Bioerodible and Biodegradable Systems:** Where the polymer erodes because of the presence of hydrolytically or enzymatically labile bonds. As the polymer erodes, the drug is released to the surrounding medium.

 - **Pendent Chain Systems:** Where the drug molecule is chemically bonded to a polymer backbone and the drug is released by hydrolytic or enzymatic cleavage. The rate of drug release is controlled by the rate of hydrolysis.
 - **Diffusion:** Diffusion of a drug from injectable and biodegradable microbeads.
- **Solvent-Activated Systems:**
 - **Osmotic Controlled Systems:** A semipermeable membrane is used to control the permeation of water. The rate of water influx controls the overall rate of drug release. The release rate remains constant as long as the drug concentration across the membrane is constant. Osmotic drug-delivery systems are capable of providing not only extended time-independent release, but also delivery rates much higher than those achievable by the solution-diffusion mechanism.
 - **Swelling-Controlled Systems:** Hydrogels consist of macromolecular chains crosslinked to create a tangled mesh structure, providing a matrix for the entrapment of drugs. When such hydrogels come in contact with a thermo-dynamically compatible solvent, polymer chains stretched. Swelling is the macroscopic evidence of this transition. The dissolved drug diffuses into the external receiving medium, crossing the swollen polymeric layer formed around the hydrogel.
- **Modulated-Release Systems:** Where the drug is released is controlled by external stimuli such as temperature, pH, ionic strength, an electric field, electromagnetic radiation or UV light, etc. Hydrogels that respond to these external stimuli can be used as controlled/modified release.

The following discussion focuses on different drug delivery systems responsive to external stimuli.

Thermo-Responsive Hydrogels

Thermo-responsive hydrogels are the most studied class of stimuli-responsive hydrogels for the drug release. They are able to swell or contract due to changes in the environmental conditions. Temperature may act as both an external and internal stimulus. Physiologically, thermal stimuli are very important e.g. during a fever there is an elevation of body temperature due to the presence of pyrogens. This elevation in temperature is mediated by an elevated concentration of prostaglandin E2 within certain areas of the brain thus altering the firing rate of neurons that control thermo-regulation (Bawa et al., 2009; Chaterji et al., 2007; Aronoff & Neilson, 2001). Changes in temperature that may trigger drug delivery can be either due to increased body temperature in a disease state, or due to modulated external temperature. A significant feature of these polymers is the presence of hydrophobic groups, e.g. methyl, ethyl and propyl groups. A unique property of temperature-responsive polymers is the presence of a critical solution temperature, which is the temperature at which the phase of polymer and solutions discontinuously changed according to their composition. In relation to the critical temperature of solubility hydrogels were divided into negative and positive thermo-sensitive.

Negative thermo-sensitive hydrogels have a lower critical solution temperature (LCST), which may be defined as the critical temperature below which the polymer swells in the solution, while above it, the polymer contracts. Below the LCST the hydrogen bonding between the polymer and water molecules, is responsible for the polymer swelling. When the temperature is raised above the LCST, a hydrophobic interaction dominates, leading to polymer contraction. The efficiency of the hydrogen bonding process has negative temperature dependency, above the LCST the hydrogen bonds between the monomer side groups and water molecules, which would be increasingly disrupted with increasing temperature (van der Linden et al., 2003).

Positive thermosensitive hydrogel has a higher critical solution temperature (HCST) or upper critical solution temperature (UCST). The hydrogel contracts upon cooling below the UCST. Positive thermosensitive drug release is much more difficult to control than negative release. A hybrid nanogel has been developed based on interpenetrating networks of p(NIPAM) and tailored nano-porous silica (Shinet al., 2001). A sustainable positive thermo-responsive drug release profile is obtained for the drug to slowly diffuse out of the porous channels. Some random copolymers based on acrylamide (AAm) and acrylic acid (AA) microgels of poly(acrylamide–acrylic acid) have also demonstrated some unique UCST properties, though nothing that can be identified as a critical temperature response (Echeverria et al., 2009). The AAm and AA polymer networks may be modified with hydrophobic or hydrophilic comonomers to shift the critical temperature, although the magnitude of collapse diminishes with increasing comonomer concentration (Katono, 1991; Xiao et al., 2003).

Thermosensitive homopolymer of p(NIPAM) has the lower critical solution temperature (LCST) at 32°C (Heskins & Guillet, 1968). This is the most frequently applied hydrogel, because its phase transition occurs at approximately body temperature for the purposes of drug targeting. The phase transition of p(NIPAM-HPMet) hydrogel was detected at 34 °C (Nizam El-Din, 2011; Cai et al., 2001). The phase behavior of linear and chemically cross-linked p(NIPAM) in water was analyzed in terms of the Flory–Huggins–Staverman theory amended with a strong concentration dependent interaction function (Afroze et al, 2000). The analysis established that p(NIPAM)/water is exemplar of Type II phase behavior, indicating that the system does not fit the classic Flory–Huggins scheme of the linear polymer. The peculiar swelling behavior is a direct consequence of the invariant interference of the swelling curve with the liquid–liquid miscibility gap (Afroze et al, 2000). Equilibrium swelling of networks capable of separating into a highly swollen and collapsed phase was discussed by Moerkerke et al (1995). The description of the solvent network binodal was good, but the predicted location of the LCST miscibility gap for linear chains deviates considerably from the measured cloud points. Due to the presence of hydrophilic HPMet monomer the influence of hydrophobic groups of NIPAM monomer was reduced which caused the LCST increase of copolymers p(NIPAM-HPMet) compared to the homopolymer p(NIPAM). The HPMet monomer incorporation in a p(NIPAM) polymer network leads to the increase of number of intramolecular hydrogen bonds in hydrogel (van der Linden et al., 2003). They can additionally be formed between the side -OH groups of HPMet and the electronegative oxygen atom of the ester functional group (of HPMet or EGDM) or electronegative nitrogen atom of the -NH group of NIPAM (Ilić-Stojanović et al., 2014a, 2014c).

Samra et al. (2003) copolymerized *N*-isopropylacrylamide, styrene and *N*-acryloyl hydroxysuccinimide by radical polymerisation. The obtained physically crosslinked copolymer, determined by ^{1}H-NMR and having a distinct phase change at its LCST when existing as a homopolymer. This reversibly crosslinked copolymer was used for a drug or enzyme delivery system. The potential use of thermo-responsive hydrogels based on NIPAM as drug carriers with the aim of modified release of non-steroidal anti-inflammatory drugs: caffeine (Nizam El-Din, 2012), paracetamol, phenacetin, ibuprofen, naproxen and piroxicam was investigated (Ilić-Stojanović et al., 2011, 2012b, 2013, 2014b). The phenacetin was successfully inserted into the p(NIPAM-HPMet) hydrogels cavity by forming intermolecular noncovalent bonds, that was confirmed in the FTIR spectrum of xerogels with loaded phenacetin (Figure 4) (Ilić-Stojanović et al., 2012b).

Figure 4. FTIR Spectra of p(NIPAM-co-HPMet), phenacetin and p(NIPAM-co-HPMet) hydrogel with loaded phenacetin

Source: Ilić-Stojanović et al. (2012b) © [2012] [Association of the Chemical Engineers of Serbia]. Used with permission.

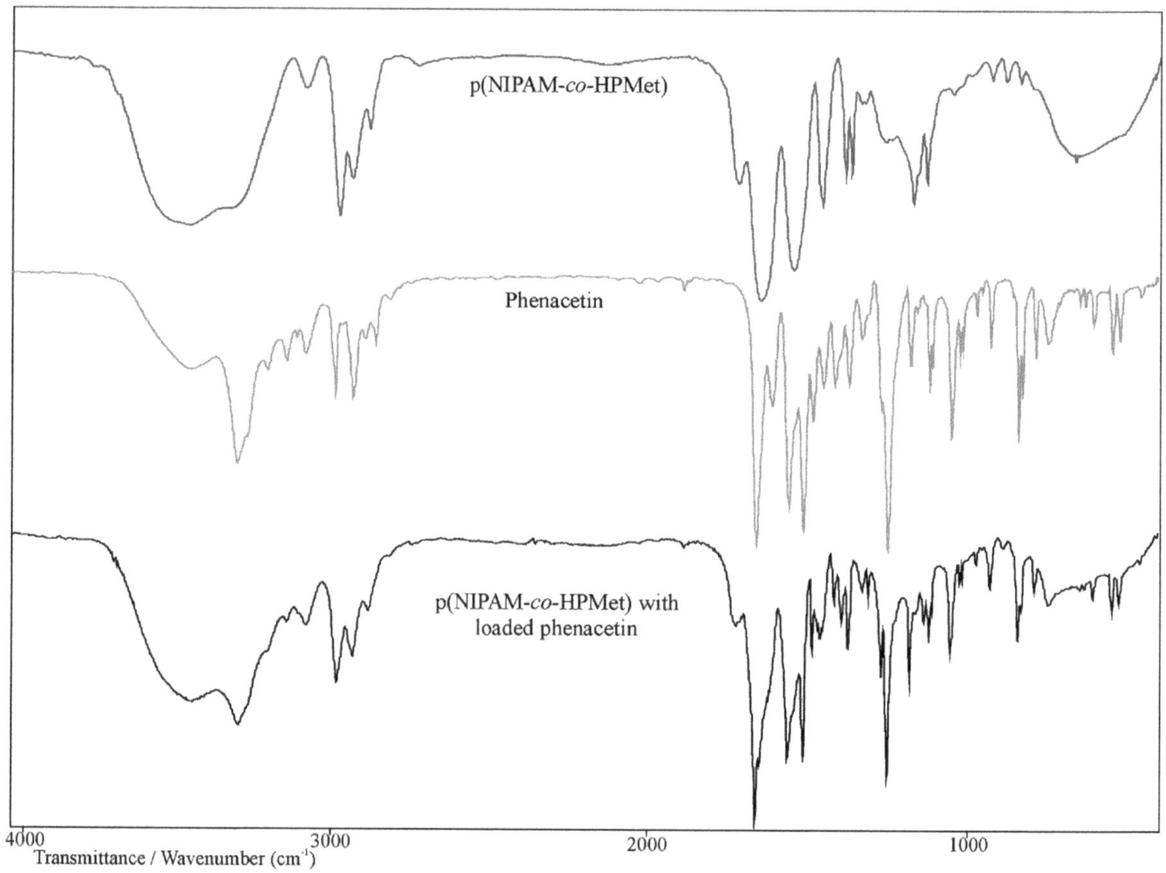

Scanning electron microscopy (SEM) was used to investigate the morphology of p(NIPAM-HPMet) hydrogel. SEM micrographs of p(NIPAM-HPMet) presentthe structure of hydrogel with the characteristic porous surface (Figure 5a) and the hydrogel morphology with the loaded particle of ibuprofen (Figure 5b) (Ilić-Stojanović et al., 2013).

The system based on thermo-responsive poly(*N*-isopropylacrylamide-*co*-acrylamide) allows the controlled release of bioactive molecules with therapeutically effective rate (Mittur, 2009). The problem of incorporation of hydrophobic drugs in hydrogels can be solved by copolymerization of hydrophilic hydrogels with hydrophobic segments, or using amphiphilic interpenetrated polymer networks (Myung et al., 2008, Liu et al., 2006c). The possible application of thermo-responsive hydrogels as carriers of chemotherapeutic agents in the cancer treatment was investigated (Armes, et al., 2007). An acoustically activated delivery of doxorubicin, embedded in the core of the polymer having hydrophobic and hydrophilic blocks, can be an effective method for the targeted drug delivery to tumors (Rapoport & Pitt, 2000). Chen et al. (2013) have designed biocompatible injectable thermoresponsive hydrogel, hyaluronic acid-*g*-chitosan-*g*-poly(*N*-isopropylacrylamide) (HA-CPN) applied as a biomimetic matrix. Embedded biphasic calcium phosphate (BCP) ceramic micoparticles were used to replace mineralized matrix. From *in vivo*

Figure 5. SEM Micrographs of p(NIPAM-co-HPMet): a) pure and b) with loaded ibuprofen
Source: Ilić-Stojanović et al. (2013) © [2013] [Association of the Chemical Engineers of Serbia]. Used with permission.

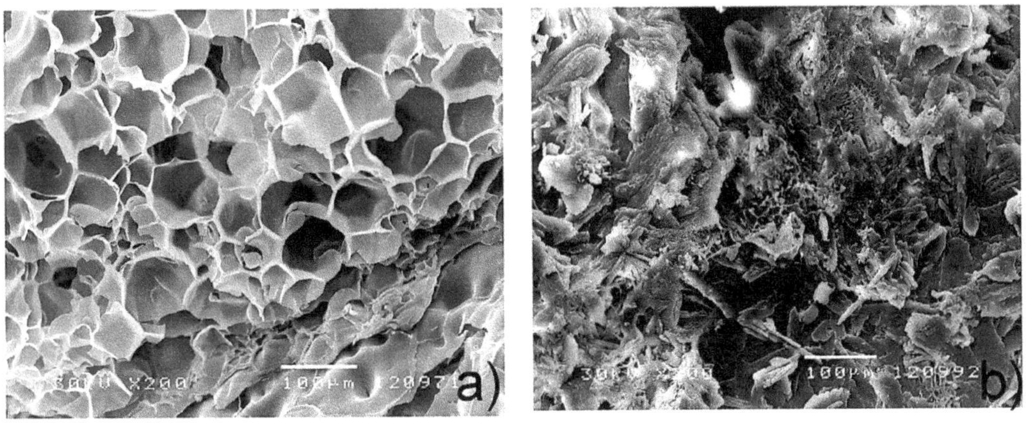

nude mice subcutaneous implantation experiments, the injected cell mass can form ectopic bone tissue in HA-CPN/BCP hydrogel composite. Thermo-responsive hydrogels as a new ocular drug delivery platform to the posterior segment of the eye were synthesized using p(NIPAM) crosslinked with poly(ethylene glycol)diacrylate and then proteins (bovine serum albumin, immunoglobulin G, bevacizumab or ranibizumab) were encapsulated (Derwent & Mieler, 2008). New applications of thermo-responsive hydrogels for ocular delivery were invented (Fedorchak et al., 2014; Ciolino et al., 2014). Anderson and Schindler (2014) disclosed an unusual and novel delivery systems: personal clothing for controlled release of actives (e.g., drug-delivery, cosmetics, alternative medicine). This invention covers a material comprising a unique combination of the thermo-responsive polymer poly(*N*-isopropylacrylamide), crosslinked and water-swollen, with embedded thin platelet-shaped solid crystals, drug-solubilizing microparticles, the drug being released at body temperature.

pH-Responsive Hydrogels

All the pH-responsive hydrogels contain the ionizable functional groups that either accept or release protons in response to changes in environmental pH. Very small changes in pH and/or ionic strength of the medium can cause a significant change in their physical properties, e.g. swelling degree. The polymers with a large number of ionizable groups are known as polyelectrolytes. Cationic hydrogels usually have a side amino group, they swell at pH-values below pKb, and they contract at pH-values above pKb (Korostynska et al., 2007). They can swell and release the drug at a low pH-value, ie. in the stomach. Anionic hydrogels usually contain carboxylic or sulfonic side groups. They swell in the solution at the pH which is above the pKa value, for a given polymer network. The amphiphilic hydrogels contain anionic and cationic side groups (Kathmann et al., 1997). Belonging to this group are polyelectrolytes containing ionized groups in primary or side chains (Koetting et al., 2015).

The pH-sensitive *N*-methacrylamido-*N*'-(6-methoxy-3-pyridazonyl)-sulfonamide was obtained by introduction of sulfonamide groups, various in pKa, to hydrophilic groups of polymers either through coupling into the hydrophilic groups, e.g, acrylamide, *N,N*-dimethylacrylamide, acrylic acid, NIPAM etc., of polymers, or copolymerization with other polymerizing monomers. These hydrogels may change solubility and swelling properties depending on pH, and may have a structure of linear polymer, grafted copolymer, hydrogel or interpenetrating network polymer, applied for a drug-delivery, bio-material, sensors, etc. (Bae & Park, 2000). Diblock copolymer of poly(ethylene oxide-*b*-methacrylic acid) was applied to the pH-dependent release of naproxen, embedded into micelles core (Jin et al., 2009). The paracetamol release from a multifunctional poly(vinilpirolidinon-*co*-polyacrylic acid) hydrogel was tested at pH 2, 6.8 and 9, as well as the thermal and pH-sensitive hydrogels based on NIPAM and itaconic acid (Krušić et al., 2009). The hydrogels based on poly[2-(dimethylamino)ethyl methacrylate] and poly(vinylamine) display basic functional groups such as primary, secondary, and tertiary amine groups that become ionized at low pH values (Kang & Bae, 2001; Korostynska et al., 2007).

Double pH- and Thermo-Responsive Hydrogels

Double pH- and thermo-responsive hydrogels are of special importance for human application, because the temperature and pH value are parameters that most often change in a living organism. They can be obtained by the copolymerization of monomers with ionization and hydrophobic functional groups, combining temperature sensitive polymers with polyelectrolytes, or by development of new monomers that respond simultaneously to both stimuli. IPN hydrogel microspheres composed of crosslinked p(NIPAM) and poly(methacrylic acid) prepared by sequential polymerization method exhibited both temperature- and pH-sensitive volume phase transitions (Ahmad et al., 2014). Spasojević et al. (2015) investigated dual thermo- and pH-responsive antibacterial Ag-poly(*N*-isopropylacrylamide/itaconic acid), p(NIPAM/IA), hydrogel nanocomposites prepared by *in situ* reduction of Ag+ ions with gamma irradiation. By introducing small amounts of itaconic acid, IA, swelling capacity increase, and the volume phase transition temperature of p(NIPAM/IA) copolymers is transferred to higher values. Ag-p(NIPAM/IA) hydrogel nanocomposites showed good antibacterial potentials. There have been many studies on the use of pH and thermo-responsive hydrogels for the drug deliveries. pH and thermo-responsive terpolymers were used for modulated delivery of streptokinase (Vakkalanka et al., 1997), for partitioning of proteins and small biomolecules (Park, 1999; Sassi et al., 1996) or in bioengineering and biotechnology fields (Zhang et al., 2004).

Biomolecule-Responsive Hydrogels

Hydrogels responsive to the biomolecules, change their swelling behavior as response to specific biomolecules (such as glucose, glutathione, antigens, enzyme, ...) and they can be modified to design smart hydroguels that respond to changes in their concentration (Miyata et al., 2002). Hydrogels responsive to glucose have great potential for self-regulated insulin release and to facilitate the construction of artificial pancreas (Bae & Kim, 1993). Many devices have been developed for this purpose and all of them have a glucose sensor built into the system. In the glucose-rich environment, the oxidation of glucose to gluconic acid catalysed by glucose oxidase can lower pH~5.8. This enzyme is probably the most widely used in glucose sensing, and makes possible to apply different types of pH-responsive hydrogels for modulated insulin delivery. Podual et al. (2000) copolymerized diethylaminoethyl methacrylate, poly(ethylene glycol)monomethacrylate and immobilized glucose oxidase and catalase in solution. Hydrogel showed pulsatile swelling behavior which can be effective in the stimulus-responsive release of insulin.

The methods for making enzyme-responsive hydrogels use peptide chains as linkers, either as crosslinks within the hydrogel, or as links between the polymer backbone and drug (Koetting et al., 2015). These peptides are typically made of short sequences chosen to be specifically digestible to certain enzymes, causing hydrogel degradation in the presence of the targeted enzyme. Hydrophilic polymers based on *N*-(2-hydroxypropyl)methacrylamide with anticancer drugs attached *via* short oligopeptide sequences were developed (Kopeček et al., 2000). Peptides have been incorporated into hydrogels as the chemical crosslinker, thus causing gel–sol degradation of the hydrogel upon cleavage by the target enzyme. The use of peptide crosslinkers has been extended to drug delivery systems (Glangchai et al., 2008). The limitations of using peptides for targeting is the difficulty of making large quantities of synthetic peptides, which result in high cost. The application of peptides as crosslinkers, enables targeted degradability. Photometric glucose measurement system was invented using glucose-sensitive hydrogel suitable for implantation to provide *in vivo* monitoring of blood glucose levels in diabetics (Han et al, 2004). The hydrogel contains both glucose binding molecules (e.g. lectin like Concanavalin A, glucokinase, xylose isomerase, isolactin I) and hexose saccharides, chemically or physically immobilized on the hydrogel backbone. Figure 6 shows an example of glucose-sensitive hydrogel filament elongation in the presence of free glucose due to competitive binding to the immobilized glucose binding molecules between the free glucose and the chemically bound glucose in the hydrogel.

Hydrogels Responsive to Electrical Impulses

Hydrogels responsive to electrical impulses are prepared from polyelectrolyte (polymers which contain relatively high concentration of ionisable group along backbone chain) and are thus pH-responsive, as well as electro-responsive (Murdan, 2003). Most of the studied polymers have been polyanions, but polycations and amphoteric polyelectrolyte have been used. The unique morphology and molecular structure of the conducting hydrogels showed unusual electric field responses. Electrically-responsive drug release is influenced by a number of factors, such as the nature of the drug and the hydrogel, the electric field magnitude, the experimental set-up, etc. Electrically controllable, pulsatile drug release from polyelectrolyte hydrogels *in vitro* and *in vivo* (in rats), in response to alternating application and removal of the electric field has been achieved (Murdan, 2003). Responsive drug release from hydrogels results from the electro-induced changes in the hydrogels, which may deswell, swell or erode in response to an electric field. The mechanisms of drug release include ejection of the drug from the gel as the fluid phase synereses out, drug diffusion along a concentration gradient, electrophoresis of charged drugs towards an oppositely charged electrode and liberation of the entrapped drug as the hydrogel complex erodes.

Figure 6. A competitive binding-type hydrogel based on Concanavalin A, and its swelling mechanism
Adapted from Han et al. (2004).

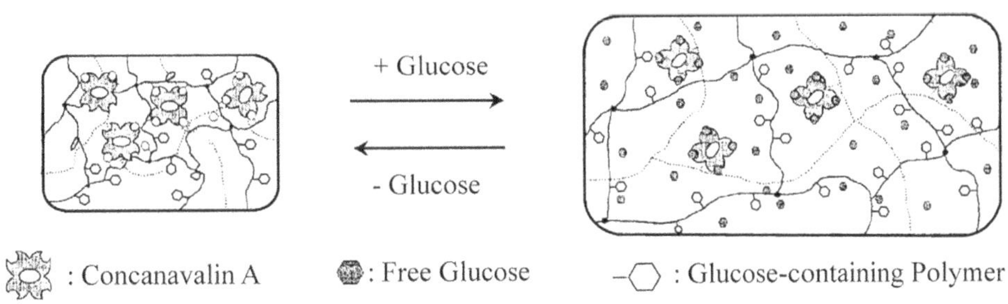

The ionization and ion exchange kinetics of the pH-responsive hydrogels can be controlled by applying an electric voltage across the hydrogel. The electrical stimulus increases the rate of drug diffusion to the target site. There have been several studies on the use of electric current *in vivo*, through iontophoresis and electroporation mechanisms, for dermal and transdermal drug deliveries. Sawahata et al. (1990) examined glucose and insulin release from pMAA gels by switching the electric field alternately on and off. The synthesis, structure and electric field sensitivity of polyacrylate/polyaniline and poly(2-acrylamido-2-methyl propylsulfonic acid-acrylic acid)/polyaniline conducting hydrogels with an interpenetrating polymer network structure was studied by Lin et al. (2009). The electric field response was improved by increasing aniline dosage, applied voltage and concentration of aqueous NaCl solution. The bending mechanism was attributed to polyelectrolyte hydrogel matrix and emeraldine polyaniline nanofibers. The development of electrically controlled release of Aloe-vera extraction, aloein, from poly(acrylamide hydrogel) system as transdermal drug delivery patch was studied by Niamlang et al. (2011). A novel electric-field responsive microsystem for controllable miniaturised drug delivery applications have been developed (Liu et al., 2011). The release rate and dose of hematoxylin as model of hydrophilic drug was accurately controlled at 37°C under voltage of 20 V. A hydrogel pharmaceutical dosage form for drug delivery (comprising polyethyleneimine and 1-vinylimidazole forming an electro-responsive matrix, polyacrylic acid and/or polyvinyl alcohol) to the target site was invented (Pillay et al., 2014). *In vivo* studies revealed a good preliminary indication, facilitating the immediate release of the entrapped indometacin into the tissues and will significantly desensitize chronic pain to the patient.

Current implantable electronic delivery systems are not biodegradable and often require additional components while extended- or controllable-release polymeric systems used not to allow switchable release profiles. The use of conductive polymers in delivery systems has been restricted due to limitations in the choice of dopant and the molecular weight of the delivered drug. Conducting polymers (e.g., polypyrrole, PPy) offers the possibility of controllable drug administration through electrical stimulation (Miller, 1988). PPy's favorable biocompatibility also makes it an ideal electroactive polymer for drug delivery (Wang et al., 2004). Polypyrrole can be made in degradable forms that enhance its value for these biomedical applications. To circumvent these barriers, a method has been developed for attaching molecules to the surface of PPy through biotin–streptavidin coupling (George et al., 2006). After attachment of streptavidin to the biotin dopant, drug release was triggered through electrical stimulation (Figure 7). This method provides a novel platform for controlled drug delivery from a conductive carrier.

Juntanon et al. (2008) studied electrically controlled release of sulfosalicylic acid from crosslinked poly(vinyl alcohol) hydrogelas the matrix/carriers. They found that the release rate of sulfosalicylic acid can be altered and controlled precisely through electric field stimulation. Electrical sensitive behavior of poly(*N*-vinylpyrrolidone-*co*-acrylic acid) hydrogel showed flexible chain nature (Jin et al., 2006). In the electric field, the gel bent toward cathode independently of the pH of buffer solution, applied voltage, crosslinking extent and polyion content in the backbone of the gel. Bending of prepared hydrogel was reinterpreted by bending theory of polyelectrolyte gel based upon the change of osmotic pressure, which is due to the difference of ion concentration between the sides facing anode and cathode. Moon et al. (2015) examined conducting poly(*N*-methylaniline)-coated crosslinked poly(methyl methacrylate) nanoparticle suspension and its steady shear response under electric fields.

Figure 7. Stimulated nerve growth factor (NGF) release. a) Voltage applied across the polymer in PBS solution causes the release of the biotin from the PPy surface. b) A 3 V stimulation of the PPy showed an increase in the amount of NGF released from the surface of the conductive polymer. Short stimulations of 30 s did not result in as much release as long stimulations of 150 s. The asterisk indicates a statistical difference versus short stimulation, no stimulation, and no biotin dopant (p< .05).
Source: George et al. (2006) © [2006] [WILEY-VCH Verlag GmbH & Co. KGaA]. Used with permission.

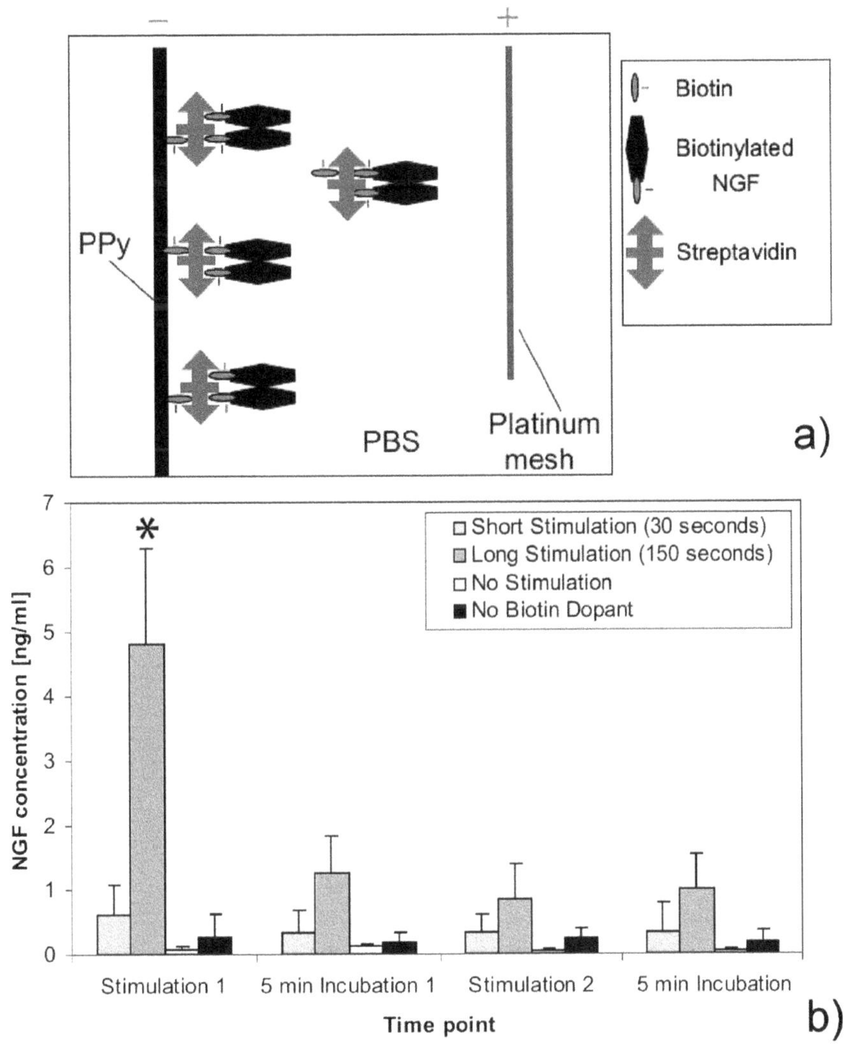

Hydrogels Responsive to Magnetic Fields

Hydrogels responsive to changes in magnetic fields, called ferrogels, include hydrogels which have the magnetic nanoparticles in their structure. They have shown the ability to trigger the drug release after applying an external magnetic stimulation (Liu et al., 2006). The magnetic hydrogels were fabricated by chemically crosslinking of gelatin hydrogels and Fe_3O_4 nanoparticles through genipin as crosslinking agent. *In vitro* release rate of vitamin B_{12} from hydrogels was considerably decreased as compared with those when the field was turned off, suggesting a close configuration of hydrogels as a result of aggregation of Fe_3O_4 nanoparticles. Based on this on-&-off mechanism, the smart magnetic hydrogels based on the gelatin-ferrite hybrid composites can be potentially developed for application in novel drug delivery systems. Materials producing strain in magnetic fields are known as magnetoelastic or magnetostrictive materials. Zrinyi et al. (1996) have prepared magnetic field responsive polymer hydrogels by introducing monodomain, magnetite nanoparticles into chemically crosslinked poly(viny1 alcohol) hydrogels. Zrinyi et al. (1997) have demonstrated the influence of a non-uniform external magnetic field on the gel tubes shape. They showed that both concentration of magnetite particles and the crosslinking density of the ferrogels play an essential role. Magnetic field responsive functional elastomers with tunable elastic modulus were analysed (Varga et al., 2006). An effective approach to creation, as targeted, nanocarriers for doxorubicin delivery using magnetic iron oxide nanoparticles coated with integrin-targeted and matrix-metalloproteinase-sensitive PEG hydrogel scaffolds was developed by Nazli et al. (2014). The functional PEG hydrogel coating has been designed for active loading as well as triggered intra-cellular release of the cancer therapeutic agent doxorubicin. Nowel starch-based hydrogel nanocomposites responding to both pH and a remote magnetic field have been designed (Lima-Tenório, et al., 2015). Supermagnetic iron oxide nanocomposite hydrogel based on graft copolymerization of poly((2-dimethylamino) ethylmethacrylate) onto salep for controlled release of drug was synthesized (Bardajee et al., 2014). The antibacterial activity and cytotoxicity studies of it suggested that the prepared hydrogel could be a promising candidate for biological dressing applications.

Hydrogels Responsive to the Light

Hydrogels responsive to the light respond to light energy by way of a reaction, which can be a variety of degradation and bonding reactions. Photo-dependent reaction rates have shown strong correlations to the energy and irradiance of light (DeForest & Anseth, 2011). Due to the inability of UV and visual electromagnetic wavelengths to penetrate tissue, these mechanisms are only really viable for *ex vivo* systems and skin level treatments in *in vivo* models. The relative response of these hydrogels can be well characterized and standardized by intensity of emitted light. The other simplification that hydrogel systems allow for photoreactive systems is the relatively low diffusion rates of molecules through the system. When a secondary molecule is involved, the rate of diffusion from the activated location can lead to bleeding over in photochemical reactions. Photo-responsive monomers can be incorporated as both crosslinkers and as pendant groups by the mechanisms of isomerization, degradation, and dimerization (Koetting et al., 2015). Isomerization monomers can be further classified as either a *cis–trans* shift or cyclization. One of the more common structures that utilizes a *cis–trans* shift in order to exhibit drastic differences in polarity and hydrophobicity are azobenzenes. Azobenzenes have been incorporated as both monomers and crosslinkers into hydrogels to induce a photo-responsive phase shift (Barrett et al., 2007). The azobenzene systems bring reversibility to their stacking, shifting from *trans* to *cis* forms and back in response to 360 and 440 nm light, respectively (Kageyama et al., 2013). Degradation depends on the breakdown of covalent bonds. The most common group utilized for photodegradable moieties is the *o*-methoxy nitro-benzene family of monomers. The wavelength of light that these monomers respond to can also be manipulated by the functionalization of the benzene group (Fomina et al., 2010). Dimerization and degradation are often both available in response to different wavelengths of light and require the presence of a catalyst. A large number of these reactions depends on cyclization of two double bonds. Coumarin is a common molecule that provides for effective dimerization route (Chujo et al., 1990).

Hydrogels responsive to the change in light intensity are used in the development of photosensitive devices, especially in systems for ophthalmic drugs delivery (Kashyap et al., 2005). Photo-crosslinked hydrogel materials based in gellan gum suitable for tissue engineering and regenerative medicine, or as drug delivery systems were invented (Figure 8) (Correia et al., 2015). The materials are capable of free radical polymerization with a photo-initiator at mild temperatures and exposure to ultraviolet light, enabling the control of reticulation and withstanding the encapsulation of human and animal cells and/ or drugs.

The potential application of photo-responsive hydrogels can be applied in the development of visible light-responsive artificial muscles, switches and memory devices (Suzuki & Tanaka, 1990), for temporal drug delivery based on the response of crosslinked hyaluronic acid hydrogels that undergo photosensitized degradation of p(NIPAM) under the influence of infrared light, in the presence of methylene blue (Zhang et al., 1995). While the action of stimulus is instantaneous, the reaction of hydrogels in response

Figure 8. The strategy for development of injectable photo-crosslinkable scaffolds, based on methacrylate modification with glycidyl methacrylate (GMA) and in situ photo-polymerization of gellan gum
Adapted from Correia et al. (2015).

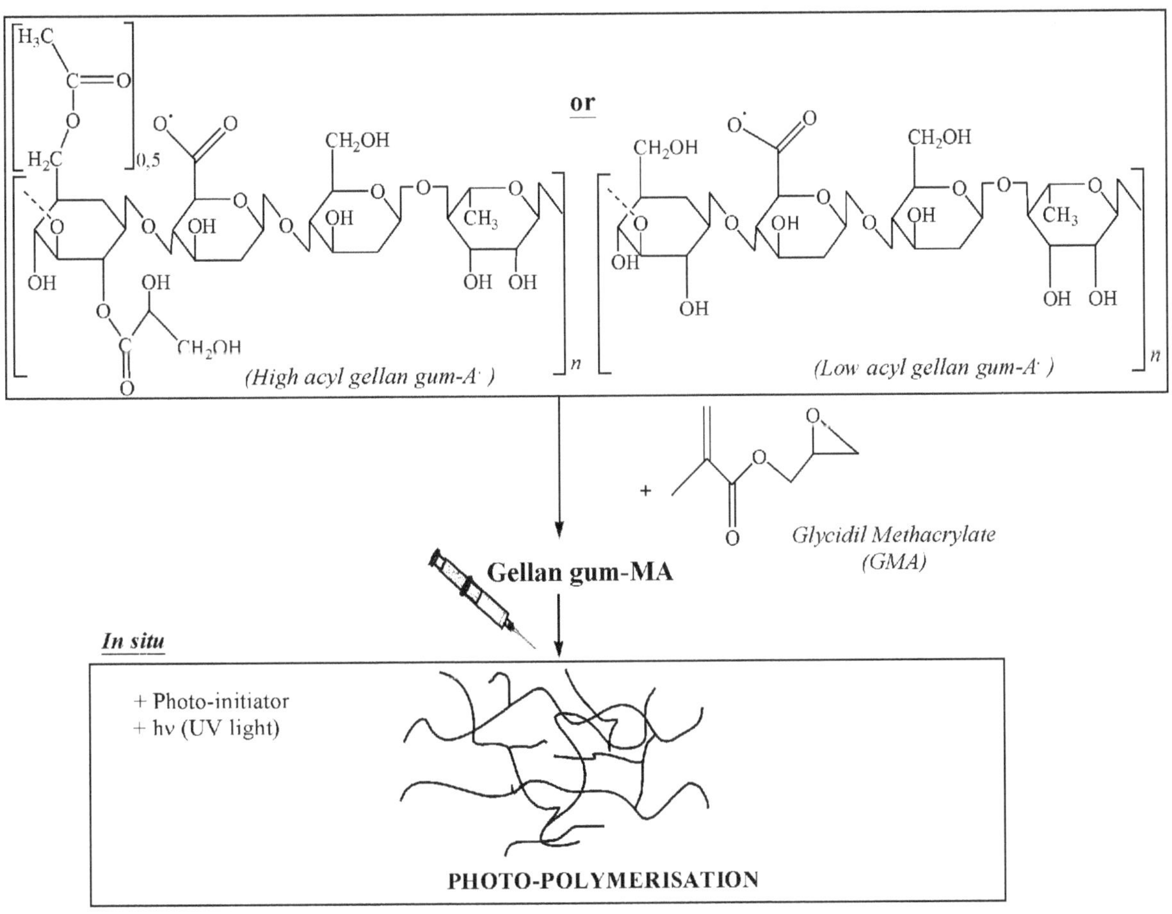

to such action is still slow. In most cases, the conversion of light into thermal energy must precede the restructuring of polymer chains upon temperature change. In addition, unless chromophores are covalently linked to the polymer backbone, they can be leached out during swelling–deswelling cycles (Qiu & Park, 2012).

Hydrogels Responsive to the Pressure

The pressure may stimulate volume phase transition of hydrogel and therefore it can be used in the drugs delivery systems sensitive to the pressure change (Kashyap et al. 2005). Stimulus responsive hydrogels can provide the actuation pressure required for both valving and dispensing functions in the device (Eddington & Beebe 2004). The microdispensing device used an array of responsive hydrogels to deform a flexible membrane above a fluid reservoir chamber. When the microvalve is open, the deformation of the membrane reduces the volume of the reservoir chamber and pushes fluid through the microvalve. When the microvalve is closed, the expanding hydrogel array generates a storable pressure source that results in fluid dispensing once the microvalve is opened.

Hydrogels sensitive to the pressure change are thermo- and/or pH-responsive where response to changes in temperature or pH is significantly altered by changing the pressure or ionic strength in the solution (Qiu & Park, 2012; Shafer-Peltier et al., 2003). According to the thermodynamic calculations based on uncharged theory, hydrogels may undergo pressure-induced volume phase transition. The swelling degree of poly(*N*-n-propylacrylamide), poly(*N,N*-diethylacrylamide) and poly(N-isopropylacrylamide) hydrogels increased under hydrostatic pressure when the temperature is close to its LCST and collapsed at low pressure (Lee et al., 1990; Zhong et al., 1996). A measurement concept has been realized for the detection of carbon dioxide, where the CO_2 induced pressure generation by an enclosed pH-sensitive hydrogel is measured with a micropressure sensor (Herber et al., 2005). The application of the sensor is the quantification of the partial pressure of CO_2 (Pco_2) in the stomach as diagnosis for gastrointestinal ischemia.

Hydrogels Responsive to Ultrasound

Ultrasound is used for drug penetration improvement through biological barriers. By using hydrogels responsive to ultrasound, "on/off" pulsatile drug delivery can be achieved. Pulsatile release of insulin after exposure to ultrasound causes a perturbation of methylene chains and release of insulin (Kashyap et al., 2005). A drug-containing polymeric monolith coated with a novel ultrasound-responsive coating was developed by Kwok et al. (2001). Ultrasound release studies showed that a copolymer of 2-hydroxyethyl methacrylate and ethylene glycol dimethacrylate coated with an ultrasound-responsive membrane maintained sufficient insulin for multiple insulin delivery. With appropriate surface coating coverage, the background leach rate can be precisely controlled. Miyazaki et al. (1988) developed a hydrophilic polymer implant capable of delivering insulin *in vivo* at increased rates on demand by an external ultrasound irradiation. When the diabetic rats, receiving implants containing insulin, were exposed to an ultrasound irradiation, a rapid rate of release of insulin was observed in the implanted site. Also, *in vitro* investigation of the ultrasound effects on degradable polymer polyanhydride matrices have been developed by D'Emanuele et al. (1992).

SOLUTIONS AND RECOMMENDATIONS

This chapter provides only an insight into the complexities and the application, striving to illustrate the versatility and potential of smart hydrogels. Researchers are increasingly paying attention to a drug delivery to a specific place in the body and once there, to be more accessible to use.

Nowadays, the concept of drugs distribution is not limited to time control of drug release. The spatial distribution control that allows the drug delivery at the target site of action is very important. The most hydrogels are capable of releasing drugs either continuously or intermittently, having accurate, but desired release rates to be a major improvement. Tissue engineering and targeted drugs delivery provide opportunities to design systems based on "intelligent" gels. The application of "smart" hydrogels for the modern medications development has growing significance, because of their availability and desired properties. The enhanced control enable ground breaking advances in healthcare, allowing for more effective treatment in a vast array of diseases.

Hydrogels responsive to biomolecules, such as glucose or antigens, can be used as biosensors in drug delivery systems. Light-responsive, magnetic field sensitive and electro-responsive hydrogels also have potential to be used in drug delivery.

The essential benefits of application of stimuli responsive hydrogels in pharmaceutical field comprise their biocompatibility, possibility for injected *in vivo* (in a whole, living organism) as a liquid, and then forms gels at body temperature, protect cells, have good transport properties, modified/controled release of drugs, easy to modify, can be biodegradable.

The main limitations for application of hydrogels are high cost, low mechanical strength, may be hard to handle, too fragile, difficult for incorporation of drugs/nutrients, may be difficult to sterilize, necessary to remove the residual reactants and impurities, non-adherent.

FUTURE RESEARCH DIRECTIONS

Novel strategies for the design and synthesis of efficient, biocompatible hydrogels will facilitate the creation of new classes of biomaterials for pharmaceutical application. Smart hydrogels have very significant role in the development of advanced drugs delivery that may effectively deliver a wide range of therapeutic molecules (e.g. proteins, nucleic acids, peptides, antibiotics). They may be used as carriers for specific drug delivery in tissue and cell.

The rapid development of novel hydrogel synthesis and the polymerization methods imply to further fast development of new generation of smart hydrogels as carriers with well designed structure which can utilize physiological signals to induce the modified drug release. Also, bone replacement therapy, soft tissue engineering are other fields where hydrogels might find plausible applications.

The next generation of stimuli-responsive hydrogels as drug carriers will have a hybrid composition that combines hydrogels with biological motifs to complementary exploit natural transport mechanisms to reach target place and natural elimination pathways. Stimuli-responsive hydrogels for pharmaceutical applications also require biocompatibility. Synthesis of new polymers and crosslinkers with more biocompatibility and better biodegradability would be essential for successful applications.

CONCLUSION

Requirements for obtaining smart gels are not only directed to formulations of therapeutic agents in biocompatible smart hydrogels, but also to research the benefits of application. This is the reason why this is a multidisciplinary research which links new intelligent materials design with fundamental disciplines, such as chemistry, biology and bioengineering. Smart hydrogels have many different physical and chemical properties, chemical structure and obtainable technology and they have a great potential for application in the pharmaceutics. The application of hydrogels is very promising and at the beginning of the development and exploitation. Although the synthesis and *in vitro* hydrogel tests look simple, from the point of *in vivo* application, they require extensive testing prior to commercial applications. Mass production and further development could reduce the cost and enable wider application in securing drug delivery systems.

REFERENCES

Afroze, F., Nies, E., & Berghmans, H. (2000). Phase transitions in the system poly (*N*-isopropylacrylamide)/water and swelling behaviour of the corresponding networks. *Journal of Molecular Structure*, *554*(1), 55–68. doi:10.1016/S0022-2860(00)00559-7

Aguilar, M. R., Elvira, C., Gallardo, A., Vázquez, B., & Román, J. S. (2007). Smart polymers and their applications as biomaterials. Topics in Tissue Engineering, 3(6).

Ahmad, H., Nurunnabi, M., Rahman, M. M., Kumar, K., Tauer, K., Minami, H., & Gafur, M. A. (2014). Magnetically doped multi stimuli-responsive hydrogel microspheres with IPN structure and application in dye removal. *Colloids and Surfaces. A, Physicochemical and Engineering Aspects*, *459*, 39–47. doi:10.1016/j.colsurfa.2014.06.038

Alvarez-Lorenzo, C., Bromberg, L., & Concheiro, A. (2009). Light-sensitive intelligent drug delivery systems. *Photochemistry and Photobiology*, *85*(4), 848–860. doi:10.1111/j.1751-1097.2008.00530.x PMID:19222790

Anderson, D., & Schindler, J. (2014). *U.S. Patent Application 14/213,808*. Washington, DC: U.S. Patent and Trademark Office.

Armes, S. P., Madsen, P. J., Vo, C.-D., & Li, C. (2007). *WO Patent Application 07/063320*.

Aronoff, D. M., & Neilson, E. G. (2001). Antipyretics: Mechanisms of action and clinical use in fever suppression. *The American Journal of Medicine*, *111*(4), 304–315. doi:10.1016/S0002-9343(01)00834-8 PMID:11566461

Ashley, G. W., Santi, D. V., & Henise, J. C. (2012). *U.S. Patent Application 14/343,819*. Washington, DC: U.S. Patent and Trademark Office.

Bae, Y. H., & Kim, S. W. (1993). *U.S. Patent No. 5,262,055*. Washington, DC: U.S. Patent and Trademark Office.

Bae, Y. H., & Park, S. Y. (2000). *U.S. Patent No. 6,103,865*. Washington, DC: U.S. Patent and Trademark Office.

Bajpai, S. K., & Saxena, S. (2004). Enzymatically degradable and pH-sensitive hydrogels for colon-targeted oral drug delivery. I. Synthesis and characterization. *Journal of Applied Polymer Science*, *92*(6), 3630–3643. doi:10.1002/app.20283

Bardajee, G. R., Hooshyar, Z., Asli, M. J., Shahidi, F. E., & Dianatnejad, N. (2014). Synthesis of a novel supermagnetic iron oxide nanocomposite hydrogel based on graft copolymerization of poly((2-dimethylamino)ethyl methacrylate) onto salep for controlled release of drug. *Materials Science and Engineering C*, *36*, 277–286. doi:10.1016/j.msec.2013.11.022 PMID:24433913

Barrett, C. J., Mamiya, J. I., Yager, K. G., & Ikeda, T. (2007). Photo-mechanical effects in azobenzene-containing soft materials. *Soft Matter*, *3*(10), 1249–1261. doi:10.1039/b705619b

Bawa, P., Pillay, V., Choonara, Y. E., & Du Toit, L. C. (2009). Stimuli-responsive polymers and their applications in drug delivery. *Biomedical Materials (Bristol, England)*, *4*(2), 022001. doi:10.1088/1748-6041/4/2/022001 PMID:19261988

Cai, W., Anderson, E. C., & Gupta, R. B. (2001). Separation of lignin from aqueous mixtures by ionic and nonionic temperature-sensitive hydrogels. *Industrial & Engineering Chemistry Research*, *40*(10), 2283–2288. doi:10.1021/ie0009435

Chalker-Scott, L. (2013). The Myth of Polyacrylamide Hydrogels. In *The informed gardener*. Washington, DC: University of Washington Press.

Chaterji, S., Kwon, I. K., & Park, K. (2007). Smart polymeric gels: Redefining the limits of biomedical devices. *Progress in Polymer Science*, *32*(8), 1083–1122. doi:10.1016/j.progpolymsci.2007.05.018 PMID:18670584

Chen, J. P., Tsai, M. J., & Liao, H. T. (2013). Incorporation of biphasic calcium phosphate microparticles in injectable thermoresponsive hydrogel modulates bone cell proliferation and differentiation. *Colloids and Surfaces. B, Biointerfaces*, *110*, 120 129. PMID:23711782

Cho, Z. K., & Hong, S. K. (2014). *Patent Application KR 2014/0115542*. Lead Biotech Co Ltd.

Chujo, Y., Sada, K., & Saegusa, T. (1990). Polyoxazoline having a coumarin moiety as a pendant group. Synthesis and photogelation. *Macromolecules*, *23*(10), 2693–2697. doi:10.1021/ma00212a017

Ciolino, J. B., Hoare, T. R., & Kohane, D. S. (2014). *Patent Application AU 2014/215997*, Massachusetts Inst. Technology.

Correia, J. C. D. S., de Oliveira, J. M. A., De Oliveira, J. M. T., De Sousa, R. P. A. R., & Dos Reis, R. L. G. (2015). *U.S. Patent No. 9,012,415*. Washington, DC: U.S. Patent and Trademark Office.

D'Emanuele, A., Kost, J., Hill, J. L., & Langer, R. (1992). An investigation of the effects of ultrasound on degradable polyanhydride matrices. *Macromolecules*, *25*(2), 511–515. doi:10.1021/ma00028a002

DeForest, C. A., & Anseth, K. S. (2011). Cytocompatible click-based hydrogels with dynamically tunable properties through orthogonal photoconjugation and photocleavage reactions. *Nature Chemistry*, *3*(12), 925–931. doi:10.1038/nchem.1174 PMID:22109271

Derwent, J. J. K., & Mieler, W. F. (2008). Thermoresponsive hydrogels as a new ocular drug delivery platform to the posterior segment of the eye. *Transactions of the American Ophthalmological Society*, *106*, 206. PMID:19277236

Dušek, K., & Prins, W. (1969). *Structure and elasticity of non-crystalline polymer networks*. Springer Berlin Heidelberg.

Echeverria, C., López, D., & Mijangos, C. (2009). UCST responsive microgels of poly (acrylamide–acrylic acid) copolymers: Structure and viscoelastic properties. *Macromolecules*, *42*(22), 9118–9123. doi:10.1021/ma901316k

Eddington, D. T., & Beebe, D. J. (2004). A valved responsive hydrogel microdispensing device with integrated pressure source. *Journal of Microelectromechanical Systems*, *13*(4), 586–593. doi:10.1109/JMEMS.2004.832190

Fedorchak, M. V., Little, S. R., Schuman, J. S., & Cugini, A. (2014). *WO Patent Application 14/138085*.

Ferry, J. D. (1980). *Viscoelastic Properties of Polymers*. New York, NY: Wiley.

Flory, P. J., & Rehner, J. Jr. (1943). Statistical mechanics of cross-linked polymer networks II. Swelling. *The Journal of Chemical Physics*, *11*(11), 521–526. doi:10.1063/1.1723792

Fomina, N., McFearin, C., Sermsakdi, M., Edigin, O., & Almutairi, A. (2010). UV and near-IR triggered release from polymeric nanoparticles. *Journal of the American Chemical Society*, *132*(28), 9540–9542. doi:10.1021/ja102595j PMID:20568765

Gao, Y., Kuang, Y., & Xu, B. (2014). *U.S. Patent No. 8,658,600*. Washington, DC: U.S. Patent and Trademark Office.

George, P. M., LaVan, D. A., Burdick, J. A., Chen, C. Y., Liang, E., & Langer, R. (2006). Electrically Controlled Drug Delivery from Biotin-Doped Conductive Polypyrrole. *Advanced Materials*, *18*(5), 577–581. doi:10.1002/adma.200501242

Ghizal, R., Fatima, G. R., & Srivastava, S. (2014). Smart Polymers and Their Applications. *International Journal of Engineering Technology. Management and Applied Sciences*, *2*(4), 104–115.

Glangchai, L. C., Caldorera-Moore, M., Shi, L., & Roy, K. (2008). Nanoimprint lithography based fabrication of shape-specific, enzymatically-triggered smart nanoparticles. *Journal of Controlled Release*, *125*(3), 263–272. doi:10.1016/j.jconrel.2007.10.021 PMID:18053607

Graham, N. B. (1992). Poly(ethylene glycol) chemistry. In J. M. Harris (Ed.), *Biotechnical and biomedical application* (pp. 1–13). New York, NY: Plenum Press.

Graham, T. (1861). On liquid transpiration in relation to chemical composition. *Philosophical Transactions of the Royal Society*, *151*, 183–224. doi:10.1098/rstl.1861.0011

Graham, T. (1864). On the properties of silicic acid and other analogous colloidal substances. *Journal of the Chemical Society of London*, *17*, 318–327.

Grant, R., & Grant, C. (Eds.). (1987). *Grant & Hackh's Chemical Dictionary* (5th ed.). New York, NY: McGraw-Hill.

Gupta, P., Vermani, K., & Garg, S. (2002). Hydrogels: From controlled release to pH-responsive drug delivery. *Drug Discovery Today*, *7*(10), 569–579. doi:10.1016/S1359-6446(02)02255-9 PMID:12047857

Han, I. S., Lew, S., & Han, M. H. (2004). *U.S. Patent No. 6,835,553*. Washington, DC: U.S. Patent and Trademark Office.

Hauser, C., & Seow, W. Y. (2014). *WO Patent Application 2014/116187*. Agency For Science, Technology and Research, SG.

Herber, S., Bomer, J., Olthuis, W., Bergveld, P., & Van Den Berg, A. (2005). A miniaturized carbon dioxide gas sensor based on sensing of pH-sensitive hydrogel swelling with a pressure sensor. *Biomedical Microdevices*, *7*(3), 197–204. doi:10.1007/s10544-005-3026-5 PMID:16133807

Heskins, M., & Guillet, J. E. (1968). Solution properties of poly (*N*-isopropylacrylamide). *Journal of Macromolecular Science. Chemistry*, *2*(8), 1441–1455. doi:10.1080/10601326808051910

Hoffman, A. S. (2012). Hydrogels for biomedical applications. *Advanced Drug Delivery Reviews*, *64*, 18–23. doi:10.1016/j.addr.2012.09.010 PMID:11755703

Ilić-Stojanović, S. (2015). *Synthesis and characterization of negatively thermosensitive hydrogels*. Saarbrücken, Germany: LAP Lambert Academic Publishing, Akademikeverlag GmbH & Co. KG.

Ilić-Stojanović, S., Mladenović-Ranisavljević, I., Nikolić, V., Takić, L., Stojiljković, D., Stojiljković, S., & Nikolić, L. (2011). Thermo-responsive hydrogels for controlled release of paracetamol, In *Proceedings of 43rd International October Conference on Mining and Metallurgy* (pp. 707-710). Kladovo, Republic of Serbia: University of Belgrade Technical Faculty in Bor.

Ilić-Stojanović, S., Nikolić, L., Nikolić, V., Petrović, S. D., & Stanković, M. (2014). *RS Patent No. 53220 B*. The Intellectual Property Office of the Republic of Serbia.

Ilić-Stojanović, S., Nikolić, L., Nikolić, V., Ristić, I., Budinski-Simendić, J., Kapor, A., & Nikolić, G. M. (2014). The structure characterization of thermosensitive poly(*N*-isopropylacrylamide-*co*-2-hydroxypropyl methacrylate) hydrogel. *Polymer International*, *63*(6), 973–981. doi:10.1002/pi.4589

Ilić-Stojanović, S. S., Nikolić, L., Nikolić, V., Stanković, M., Stamenković, J., Mladenović-Ranisavljević, I., & Petrović, S. D. (2012). Influence of monomer and crosslinker molar ratio on the swelling behaviour of thermosensitive hydrogels. *Chemical Industry & Chemical Engineering Quarterly*, *18*(1), 1–9. doi:10.2298/CICEQ110711040I

Ilić-Stojanović, S. S., Nikolić, L. B., Nikolić, V. D., Milić, J. R., Petrović, S. D., Nikolić, G. M., & Kapor, A. J. (2012). Potential application of thermo-sensitive hydrogels for controlled release of phenacetin. *Hem. Ind.*, *66*(6), 831–839. doi:10.2298/HEMIND120222089I

Ilić-Stojanović, S. S., Nikolić, L. B., Nikolić, V. D., Milić, J. R., Stamenković, J., Nikolić, G. M., & Petrović, S. D. (2013). Synthesis and characterization of thermosensitive hydrogels and the investigation of modified release of ibuprofen. *Hem. Ind.*, *67*(6), 901–912. doi:10.2298/HEMIND130119038I

Ilić-Stojanović, S. S., Nikolić, L. B., Nikolić, V. D., Petrović, S. D., Zdravković, A. S., & Stamenković, J. V. (2014). The effect of the crosslinker content on the swelling properties of intelligent gels. *Advanced Technologies*, *3*(2), 10–15.

Jagur-Grodzinski, J. (2010). Polymeric gels and hydrogels for biomedical and pharmaceutical applications. *Polymers for Advanced Technologies*, *21*(1), 27–47.

Jin, G. W., Ji, X. Y., & Choi, J. S. (2009). Preparation of naproxen-loaded poly(ethylene oxide-b-methacrylic acid) micelle and its pH-dependent drug release behavior. *Bulletin of the Korean Chemical Society*, *30*(4), 931–934. doi:10.5012/bkcs.2009.30.4.931

Jin, S., Gu, J., Shi, Y., Shao, K., Yu, X., & Yue, G. (2013). Preparation and electrical sensitive behavior of poly(*N*-vinylpyrrolidone-co-acrylic acid) hydrogel with flexible chain nature. *European Polymer Journal*, *49*(7), 1871–1880. doi:10.1016/j.eurpolymj.2013.04.022

Jones, R. G., Wilks, E. S., Metanomski, W. V., Kahovec, J., Hess, M., Stepto, R., & Kitayama, T. (2009). *Compendium of Polymer Terminology and Nomenclature: IUPAC Recommendations 2008* (p. 443). Cambridge, UK: Royal Society of Chemistry. doi:10.1039/9781847559425

Jordan-Lloyd, D. (1926). Article. In J. Alexander (Ed.), Colloid Chemistry (Vol. 1, pp. 767–782). New York, NY: The Chemical Catalogue Company.

Juntanon, K., Niamlang, S., Rujiravanit, R., & Sirivat, A. (2008). Electrically controlled release of sulfosalicylic acid from crosslinked poly(vinyl alcohol) hydrogel. *International Journal of Pharmaceutics*, *356*(1), 1–11. doi:10.1016/j.ijpharm.2007.12.023 PMID:18242901

Kabiri, K., Hesarian, S., Jamshidi, A., Zohuriaan-Mehr, M. J., Boohendi, H., Poorheravi, M. R., & Ahmad-Khanbeigi, F. et al. (2011). Minimization of residual monomer content of superabsorbent hydrogels *via* alteration of initiating system. *Journal of Applied Polymer Science*, *120*(5), 2716–2723. doi:10.1002/app.33431

Kageyama, Y., Tanigake, N., Kurokome, Y., Iwaki, S., Takeda, S., Suzuki, K., & Sugawara, T. (2013). Macroscopic motion of supramolecular assemblies actuated by photoisomerization of azobenzene derivatives. *Chemical Communications*, *49*(82), 9386–9388. doi:10.1039/c3cc43488e PMID:23793067

Kang, S. I., & Bae, Y. H. (2001). pH-induced volume-phase transition of hydrogels containing sulfonamide side group by reversible crystal formation. *Macromolecules*, *34*(23), 8173–8178. doi:10.1021/ma0021949

Kashyap, N., Kumar, N., & Kumar, M. N. V. R. (2005). Hydrogels for pharmaceutical and biomedical applications. *Critical Reviews™ in Therapeutic Drug Carrier Systems, 22*(2), 107-150.

Kathmann, E. E., White, L. A., & McCormick, C. L. (1997). Water-Soluble Polymers. 73. Electrolyte- and pH-responsive zwitterionic copolymers of 4-[(2-acrylamido-2-methylpropyl)-dimethylammonio] butanoate with 3-[(2-acrylamido-2-methyl-propyl)dimethylammonio] propanesulfonate. *Macromolecules*, *30*(18), 5297–5304. doi:10.1021/ma961214x

Katono, H., Maruyama, A., Sanui, K., Ogata, N., Okano, T., & Sakurai, Y. (1991). Thermo-responsive swelling and drug release switching of interpenetrating polymer networks composed of poly(acrylamide-co-butyl methacrylate) and poly(acrylic acid). *Journal of Controlled Release*, *16*(1), 215–227. doi:10.1016/0168-3659(91)90045-F

Koetting, M. C., Peters, J. T., Steichen, S. D., & Peppas, N. A. (2015). Stimulus-responsive hydrogels: Theory, modern advances, and applications. *Materials Science and Engineering R Reports*, *93*, 1–49. doi:10.1016/j.mser.2015.04.001 PMID:27134415

Koh, Y. J., Kim, H. K., Kim, S. W., & Yeo, G. D. (2012). *U.S. Patent Application 14/363,022*. Washington, DC: U.S. Patent and Trademark Office.

Kopeček, J., Kopečková, P., Minko, T., & Lu, Z. R. (2000). HPMA copolymer–anticancer drug conjugates: Design, activity, and mechanism of action. *European Journal of Pharmaceutics and Biopharmaceutics*, *50*(1), 61–81. doi:10.1016/S0939-6411(00)00075-8 PMID:10840193

Korostynska, O., Arshak, K., Gill, E., & Arshak, A. (2007). Review on State-of-the-art in Polymer Based pH Sensors. *Sensors (Basel, Switzerland)*, *7*(12), 3027–3042. doi:10.3390/s7123027

Kostić, M., Krunić, N., Nikolić, L., Nikolić, V., & Najman, S., Kostić, … Petković, D. (2011). Influence of residual monomer reduction on acrylic denture base resins quality. *Hem. Ind.*, *65*(2), 171–177. doi:10.2298/HEMIND101103008K

Kostić, M., Krunić, N., Nikolić, L., Nikolić, V., Najman, S., & Kocić, J. (2009). Residual monomer content determination in some acrylic denture base materials and possibilities of its reduction. *Vojnosanitetski Pregled. Military-Medical and Pharmaceutical Review*, *66*(3), 223–227. doi:10.2298/VSP0903223K PMID:19341229

Krušić, M. K., Ilić, M., & Filipović, J. (2009). Swelling behaviour and paracetamol release from poly(*N*-isopropylacrylamide-itaconic acid) hydrogels. *Polymer Bulletin*, *63*(2), 197–211. doi:10.1007/s00289-009-0086-3

Kumar, A., Srivastava, A., Galaev, I. Y., & Mattiasson, B. (2007). Smart polymers: Physical forms and bioengineering applications. *Progress in Polymer Science*, *32*(10), 1205–1237. doi:10.1016/j.progpolymsci.2007.05.003

Kwok, C. S., Mourad, P. D., Crum, L. A., & Ratner, B. D. (2001). Self-assembled molecular structures as ultrasonically-responsive barrier membranes for pulsatile drug delivery. *Journal of Biomedical Materials Research*, *57*(2), 151–164. doi:10.1002/1097-4636(200111)57:2<151::AID-JBM1154>3.0.CO;2-5 PMID:11526905

Langer, R., & Peppas, N. (1983). Chemical and physical structure of polymers as carriers for controlled release of bioactive agents: A review. *Journal of Macromolecular Science-Reviews in Macromolecular Chemistry and Physics*, *23*(1), 61–126. doi:10.1080/07366578308079439

Lee, K. K., Cussler, E. L., Marchetti, M., & McHugh, M. A. (1990). Pressure-dependent phase transitions in hydrogels. *Chemical Engineering Science*, *45*(3), 766–767. doi:10.1016/0009-2509(90)87019-O

Lima-Tenório, M. K., Tenório-Neto, E. T., Guilherme, M. R., Garcia, F. P., Nakamura, C. V., Pineda, E. A., & Rubira, A. F. (2015). Water transport properties through starch-based hydrogel nanocomposites responding to both pH and a remote magnetic field. *Chemical Engineering Journal*, *259*, 620–629. doi:10.1016/j.cej.2014.08.045

Lin, J., Tang, Q., Hu, D., Sun, X., Li, Q., & Wu, J. (2009). Electric field sensitivity of conducting hydrogels with interpenetrating polymer network structure. *Colloids and Surfaces. A, Physicochemical and Engineering Aspects*, *346*(1), 177–183. doi:10.1016/j.colsurfa.2009.06.011

Lin, Y., Chen, Q., & Luo, H. (2007). Preparation and characterization of N-(2-carboxybenzyl) chitosan as a potential pH-sensitive hydrogel for drug delivery. *Carbohydrate Research*, *342*(1), 87–95. doi:10.1016/j.carres.2006.11.002 PMID:17125756

Liu, T. Y., Hu, S. H., Liu, K. H., Liu, D. M., & Chen, S. Y. (2006). Preparation and characterization of smart magnetic hydrogels and its use for drug release. *Journal of Magnetism and Magnetic Materials*, *304*(1), e397–e399. doi:10.1016/j.jmmm.2006.01.203

Liu, Y., Servant, A., Guy, O. J., Al-Jamal, K. T., Williams, P. R., Hawkins, K. M., & Kostarelos, K. (2011). An electric-field responsive microsystem for controllable miniaturised drug delivery applications. *Procedia Engineering*, *25*, 984–987. doi:10.1016/j.proeng.2011.12.242

Liu, Y. Y., Shao, Y. H., & Lü, J. (2006). Preparation, properties and controlled release behaviors of pH-induced thermosensitive amphiphilic gels. *Biomaterials*, *27*(21), 4016–4024. doi:10.1016/j.biomaterials.2006.02.042 PMID:16563494

Loh, X. J., Lee, T.-C., & Ito, Y. (2012). Hydrogels for Biomedical Applications. In Polymeric and Self Assembled Hydrogels: From Fundamental Understanding to Applications (No. 8, pp. 167-209). Cambridge, UK: The Royal Society of Chemistry.

Mellin, L., Borg, N., & Kaellrot, M. J. (2014). *Patent Application JP 2014177460*.

Merrigan, S. R., Schechtman, L. A., Goldman, S. A., Beck, M., Gorth, F. C., Weidl, … Stephan, O. (2004). *U.S. Patent Application 2004/0068093*. Washington, DC: U.S. Patent and Trademark Office.

Milić, J., & Petrović, S. D. (2003). The characteristics of novel dosage forms. *Hem. Ind.*, *57*(10), 424–436. doi:10.2298/HEMIND0310424M

Miller, L. L. (1988). Electrochemically controlled release of drug ions from conducting polymers. *Molecular Crystals and Liquid Crystals*, *160*(1), 297–301.

Mittur, A. (2005). *U.S. Patent Application 11/304,335*. Washington, DC: U.S. Patent and Trademark Office.

Miyata, T., Uragami, T., & Nakamae, K. (2002). Biomolecule-sensitive hydrogels. *Advanced Drug Delivery Reviews*, *54*(1), 79–98. doi:10.1016/S0169-409X(01)00241-1 PMID:11755707

Miyazaki, S., Yokouchi, C., & Takada, M. (1988). External control of drug release: Controlled release of insulin from a hydrophilic polymer implant by ultrasound irradiation in diabetic rats. *The Journal of Pharmacy and Pharmacology*, *40*(10), 716–717. doi:10.1111/j.2042-7158.1988.tb07001.x PMID:2907539

Moerkerke, R., Koningsveld, R., Berghmans, H., Dusek, K., & Solc, K. (1995). Phase transitions in swollen networks. *Macromolecules*, *28*(4), 1103–1107. doi:10.1021/ma00108a043

Moon, I. J., Kim, H. Y., & Choi, H. J. (2015). Conducting poly(*N*-methylaniline)-coated cross-linked poly(methyl methacrylate) nanoparticle suspension and its steady shear response under electric fields. *Colloids and Surfaces. A, Physicochemical and Engineering Aspects*, *481*, 506–513. doi:10.1016/j.colsurfa.2015.05.051

Murdan, S. (2003). Electro-responsive drug delivery from hydrogels. *Journal of Controlled Release*, *92*(1), 1–17. doi:10.1016/S0168-3659(03)00303-1 PMID:14499181

Myung, D., Waters, D., Wiseman, M., Duhamel, P. E., Noolandi, J., Ta, C. N., & Frank, C. W. (2008). Progress in the development of interpenetrating polymer network hydrogels. *Polymers for Advanced Technologies*, *19*(6), 647–657. doi:10.1002/pat.1134 PMID:19763189

Nazli, C., Demirer, G. S., Yar, Y., Acar, H. Y., & Kizilel, S. (2014). Targeted delivery of doxorubicin into tumor cells via MMP-sensitive PEG hydrogel-coated magnetic iron oxide nanoparticles (MIONPs). *Colloids and Surfaces. B, Biointerfaces*, *122*, 674–683. doi:10.1016/j.colsurfb.2014.07.049 PMID:25183059

Niamlang, S., Buranut, T., & Niansiri, A. (2011). Electrically controlled Aloe-vera extraction release from polyacrylamide hydrogel. *Energy Procedia*, *9*, 468–473. doi:10.1016/j.egypro.2011.09.053

Nizam El-Din, H. M. (2011). Characterization and caffeine release properties of N-isopropylacrylamide/hydroxypropyl methacrylate copolymer hydrogel synthesized by gamma radiation. *Journal of Applied Polymer Science*, *119*(1), 577–585. doi:10.1002/app.32675

Omidian, H., Gavrilas, C., Han, W., Li, G., & Rocca, J. G. (2008). *U.S. Patent Application 12/036,680*. Washington, DC: U.S. Patent and Trademark Office.

Pal, K., Banthia, A. K., & Majumdar, D. K. (2009). Polymeric hydrogels: Characterization and biomedical applications. *Designed Monomers and Polymers*, *12*(3), 197–220. doi:10.1163/156855509X436030

Park, T. G. (1999). Temperature modulated protein release from pH/temperature-sensitive hydrogels. *Biomaterials*, *20*(6), 517–521. doi:10.1016/S0142-9612(98)00197-5 PMID:10213354

Peppas, N. A. (1986). Hydrogels of poly(vinyl alcohol) and its copolymers. In N. A. Peppas (Ed.), *Hydrogels in medicine and pharmacy* (Vol. 2, pp. 1–48). Boca Raton, FL: CRC Press.

Peppas, N. A. (1991). Physiologically responsive hydrogels. *Journal of Bioactive and Compatible Polymers*, *6*(3), 241–246. doi:10.1177/088391159100600303

Peppas, N. A., Bures, P., Leobandung, W., & Ichikawa, H. (2000). Hydrogels in pharmaceutical formulations. *European Journal of Pharmaceutics and Biopharmaceutics*, *50*(1), 27–46. doi:10.1016/S0939-6411(00)00090-4 PMID:10840191

Peppas, N. A., & Khare, A. R. (1993). Preparation, structure and diffusional behavior of hydrogels in controlled release. *Advanced Drug Delivery Reviews*, *11*(1), 1–35. doi:10.1016/0169-409X(93)90025-Y

Pillay V., Indermun S., Du Toit L. C., Choonara Y. E., & Kumar P. (2014). *WO Patent Application, WO 2014/191979*.

Podual, K., Doyle, F. J., & Peppas, N. A. (2000). Preparation and dynamic response of cationic copolymer hydrogels containing glucose oxidase. *Polymer*, *41*(11), 3975–3983. doi:10.1016/S0032-3861(99)00620-5

Qiu, Y., & Park, K. (2012). Environment-sensitive hydrogels for drug delivery. *Advanced Drug Delivery Reviews*, *64*, 49–60. doi:10.1016/j.addr.2012.09.024 PMID:11744175

Ratner, B. D., & Hoffman, A. S. (1976). Synthetic hydrogels for biomedical applications. In J. D. Andrade (Ed.), *Hydrogels for medical and related applications* (Vol. 31, pp. 1–36). Washington, DC: American Chemical Society. doi:10.1021/bk-1976-0031.ch001

Rosenblatt, J., Devereux, B., & Wallace, D. G. (1994). Injectable collagen as a pH-sensitive hydrogel. *Biomaterials*, *15*(12), 985–995. doi:10.1016/0142-9612(94)90079-5 PMID:7841296

Samra, B., Galaev, I., & Mattiasson, B. (2003). *U.S. Patent No. 6,538,089*. Washington, DC: U.S. Patent and Trademark Office.

Sassi, A. P., Shaw, A. J., Han, S. M., Blanch, H. W., & Prausnitz, J. M. (1996). Partitioning of proteins and small biomolecules in temperature-and pH-sensitive hydrogels. *Polymer*, *37*(11), 2151–2164. doi:10.1016/0032-3861(96)85860-5

Sawahata, K., Hara, M., Yasunaga, H., & Osada, Y. (1990). Electrically controlled drug delivery system using polyelectrolyte gels. *Journal of Controlled Release*, *14*(3), 253–262. doi:10.1016/0168-3659(90)90165-P

Shafer-Peltier, K. E., Haynes, C. L., Glucksberg, M. R., & Van Duyne, R. P. (2003). Toward a glucose biosensor based on surface-enhanced Raman scattering. *Journal of the American Chemical Society*, *125*(2), 588–593. doi:10.1021/ja028255v PMID:12517176

Shin, Y., Chang, J. H., Liu, J., Williford, R., Shin, Y. K., & Exarhos, G. J. (2001). Hybrid nanogels for sustainable positive thermosensitive drug release. *Journal of Controlled Release*, *73*(1), 1–6. doi:10.1016/S0168-3659(01)00247-4 PMID:11337054

Slomkowski, S., Alemán, J. V., Gilbert, R. G., Hess, M., Horie, K., Jones, R. G., & Stepto, R. F. (2011). Terminology of polymers and polymerization processes in dispersed systems (IUPAC Recommendations 2011). *Pure and Applied Chemistry*, *83*(12), 2229–2259. doi:10.1351/PAC-REC-10-06-03

Sojka, R. E., Bjorneberg, D. L., Entry, J. A., Lentz, R. D., & Orts, W. J. (2007). Polyacrylamide in agriculture and environmental land management. *Advances in Agronomy*, *92*, 75–162. doi:10.1016/S0065-2113(04)92002-0

Spasojević, J., Radosavljević, A., Krstić, J., Jovanović, D., Spasojević, V., Kalagasidis-Krušić, M., & Kačarević-Popović, Z. (2015). Dual responsive antibacterial Ag-poly(*N*-isopropylacrylamide/itaconic acid) hydrogel nanocomposites synthesized by gamma irradiation. *European Polymer Journal*, *69*, 168–185. doi:10.1016/j.eurpolymj.2015.06.008

Sperling, L. H., & Mishra, V. (1996). The current status of interpenetrating polymer networks. *Polymers for Advanced Technologies*, *7*(4), 197–208. doi:10.1002/(SICI)1099-1581(199604)7:4<197::AID-PAT514>3.0.CO;2-4

Suzuki, A., & Tanaka, T. (1990). Phase transition in polymer gels induced by visible light. *Nature, 346*(6282), 345-347.

Tanaka, T., & Fillmore, D. J. (1979). Kinetics of swelling of gels. *The Journal of Chemical Physics, 70*(3), 1214–1218. doi:10.1063/1.437602

The Chemical Industry and its Development. (1950). *Nature, 165*, 413-415.

Vakkalanka, S. K., Brazel, C. S., & Peppas, N. A. (1997). Temperature-and pH-sensitive terpolymers for modulated delivery of streptokinase. *Journal of Biomaterials Science. Polymer Edition, 8*(2), 119–129. doi:10.1163/156856296X00192 PMID:8957708

van der Linden, H. J., Herber, S., Olthuis, W., & Bergveld, P. (2003). Stimulus-sensitive hydrogels and their applications in chemical (micro) analysis. *Analyst (London), 128*(4), 325–331. doi:10.1039/b210140h PMID:12741636

Varga, Z., Filipcsei, G., & Zrínyi, M. (2006). Magnetic field sensitive functional elastomers with tuneable elastic modulus. *Polymer, 47*(1), 227–233. doi:10.1016/j.polymer.2005.10.139

Wang, X., Gu, X., Yuan, C., Chen, S., Zhang, P., Zhang, T., & Chen, G. et al. (2004). Evaluation of biocompatibility of polypyrrole *in vitro* and *in vivo*. *Journal of Biomedical Materials Research. Part A, 68*(3), 411–422. doi:10.1002/jbm.a.20065 PMID:14762920

Xiao, X. C., Chu, L. Y., Chen, W. M., Wang, S., & Li, Y. (2003). Positively thermo-sensitive monodisperse core–shell microspheres. *Advanced Functional Materials, 13*(11), 847–852. doi:10.1002/adfm.200304513

Zhang, X., Li, Y., Hu, Z., & Littler, C. L. (1995). Bending of *N*-isopropylacrylamide gel under the influence of infrared light. *The Journal of Chemical Physics, 102*(1), 551–555. doi:10.1063/1.469434

Zhang, X., Wu, D., & Chu, C. C. (2004). Synthesis and characterization of partially biodegradable, temperature and pH sensitive Dex–MA/PNIPAAm hydrogels. *Biomaterials, 25*(19), 4719–4730. doi:10.1016/j.biomaterials.2003.11.040 PMID:15120518

Zhong, X., Wang, Y. X., & Wang, S. C. (1996). Pressure dependence of the volume phase-transition of temperature-sensitive gels. *Chemical Engineering Science, 51*(12), 3235–3239. doi:10.1016/0009-2509(95)00344-4

Zrinyi, M., Barsi, L., & Büki, A. (1996). Deformation of ferrogels induced by non uniform magnetic fields. *The Journal of Chemical Physics, 104*(21), 8750–8756. doi:10.1063/1.471564

Zrinyi, M., Barsi, L., & Büki, A. (1997). Ferrogel: A new magneto-controlled elastic medium. *Polymer Gels and Networks, 5*(5), 415–427. doi:10.1016/S0966-7822(97)00010-5

KEY TERMS AND DEFINITIONS

Biomolecule-Responsive: The specific behavior by changing the properties as result in some biomolecule change.

Drug Carrier: The substance that serves as mechanism to improve delivery and to increase the effectiveness of drug delivery to the target site of pharmacological action. It is used for prolonged, delayed, or pulsatile release of drug; reducing drug toxicity and to decrease drug metabolism.

Field-Sensitive: The specific ability of a specific system/functional unit/molecule (e.g. hydrogel) to react in slight differences or small changes in the various surrounding field (electric, magnetic, ultrasound).

Hydrogel Synthesis: A combination of two or more entities (compounds, monomers and croslinkers) that together form a new three-dimensional solid network structure. The internal network structure may form physical bonds or chemical bonds.

Modified Drug Release: Place and/or the release rate of active substance/drug are different compared to conventional pharmaceutical form of the same drug administered through the same application.

pH-Responsive: Ability of a system or functional unit to reversible react in small changes in the pH value of surrounding fluid.

Stimuli Responsive: Noticeable changes of features in a reversible manner with environmental stimulus variations (e.g., pH, temperature, redox potential, ultrasound, glucose, electric' magnetic field, light, or a combination thereof).

Thermo-Responsive: Reaction caused by change in the external temperature.

Chapter 12
Rational Design of Polymeric Micelle for Cancer Therapy

Yixian Huang
University of Pittsburgh, USA

Jingjing Sun
University of Pittsburgh, USA

Song Li
University of Pittsburgh, USA

ABSTRACT

Clinical application of anticancer drugs is limited by problems such as low water solubility, lack of tissue-specificity and toxicity. Formulation development represents an important approach to these problems. Among the many delivery systems studied, polymeric micelles are an attractive nano-scaled delivery system due to their simplicity, ability to solubilize water-insoluble drugs, and small size (10-100 nm) that can take advantage of enhanced permeability and retention effect to specifically accumulate in tumors. This book chapter provides a brief review of recent advancements in developing environmentally responsive micellar systems for controlled delivery of chemotherapeutic agents to tumor tissues. The emphasis is placed on the discussion of several dual functional nanomicellar systems that were recently developed in our laboratory as well as a new strategy of improving micellar formulations via incorporation of an interfacial drug-interactive motif(s).

INTRODUCTION

Cancer is a major cause of death around the world, especially in USA. The most common cancer treatments are surgery, radiation and chemotherapy, with chemotherapy being the major treatment modality. However, the chemotherapeutic agents are limited by their unsuitable properties, such as low water solubility, toxicity and drug resistance (Mishra et al., 2010; Alexis, et al., 2008; Shapria, et al., 2011). Currently, nanotechnology has been extensively studied for their potential applications in cancer diagnosis and treatment. Various nanocarriers have been developed including liposomes, micelles, dendrimers and nanocrystals.

DOI: 10.4018/978-1-5225-0751-2.ch012

Most of the nanoparticles use enhanced permeability and retention (EPR) effect which is a property by which molecules of certain sizes (typically liposomes, micelles and macromolecular drugs) tend to accumulate in tumor tissue much more than they do in normal tissues (Matsumura, & Maeda 1986; Duncan, & Sat 1998). In addition, a tumor-specific ligand can be introduced onto the surface of nanoparticles to further facilitate their interaction with tumor cells following accumulation at tumor sites (Michalet, et al., 2005; van Vlerken, et al., 2007). The development of tumor-targeting nano delivery systems has revived the therapeutic uses of many potent chemotherapeutics that are too toxic to be applied in human body directly. In the past decade, polymeric micelles have been utilized as a novel promising colloidal carrier for the targeted delivery and controlled release of drugs, proteins and genes in the cancer diagnosis and therapy. Micelles have a size of 10-200 nm, a structure with the hydrophobic core for efficient loading of poorly water soluble drugs and a layer of hydrophilic shells to warrant excellent colloidal stability and more importantly intrinsic stealth effect (Davis, et al., 2008).

One major advantage of polymeric micellar systems is their simplicity. However, conventional micellar systems suffer from limited drug loading capacity and colloidal stability in the blood circulation. Accordingly, significant efforts have been devoted to resolve these problems. In addition, significant progress has been made in developing intelligent micellar systems that are stable in blood but become destabilized and release payload drug in response to "tumor-specific" microenvironment. This review summarizes recent progress in targeted delivery of chemotherapeutic agents via polymeric systems.

Polymeric Micelles

Most polymeric systems involve the use of polymers as the hydrophobic domain including polyesters such as poly(lactic acid) (PLA) and polyamides such as poly (L-aspartic acid) (PAPS) and poly (beta-amino ester). One critical consideration for clinical application of micellar carriers is the biocompatibility and biodegradability. Polyesters and polyamides can be hydrolyzed by enzymes in vivo and are considered biodegradable. There are several polymeric micelle systems that have been studied in clinical phase. For example, Genexol-PM is a polymeric micelle formulation of PTX that is based on monomethoxy poly(ethylene glycol)-block-poly(D,L-lactide) (mPEG-PDLLA) (Jones, et al., 1999; Kim, et al., 2004, Lee, et al., 2008). It has a mPEG molecular weight of 2000 g/mol and a PDLLA molecular weight of 1750 g/mol. In this system, the drug loading was as high as 16.7% (w/w) and the size was smaller than 50 nm. The solution can be stable for 2 months at 4 °C and 1 day at room temperature, respectively. Genexol-PM has been in market in Korea and Europe (see Figure 1).

NK-105 used poly(ethylene glycol)-poly(aspartic acid) (PEG-P(Asp)) that was modified with 4-phenyl-1-butanol to increase the hydrophobicity (Hamaguchi, et al., 2007). The micelle system could effectively load PTX via hydrophobic interaction with a drug loading of about 23% (w/w) and particle size of around 85 nm. NK105 can be readily dissolved in 5% glucose solution and is stable for more than 1 day at room temperature. NK-105 has been examined in a phase I study in patients suffering from pancreatic, bile duct, gastric, and colonic cancers. NK-105 was administered intravenously for 1 h every 3 weeks, and the recommended dose of 150 mg/m^2 was well-tolerated with less hypersensitivity reactions than Taxol. Currently, a phase II study in patients with advanced stomach cancer is underway.

NC-6004 is another polymeric micelle formation that is loaded with cisplatin. Cisplatin (cis-dichlorodiammineplatinum (II), CDDP) is an important anti-tumor agent and is frequently used for the treatment of many cancers (Alami, et al., 2005). Due to its water solubility, CDDP was rapidly cleared from circulation after i.v. injection and excreted through the kidney filtration within a few minutes. NC-6004

Figure 1. Composition of polymeric micelles

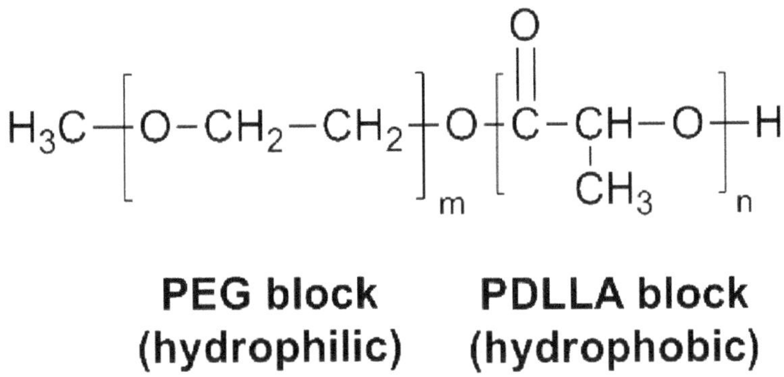

is a polymeric micellar formulation of cisplatin. It consists of a outer shell of PEG and an inner core of the coordinate complex of poly (glutamic acid) (P(Glu)) and CDDP. The size of NC-6004 is about 30 nm with narrow distribution. The loading capacity of NC-6004 is as high as 39%. NC-6004 is extremely stable in distilled water even under much diluted condition, with a critical micelle concentration (CMC) less than 5×10^{-7} M. Nevertheless, CDDP showed sustained release in physiological saline due to an inverse ligand substitution of the Pt (II) atom from a Glu residue of PEG–P(Glu) to chloride. The affinity between the Pt (II) atom and Glu residue is optimal in terms of the anti-tumor effect and toxicity of CDDP because a highly stable complex, such as CDDP-DNA, may weaken and even eliminate the anti-tumor effect of CDDP, while a low affinity complex, such as CDDP-hyaluronic acid, may possess the same toxicity as CDDP (Plummer, et al., 2011). SN-38 (7-ethyl-10-hydroxy-camptothecin) is a biologically active metabolite of irinotecan hydrochloride (CPT-11), and shows a superior cytotoxicity over CPT-11 against various cancer cells *in vitro*, but is unavailable in the market because of its poor solubility. (Lavelle, et al., 1996). NK-012 is a micellar formulation of SN-38 that is based on the amphiphilic copolymer, PEG–PGA (poly L-glutamic acid) (Matsumura, et al., 2011).

The hydrophobic SN-38- bound PGA forms the core of the micelle and is protected from nonspecific uptake by RES and degradation. The drug loading of NK-012 is about 20% (w/w). The release rates of SN-38 from NK-012 in PBS (pH 7.4) at 37 °C are 57% and 74% at 24 and 48 h, respectively, ensuring the stability for clinical use after reconstitution. Besides, the release behavior of SN-38 from NK-012 is a nonenzymatic manner, which is regardless of the inter individual variability of carboxylesterase activity. Like other PM formulation, the PK of NK-012 was characteristic of slow clearance and tumor accumulation. CPT-11 was significantly distributed in the epithelium of the small intestine whereas NK-012 tended to be distributed weakly and uniformly in the mucosal interstitium, consistent with the less intestinal toxicity observed in NK-012 group. NK-012 has been studied in two phase I trials. The first examined pharmacokinetics and toxicity in 24 patients with advanced solid tissue malignancies refractory to standard therapy. A second phase I study found similar results with an MTD of 37 mg/m^2. Several other phase I trials have been completed with results pending.

NK-911 is a polymeric micelle formulation of doxorubicin (DOX) containing PEG as hydrophilic segment and DOX conjugated P(Asp) (P(Asp)(DOX)) as hydrophobic segment with both free DOX and DOX derivatives in this system (Matsumura, et al., 2004). This formulation displayed a better antitumor activity in vivo as well as an increased tumor accumulation and prolonged circulation in blood. Further study showed that the loaded free DOX was largely responsive for the antitumor activity while the conjugated DOX played a major role in facilitating the interaction with loaded DOX. Interestingly, it was found that the free DOX existed as both monomer and dimer. DOX monomer is the active component for the cytotoxicity. However, the dimer helps to stabilize the drug-loaded micelles. Comparative study with DOXIL also suggested that DOXIL may be more efficient at delivering drugs to tumors near the vasculature, whereas NK-911 may have better accessibility to tumor cells further away from the blood vessels through improved diffusion. The phase I clinical trial of NK911 began in July 2001.

Lipid-Core Micelles

A special group of polymeric micelles is lipid-core micelles, i.e., micelles formed by conjugates of water-soluble polymers with lipids such as poly(ethylene glycol)-phosphatidylethanolamine conjugate (PEG-PE) (Trubetskoy, et al., 1995). The use of lipid moieties as hydrophobic blocks provides a very high stability of the micelles because of very strong hydrophobic interactions between double acyl chains of the phospholipid molecules. Similar to long circulating liposomes, the exposure of PEG residues on the surface prevents the rapid uptake of the micelles by the reticuloendothelial system. Micelle preparation from PEG–PE conjugates with a molecular weight of PEG chains from 750 to 5000 Da is a simple process since such conjugates spontaneously form micelles in an aqueous medium. All versions of PEG-PE conjugates form micelles with the size of 7-35 nm. The use of conjugates with PEG blocks of higher molecular weight results in the formation of slightly larger micelles thus indicating that the micelle size may be tailored for a particular application by varying the length of PEG. Preparation of PEG-PE micelles by a detergent or water-miscible solvent removal method results in formation of particles with very similar diameters. Usually, micelles have a spherical shape and uniform size distribution. Lipid-core micelles can be loaded with a variety of poorly soluble drugs, and are very stable both in terms of the ability to preserve their morphology and retain encapsulated material upon conditions modeling parenteral administration (Lukyanov, et al., 2004).

The last decade has seen significant progress in the development of various micellar systems for targeted delivery of anticancer agents. However, much improvement is still needed for the existing systems with respect to drug-loading capacity and formulation stability. Despite the structural differences among the reported micellar systems, most of them mainly rely on hydrophobic/hydrophobic interaction for drug incorporation into the hydrophobic cores. Such mechanism, while working well for some highly lipophilic drugs, may not provide sufficient drug/carrier interaction to effectively load other drugs. Various new strategies have been attempted to improve the performance of micellar systems. Lam and colleagues have developed a series of micellar systems composed of PEG-cholic acid (CA) conjugates. A conjugate of eight CA molecules with one PEG 5K chain (PEG_{5K}-CA_8) was shown to load paclitaxel with high loading capacity and a size of 20–60 nm paclitaxel-loaded PEG_{5K}-CA_8 micelles achieved improved antitumor effect and showed less toxicity in a murine model of ovarian cancer compared to Taxol and Abraxane at equivalent paclitaxel doses nm (Xiao, et al., 2009). Phase I clinical trial of paclitaxel-loaded PEG_{5K}-CA_8 micelles demonstrated anticancer efficacy and tolerance. In addition, compared to PEG_{5K}-CA_8 micelles, a similar micellar carrier, PEG_{2K}-CA_4, was shown to have higher loading capacity and more sustained drug release profile for doxorubicin (Xiao, et al., 2011). Another strategy to improve the micellar systems involves introduction of additional drug-interactive domains to enhance the overall carrier/drug interaction. In addition, progress has been made in developing dual-functional carriers that demonstrate both delivery function and antitumor activity. Detailed discussion of these approaches is provided in the later part of this chapter.

"SMART" POLYMERIC MICELLES

pH Sensitive Polymeric Micelles

Intracellular compartments are characterized by various *p*H values, while pH stabilizes around 7.4 in normal extracellular matrices and blood. The pH in early endosomes is around 6, followed by late endosomes that rapidly acidify to pH 5–6 due to the action of an ATPase proton-pump enzyme in the vesicle membrane (Xiao, et al., 2011). The carriers can subsequently encounter lysosomes, which further acidify to pH ~4.5 and contain various degradative enzymes. Tumors, in general, have a mildly acidic microenvironment (Cain, et al., 1989; Mellman, 1986). This is mainly a consequence of irregular angiogenesis in fast-growing tumors, which causes a rapid deficit to both nutrients and oxygen and thus a shift towards a glycolytic metabolism, therefore leading to the production of acidic metabolites in the tumor interstitium. Accordingly, *p*H-responsive micelles with acid-cleavable links are usually designed to rapidly destroy the integrity of vehicles by the *p*H variation in tumor tissues or in endosome following intracellular delivery, which facilitates the prompt release of encapsulated cargoes within the tumor tissues/cells.

Efficient pH-sensitive systems should show a sharp response to a subtle change of *p*H in the tumor extracellular microenvironment and/or endosome. There has been extensive application of various acid-cleavable covalent links, such as acetal, orthoester, hydrazone, imine, cis-acotinyl, and oxime, which hydrolyze rapidly in a *p*H of ~5 (Figure 2). These have been placed in the polymer structure, either in the backbone, or at the side chain, leading to the facile and robust development of new strategies toward the preparation of *p*H-responsive polymeric drug carriers.

Acid-Cleavable Backbones

*p*H-responsive polymers with acid-cleavable backbones are designed to remain stable at the physiological *p*H (7.4), but degrade quickly into several low molecular weight compounds and/or many small molecules at *p*H 5.0–6.0, corresponding to the mildly acidic environment in lysosomes, endosomes, or tumor tissues. Upon lowering the *p*H, the degradation of polymer along the backbone will result in the structural destruction of polymer-based drug containers, leading to the prompt dissociation of biotherapeutics from the polymer matrix, as well as facilitated endosomal escape of drug carriers due to the membrane destabilization induced by the acidic *p*H-triggered deformation of polymer structure. Brocchini et al. developed water-soluble, biocompatible, amino-functionalized polyacetals that display *p*H-dependent degradation and, moreover, are suitable for drug conjugation (Tomlinson, et al., 2002). In their study, polyacetals were first prepared by the reaction of a diol (e.g., PEG) and a divinyl ether (e.g., tri(ethylene glycol) divinyl ether) using an acid catalyst. Using PEG3400, the resulting polyacetals had Mw of 36,000–43,000 g/mol and displayed pH-dependent degradation (Tomlinson, et al., 2002). Heffernan and Murthy reported another interesting family of acid-degradable polymers, poly-(1,4- phenyleneacetone dimethylene ketal) (PPADK), containing ketal links in their backbone (Heffernan, et al., 2005).

Figure 2. Functional groups for generation of pH responsive micelles

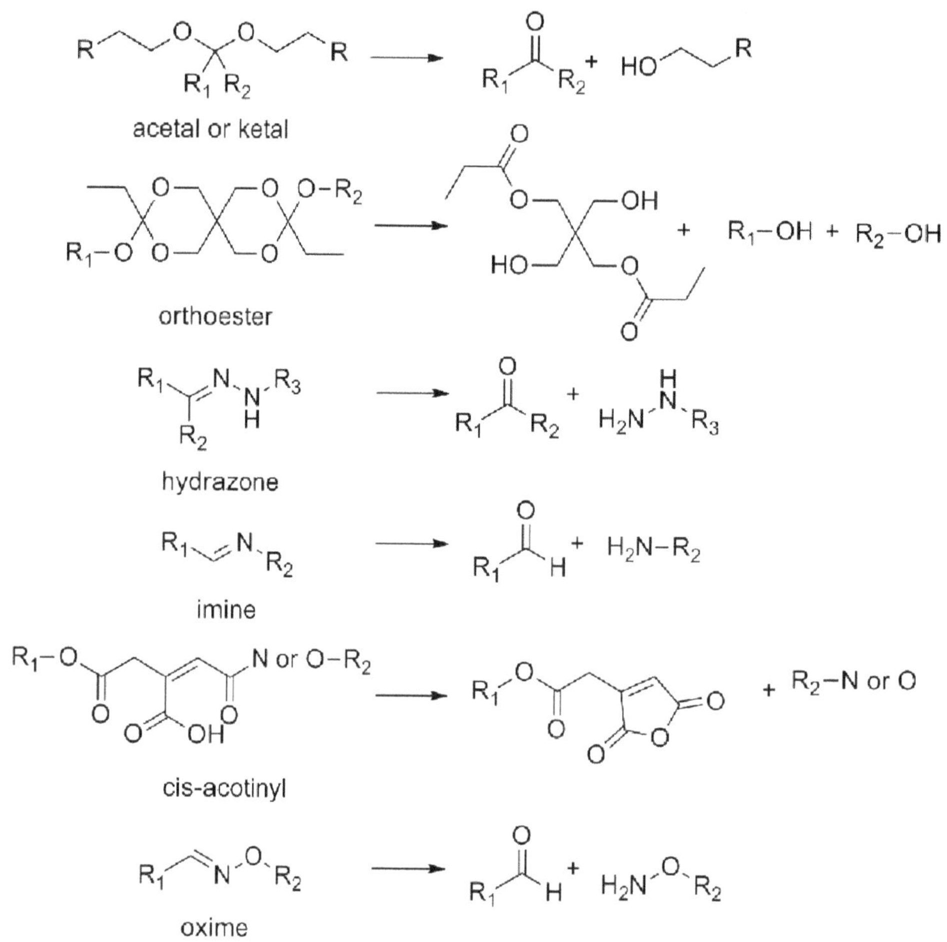

The hydrolysis half-life of PPADK was 102 h at pH 7.4 and 35 h at pH 5.0. The micro- and nanoparticles formed by PPADK via an emulsion procedure can be used for the delivery of hydrophobic drugs and potentially, proteins. In contrast to polyester-based biomaterials, the hydrolysis of polyketal nanoparticles did not generate acidic degradation products. Dexamethasone-loaded nanoparticles with diameter around 200–600 nm were fabricated, suitable for applications involving phagocytosis by macrophages.

Recently, Fréchet and co-workers reported the preparation of various acid-degradable difunctional monomers containing acetal or ketal links. They incorporated these monomers into the backbone of different polymers to generate various pH-sensitive polymers including a family of poly(amidoamine)s and a library of polyurethanes and polyureas, with tunable hydrophobicity and enhanced degradability (Jain, et al., 2007; Paramonov, et al., 2008). All of the polymers exhibited a *p*H-dependent degradation profile with a very significant increase in hydrolysis rate as the *p*H was lowered from 7.4 to 5.0. The library of polyurethanes and polyureas was further screened for the formation of microparticles using a double emulsion technique. A study of the hydrolysis of selected microparticles indicated that their degradation afforded only small molecules, without any polymeric byproduct possessing high molecular weight. In vitro studies demonstrated the ability of the FITC-BSA-loaded microparticles to be phagocytosed by macrophages resulting in a 10-fold increase in the protein uptake, compared to a free protein control. Such acid-sensitive, fully degradable polymers and corresponding microparticles may find great potential for the delivery of various therapeutic agents or vaccines.

Yang et al. prepared an amphiphilic PEG-*b*-(noctadecane amine) copolymer by conjugating two blocks via a novel *p*H-responsive benzoic-imine bond (Ding, et al., 2009). The benzoic-imine linker is stable at physiological *p*H and cleavable with increasing magnitude following the decrease of *p*H to the levels of tumor and endosomal *p*Hs. The polymer can self-assemble into non-charged micellar aggregates in aqueous solution at physiological *p*H. These particles gain a positive surface charge at tumor pH and dissociate at endosomal *p*H. As a result, these particles were more easily taken up by tumor cells upon reaching tumor site and had an enhanced membrane disrupting capability in endosomes. Their study indicated that the incorporation of benzoic-imine bond was a powerful tool for the design of drug delivery systems with both tumor-specific uptake and intracellular delivery abilities (Ding, et al., 2009).

To obtain a stepwise controllable biodegradable polymer for multifunctional anti-tumor drug carriers, the group of Fu and Tan synthesized *p*H-sensitive biodegradable polyurethanes using PCL and *p*H-sensitive PEG-hydrazone-PCL macrodiol (PCLH) as the soft segment; l-lysine ethyl ester diisocyanate (LDI), l-lysine derivative tripeptide and 1,4-butandiol (BDO) as the hard segment; and hydrazone-linked methoxyl-PEG (mPEG-Hyd) as the end-capper. A tunable content of hydrazone bonds in these polymers could be achieved by varying the ratio of PCLH and PCL. The *in vivo* biocompatibility was evaluated in an intramuscular implantation model on Sprague-Dawley rats. The results showed that the prepared polyurethanes can be easily degraded and the degradation products did not induce any adverse response from surrounding muscle tissues (Zhou, et al., 2012). Such *p*H-sensitive polyurethanes could be promising materials as controllable biodegradable and nontoxic multifunctional carriers for intracellular drug delivery.

Acid-Cleaved Side Chain

A new approach to the preparation of acid-degradable micelles was developed by Fréchet and co-workers (Gillies, et al., 2003). This approach involved attachment of hydrophobic groups to one block of a linear di-block copolymer via a highly acid sensitive cyclic acetal link. It was found that upon hydrolysis of such a link, the hydrophobic block became more hydrophilic, thus the loaded drug in the micelles can easily escape from the micellar compartment. The resulting system based on a di-block copolymer of PEG and reversibly hydrophobilized poly(aspartic acid) (P(Asp)) showed promise for the selective release of drugs in an acidic environment (pH 5.0), as that in tumor tissue or cellular compartments such as endosomes or lysosomes. They further applied this approach to acid-degradable micelles based on PEO–dendrimer hybrids as backbones (Gillies, et al., 2004)

The hydrophobic groups were conjugated to the periphery of the core-forming dendrimer block by acetal links. Hydrolysis of the acetal link at mildly acidic pH was designed to reveal polar groups on the core-forming block, thus changing its solubility and disrupting the micelle, leading to drug release (Gillies, et al., 2004). Inspired by Fréchet's work, Zhong et al. prepared pH responsive biodegradable micelles from block copolymers comprising a novel acid-labile polycarbonate hydrophobe and PEG (Chen, et al., 2009). These block copolymers were synthesized by ROP of cyclic aliphatic carbonate monomer in the presence of methoxy PEG as a macro-initiator. The hydrolysis study of the acetal groups of the polycarbonate showed that the acetals of micelles, while stable at pH 7.4, were prone to rapid hydrolysis at mildly acidic *p*H of 4.0 and 5.0, with a half-life of 1 and 6.5 h, respectively. The hydrolysis of acetal groups led to significant swelling of micelle structure, resulting from the transition of polycarbonate from hydrophobic to hydrophilic state. Both PTX and DOX could be efficiently encapsulated into the micelles with high drug loading content (13.0 and 11.7 wt%, respectively) (Chen, et al., 2009).

Zhang et al. reported the fabrication of novel stimuli-responsive non-covalently connected micelles (NCCMs) with cleavable PEG side chain (Quan, et al., 2010). In their work, PEG side chains were connected to the polymer backbone through a benzoic-imine bond. This link was stable under physiological *p*H but hydrolyzed when the *p*H decreased below 6.8, corresponding to the *p*H of extracellular environment in the solid tumor tissues. A RGD targeting ligand was also conjugated to the polymer but buried in the PEG hydrophilic shell. The presence of PEG facilitated the accumulation of the particles at the tumor tissues via EPR effect. However, upon arrival at the tumor sites, the acid- triggered hydrolysis of benzoic-imine bond enabled the detachment of PEG outer corona, leading to the exposure of the RGD peptide, which can achieve active targeting and increase targeting efficacy to tumor cells. Therefore, the active targeting by RGD was switched off before reaching the tumor sites and switched on in the tumor sites, which was defined as "tumor triggered targeting". Moreover, the detachment of the PEG shell facilitated rapid release of loaded drugs from NCCMs due to the thermo-induced phase transition (Quan, et al., 2010).

Wang et al. prepared a new amphiphilic block copolymer by ATRP from a PEG macro-initiator, consisting of PEG and a poly methacrylate derivative, poly(2- ethoxytetrahydrofuran-2-yloxyethyl methacrylate), PEYM, bearing acid-labile ortho ester side chains (Tang, et al., 2011). The resulting PEG-*b*-PEYM copolymer can self-assemble into core–shell micelles with the ortho ester side chains buried in the hydrophobic cores in aqueous phase at physiological *p*H, which became hydrophilic upon rapid hydrolysis of the ortho ester at slightly acidic *p*H. Dox was successfully loaded into the micelles at *p*H 7.4 and released at a much higher rate in response to slight acidification to *p*H 5. They investigated the in vitro uptake of Dox-loaded micelles using a line of multi-drug resistant human glioma cells (T98G) and found that micelles containing DOX were rapidly taken up by human glioma cells, accumulating in the endo-lysosome and subsequently in the nucleus in a few hours, in contrast to the very low uptake of free drug at the same dose. The cytotoxicity of Dox-loaded micelles against the human glioma cells was further determined by MTT assay. While the empty micelles themselves were not toxic, the IC_{50} values of the Dox-loaded micelles were approximately ten-times (by 24 h) and three-times (by 48 h) lower than those of the free drug. The much enhanced potency in killing the multi-drug-resistant human glioma cells by Dox loaded in the micelles could be attributed to high intracellular drug concentration and the subsequent pH-triggered drug release. These results established the PEG-*b*-PEYM block copolymer with acid-labile ortho ester side-chains as a novel and effective pH-responsive nano-carrier for enhanced tumor-targeted drug delivery.

Redox-Sensitive Polymeric Micelles

Disulphide bonds, prone to rapid cleavage by glutathione (GSH), can be used to achieve redox sensitivity. The cytosolic release of drugs can then be triggered by the different concentrations of GSH found in extracellular (~2-10 μM) and intracellular (~2-10 mM) (Ballatori, et al., 2009; Estrela, et al., 2006; Franco, et al., 2007; Franco, et al., 2009; Schafer, et al., 2001).

Moreover, it has been found that tumor cells generally have elevated levels of cytosolic GSH, several times higher than that in normal cells. Therefore, disulfide bonds are stable under physiological conditions in the circulation, as well as in extracellular interstitium due to a low concentration of GSH, but can quickly degrade in a highly reductive environment within cells, facilitating intracellular rapid release and accumulation of the loaded drugs. Over the past few years, redox-responsive polymers, bioconjugates and nano-carriers containing disulfide bonds have drawn great attention for diverse biomedical applications including intracellular delivery of drug, protein, DNA and siRNA (Saito, et al., 2003).

Recent development in the field of reduction responsive micelles for controlled delivery of various therapeutic agents is discussed in the following section. The combination of unique disulfide and thiol chemistries with robust controlled living radical polymerization (CLRP) techniques, such as atom transfer free radical polymerization (ATRP) and reversible addition fragmentation chain transfer (RAFT), has enabled novel and versatile design of multifunctional delivery systems to overcome both extra- and intra-cellular barriers.

Redox-Cleavable Backbones

The development of micelles with reduction-responsive links at the junction of hydrophobic and hydrophilic blocks has been recognized as a powerful and efficient strategy for tumor-targeted drug delivery. The disulfide links are stable in the blood circulation, but can be cleaved rapidly in the intracellular reductive environment or under tumor-relevant GSH level. The shedding of hydrophilic shells on the cleavage of SS links will make the micelles lose colloidal stability, leading to the disassembly of micelles and reformation of aggregates by hydrophobic segments, which enables prompt release of encapsulated drugs. Yan et al. designed a series of biodegradable micelles based on hyperbranched polymers for GSH-mediated intracellular drug delivery (Liu, et al., 2011; Huang, et al., 2011).

They prepared amphiphilic hyperbranched multi-arm copolymers, such as H40-star-PLA-SS-PEP and copolyphosphates (HPHSEP-star-PEPx) with redox-responsive backbones containing disulfide links. The resulting hyperbranched multi-arm copolymers were able to self-assemble into nano-sized micelles in aqueous solution with tunable dimensions. The GSH-mediated intracellular drug delivery was examined with HeLa cells by pretreating these cells with either glutathione monoester (GSH-OEt) or buthionine sulfoximine (BSO), which could increase or decrease the concentration of GSH in the cytoplasm, respectively. The results demonstrated a faster drug release in GSH-OEt pretreated HeLa cells than that in the non-pretreated cells. Cytotoxicity study of the DOX-loaded micelles indicated higher cellular proliferation inhibition against HeLa cells pretreated with 10 mM of GSH-OEt and lower inhibition against cells pretreated with 0.1 mM of BSO, demonstrating an accelerated DOX release in response to intracellular GSH, leading to more effective cell proliferation inhibition.

Zhong et al. prepared biodegradable micelles with sheddable PEG shells based on disulfide-linked PEG-SS-PCL di-block copolymer and applied the resulting self-assembled micelles for rapid intracellular release of DOX (Sun, et al., 2009). The PEG-SS-PCL di-block copolymer with tailored block lengths was synthesized via exchange reaction between PEG orthopyridyl disulfide and mercapto PCL. The resultant micelles exhibited sufficient stability in water, however, were prone to rapid aggregation in the presence of 10 mM dithiothreitol (DTT) due to shedding of the PEG shells through reductive cleavage of the intermediate disulfide bonds. In vitro drug release study revealed that DOX was released from these shell-sheddable micelles quantitatively within 12 h under a reductive environment similar to that of the intracellular compartments such as cytosol and the cell nucleus. In contrast, minimal drug release (<20%) was observed within 24 h for the reduction insensitive PEG–PCL micelles under the same conditions, as well as for PEG-SS-PCL micelles under the non-reductive conditions. Further cell experiments using mouse leukemic monocyte macrophage cell line (RAW264.7) confirmed that these shell-sheddable micelles exhibited much faster release of DOX inside cells and more effective cell proliferation inhibition as compared to the reduction insensitive control. Following the same synthetic procedure, they further prepared disulfide-linked dextran-b-poly(-caprolactone)di-block copolymer (Dex-SS-PCL) with similar results (Sun, et al., 2010).

Liu et al. (2011) reported the preparation of disulfide linked mPEG-SS-PzLL block copolymer by ring opening polymerization (ROP) of ε-benzyloxycarbonyl-l-lysine N-carboxyanhydride (zLL-NCA) monomer using amino-terminated PEG containing disulfide bond as a macroinitiator (Wen, et al., 2011). The resulting self-assembled micelles consist of a sheddable PEG shell and a PzLL core. Cell proliferation assays with MCF-7 cells demonstrated the pharmacological activity of DOX released from mPEG-SS-PzLL micelles in the presence of elevated GSH. Following the same synthetic approach, they developed reduction-sensitive sheddable micelle based on disulfide-linked hybrid PEG–polypeptide (mPEG-SS-Pleu) for intracellular drug delivery (Ren, et al., 2011). In addition, they synthesized star-shaped amphiphilic block copolymer 6sPCL-SS-PEG using a DCC/DMAP coupling reaction between 6sPCL-OH and COOH-terminated SS-labeled PEG (PEG-SS-COOH). Both systems exhibited rapid destabilization under a reduction environment and GSH-dependent cytotoxicity of DOX-loaded formulations against cancer cells.

Sun et al. (2010) constructed disassemblable micelles for intracellular delivery of DOX based on a reduction-degradable amphiphilic poly(amide amine) (PAA)-*g*-PEG graft copolymer containing disulfide links throughout the main chain. The drug release of the micelles in normal conditions was less than 25% within 24 h, whereas in the presence of reductive agent, DTT, the micelles can quickly release the entire loaded drug within 10 h. They further confirmed that the micelles could effectively deliver the drug cargo into nuclei after endocytosis by CLSM observation using HeLa cells (Sun, et al., 2010).

Fan et al. (2010) prepared camptothecin (CPT)-conjugated reduction-sensitive polymer mPEG-g-SS-PAA-CPT by combination of Michael addition polymerization and click chemistry. As compared with CPT free drug, mPEG-g-SS-PAA-CPT micelles showed improved solubility and enhanced stability for CPT in aqueous media. Most importantly, the reduction-responsive cleavage of disulfide links in the main chain of mPEG-*g*-SS-PAA-CPT in the presence of DTT led to gradual degradation of polymer backbone as well as sustained release of conjugated CPT, while almost no change was observed at the normal conditions corresponding to extracellular environment (Fan et al., 2010)

Zhong et al. designed and synthesized a series of novel copolymers based on PEG and reducible poly(L-amino ester)s containing disulfide bonds in the backbone of poly(amino ester)s, via Michael addition polymerization from 2,2-dithiodiethanol diacrylate, 4,4-trimethylene dipiperidine, and methoxy-PEG-NH2 (Chen, et al., 2011).

The resulting copolymers can self-assemble into stable micelles in a physiological environment, with a poly(amino ester)s-based core and a PEG-based shell. DOX release was faster from the micelles in a weakly acidic environment (pH 6.5) than at pH 7.4 or in the presence of a higher concentration (5 mM) of reducing agent (DTT). The release was even more effective upon exposure to both stimuli (pH 6.5 and 5 mM DTT), analogous to the pH and reduction conditions in the endosomes, therefore demonstrating great potential for tumor-targeted intracellular drug delivery.

Wang et al. reported the synthesis of a disulfide-linked biodegradable di-block copolymer of PCL and poly(ethyl ethylene phosphate), PEEP, by a coupling reaction between the thiol end group-functionalized PCL, PCL-SH, and the pyridyl disulfide group at the end of PEEP, PEEP-Py. PCL-SS-PEEP formed biocompatible micelles loaded with DOX in aqueous solution, but detached the PEEP shell under GSH stimulus, resulting in the destruction of micellar structure as well as rapid drug release profile, which led to enhanced growth inhibition against A549 tumor cells (Tang, et al., 2009)

Most of the disulfide-incorporated amphiphilic block copolymers discussed above were generated using a coupling reaction between two macromolecules, which often required extra separation or purification steps to get rid of excess homopolymers from the targeted block copolymers. Therefore, the development of facile approaches leading to novel sheddable micelles is highly desirable. In this regard, Oh et al. designed a new method for the synthesis of well-controlled biodegradable PLA-based amphiphilic block copolymers with SS links located at the block junctions (Sourkohi, 2011).

The method employed combined ROP and ATRP, as well as the synthesis of a new disulfide-functionalized double-head initiator having both terminal OH and Br groups (OH-SS-iBuBr). In the presence of OH-SS-iBuBr, both ROP of LA and ATRP of oligo(ethylene glycol) methyl ether methacrylate (OEGMA) were well controlled, resulting in well-defined PLA-SS-iBuBr and PLA-SS-POEGMA-Br with narrow-distributed molecular weight (Mw/Mn < 1.2). Aqueous micellization of PLA-SSPOEGMA resulted in core/shell micelles with SS links positioned at the interface between PLA cores and POEGMA coronas. Most importantly, POEGMA coronas were shed from the PLA cores upon the cleavage of SS links in the presence of DTT, analogous to the intracellular level of reducing potential, causing the precipitation of PLA core due to the loss of colloidal stability. In addition, these micelles were essentially nontoxic to cells. These results suggested that the biodegradable PLA-based sheddable micelles could be useful as novel drug delivery systems for intracellular drug delivery.

Reduction-Cleavable Side Chains

Thayumanavan et al. prepared amphiphilic polymers of different hydrophilic–hydrophobic ratios by free radical polymerization using two monomers consisting of tri(ethylene glycol) as the hydrophilic part and an alkyl chain connected by a disulfide bond as the hydrophobic part (Ryu, et al., 2010). These polymers formed micelle-type nano-assemblies in aqueous media and can encapsulate hydrophobic drug molecules up to 14% of their mass. In a reducing environment, these polymeric micelles disassembled and dissolved in water due to the conversion of amphiphilic polymers into hydrophilic polymers upon cleavage of the disulfide bonds and detachment of the lipophilic alkyl chains. This disassembly event resulted in the release of hydrophobic guest molecules that had been encapsulated inside the micelles, the rate of which was found to be dependent on the concentration of the reducing agent, GSH. In vitro experiments also showed that the GSH-dependent release of the DOX exerted cytotoxicity on MCF-7 cells.

Cross-Linked Polymeric Micelles

In blood circulation, blood proteins and lipoproteins such as high density lipoprotein (HDL), low density lipoprotein (LDL), very low density lipoprotein (VLDL) and chylomicron may interact with the polymeric micellar nanoparticles (Li, et al., 2012). This process can result in the early disintegration or aggregation of micelles and premature drug release (Rijcken, 2007).

Besides, polymeric micelles are a thermodynamically self-assembling system that has a well-known equilibrium existed between micelles and unimers (assembly unit) in aqueous condition. After being injected into the blood stream, conventional self-assembled polymeric micelles are susceptible to dilution below the critical micelle concentration (CMC). This may lead to the dissociation of micelles into unimers. Cross-linking strategy has been utilized to solve the above- mentioned stability problems following the pioneer work by Wooley's group (Jacksona, et al., 2013). Since then, this strategy has been exploited by a number of other groups (Huang, et al., 2012; Li, et al., 2009; Li, et al., 2012; Meng, et al., 2012; Popescu, et al., 2012; Wang, et al., 2013). Covalent cross-links between specific domains of the micelles are formed in order to improve the micelles' structural stability in the blood circulation. However, while the micelles need to be stable before they reach tumor site, they also need to be disassembled to facilitate the drug release once they are accumulated at tumor tissues or taken up by tumor cells. Excessively stabilized micelles may prevent the drug from releasing to target sites, thus reducing the therapeutic efficacy. Stimuli-responsive cross-linked micelles (SCMs) are introduced to achieve such a balance. SCMs exhibit unique stability in blood circulation and can better retain the drug contents. The utilization of environmentally sensitive cross-linkers or assembling units makes SCMs responsive to single or multiple stimuli in the microenvironment of tumor site or inside the tumor cells or the application of exogenous stimuli. The cleavage of the intra-micellar cross-linkage or disassembly of the micelles responding to stimuli leads to exclusively drug release in the target site.

Acid-Cleavable Cross-Linkers

Li et al. fabricated a novel cross-linked micelle using an acid-labile di-functional PEG containing two symmetrical cyclic ortho-esters for cross-linking (Yuan, et al., 201). Detachment of PEG side chains upon cleavage of ortho-ester groups at mildly acidic *p*H further led to the formation of a vesicle due to alteration of the hydrophilic/hydrophobic ratio in micelle structure. PTX-loaded cross-linked micelles showed *p*H-controlled drug release behaviors, namely, the drug release was accelerated dramatically at *p*H 5.4 and 6.4 as compared with that at *p*H 7.4 (Yuan, et al., 201). The results demonstrated that the resulting cross-linked micelle with acid-labile cross-linker could be a good candidate for intracellular tumor-targeted drug delivery.

Bulmus et al. (2004) described the combined use of acid-labile microgel approach and RAFT-mediated seeded dispersion polymerization technique to prepare an acid-cleavable core–shell polymeric colloidal system for delivery of hydrophobic drugs at slightly acidic sites (Chan, et al., 2008). In their design, a new divinyl cross-linker having acetal bonds, cleavable at mildly acidic *p*Hs, was copolymerized with n-butyl acrylate (BA) in the presence of a RAFT agent to produce cross-linked poly(BA) particles with surface RAFT groups (Chan, et al., 2008). The RAFT agent-functionalized particles were then modified via graft polymerization of poly (ethylene glycol) acrylate monomer (PEG-A) to mask the hydrophobicity of the surface. The acidic-site selective delivery potential of the poly (BA)-*g*-poly (PEG-A) particles was assessed in vitro using a lipophilic fluorescent dye as a model hydrophobic drug. Approximately 73% and 34% of the total dye loaded in the particles were found to be released at pH 5.0 and 7.4 in 24 h, respectively. The physicochemical and the functional features supported the potential value of the acid-cleavable poly (BA) core–poly (PEG-A) shell particles as carriers for the delivery of hydrophobic drugs at acidic sites. By copolymerization of the same acid-degradable cross-linker from the living RAFT-end groups of polymer chain, they further prepared acid-labile, core cross-linked (CCL) micelles based on amphiphilic poly (hydroxyethyl acrylate)-b-poly (n-butyl acrylate) (PHEA-*b*-PBA) copolymer. The resulting CCL micelles exhibited high DOX loading capacities (60 wt%), and *p*H-dependent control of drug release. Hydrolysis of less than half of the cross-linkers in the core was found to be sufficient to release DOX faster at acidic *p*H compared to neutral *p*H. Two important aspects should be considered when a specific acid-degradable cross-linker is chosen to fabricate acid-responsive nano-carriers, i.e., the incorporation strategy and the degradability of the acid-cleavable cross-linker.

Bulmus et al. (2006) reported that the hydrolysis half-life of the ketal-based cross-linker increased significantly with increasing *p*H (7 min at *p*H 4.5, 50 min at *p*H 6.1, and 44 h at *p*H 7.4), and their hydrolysis rate was faster than that of acetals, the half-life of which was in the range of several hours at *p*H 5.0 (Grillies, et al., 2006). The degradation half-lives of different acid cleavable links vary from less than 1 h to dozens of days at pH 5.0. The time frame desired for drug delivery applications relies on the characteristics of different diseases. A short hydrolysis half-life usually results in prompt dissociation of drug-carriers, leading to fast drug release with high efficacy, which is beneficial for the treatment of acute diseases, while retardant drug release resulting from longer hydrolysis duration should be highly desirable for chronic diseases, such as diabetes. Therefore, both release behaviors are necessary practice. In the case of tumor-targeted drug delivery a prompt destabilization of drug carriers inside cells and rapid release of the loaded therapeutics is preferred to significantly enhance drug efficacy, overcome multi-drug resistance (MDR), and minimize drug and carrier-associated side effects.

Reduction-Cleavable Cross-Linkers

Stenzel et al. explored the synthesis of reduction sensitive micelles using nucleosides containing block copolymer POEGMA-b-poly (5-O-methacryloyluridine), POEGMA30-*b*-PMAU80. The block copolymer underwent self-assembly into micelles in aqueous solution. Subsequent chain extension of the block co-polymer via RAFT process using a disulfide containing cross-linking agent, bis (2-methacryloyloxyethyl) disulfide, afforded CCL micelles with a P(OEGMA) shell and a polynucleotide core, which can further degrade under reductive conditions. As expected, the resulting CCL micelles readily dissociated into free block copolymer chains in the presence of DTT in less than 1 h, depending on the concentration of the reducing agent and the amount of cross-linker in the micelles. An *in vitro* drug loading and release study using vitamin B2 as a model drug indicated that the loading capacity increased with increasing cross-linking degree and the amount of drug released could reach 60–70% after 7 h in the presence of DTT (0.65 mM), while the release in the absence of DTT was significantly delayed. MTT assay revealed that the cross-linked micelles as well as the residues after reduction exhibited no cytotoxicity against COS-1 cell line, confirming their biocompatibility for intracellular drug delivery (Zhang, et al., 2008).

Wang et al. fabricated reversibly cross-linked core–shell-corona (CSC) micelles based on the triblock copolymer PCL-*b*-poly((2,4-dinitrophenyl) thioethyl ethylene phosphate)-*b*-PEG. The triblock copolymer was synthesized via consecutive ROP of CL and 2,4-dinitrophenylthioethyl ethylene phosphate, followed by coupling reaction with PEG. After deprotection, the middle block polyphosphoester exhibited free thiol side groups, which enabled further cross-linking of self-assembled micelles via disulfide link. The resulting CSC micelles with cross-linked shell layer displayed reduced CMC and enhanced stability against dilution. An in vitro drug release study demonstrated that DOX release was retarded by the cross-linked micellar structure, but was accelerated under simulated intracellular reductive environment due to the cleavage of cross-linking sites. Wang et al. (2008) reported the synthesis of an amphiphilic block copolymer of PEG and PCL that contained two pendent lipoyl functional groups at the block junctions (PEG-L2-PCL).

Xu, et al. (2009) reported PEG-L2-PCL formed micelles with sizes varying from 20 to 150 nm in aqueous solutions. These micelles were conveniently cross-linked in PBS (pH 7.4) by introducing

7.6 mol% of DTT relative to lipoyl moieties. The cross-linking mechanism is based on thiol-disulfide exchange. Under the catalysis of DTT, part of the lipoyl rings open to yield dihydrolipoyl groups (i.e., the reduced form of the lipoyl groups). The dihydrolipoyl groups readily exchange with the disulfide bonds of other lipoyl rings, which result in the formation of linear disulfide bonds between different lipoyl groups. As expected, these disulfide cross-linked micelles demonstrated a markedly enhanced stability against dilution, physiological salt concentration, and organic solvent, but were prone to dissociation under a reductive environment that mimics intracellular conditions. They further applied such reduction-responsive reversibly cross-linked biodegradable micelles for triggered release of DOX, and investigated the in vitro drug release behavior. The results showed minimal release of DOX from cross-linked micelles at a concentration of 10 mg/L (lower than CMC (16 mg/L), analogous to an intravenous injection), wherein less than 15% of the DOX was released in 10 h. In contrast, rapid drug release was recorded for DOX-loaded non-cross-linked micelles under otherwise the same conditions (~80% drug release in 0.5 h). In the presence of 10 mM DTT mimicking the intracellular reductive environment, sustained release of DOX from cross-linked micelles was achieved, in which 75% of the DOX was released in 9 h (Xu, et al., 2009).

N-acryloxysuccinimide (NAS) with activated pendant ester group provides optimized accessibility toward compound containing amino groups. Cystamine is a disulfide containing difunctional primary amine. The combined use of NAS and cystamine, namely, the incorporation of NAS monomer into polymer structure as the cross-linking sites via copolymerization followed by cross-linking of resultant polymer-based self-assembly using cystamine, represents a facile approach to fabricate reversible cross linked micelles with reduction-sensitivity. Similarly, Liu et al. synthesized the di-block copolymer PEO-*b*-P (NIPAAm-co-NAS) via RAFT polymerization using a PEO-based macro-RAFT agent. Such block copolymers self-assembled into micelles consisting of thermo-sensitive P (NIPAAm-*co*-NAS) cores and PEO coronas above the LCST (lower critical solution temperature) of P (NIPAAm-*co*-NAS) block. Further reaction of NAS residues in the micellar core with cystamine led to the formation of reversible CCL micelles. The cross-linking was conveniently cleaved in the presence of DTT and re-formed again upon addition of cystamine as a thiol/disulfide exchange promoter (Zhang, et al., 2007). In another paper, Liu et al. prepared CCL micelles composed of well-solvated poly (2-aminoethylmethacrylamide) (PAEMA) coronas and thermo-responsive cores in a one-pot manner via RAFT copolymerization of NIPAAm and a di-functional monomer bis(2-methacryloyloxyethyl) disulfide (DSDMA) by employing PAEMA as the macro-RAFT agent. In the presence of 15.4 mM DTT, the CCL micelles obtained could be disintegrated into unimers due to the cleavage of disulfide links, whereas deswelling of micellar cores could be achieved via heating above the LCST of PNIPAAm. Therefore, the release profiles of this type of nano carriers could be controlled by temperature and thiols or a combination of both stimuli. Due to the location of primary amine residues on the coronas of the CCL micelles, they further explored the possibility of surface-decoration by conjugating biotin and galactose moieties to the micellar shell as the targeting ligands for potential targeted drug delivery (Jiang, et al., 2009)

Lee et al. reported the synthesis of PEG-b-poly (L-lysine)-*b*-poly(l-phenylalanine), PEG-*b*-PLL-*b*-PPha, triblock copolymers by the sequential one-pot two-step ring opening polymerization in the presence of a CH3OPEG-NH2 macro-initiator and the subsequent deprotection process (Koo, et al., 2008). Based on such tri-block copolymers, they further prepared SCL (shell cross-linked) micelles by cross-linking the PLL middle shells with 3,3-dithiobis(sulfosuccinimidylpropionate), DTSSP. These SCL micelles demonstrated enhanced stability against sodium dodecyl sulfate (SDS) and the release of methotrexate (MTX) was greatly retarded as compared with the non-cross-linked analogs. An in vitro drug release study showed that the rate of drug release from SCL micelles increased with increasing GSH concentrations. They further investigated the cytotoxicity of MTX-loaded SCL micelles in A549 cells. The GSH dose-dependent cellular toxicity indicated clearly that GSH was responsible for modulating the MTX release from the SCL micelles with GSH-reducible cross-linked structures (Koo, et al., 2008).

Bronich et al. developed novel hybrid polymeric micelles with ionic cores containing biodegradable crosslinks for delivery of chemotherapeutic agents (Kim, et al., 2010). In their study, block ionomer complexes (BIC) of PEG-bpoly(methacrylic acid), PEO-*b*-PMA, and divalent metal cations (Ca2+) were used as the template. Disulfide bonds were further introduced in the ionic cores using cystamine as a biodegradable cross-linker. The resulting CCL hybrid micelles with disulfide bonds formed soft, hydrogel-like nanospheres and demonstrated time-dependent degradation in the conditions mimicking the intracellular reducing environment. Very interestingly, the ionic character of the cores facilitated a very high level of DOX loading (50%, w/w) into the CCL micelles. An in vitro drug release study demonstrated significant acceleration of DOX release from CCL micelles in the presence of GSH or cysteine in the release media, wherein about 75% of DOX was released within 1 h in the presence of 10 mM GSH. MTT assay indicated that the DOX-loaded degradable CCL micelles exhibited more potent cytotoxicity against human A2780 ovarian carcinoma cells, with IC_{50} value at least six times lower, as compared with the counterpart formulations without disulfide links (Kim, et al., 2010).

Dual Functional Polymeric Micelles

Vitamins E and its derivatives have been shown to have various biological activities such as antioxidant and enzymatic activity regulator. Due to their structures, they can also serve as hydrophobic domains to form dual functional drug carriers, i.e., carriers that can be used to deliver other therapeutic agents in addition to possessing biological activity themselves. Feng's group reported PEG conjugated Vitamin E (TPGS) based micelles (Mi, et al., 2011). TPGS is a water-soluble derivative of natural Vitamin E, which is formed by esterification of PEG with Vitamin E. As such it has advantages of PEG and Vitamin E in application of various drug delivery systems, including extending the half-life of the drug in plasma and enhancing the cellular uptake of the drug. TPGS has amphiphilic structure of lipophilic alkyl tail and hydrophilic polar head with a hydrophile-lipophile balance (HLB) value of 13.2 and a critical micelle concentration (CMC) of 0.02% w/w (Zhang. et al., 2012). US FDA has approved TPGS as a safe pharmaceutical adjuvant used in drug formulation. TPGS has also been used as the excipient for overcoming multidrug resistance (MDR) and for increasing the oral bioavailability of anticancer drugs through inhibition of P-glycoprotein (P-gp) (Zhang, et al., 2012). The CMC of TPGS is relatively high as mentioned above, which means TPGS micelles dissociate rapidly in the plasma. Thus TPGS was usually used together with other micellar materials to form mixed micelles to increase the micelle stability and the drug solubilization. Mu et al. prepared mixed micelles from poly (ethylene glycol)-phosphatidylethanolamine conjugate (PEG-PE) and TPGS with a molar ratio of 2:1 (Mu, et al., 2005). The CMC of the mixture was within 10^{-6} to 10^{-5} M and the solubility of camptothecin (CPT) was improved by at least 50% compared to the PEG-PE micelles due to the increased inner micelle core volume through the large vitamin E head. The anticancer efficiency of the mixed micelles was quite high because of their enhanced CPT solubility, permeability and stability as well as improved cellular uptake ability. This PEG-PE/TPGS system was further used to encapsulate anticancer drugs PTX and gossypol with a 1:1 carrier/drug molar ratio. PTX-loaded TPGS-lipid mixed micelles were found to be quite stable with only about 20% of drug release after 48 h at 37 ^{0}C.

The PEG–VE conjugates with variations in the average molecular weight (Mn) of PEG (2000 or 5000) and the molar ratio of PEG/VE (1: 1 or 1: 2) were independently synthesized by He, Sun et al., and Li et al. for DOX and PTX delivery, respectively (Wang, et al., 2012; Lu, et al., 2013).

All the PEG–VE conjugates could suppress the P-glycoprotein (P-gp) function effectively. The DOX-loaded micelles with a DLE as high as 94.5 wt% were revealed to be effectively internalized into P-gp-overexpressed adriamycin-resistant MCF-7 cells (MCF-7/ADR) through micropinocytosis and caveolin-dependent endocytosis, and showed enhanced cytotoxicity. Interestingly, the PTX-loaded PEG_{5K}–VE_2 micelles gave the best tumor growth inhibitory effect compared with PTX-encapsulated PEG_{2K}–VE and PEG_{2K}–VE_2 as well as Taxol in a syngeneic mouse model of breast cancer. Embelin is a natural product containing alkyl-substituted hydroxyl benzoquinone structure discovered from the Japanese Ardisia Herb (Herba Ardisiae Japonicae). Embelin has a broad spectrum of biological activities including antidiabetic, anti-inflammatory, and hepato-protective effects. In addition, embelin exhibits antitumor activity in many types of cancers such as breast, colon, prostate, and pancreatic cancer. Through computational structure-based computer screening, Wang and colleagues discovered that embelin is a potent inhibitor of X-linked inhibitor of apoptosis protein (XIAP), which partially explained its anticancer mechanism. XIAP is over-expressed in various types of cancer cells, particularly in drug-resistant cancer cells, while it plays a minimal role in normal cells (Chitra, et al., 1994; Bhandari, et al., 2007; Singh, et al., 2009).

Inhibition of XIAP has been demonstrated as an effective approach to selectively inhibit the growth of cancer cells. Embelin also inhibits NF-κB activation, which mediates the downregulation of several genes including surviving, XIAP, IAP1/2, TRAF1, cFLIP, Bcl-2 and Bcl-xL. Bearing a long lipophilic chain, embelin is extremely hydrophobic and water-insoluble (Singh, et al., 2009). In an attempt to explore the PEG modification as an approach to increase its water solubility, we have found that PEG-derivatized embelin forms micelles in aqueous solution (Lu, et al., 2013; Weisz, et al., 1999).

This is not a surprise considering the structural similarity between embelin and vitamin E. Interestingly, the antitumor activity of embelin was well retained after coupling with PEG chain. In addition, the PEG-embelin micelles are highly efficient in solubilizing various types of anticancer agent such as paclitaxel. Furthermore, PEG-embelin, at nanomolar range, showed synergistic effect with paclitaxel in several cancer cell lines tested. In vitro and in vivo studies have shown that the conjugates with two embelin molecules linked with one PEG chain were significantly more effective for loading paclitaxel than the conjugate with a 1:1 molar ratio of PEG and embelin. In addition, the PEG-embelin conjugates with a longer PEG chain were shown to be more advantageous compared with the counterparts with a shorter PEG chain. Near-infrared fluorescence (NIRF) imaging of PC-3 xenograft-bearing mice showed that PEG_{5K}-EB_2 micelles were selectively accumulated at tumor site with minimal distribution in major organs including liver and spleen. Delivery of paclitaxel via PEG_{5K}-$embelin_2$ micelles leads to superior antitumor activity compared to Taxol in murine models of breast and prostate cancers (Lu, et al., 2013; Weisz, et al., 1999). S-trans, trans farnesylthiosalicylic acid (Salirasib, or FTS) is a synthetic antagonist of Ras protein (Weisz, et al., 1999). By disrupting the anchorage of Ras on cell membrane, FTS is designed to inhibit Ras-dependent growth of cancer cells. Approximately 20% to 30% of human tumors express permanently active oncogenic Ras, and the mutationally activated Ras was most commonly found in adenocarcinomas of the pancreas, colon, lung, thyroid tumors, and myeloid leukemia. Accordingly, FTS exhibited potent antitumor effect in various tumors such as pancreatic cancer, colon cancer, melanoma, and neurofibromatosis. In addition, Ras inhibitors demonstrated synergistic effect with other chemotherapeutics, which validated their application in combination therapy. For example, treatment of the resistant SW480 cells with FTS dramatically enhanced the sensitivity to gemcitabine and led to improved inhibition of tumor growth in vivo (Gana-Weisz, et al., 2002).

Similar to vitamin E and embelin, FTS is also a hydrophobic small molecule with a long hydrophobic chain and a functional group (–COOH) that can be readily used for further modification. The biological activity and chemical structure of FTS has prompted us to design the PEG derivatized FTS conjugate as another dual-function micellar drug carrier. A labile ester linkage was used to facilitate the release of FTS and disassembly of the drug-loaded micelles following intracellular delivery to tumor cells. Our data have shown that the PEG-FTS2 readily forms micelles in aqueous solution with a CMC of 0.68 μM. Paclitaxel can be efficiently loaded into those micelles, which are spherical in morphology with a uniform size of 20–30 nm. Ras protein downregulation and cytotoxicity by PEG-FTS2 were comparable to free FTS as shown in 4T1.2 and HCT-116 cancer cell lines. The antitumor activity of paclitaxel-loaded PEG-FTS2 micelles was shown to be significantly higher than that of Taxol in a syngeneic murine breast cancer model (Zhang, et al., 2013) (see Figure 3).

Micellar Systems with Drug-Interactive Domains

Typically, the hydrophobic segments of amphiphilic copolymers incline to hide from the aqueous phase becoming the micellar core, while the hydrophilic segments tend to combine with water molecules forming the micellar shell. However, the amphiphilicity is often too weak and restricted for preparation of stable micelles that exhibit a broad application in the field of drug delivery. The carrier/drug incompatibility may account for, among others, the limited drug loading capacity and formulation stability. Park's group

Figure 3. Dual functional polymeric micelles

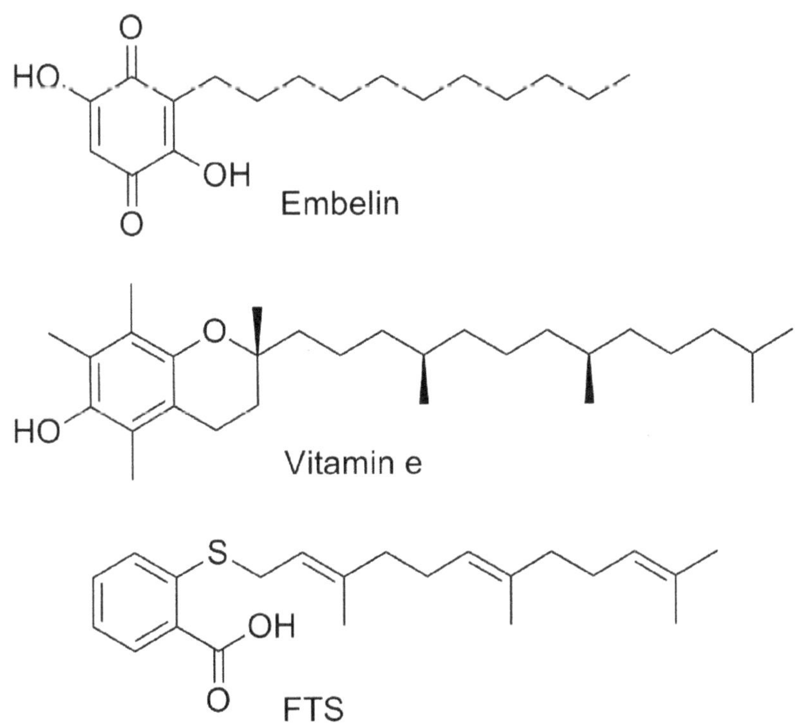

has shown that inclusion of less hydrophobic and hydrogen bond-forming "hydrotropic motifs" into the hydrophobic domain of polymeric micelles significantly improved the compatibility of the core-forming blocks with the drugs that were not entirely hydrophobic/lipophilic, leading to significant improvement in both drug loading capacity and the colloidal stability of drug-loaded micelles (Huh, et al., 2005; Kim, et al., 2011). Interestingly, pegylated surfactants with Vitamin E, embelin, or FTS as a hydrophobic domain work significantly better than those with simple lipids as micellar formulations. Vitamin E, embelin, and FTS all have an interfacial aromatic ring linked to an acyl chain. The π-π stacking between drug and carrier molecules as well as among carrier molecules themselves may contribute significantly to the improved formulation properties over the surfactants with simple lipid chains. These studies highlight the benefit of introducing additional structural variables to the traditional lipid-based excipients. We recently hypothesized that incorporation into a surfactant a drug-interactive motif at interfacial region will introduce additional carrier/drug interaction mechanism, which shall lead to improvement in both drug-loading capacity and formulation stability. This concept was tested with JP4-039, a mitochondria-targeted antioxidant and also a poorly water-soluble agent. A simple screening process was developed to identify agents that have potential drug-interactive activities based on the ability that prevents the formation of JP4-039 crystals in aqueous solution. Among several motifs screened, 9-Fluorenylmethoxy-carbony (Fmoc) moiety, a functional group that is routinely used for amino acid protection, was the most potent one (Gao, et al., 2013). A new micelle-forming PEG-lipopeptide conjugate was then synthesized. It has a lysine branching segment and two Fmoc groups located at the interfacial region, and two oleoyl chains as the hydrophobic core. It was found that incorporation of Fmoc motifs into a PEG-lipopeptide conjugate led to a significantly improved formulation with respect to both JP4-039 loading capacity and the stability of JP4-039-loaded micelles. More recently, we have shown that incorporation of an interfacial Fmoc group similarly improved the performance of PEG-Vitamin E- and PEG-FTS-based dual functional carriers. Delivery of PTX or DOX via PEG-Fmoc-Vitamin E or PEG-Fmoc-FTS led to significant inhibition of tumor growth in both breast and prostate cancer mouse models (Zhang, et al., 2014; Lu, et al., 2014; Zhang, et al., 2014) (see Figure 4).

Figure 4. Micellar systems with drug-interactive domains

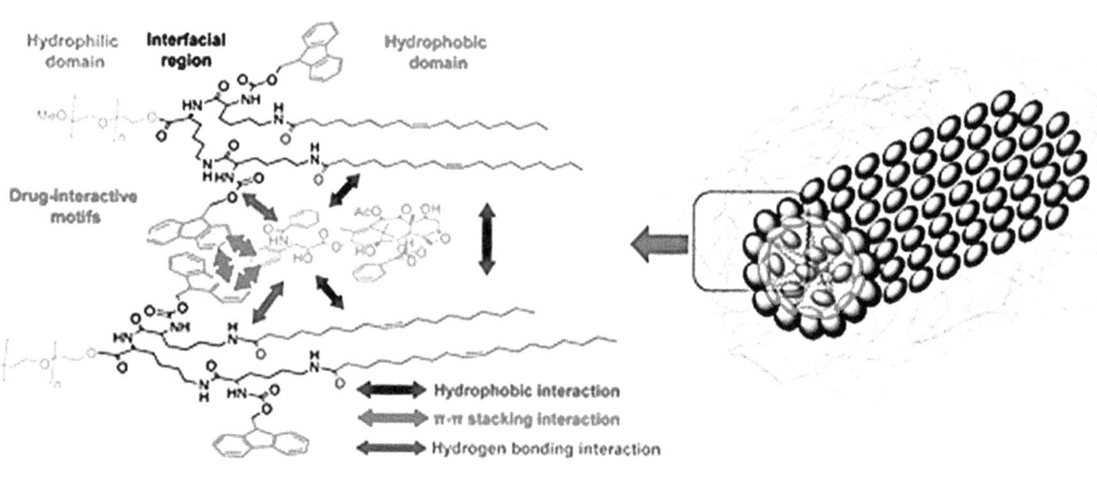

CONCLUSION

The last decade has seen tremendous progress in the field of polymeric micellar systems in the application of targeted cancer therapy. Several polymeric formulations have already entered into clinical phase. In addition, significant progresses have been made in the development of intelligent systems that can selectively respond to tumor microenvironment, leading to controlled and selective release of loaded drugs at tumor site. Future progress in this field shall rely on our better understanding of cellular barriers in delivery and the advancement of tumor biology and immunology. In addition, the biocompatibility of various new biomaterials needs to be thoroughly investigated. Finally, new strategies need to be developed to better incorporate targeted chemotherapy with other approaches such as immunotherapy to further improve the outcome of cancer treatment.

REFERENCES

Alami, N., Banerjee, K., Page, V., Hayashi, T., Igarashi, E., & Leyland-Jones, B. (2005). Long term survival with no apparent toxicity observed with a novel cisplatin-incorporated polymeric micelle, NC-6004, in the MCF-7 breast cancer model. *Breast Cancer Research and Treatment*, *94*, S64–S65.

Alexis, F., Rhee, J. W., Richie, J. P., Radovic-Moreno, A. F., Langer, R., & Farokhzad, O. (2008). New frontiers in nanotechnology for cancer treatment. *Urologic Oncology*, *26*(1), 74–85. doi:10.1016/j.urolonc.2007.03.017 PMID:18190835

Ballatori, N., Krance, S. M., Notenboom, S., Shi, S., Tieu, K., & Hammond, C. L. (2009). Glutathione dysregulation and the etiology and progression of human diseases. *Biological Chemistry*, *390*(3), 191–214. doi:10.1515/BC.2009.033 PMID:19166318

Bhandari, U., Jain, N., & Pillai, K. K. (2007). Further studies on antioxidant potential and protection of pancreatic beta-cells by Embelia ribes in experimental diabetes. *Experimental Diabetes Research*, 15803–15808. PMID:17641739

Cain, C. C., Sipe, D. M., & Murphy, R. F. (1989). Regulation of endocytic pH by the Na+/K+-ATPase in living cells. *Proceedings of the National Academy of Sciences of the United States of America*, *86*(2), 544–548. doi:10.1073/pnas.86.2.544 PMID:2536168

Chan, Y. N., Bulmus, V., Zareie, M. H., Byrne, F. L., Barner, L., & Kavallaris, M. (2006). Acid-cleavable polymeric core–shell particles for delivery of hydrophobic drugs. *Journal of Controlled Release*, *115*(2), 197–207. doi:10.1016/j.jconrel.2006.07.025 PMID:16996635

Chan, Y. N., Wong, T., Byrne, F., Kavallaris, M., & Bulmus, V. (2008). Acid-labile core cross-linked micelles for pH-triggered release of antitumor drugs. *Biomacromolecules*, *9*(7), 1826–1836. doi:10.1021/bm800043n PMID:18564874

Chen, J., Qiu, X. Z., Ouyang, J., Kong, J. M., Zhong, W., & Xing, M. M. Q. (2011). pH and reduction dual-sensitive copolymeric micelles for intracellular doxorubicin delivery. *Biomacromolecules*, *12*(10), 3601–3611. doi:10.1021/bm200804j PMID:21853982

Chen, W., Meng, F. H., Li, F., Ji, S. J., & Zhong, Z. Y. (2009). pH-responsive biodegradable micelles based on acid-labile polycarbonate hydrophobe: Synthesis and triggered drug release. *Biomacromolecules, 10*(7), 1727–1735. doi:10.1021/bm900074d PMID:19469499

Chitra, M., Sukumar, E., Suja, V., & Devi, C. S. (1994). Antitumor, anti-inflammatory and analgesic property of embelin, a plant product. *Chemotherapy, 40*(2), 109–113. doi:10.1159/000239181 PMID:7510605

Davis, M. E., Chen, Z., & Shin, D. M. (2008). Nanoparticle therapeutics: An emerging treatment modality for cancer. *Nature Reviews. Drug Discovery, 7*(9), 771–782. doi:10.1038/nrd2614 PMID:18758474

Ding, C. X., Gu, J. X., Qu, X. Z., & Yang, Z. Z. (2009). Preparation of multifunctional drug carrier for tumor-specific uptake and enhanced intracellular delivery through the conjugation of weak acid labile linker. *Bioconjugate Chemistry, 20*(6), 1163–1170. doi:10.1021/bc800563g PMID:19472997

Duncan, R., & Sat, Y. N. (1998). Tumour targeting by enhanced permeability and retention (EPR) effect. *Annals of Oncology, 9*(Suppl.2), 39–44. doi:10.1023/A:1008418325819

Estrela, J. M., Ortega, A., & Obrador, E. (2006). Glutathione in cancer biology and therapy. *Critical Reviews in Clinical Laboratory Sciences, 43*(2), 143–181. doi:10.1080/10408360500523878 PMID:16517421

Fan, H. L., Huang, J., Li, Y. P., Yu, J. H., & Chen, J. H. (2010). Fabrication of reduction-degradable micelle based on disulfide-linked graft copolymer–camptothecin conjugate for enhancing solubility and stability of camptothecin. *Polymer, 51*(22), 5107–5114. doi:10.1016/j.polymer.2010.09.004

Franco, R., & Cidlowski, J. A. (2009). Apoptosis and glutathione: Beyond an antioxidant. *Cell Death and Differentiation, 16*(10), 1303–1314. doi:10.1038/cdd.2009.107 PMID:19662025

Franco, R., Schoneveld, O. J., Pappa, A., & Panayiotidis, M. I. (2007). The central role of glutathione in the pathophysiology of human diseases. *Archives of Physiology and Biochemistry, 113*(4-5), 234–258. doi:10.1080/13813450701661198 PMID:18158646

Gana-Weisz, M., Halaschek-Wiener, J., Jansen, B., Elad, G., Haklai, R., & Kloog, Y. (2002). The Ras inhibitor S-trans, trans-farnesylthiosalicylic acid chemosensitizes human tumor cells without causing resistance. *Clinical Cancer Research, 8*(2), 555–565. PMID:11839677

Gao, X., Huang, Y., Makhov, A. M., Epperly, M., Lu, J., Grab, S., & Li, S. et al. (2013). Nanoassembly of surfactants with interfacial drug-interactive motifs as tailor-designed drug carriers. *Molecular Pharmaceutics, 10*(1), 187–198. doi:10.1021/mp300319m PMID:23244299

Gillies, E. R., & Fréchet, J. M. J. (2003). A new approach towards acid sensitive copolymer micelles for drug delivery. *Chemical Communications, 14*(14), 1640–1641. doi:10.1039/B304251K PMID:12877480

Gillies, E. R., Jonsson, T. B., & Fréchet, J. M. J. (2004). Stimuli-responsive supramolecular assemblies of linear-dendritic copolymers. *Journal of the American Chemical Society, 126*(38), 11936–11943. doi:10.1021/ja0463738 PMID:15382929

Hamaguchi, T., Kato, K., Yasui, H., Morizane, C., Ikeda, M., Ueno, H., & Matsumura, Y. et al. (2007). A phase I and pharmacokinetic study of NK105, a paclitaxel-incorporating micellar nanoparticle formulation. *British Journal of Cancer, 97*(2), 170–176. doi:10.1038/sj.bjc.6603855 PMID:17595665

Heffernan, M. J., & Murthy, N. J. (2005). Polyketal nanoparticles: A new pHsensitive biodegradable drug delivery vehicle. *Bioconjugate Chemistry*, *16*(6), 1340–1342. doi:10.1021/bc050176w PMID:16287226

Huang, Y., Lu, J., Gao, X., Li, J., Zhao, W., Sun, M., & Li, S. et al. (2012). PEGderivatized embelin as a dual functional carrier for the delivery of paclitaxel. *Bioconjugate Chemistry*, *23*(7), 1443–1451. doi:10.1021/bc3000468 PMID:22681537

Huang, Y. C., Yang, Y. S., Lai, T. Y., & Jan, J. S. (2012). Lysine-block-tyrosine block copolypeptides: Self-assembly, cross-linking, and conjugation of targeted ligand for drug encapsulation. *Polymer*, *53*(4), 913–922. doi:10.1016/j.polymer.2012.01.010

Huh, K. M., Lee, S. C., Ch, Y. W., Lee, J., Jeong, J. H., & Park, K. (2005). Hydrotropic polymer micelle system for delivery of paclitaxel. *Journal of Controlled Release*, *101*(1–3), 59–68. doi:10.1016/j.jconrel.2004.07.003 PMID:15588894

Jacksona, A. W., & Fulton, D. A. (2013). Making polymeric nanoparticles stimuli-responsive with dynamic covalent bonds. *Polymer Chemistry*, *4*(1), 31–45. doi:10.1039/C2PY20727C

Jain, R., Standley, S. M., & Fréchet, J. M. J. (2007). Synthesis and degradation of pH-sensitive linear poly(amidoamine)s. *Macromolecules*, *40*(3), 452–457. doi:10.1021/ma062319v

Jiang, X. Z., Liu, S. Y., & Narain, R. (2009). Degradable thermoresponsive core cross-linked micelles: Fabrication, surface functionalization, and biorecognition. *Langmuir*, *25*(23), 13344–13350. doi:10.1021/la9034276 PMID:19928937

Jones, M. C., & Leroux, J. C. (1999). Polymeric micelles - a new generation of colloidal drug carriers. *European Journal of Pharmaceutics and Biopharmaceutics*, *48*(2), 101–111. doi:10.1016/S0939-6411(99)00039-9 PMID:10469928

Kim, J. O., Sahay, G., Kabanov, A. V., & Bronich, T. K. (2010). Polymeric micelles with ionic cores containing biodegradable cross-links for delivery of chemotherapeutic agents. *Biomacromolecules*, *11*(4), 919–926. doi:10.1021/bm9013364 PMID:20307096

Kim, J. Y., Kim, S., Pinal, R., & Park, K. (2011). Hydrotropic polymer micelles as versatile vehicles for delivery of poorly water-soluble drugs. *Journal of Controlled Release*, *152*(1), 13–20. doi:10.1016/j.jconrel.2011.02.014 PMID:21352878

Kim, T. Y., Kim, D. W., Chung, J. Y., Shin, S. G., Kim, S. C., Heo, D. S., & Bang, Y. J. et al. (2004). Phase I and pharmacokinetic study of Genexol-PM, a cremophor-free, polymeric micelle-formulated paclitaxel, in patients with advanced malignancies. *Clinical Cancer Research*, *10*(11), 3708–3716. doi:10.1158/1078-0432.CCR-03-0655 PMID:15173077

Koo, A. N., Lee, H. J., Kim, S. E., Chang, J., Park, C. Y., Kim, C. H., & Lee, S. C. et al. (2008). Disulfide-cross-linked PEG–poly(amino acid)s copolymer micelles for glutathione-mediated intracellular drug delivery. *Chemical Communications*, *48*(48), 6570–6572. doi:10.1039/b815918a PMID:19057782

Lavelle, F., Bissery, M. C., Andre, S., Roquet, F., & Riou, J. F. (1996). Preclinical evaluation of CPT-11 and its active metabolite SN-38. *Seminars in Oncology*, *23*(1), 11–20. PMID:8633248

Lee, K. S., Chung, H. C., Im, S. A., Park, Y. H., Kim, C. S., Kim, S. B., & Ro, J. et al. (2008). Multicenter phase II trial of Genexol-PM, a Cremophor-free, polymeric micelle formulation of paclitaxel, in patients withmetastatic breast cancer. *Breast Cancer Research and Treatment*, *108*(2), 241–250. doi:10.1007/s10549-007-9591-y PMID:17476588

Li, Q. M., Zhu, L. J., Liu, R. G., Huang, D., Jin, X., Che, N., & Huang, Y. et al. (2012). Biological stimuli responsive drug carriers based on keratin for triggerable drug delivery. *Journal of Materials Chemistry*, *22*(37), 19964–19973. doi:10.1039/c2jm34136k

Li, Y., Budamaguta, M. S., Luo, J., Xiao, W., Voss, J. C., & Lam, K. S. (2012). Probing of the assembly structure and dynamics within nanoparticls during interaction with bold proteins. *ACS Nano*, *6*(11), 9486–9495. doi:10.1021/nn302317j

Li, Y. L., Zhu, L., Liu, Z. Z., Chemg, R., Meng, F. H., Cui, J. H., & Zhong, Z. Y. et al. (2009). Reversibly Stabilized Multifunctional Dextran Nanoparticles Efficiently Deliver Doxorubicin into the Nuclei of Cancer Cells. *Angewandte Chemie*, *48*(52), 9914–9918. doi:10.1002/anie.200904260 PMID:19937876

Liu, J. Y., Pang, Y., Huang, W., Huang, X. H., Meng, L. L., Zhu, X. Y., & Yan, D. Y. et al. (2011). Bioreducible micelles self-assembled from amphiphilic hyperbranched multiarm copolymer for glutathione-mediated intracellular drug delivery. *Biomacromolecules*, *12*(5), 1567–1577. doi:10.1021/bm200275j PMID:21456627

Liu, J. Y., Pang, Y., Huang, W., Huang, X. H., Meng, L. L., Zhu, X. Y., & Yan, D. Y. et al. (2011). Redox-responsive polyphosphate nanosized assemblies: A smart drug delivery platform for cancer therapy. *Biomacromolecules*, *12*(6), 2407–2415. doi:10.1021/bm2005164 PMID:21557536

Lu, J., Huang, Y., Zhao, W., Chen, Y., Li, J., Gao, X., & Li, S. et al. (2013). Design and characterization of PEG-derivatized vitamin E as a nanomicellar formulation for delivery of paclitaxel. *Molecular Pharmaceutics*, *10*(8), 2880–2890. doi:10.1021/mp300729y PMID:23768151

Lu, J., Huang, Y., Zhao, W., Marquez, R. T., Meng, X., Li, J., & Li, S. et al. (2013). PEGderivatized embelin as a nanomicellar carrier for delivery of paclitaxel to breast and prostate cancers. *Biomaterials*, *34*(5), 1591–1600. doi:10.1016/j.biomaterials.2012.10.073 PMID:23182923

Lu, J., Zhao, W., Liu, H., Marquez, R., Huang, Y., Zhang, Y., & Li, S. et al. (2014). …Li, S. (2014). An improved d-alpha-tocopherol-based nanocarrier for targeted delivery of doxorubicin with reversal of multidrug resistance. *Journal of Controlled Release*, *196*, 272–286. doi:10.1016/j.jconrel.2014.10.016 PMID:25456831

Lukyanov, A. N., & Torchilin, V. P. (2004). Micelles from lipid derivatives of water-soluble polymers as delivery systems for poorly soluble drugs. *Advanced Drug Delivery Reviews*, *56*(9), 1273–1289. doi:10.1016/j.addr.2003.12.004 PMID:15109769

Matsumura, Y. (2011). Preclinical and clinical studies of NK012, an SN-38-incorporating polymeric micelles, which is designed based on EPR effect. *Advanced Drug Delivery Reviews*, *63*(3), 184–192. doi:10.1016/j.addr.2010.05.008 PMID:20561951

Matsumura, Y., Hamaguchi, T., Ura, T., Muro, K., Yamada, Y., Shimada, Y., & Watanabe, N. et al. (2004). Phase I clinical trial and pharmacokinetic evaluation of NK911, a micelle-encapsulated doxorubicin. *British Journal of Cancer*, *91*(10), 1775–1781. doi:10.1038/sj.bjc.6602204 PMID:15477860

Matsumura, Y., & Maeda, H. (1986). A new concept formacromolecular therapeutics in cancer chemotherapy: Mechanism of tumouritropic accumulation of proteins and the antitumour agent smancs. *Cancer Research*, *46*, 6387–6392. PMID:2946403

Mellman, I., Fuchs, R., & Helenius, A. (1986). Acidification of the endocytic and exocytic pathways. *Annual Review ofBiochemistry*, *55*(1), 663–700. doi:10.1146/annurev.bi.55.070186.003311 PMID:2874766

Meng, F. H., Cheng, R., Deng, C., & Zhong, Z. Y. (2012). Intracellular drug release nanosystems. *Materials Today*, *15*(10), 436–442. doi:10.1016/S1369-7021(12)70195-5

Mi, Y., Liu, Y., & Feng, S. S. (2011). Formulation of docetaxel by folic acid conjugated D-α-tocopheryl polyethylene glycol succinate 2000 (Vitamin E TPGS2k) micelles for targeted and synergistic chemotherapy. *Biomaterials*, *32*(16), 4058–4066. doi:10.1016/j.biomaterials.2011.02.022 PMID:21396707

Michalet, X., Pinaud, F. F., Bentolila, L. A., Tsay, J. M., Doose, S., Li, J. J., & Weiss, S. et al. (2005). Quantum dots for live cells, in vivo imaging, and diagnostics. *Science*, *307*(5709), 538–544. doi:10.1126/science.1104274 PMID:15681376

Misra, R., Acharya, S., & Sahoo, S. K. (2010). Cancer nanotechnology: Application of nanotechnology in cancer therapy. *Drug Discovery Today*, *15*(19-20), 842–850. doi:10.1016/j.drudis.2010.08.006 PMID:20727417

Mu, L., Elbayoumi, T. A., & Torchilin, V. P. (2005). Mixed micelles made of poly(ethylene glycol)–phosphatidylethanolamine conjugate and d-α-tocopheryl polyethylene glycol 1000 succinate as pharmaceutical nanocarriers for camptothecin. *International Journal of Pharmaceutics*, *306*(1–2), 142–149. doi:10.1016/j.ijpharm.2005.08.026 PMID:16242875

Paramonov, S. E., Bachelder, E. M., Beaudette, T. T., Standley, S. M., Lee, C. C., Dashe, J., & Fréchet, J. M. J. (2008). Fully acid-degradable biocompatible polyacetal microparticles for drug delivery. *Bioconjugate Chemistry*, *19*(4), 911–919. doi:10.1021/bc7004472 PMID:18373356

Plummer, R., Wilson, R. H., Calvert, H., Boddy, A. V., Griffin, M., Sludden, J., & Nishiya, T. et al. (2011, February15). …Nishiya, T. A Phase I clinical study of cisplatin-incorporated polymeric micelles (NC-6004) in patients with solid tumours. *British Journal of Cancer*, *104*(4), 593–598. doi:10.1038/bjc.2011.6 PMID:21285987

Popescu, M. T., Tsitsilianis, C., Papadakis, C. M., Adelsberger, J., Balog, S., Busch, P., & Patrickios, C. S. et al. (2012). Stimuli-Responsive Amphiphilic Polyelectrolyte Heptablock Copolymer Physical Hydrogels: An Unusual pH-Response. *Macromolecules*, *45*(8), 3523–3530. doi:10.1021/ma300222d

Quan, C. Y., Chen, J., Wang, H.-Y., Li, C., Chang, C., Zhang, X.-Z., & Zhuo, R.-X. (2010). Core–shell nanosized assemblies mediated by the cyclodextrindimer with a tumor-triggered targeting property. *ACS Nano*, *4*(7), 4211–4219. doi:10.1021/nn100534q PMID:20521828

Ren, T. B., Feng, Y., Zhang, Z. H., Lia, L., & Li, Y. Y. (2011). Shell-sheddable micelles based on star-shaped poly(3-caprolactone)-SS-poly(ethylglycol) copolymer for intracellular drug release. *Soft Matter*, *7*(6), 2329–2331. doi:10.1039/c1sm05020f

Ren, T. B., Xia, W. J., Dong, H. Q., & Li, Y. Y. (2011). Sheddable micelles based on disulfide-linked hybrid PEG–polypeptide copolymer for intracellular drug delivery. *Polymer*, *52*(16), 3580–3586. doi:10.1016/j.polymer.2011.06.013

Rijcken, C. J., Snel, C. J., Schiffelers, R. M., van Nostrum, C. F., & Hennink, W. E. (2007). Hydrolysable core-crosslinked thermosensitive polymeric micelles: Synthesis, characterization and in vivo studies. *Biomaterials*, *28*(36), 5581–5593. doi:10.1016/j.biomaterials.2007.08.047 PMID:17915312

Ryu, J. H., Roy, R., Ventura, J., & Thayumanavan, S. (2010). Redox-sensitive disassembly of amphiphilic copolymer based micelles. *Langmuir*, *26*(10), 7086–7092. doi:10.1021/la904437u PMID:20073533

Saito, G., Swanson, J. A., & Lee, K. D. (2003). Drug delivery strategy utilizing conjugation via reversible disulfide links: Role and site of cellular reducing activities. *Advanced Drug Delivery Reviews*, *55*(2), 199–215. doi:10.1016/S0169-409X(02)00179-5 PMID:12564977

Schafer, F. Q., & Buettner, G. R. (2001). Redox environment of the cell as viewed through the redox state of the glutathione disulfide/glutathione couple. *Free Radical Biology & Medicine*, *30*(11), 1191–1212. doi:10.1016/S0891-5849(01)00480-4 PMID:11368918

Shapria, A., Livney, Y. D., Broxterman, H. J., & Assaraf, Y. G. (2011). Nanomedicine for targeted cancer therapy: towards the overcoming of drug resistance. *Drug Resistance Updates: Reviews and Commentaries in Antimicrobial and Anticancer Chemotherapy, 14*(3), 150-163.

Singh, D., Singh, R., Singh, P., & Gupta, R. S. (2009). Effect of embelin on lipid peroxidation and free radical scavenging activity against liver damage in rats. *Basic & Clinical Pharmacology & Toxicology*, *105*(4), 243–248. doi:10.1111/j.1742-7843.2009.00429.x PMID:19496777

Sourkohi, B. K., Cunningham, A., Zhang, Q., & Oh, J. K. (2011). Biodegradable block copolymer micelles with thiol-responsive sheddable coronas. *Biomacromolecules*, *12*(10), 3819–3825. doi:10.1021/bm2011032 PMID:21879701

Sun, H. L., Guo, B. N., Cheng, R., Meng, F. H., Liu, H. Y., & Zhong, Z. Y. (2009). Biodegradable micelles with sheddable poly(ethylene glycol) shells for triggered intracellular release of doxorubicin. *Biomaterials*, *30*(31), 6358–6366. doi:10.1016/j.biomaterials.2009.07.051 PMID:19666191

Sun, H. L., Guo, B. N., Cheng, R., Meng, F. H., Liu, H. Y., & Zhong, Z. Y. (2010). Shellsheddable micelles based on dextran-SS-poly(ε-caprolactone) diblock copolymer for efficient intracellular release of doxorubicin. *Biomacromolecules*, *11*(4), 848–854. doi:10.1021/bm1001069 PMID:20205476

Sun, Y., Yan, X. L., Yuan, T. M., Liang, J., Fan, Y. J., Gu, Z. W., & Zhang, X. D. (2010). Disassemblable micelles based on reduction-degradable amphiphilic graft copolymers for intracellular delivery of doxorubicin. *Biomaterials*, *31*(27), 7124–7131. doi:10.1016/j.biomaterials.2010.06.011 PMID:20580429

Tang, L. Y., Wang, Y. C., Li, Y., Du, J. Z., & Wang, J. (2009). Shell-detachable micelles based on disulfide-linked block copolymer as potential carrier for intracellular drug delivery. *Bioconjugate Chemistry*, *20*(6), 1095–2009. doi:10.1021/bc900144m PMID:19438224

Tang, R., Ji, W., Panus, D., Palumbo, R. N., & Wang, C. (2011). Block copolymer micelles with acid-labile ortho ester side-chains: Synthesis, characterization, and enhanced drug delivery to human glioma cells. *Journal of Controlled Release*, *151*(1), 18–27. doi:10.1016/j.jconrel.2010.12.005 PMID:21194551

Tomlinson, R., Klee, M., Garrett, S., Heller, J., Duncan, R., & Brocchini, S. (2002). Pendent chain functionalized polyacetals that display pH-dependent degradation: A platform for the development of novel polymer therapeutics. *Macromolecules*, *35*(2), 473–480. doi:10.1021/ma0108867

Trubetskoy, V. S., & Torchilin, V. P. (1995). Use of polyoxyethylene-lipid conjugates as long-circulating carriers for delivery of therapeutic and diagnostic agents. *Advanced Drug Delivery Reviews*, *16*(2–3), 311–320. doi:10.1016/0169-409X(95)00032-3

Van Vlerken, L. E., Vyas, T. K., & Amiji, M. M. (2007). Poly(ethylene glycol)-modified nanocarriers for tumor-targeted and intracellular delivery. *Pharmaceutical Research*, *24*(8), 1405–1414. doi:10.1007/s11095-007-9284-6 PMID:17393074

Wang, J., Sun, J., Chen, Q., Gao, Y., Li, L., Li, H., & He, Z. (2012). Star-shape copolymer of lysine linked di-tocopherol polyethylene glycol 2000 succinate for doxorubicin delivery with reversal of multidrug resistance. *Biomaterials*, *28*(28), 6877–6888. doi:10.1016/j.biomaterials.2012.06.019 PMID:22770799

Wang, K., Liu, Y., Yi, W. J., Li, C., Li, Y. Y., Zhuo, R. X., & Zhang, X. Z. (2013). Novel shell-cross-linked micelles with detachable PEG corona for glutathione-mediated intracellular drug delivery. *Soft Matter*, *9*(3), 692–699. doi:10.1039/C2SM27028E

Wang, Y. C., Li, Y., Sun, T. M., Xiong, M. H., Wu, J. J., Yang, Y. Y., & Wang, J. (2010). Core–shell-corona micelle stabilized by reversible cross-link for intracellular drug delivery. *Macromolecular Rapid Communications*, *31*(13), 1201–1206. doi:10.1002/marc.200900863 PMID:21590876

Weisz, B., Giehl, K., Gana Weisz, M., Egozi, Y., Ben-Baruch, G., Marciano, D., & Kloog, Y. et al. (1999). A new functional Ras antagonist inhibits human pancreatic tumor growth in nude mice. *Oncogene*, *18*(16), 2579–2588. doi:10.1038/sj.onc.1202602 PMID:10353601

Wen, H. Y., Dong, H. Q., Xie, W. J., Li, Y. Y., Wang, K., Pauletti, G. M., & Shi, D. L. (2011). Rapidly disassembling nanomicelles with disulfide-linked PEG shells for glutathione-mediated intracellular drug delivery. *Chemical Communications*, *47*(12), 3550–3562. doi:10.1039/c0cc04983b PMID:21327187

Xiao, K., Luo, J., Fowler, W. L., Li, Y., Lee, J. S., Xing, L., & Lam, K. S. et al. (2009). A self-assembling nanoparticle for paclitaxel delivery in ovarian cancer. *Biomaterials*, *30*(30), 6006–6016. doi:10.1016/j.biomaterials.2009.07.015 PMID:19660809

Xiao, K., Luo, J., Li, Y., Lee, J. S., Fung, G., & Lam, K. S. (2011). PEG-oligocholic acid telodendrimer micelles for the targeted delivery of doxorubicin to B-cell lymphoma. *Journal of Controlled Release*, *155*(2), 272–281. doi:10.1016/j.jconrel.2011.07.018 PMID:21787818

Xu, Y. M., Meng, F. H., Cheng, R., & Zhong, Z. Y. (2009). Reduction-sensitive reversibly crosslinked biodegradable micelles for triggered release of doxorubicin. *Macromolecular Bioscience*, *9*(12), 1254–1261. doi:10.1002/mabi.200900233 PMID:19904724

Yuan, Z. F., Huang, J. Y., Liu, J., Cheng, S. X., Zhuo, R. X., & Li, F. (2011). PEG-detachable and acid-labile cross-linked micelles based on orthoester linked graft copolymer for paclitaxel release. *Nanotechnology*, *22*(33), 335601. doi:10.1088/0957-4484/22/33/335601 PMID:21788685

Zhang, J. Y., Jiang, X. Z., Zhang, Y. F., Li, Y. T., & Liu, S. Y. (2007). Facile fabrication of reversible core cross-linked micelles possessing thermosensitive swellability. *Macromolecules*, *40*(25), 9125–9132. doi:10.1021/ma071564r

Zhang, L., Liu, W. G., Lin, L., Chen, D. Y., & Stenzel, M. H. (2008, November10). (208). Degradable disulfide core-cross-linked micelles as a drug delivery system prepared from vinyl functionalized nucleosides via the RAFT process. *Biomacromolecules*, *9*(11), 3321–3331. doi:10.1021/bm800867n PMID:18842025

Zhang, X., Huang, Y., Zhao, W., Liu, H., Marquez, R., Lu, J., & Li, S. et al. (2014). Targeted delivery of anticancer agents via a dual function nanocarrier with an interfacial drug-interactive motif. *Biomacromolecules*, *10*(15), 4326–4335. doi:10.1021/bm501339j PMID:25325795

Zhang, X., Lu, J., Huang, Y., Zhao, W., Li, J., Gao, X., & Li, S. et al. (2013). PEGfarnesylthiosalicylate conjugate as a nanomicellar carrier for delivery of paclitaxel. *Bioconjugate Chemistry*, *24*(3), 464–472. doi:10.1021/bc300608h PMID:23425093

Zhang, Y., Huang, Y., Zhao, W., Lu, J., Zhang, P., Zhang, X., & Li, S. et al. (2014). Design and evaluation of a PEGylated lipopeptide equipped with drug-interactive motifs as an improved drug carrier. *The AAPS Journal*, *16*(1), 114–124. doi:10.1208/s12248-013-9536-9 PMID:24281690

Zhang, Y., Huang, Y., Zhao, W., Lu, J., Zhang, P., Zhang, X., & Li, S. et al. (2014). Fmoc-conjugated PEG-vitamin E micelles for tumor-targeted delivery of paclitaxel: Enhanced drug–carrier interaction and loading capacity. *The AAPS Journal*, *16*(6), 1282–1291. doi:10.1208/s12248-014-9651-2 PMID:25193267

Zhang, Z., Tan, S., & Feng, S. S. (2012). Vitamin E TPGS as a molecular biomaterial for drug delivery. *Biomaterials*, *33*(19), 4889–4906. doi:10.1016/j.biomaterials.2012.03.046 PMID:22498300

Zhou, L. J., Liang, D., He, X., Li, J., Tan, H., Li, J., & Gu, Q. et al. (2012). The degradation and biocompatibility of pH-sensitive biodegradable polyurethanes for intracellular multifunctional antitumor drug delivery. *Biomaterials*, *33*(9), 2734–2745. doi:10.1016/j.biomaterials.2011.11.009 PMID:22236829

Section 10
Nanotechnology

Chapter 13
Pharmaceutical and Medical Applications of Nanofibers

Khosro Adibkia
Tabriz University of Medical Sciences, Iran

Shadi Yaqoubi
Tabriz University of Medical Sciences, Iran

Solmaz Maleki Dizaj
Tabriz University of Medical Sciences, Iran

ABSTRACT

Nanofibers as a main group of nanoparticles have a vast range of applicability for therapeutic purposes, duo to their outstanding attributes such as very large surface to volume ratio and high porosity. These types of nanoparticles are more known as tissue scaffolds and drug delivery carriers. Nanofiber-based carriers are able to control the release pattern of drugs. In addition, they can act as multidrug-loaded materials with programed dual release profile. Electrospinning is a simple method, which is recognized as the most efficient approach for the fabrication of nanofibers. Production of ultrafine fibers based on various natural or synthetic polymers is possible by means of electrospinning. In this chapter, a comprehensive review is presented on various medical applications of electrospun nanofibers in the case of tissue engineering and drug delivery. Several investigations on therapeutic nanofibers and their processing methods are also summarized in this chapter.

INTRODUCTION

During recent years, the science of nanoparticles has received great importance owing to their applications in various aspects of medical and pharmaceutical sciences, engineering, and other areas of human life (Barzegar-Jalali et al., 2008; Burgess et al., 2010; Kamaly, Xiao, Valencia, Radovic-Moreno, & Farokhzad, 2012; Mohanraj & Chen, 2007). To reach a successful treatment process for various diseases and abnormalities in human body, the key factor is to smartly use of the therapeutic agents (either pharmaceuticals or other medical applications). In order to deliver the therapeutic agents to the site of

DOI: 10.4018/978-1-5225-0751-2.ch013

action and to control their fate in patients' body, nanotechnology and more specifically nanomedicine is a promising approach because of the unique and outstanding physicochemical properties of the nanoparticles (Yang, Chang, Yang, & Lin, 2010). Biomedical nanoparticles, with a diameter in the nanometer size range and modified physicochemical properties, are appropriate for several biomedical purposes. Nanoparticles could be applied as targeted delivery systems (Brannon-Peppas & Blanchette, 2012; Cho, Wang, Nie, & Shin, 2008), as tissue scaffolds (Berry & Curtis, 2003; Goldberg, Langer, & Jia, 2007; Hans & Lowman, 2002; Qian et al., 2008; Zhang et al., 2008), and for improving the bioavailability of drugs (Li & Huang, 2008). Nanoparticles also have some other advantages like high capacity of drug loading due to their porosity and reduced size, which improves water-solubility of the poor soluble drugs. This submicron diameter also enhances their membrane permeation in order to modify the absorption profile of the drug via different tissues. In addition, reduced dose, less toxicity, less adverse effects, and also better patient compliance are other attributes which draw attention toward apprising nanoparticles as an interesting novel drug delivery system (Adibkia, 2014; Dizaj, Barzegar-Jalali, Zarrintan, Adibkia, & Lotfipour; Jahangiri et al., 2014). With the purpose of improving controlled drug delivery devices, nanofibers made of biocompatible materials as well as other nanomedicines are of the most highly considered choices, which are used as ideal carriers or vehicles for therapeutic agents. They profit all the advantages mentioned for nanoparticles beside some unique specificities, which makes them play a potential promising role in various biomedical applications including medical prostheses, tissue template, wound dressing, and cosmetics (Huang, Zhang, Kotaki, & Ramakrishna, 2003).

BACKGROUND

Nanofibers are ultrafine fibers with nano-scaled diameter and very large surface area. High porous structure is also one of the outstanding properties of the nanofibers. They have many different applications in various fields; they can be used as filters to remove particles via different mechanisms, may act as vehicles for catalysts and enzymes, may be used as sensors, or may be applied to store energy (Fang, Niu, Lin, & Wang, 2008). Therapeutic applications of the nanofibers, as another advantageous aspect of these ultrafine fibers, have become the field of interest by many researchers who work on biomedical devices. Nanofibers with therapeutic purposes have shown a promising potential in the case of both drug delivery and tissue engineering (Fang et al., 2008; Sill & von Recum, 2008; Vasita & Katti, 2006).

Nanofibers for medical purposes can be produced using biodegradable materials (e. g. polymers) along with various additives in order to gain the planned functionality. Biopolymer-based nanofibers can be used as a carrier for bioactive materials or drugs. Consequently, nanofibers can provide improved bioavailability, especially for the poorly soluble drugs. Furthermore, their structure and size can be optimized for tissue engineering studies. Nanofibers prepared from biopolymers such as collagen, polylactic acid (PLA), and polycaprolactone (PCL) are potential substrates for growing the cells. It has been shown that electrospun collagen, for example, promotes cell growth and penetration of the cells into the engineered scaffold. Special properties (structural, material, and biological) of the electrospun collagen propose this material as a nearly ideal tissue-engineering scaffold. Preparation of the scaffolds that are appropriate for implanting by different types of the cells is possible by means of biomaterial-based nanofibers. During the preparation of nanofiber-based scaffolds, the incorporation of different bioactive materials such as growth factor and the drugs such as an immunosuppressant is possible.

Nanofibers have also been utilized in other main areas of healthcare. For example, barrier textiles containing hydrophobic nanofiber layers (such as polyurethane or polyvinyldenfluorid) are an effective barrier for microorganism penetration (viruses, bacteria, and molds). Nanofiber layers composed of biopolymers (such as chitosan, gelatin, collagen, and PCL) can be used as a wound dressing for significant support of the wound healing process.

Several available methods for producing the nanofibers include drawing, self-assembly, phase separation, melt blown, template, and the most common method, electrospinning. Electrospinning is the most efficient method for preparing the continuous nanofibers. In addition, this method is simple, cost-effective, applicable to a wide range of polymers, and flexible in forming the fibers with various properties. Nanofibers can be obtained from polymer solutions or even molten polymers by electrospinning method (Adibkia, 2014).

1. NANOFIBERS

A vehicle can significantly influence the biopharmaceutical fate of the administered drug in patients' body by affecting its absorption, distribution, metabolism, and excretion. Furthermore, the toxicological and immunological effects of a drug delivery system depend on the nature of vehicle or drug vehicle complex. A drug delivery vehicle also influences the pharmacokinetic and pharmacodynamics properties of the loaded drug. An ideal vehicle must meet the purpose of its application. It must be nontoxic, non-immunogenic, biocompatible, biodegradable, and pharmacologically inert, while it must protect the active ingredient via enzymatic or physicochemical degradations in the body. A vehicle also must improve diffusion and permeation among various biological barriers. The enhancement of penetration into the target cells is another important role of an ideal vehicle (Kumar, 2000; Mainardes & Silva, 2004).

Nowadays, nanotechnology has gained significant interest due to its various applications in medical and pharmaceutical sciences. The nano-scaled technology, used in therapeutic fields, is recognized as "nanomedicine" and according to the National Institute of Health (Bethesda, MD, USA), nanomedicine is the biological application of nanoparticles that involves several biomedical claims like diagnosis, prevention, treatment, monitoring, and control of diseases. The widespread area of nanomedicine applications includes nanomachines such as DNA scaffolds, mimesis of the biological components, and nanotubes of the functionalized carbon, nano-scaled devices like nano-vehicles for the drug targeting, laboratorial disease classification devises, and nano-sensors, as well as nanostructures as biomaterials like nanofibers of peptides or proteins for tissue engineering, nanoporous membrane, etc. (Moghimi, Hunter, & Murray, 2005).

Nanoparticles with increased surface area can improve the rate and extent of solubility of lipophilic drugs, which in turn results in increasing the bioavailability of the drugs classified in class II of Biopharmaceutical Classification System (BCS). In addition, nano-sized delivery systems are able to improve physicochemical properties and pharmacokinetics of either water-soluble or -insoluble drugs in the case of both local and systemic drug delivery approaches. Nanoparticles are very beneficial for drug delivery because of their several outstanding attributes such as: a) reduced size of particles, which causes the enhancement of surface area; the improved surface increases the solubility of insoluble drugs and also enhances the capability of drug delivery system to penetrate more efficiently into the epithelial surface of different organs or diffuse through various physical barriers; b) efficient drug transport results in the reduction of administered doses and, therefore, less adverse effects and/or less toxicological effects. Dose reduction can also make drug therapy more cost-effective and, thereby, enhance patient compliance and convenience; c) the aptitude to target various cells, extracellular origins, or special organs in the body to deliver drugs, imaging, diagnostic means, and genetic material, which makes this drug delivery system more efficient for the treatment of malignancies or genetic disease; and d) avoidance of unwanted mucociliary clearance and epithelial phagocytosis as well as reduction of undesirable reticuloendothelial uptake while providing a prolonged release pattern. Hence, drug delivery via nanoparticles, with novel and desired properties, has the potential for a vast range medical and pharmaceutical applications (Barzegar-Jalali et al., 2008; Gelperina, Kisich, Iseman, & Heifets, 2005; Kumari, Yadav, & Yadav, 2010; Labhasetwar, Song, & Levy, 1997).

2. NANOFIBERS BIOMEDICAL APPLICATIONS

In the last few decades, application of the nanofibers in various drug delivery systems has gained significant interest, like other nanoparticles. Biodegradable and biocompatible nanofibers are well known as biological scaffolds and drug delivery vehicles. The most recognized use of nanofibers is their application as scaffolds in several tissues such as bone, cartilage, blood vessels, tendons, and muscles, which is due to the nanofibrous shape or structure of almost all of the tissues and organs in the human body (Huang et al., 2003). In order for wound healing or restoration of the physically or structurally damaged tissues, nanofibers as a tissue scaffold are very favorable because of their large surface area, which causes high capability in supporting the cell adhesion and cell growth on the scaffold, and also really rapid and efficient renovation of the damaged organ by proliferation of the cells with accurate properties, similar to those in natural organs. In addition, the improved surface area of nanofibers makes them suitable and highly advantageous for several other pharmaceutical and therapeutic purposes such as designing the medical prosthesis loaded with a drug and a novel targeted or controlled release drug delivery system, etc. (Jahangiri et al., 2014; Thandavamoorthy, Gopinath, & Ramkumar, 2006). Further findings have suggested that the nanofibers can modulate specific gene expression or they involve the guidance of growth and proliferation of various organ cells with sizes and orientations similar to those of natural organs (Melanko, Pearce, & Salem, 2009; Moghimi et al., 2005; Thassu, Deleers, & Pathak, 2007).

3. TISSUE ENGINEERING SCAFFOLDS

All through the recent years, there has been a rise in terms of focus on bioengineering, which is because of the potential resemblance of synthetic tissues to natural ones. It has been demonstrated that almost all tissues and organs in the human body (including bone, muscle, cartilage, skin, etc.) have a fibrous structure with fibers in nanometer size range; hence, in order to reach various therapeutic purposes, nanofibers are potentially promising. Some of the most important issues with nanofiber-based tissue engineering are to repair the injured tissue, heal wounds, maintain functionality of a damaged or abnormal organ, or either enhance or normalize the reduced functionalities of the organs. There are some main technologies in the case of tissue engineering, which include scaffold contrast technology with a focus on the improvement of three-dimensional tissue scaffolds in order for the subsequent cell attachment, either *in vitro* or *in vivo* culturing. Cell technology is another technology for *in vivo* synthesis, which is the most widely used technique in the case of tissue engineering (Fang et al., 2008; Pham, Sharma, & Mikos, 2006; Sill & von Recum, 2008; Yoshimoto, Shin, Terai, & Vacanti, 2003).

Tissue engineering has three main requirements; the first and most important parameter necessary for all tissue engineering purposes is cell, which can be either stem or other tissue cells. The second and also vital requirement is scaffold which has a determining role in successful cell engineering. Finally, the last important key requirement in the case of tissue engineering is "signal" that refers to molecular signaling and is known as growth factor. To design an ideal nanofiber scaffold, various important factors must be taken into account. For this purpose, a biomedical scaffold must be highly biocompatible, non-toxic, and biodegradable with a degradation rate suitable for *in vivo* neo-tissue improvement. It must also have a very large surface area to be capable of adhering to the cells and stimulating cell proliferation, migration, and differentiation of cell functions by generating all the needed signals for cell growth. In addition, other properties such as surface specificities, high porosity, and size and morphology of the pores are important parameters so that an appropriate scaffold should have an integrant structure to avoid pore collapse during the formation of neo-tissues. The mechanical properties and stability should also be considered. Nanofibers with desired properties such as large surface area, large pore size, and high porosity can be fabricated by means of electrospinning. It must also be considered that the high porous nanofibers have poor mechanical properties, where the anisotropic mechanical properties are very important parameters and the kind of direction (parallel, perpendicular, etc.) can significantly determine the mechanical properties of the fabricated fibers (Lim, Tan, & Ng, 2008). Another specificity of nanofibers is their hydrophobic nature, which is a limitation and causes reduction of cell attachment. Similarity of the fabricated nanofibrous scaffold to the native extracellular matrix has an important role in achieving successful results in tissue engineering. It is well known that cellular structures in body and extracellular matrix compounds mostly have nano-scaled fibrous natives (Fang et al., 2008; Hay, 2013). Thus, in order to obtain a suitable scaffold with the promising potential for cell support, similarity of physical and chemical properties of the scaffold to natural extracellular matrix is very important. This similarity is a key parameter in the case of successful tissue engineering. Hence, the importance of material nature, from which the nanofiber is made, is negligible. Furthermore, due to the wide range of mats suitable for nanofiber fabrication (either natural or synthetic), one must choose the material very precisely to avoid unsuccessful procedures. Collagen, plasma serum protein fibrinogen, elastin, hyaluronic acid, DNA, agarose, starch, alginate gum, silk, chitosan, and dextran are some examples of natural materials. Natural mats have the superiority of being highly biocompatible; in addition, the ability of these materials to create a biological scaffold with significant similarity to those in natural extracellular matrix makes them ideal for biomedical uses. Various polymers with different hydrophilic or lipophilic manners and also different thermo-dependent behaviors (like thermoplastic polymers) are used in this regard. Some examples of commonly used synthetic polymers are PGA, PLA, PCL, and PLGA. Very high porosity of electrospun nanofibers prepared via PLGA (with the porosity more than 90%), which can cause more cell attachment via many focal adhesion points on several fibers as well as acceptable mimesis of extracellular matrix, makes these nano-scaled fibers a very suitable choice for tissue engineering (Pham et al., 2006).

Nowadays, there is significant attraction to the scaffolds made of electrospun or self-assembled nanofibers. Nanofibrous scaffolds fabricated via different methods are applicable as tissue prosthesis for either soft tissues (such as muscles, blood vessels, breast, bladder, skin, etc.) or hard tissues like bone, tooth, etc. According to the natural specificities of the utilized polymer, nanofiber-based scaffolds have the potential to use in both two- and three-dimensional cell cultures. In order to obtain a promising cell culture, some basic principles should be considered; the first one is the reproducibility of scaffold, which must be ensured by the modification of physical and chemical process parameters. The second important consideration is the mechanical stability of the scaffold, which avoids its rapid fragmentation during culture, and the third is the architectural and surface properties of scaffold, which can directly influence cell phenotype. The fourth and last important parameter is the hydrophobicity of the prepared scaffold, which has a significant effect on cell attachment (Baker et al., 2006; Li et al., 2005).

3.1. Muscle

An investigation on the application of nanofibrous scaffolds as tissue templates was done by Matthews et al (2002). They assessed the feasibility of culturing smooth muscles using collagen nanofibers. According to their results, smooth muscle cells were successfully adhered to the collagen nanofibers within 7 days and the collagen scaffold could effectively promote cell proliferation and cell growth (Matthews, Wnek, Simpson, & Bowlin, 2002). Further studies have illustrated that nanofibers fabricated by synthetic polymers (such as PCL, polystyrene, polyethylene glycol, polyethylene-co-vinyl alcohol, polyester urethane urea (PEUU)/collagen blend, and poly(L-lactide-co-ε-caprolactone) (PLLA-CL)) are also potential for adherence to the smooth muscle cells and promoting their proliferation. On the other hand, it has been illustrated that the incorporation of collagen into nanofibers makes the scaffold more elastic (increasing modulus elasticity) and enhances the adhesion of cells on the scaffold (Baker et al., 2006; Stankus, Guan, & Wagner, 2004; Venugopal, Zhang, & Ramakrishna, 2005).

3.2. Bone

Several studies have been done on the engineering of bone tissues along with muscle. Various polymer bases have been found to be suitable for the improvement of scaffolds to implant in the bones. Several investigations have been done on the functionality of PCL nanofibers hybridized with calcium carbonate or hydroxyapatite nanoparticles, or mixtures containing gelatin and PCL. All of these studies have confirmed the suitability of PCL-based nanofibers for application in bone engineering because of the integrity of these scaffolds. Other natural or synthetic polymers which have been studied in order to fabricate the bone scaffolds are PLGA, silk, polyester urethanes (PEU), polyphosphazenes, PLA, PLLA containing montmorillonite (MMT) nanoplatelets, silicate fibers, etc. (Henry, Simonet, Pandit, & Neuenschwander, 2007; Jin, Chen, Karageorgiou, Altman, & Kaplan, 2004; Kim et al., 2005; Sakai, Yamada, Yamaguchi, & Kawakami, 2006).

3.3. Cartilage

Collagen-based nanofibers are the best choice for cartilage tissue engineering, because natural collagen (especially type II collagen) is the main component of articular cartilage. Acceptability of collagen-based tissue scaffolds has been illustrated in several studies due to the natural manner of collagen and its compatibility with chondrocytes. It has been shown that collagen nanofibers can successfully mimic the extracellular matrix and can simulate the proliferation of chondrocytes. On the other hand, it has been demonstrated that PCL-based nanofibers are also suitable for cartilage tissue engineering. During a study, Li et al. observed that PCL nanofibers were capable to be used as cartilage scaffolds and

PCL matrix had significant proliferation effects on the phenotypic differentiations of chondrocytes (Li, Danielson, Alexander, & Tuan, 2003; Matthews, Boland, Wnek, Simpson, & Bowlin, 2003; Matthews et al., 2002; Shields, Beckman, Bowlin, & Wayne, 2004).

3.4. Skin

The employed polymers in the fabrication of scaffolds for tissue engineering must be compatible to fibroblast and/or keratinocytes. The importance of skin as the biggest protective tissue in the body and the beauty aspects related to skin make this field of tissue engineering a very interesting one. Polymers reported as suitable vehicles for skin tissue engineering are collagen, gelatin, silk, chitosan, hyaluronic acid, PLGA, PLLA, PCL, and many others. Most of these polymers have shown good performance as a scaffold, successfully attached to the cells, and stimulated cell growth and proliferation (Fang et al., 2008; Ki et al., 2007; Min et al., 2004).

4. NANOFIBERS AS DRUG DELIVERY DEVICES

As mentioned above, nanofibers have several outstanding physical and structural attributes such as a very large surface to volume ratio and high degree of porosity. In addition, nanofibers could mimic the extracellular matrix in terms of biological functions and both physical and chemical structures (Mickova et al., 2012; Sill & von Recum, 2008). Beside the mentioned advantages, nanofibers are capable of being more useful if they are fabricated as sheets with high mechanical strength and elastic properties (made up of lipophilic polymers). Loading of various pharmaceutical agents within or on the surface of nanofibers also make them more valuable in the case of therapeutic applications (Kim, 2008; Lim et al., 2008).

Drug-loaded nanofibers are able to release the loaded drug with a controlled release pattern in the site of action. There are various researches which confirm that nanofibrous structures containing a pharmaceutical agent may cause to more efficient treating processes in the case of wound healing and transdermal drug delivery systems (Meinel, Germershaus, Luhmann, Merkle, & Meinel, 2012). Considering that infection is the major cause of failure in the Guided tissue or bone regeneration (Xue et al., 2014), thus application of antimicrobial agents will minimize the risk of bacterial infection and it will lead to successful regenerative operations (Meinel et al., 2012). Other investigations have confirmed the promising efficacy of drug-loaded nanofibers in the case of repairing deficiencies of nervous system (Madduri, Papaloizos, & Gander, 2010).

The complex of drug and carrier can illustrate various types of prolonged or extended release patterns. A wide range of pharmaceutical agents, either large molecular peptides and proteins (Chew, Wen, Yim, & Leong, 2005; Jiang et al., 2005; Jiang, Hu, Zhao, Li, & Zhu, 2006) or small molecular drugs including antibiotics (Bölgen, Vargel, Korkusuz, Menceloğlu, & Pişkin, 2007; Huang et al., 2006; Kenawy et al., 2002), anti-inflammatory drugs (Taepaiboon, Rungsardthong, & Supaphol, 2006), vitamins (Taepaiboon, Rungsardthong, & Supaphol, 2007), anticancer drugs (Burger & Chu, 2007; Xie & Wang, 2006; Xu et al., 2006), and DNA (Nie & Wang, 2007), can be loaded to nanofibers via different loading approaches. Sometimes, electrospun nanofibers can illustrate a faster release than untreated drugs (Jafari-Aghdam et al., 2014). The mechanism of drug release varies according to the loading method, physical and structural characteristics of nanofiber, nature of the loaded drug, and other parameters.

However, the large surface area of nanofibers makes them suitable for drug loading in order to reach various controlled release patterns. It can also lead to an unwanted initial burst release effect. The initial burst release, prolonged or delayed release, multi-stage release profile, multi-drug loading, and overall kinetics of drug release can be managed by the application of different nanofiber production techniques or by changing the drug loading method. For example, the application of co-axial nozzle electrospinning (Liao, Chew, & Leong, 2006), instead of single nozzle method, can be used in order to avoid unwanted burst release effect. There are many techniques for the production of drug-loaded nanofibers; they may be produced by simply mixing of the polymer solution with the drug either at the same time or before the nanofiber fabrication. Other methods are chemical or physical surface immobilization or indirect drug loading after the nanofiber fabrication (Huang et al., 2006; Moghimi et al., 2005). Kenawy et al. (2002) designed the first drug loaded nanofibers of tetracycline in order to treat the infected wounds. They investigated the release of the loaded tetracycline from the electrospun nanofibers based on poly (ethylene-co-vinyl acetate), PLA, and a mixture of these two polymers (Kenawy et al., 2002).

As mentioned above, the nature of the drug and the expected release pattern of drug delivery system are two main factors which should be considered for selecting the suitable drug-loading approach. As the drug and the polymer can be mixed during this method, four different types of drug loading can occur. The first type of drug loading during this method is the attachment of drug particulates to the surface of the fabricated nanofibers, which may cause an initial, fast and immediate release of the drug. The second type is the fabrication of a mixture of nanofibers, containing drug nanofibers and carrier nanofibers; the third type is the electrospinning of a blend mixture of drug and polymer, which causes the production of nanofibers of dispersed drug in the base of polymer. Finally, the fourth type is encapsulating the drug in the electrospun fiber; the latter two types are the most favorable types (Huang et al., 2003).

Nanofibers and more specifically core sheath nanofibers have the capability to provide biphasic drug release profiles in which an immediate release is followed by a sustained release (Jiang, Mo, & Yu, 2012; Yu et al., 2013; Yu, Jia, Yao, & Lu, 2014).

5. ELECTROSPINNING

5.1. Historical Background

Electrospinning method is a simple, one step, surfactant-free, and cost-effective approach which is now the most common technique for improving the nanofibers (Payab et al., 2014). The electrostatic spraying of the liquids dates back to the mid-1700s (Jean-Antoine Nollet, 1750), long before the invention of the term electrospinning; but, the first documented data of forming fibers via electrostatic spraying were described by J. F. Cooley and W. J. Morton in 1902. A viscose polymer solution was introduced to a positively charged electrode nearby a negatively charged electrode in order to produce the fibers. They presumed that this process was the result of "electrical disruption of the fluid". It is interesting to know that the described method in that early, primitive patent has changed just a little over time. Another related patent was worked on a quarter of century later by Formhals in 1934. He also used electrical charge to form the fibers applying cellulose acetate. His process included moveable fiber collection, which allowed the fibers to have some degrees of orientation. During later years, he improved his patent and claimed different methods about electrostatic spinning. Mostly, the described process by Formhals has been known as the first patent for the production of the fibers via electrostatic spinning. C. L. Norton

(1936) provided an innovative method called "transverse intermittent electromotive force" to improve the properties of the fabricated fibers. During 1960s, Sir Geoffrey Taylor carried out his substantial studies based on the jet formation process to understand the behavior of droplets placed in an electric field; thus, further observed conical shape of the jet has been referred to as "Taylor cone" by other researchers. Later studies have been mostly focused on the morphological investigations of nanofibers due to the development of some reliable morphological tools based on microscopy such as atomic force microscopy (AFM), transmission electron microscopy (TEM), and scanning electron microscopy (SEM).

H. L. Simons (1966) investigated the important role of some key parameters such as polymer solution viscosity, conductivity, and dielectric constant as well as the nature of organic solvent used to dissolve the polymer (like the volatility of the solvent) on the physicochemical properties and size of the fabricated fibers. Further studies on the size and other morphological aspects of the nanofibers have illustrated that the enhanced concentration of the polymer solution leads to the enhancement of viscosity and causes the increase of nanofibers diameter (Baumgarten 1971). On the other hand, it has been shown that the lower temperature of polymer solution will result in the larger fibers, which is probably due to the increased viscosity followed by decreased temperature (Andrady, 2008; Martins, Reis, & Neves, 2008). Finally, almost recently in 1994, the term "electrospinning" was derived from "electrostatic spinning", and since then, it became one of the most interesting research fields because of its applicability for a wide range of polymeric materials in order to produce ultrafine fibers (Adibkia, 2014; Yoo, Kim, & Park, 2009)

5.2. Process Definition of Electrospinning

Briefly, electrospinning can be defined as a process in which the application of high voltage electric energy to a capillary field of polymer solution causes the formation of fine filaments. A basic electrospinning apparatus made of 1) a high voltage electric force supplier, 2) a capillary tube with a needle or pipette (referred to as syringe or nozzle), and 3) an electrode collector (or target) (Figure 1). This simple apparatus can be used in order to prepare droplets, beads, and fibers; each of these shapes can be obtained by optimizing the process parameters. There are several choices to be utilized as targets, e.g. copper plates, aluminum foil or plates, rotating drums, and human hands (Gopal et al., 2007; Kenawy et al., 2003; Li, Bellan, Craighead, & Frey, 2006; Matthews et al., 2002). As is obvious in Figure 1, the capillary tube containing the polymer solution and the collector are connected to the power supply. The capillary tube and collector must be almost close to each other and the distance between these two parts is one of the key parameters that maintains the shape and morphological properties of the fabricated fibers. Application of high voltage to viscose polymer fluid by the electrical field leads to the foundation of a force opposite to the surface tension force of the polymer solution, which in turn transverses the solution to a liquid jet. Enhancement in the power force of the electrical field elongates the spherical droplet at the top of the capillary tube and forms a conical shape which is known as "Taylor cone". Due to the enhancement of the power supplied by electrical field, at a critical power value, the repulsion force generated by electrical field becomes stronger than the surface tension of the polymer fluid and leads to the ejection of a charged jet from the top of the Taylor cone (shaped previously on the top of the capillary tube) toward the collector electrode. Because of the interaction between the charge inside the jet and the external electrical field, the jet becomes thinner and a long filament with a small diameter is formed.

As mentioned above, the wide-range applicability of electrospinning process is one of the most important beneficial aspects of this approach. There are more than 100 polymers and other starting materials that are electrospun up to now and, among the whole electrospun materials, those made up of

Figure 1. A schematic view of electrospinning procedure

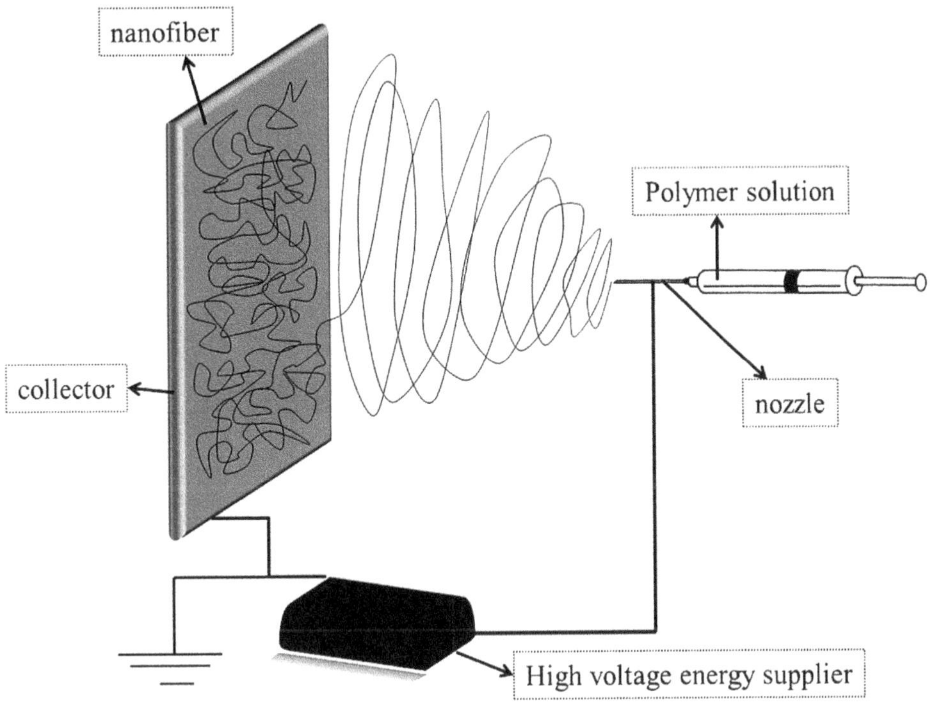

biodegradable polymers (such as PCL, PLA, polyglycolic acid (PGA), and poly(lactic-co-glycolic acid) (PLGA)), have received the highest attention. Synthetic mats, natural biopolymers, can also be used to fabricate the nanofibers. Some examples for the mostly used natural mats are polysaccharides (including cellulose, chitin, chitosan, and dextrose), DNA, and proteins (such as collagen, gelatin, silk, etc.) (Fang et al., 2008; Martins et al., 2008; Schiffman & Schauer, 2008).

Electrospinning as a fast and efficient method can be used to selectively deposit polymers either in a random fashion or along a programmed axis. Studies have demonstrated that it is possible to modify the mechanical properties by controlling fiber orientation.

6. DRUG LOADING TECHNIQUES

6.1. Co-Electrospinning of the Drugs and Polymer

Dissolving the drug and polymer in the same solvent and electrospinning of the resulted solution are the simplest method of drug loading into nanofibers. Figure 2 illustrates a schematic view of co-electrospinning process. By means of this method, the drug will be loaded within the nanofibers. The mechanism of drug release will be the simple diffusion mechanism at the initial stages, while at the following stages; the release mechanism is polymer degradation. This profile of drug release will probably illustrate an initial burst release that will slow down over time. Simplicity of electrospinning and wide range of the polymers, which can be applied, make this approach a very useful and comprehensive method to form

Figure 2. Schematic diagram of simple drug loading method within the nanofiber via co-electrospinning

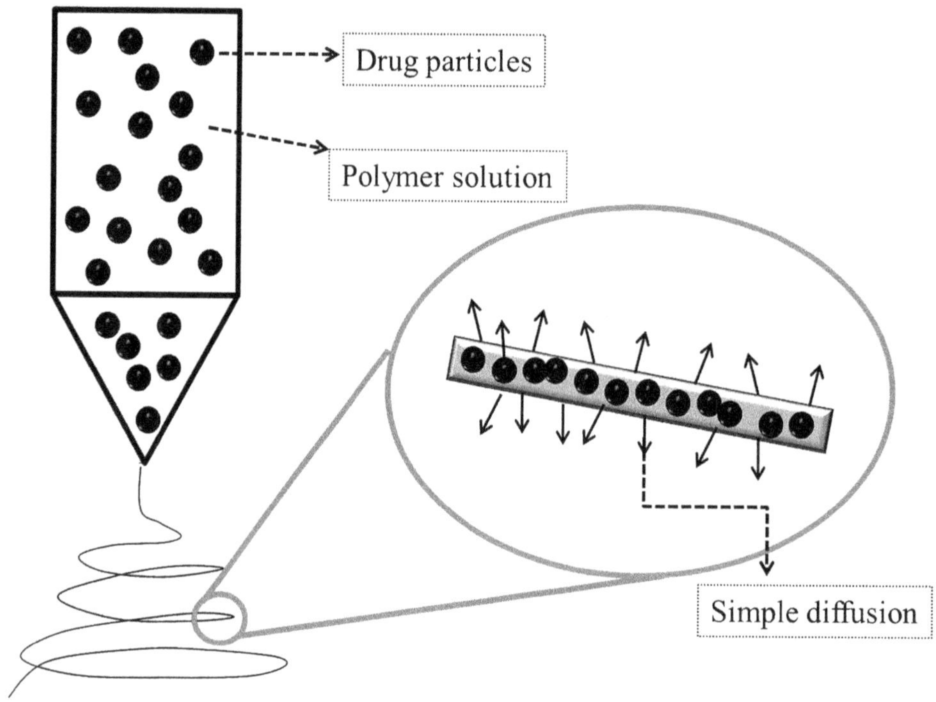

the drug-loaded matrices and design controlled drug delivery systems. However, it is possible that the dissolution of drug in an organic solvent and further application of high voltages during the electrospinning process will cause drug degradation, which will be especially harmful for bioactive drugs such as proteins, peptides, and DNA. Nevertheless, several studies have shown that no remarkable changes including degradation and hydrolysis occur to drugs or polymers by electrospinning process (Taepaiboon et al., 2006; Yang, Li, Qi, Zhou, & Weng, 2008). These investigations have assured the applicability of simple mixing method for a wide range of drugs. An instance for antibiotic loading within nanofibers with the purpose of treating bacterial infections was studied by Kenawy et al. (2002). Kenawy et al. used this simple mixing method for the first time to improve a novel controlled release drug delivery system of tetracycline-loaded electrospun polymer nanofibers based on (Poly(ethylene-covinylacetate) (PEVA) and PLA and a mixture of these two polymers. Tetracycline hydrochloride was co-electrospun with polymer solution to produce the tetracycline-polymer monolithic fibers. Consequently, the release of tetracycline from electrospun mats was studied to determine the profile of drug release, and it was found that electrospun nanofibers, based on PEVA and a 50/50 mixture of PEVA and PEA, showed a burst release effect which was followed by a slow release over 5 days (Kenawy et al., 2002). The result confirmed the expected sustained profile of release by means of drug loading within nanofibers via simple mixing process. Kim et al. (2004) designed an investigation on the controlled release of the electrospun nanofibers based on PLGA and poly (lactic-co-glycolic acid) block polylactic acid (PEG-b-PLA) loaded with Cefoxitin (mofexin®) (Kim et al., 2004). It has been demonstrated that the loaded drug influenced morphological characteristics of the electrospun nanofibers; e.g. drug loading changed the shape of nanoparticles from a string and bead shape to completely fibrous forms and also the presence of the drug in the component of electrospun nanofiber reduced the fibers diameter. This reduction in the size of nanofibers occurs probably due to the hydrophilic nature of mofexin, which enhances the electrical conductivity of drug: polymer solution. In addition, high ionic strength of mofexin causes a difference between the loading mechanisms of PLGA and PLGA-b-PLA nanofibers. Low physical interaction between drug and PLGA leads to the attachment of the drug only to the surface of fibers, while the incorporation of the drug with PLGA-b-PLA embeds the drug within the nanofiber, which in turn leads to illustrating a more sustained release by PLGA-b-LGA than PLGA. Additionally, both UV-Vis and HNMR methods confirmed that, despite the application of electrical force, antibiotic remained in its bioactive manner (Sill & von Recum, 2008).

Katti et al. (2004) mixed cefazolin and PLGA in the same solvent and fabricated electrospun nanofibers with the purpose of treating infected wounds. Further studies have been designed on various types of drugs such as proteins, anticancer drugs, etc. During an investigation by Zeng et al. (2005), protein loaded nanofibers were provided via electrospinning of bovine serum albumin or luciferase within the nanofibers of poly (vinyl alcohol) (PVA) and the release profile was monitored. Moreover, in previous studies, an initial burst release pattern caused by the large surface area of nanofibers was observed (Zeng et al., 2005). Another study on porous electrospun PLA nanofibers loaded with a non-steroidal anti-inflammatory agent (ketoprofen) was designed by Park et al. (2011). PLA fibers were produced by phase separation during electrospinning method and the drug release profile was monitored; similar to others, an initial burst release for few first hours was observed which was followed by slower release rates (Park & Lee, 2011). Taepaiboon et al. (2006) also worked on the non-steroidal anti-inflammatory drugs before the mentioned research; PVA fibers were co-electrospuan with four different non-steroidal anti-inflammatory drugs with different solubility in water, i.e. sodium salicylate (freely soluble in water), diclofenac sodium (sparingly soluble in water), naproxen, and indomethacin (both insoluble in water), were selected as model drugs. Further investigations have illustrated that the nature of the model drug significantly influenced the morphological aspects of the drug loaded nanofibers, e.g. sodium salicylate formed hydrogen bonds with PVA molecules and affected the molecular packing of PVA, while there was no interaction between other drug models with PVA. Besides, it was shown that both rate and extent of drug release were dependent on the molecular weight of model drugs; so that both rate and total amount of released drug were decreased as a result of enhancing molecular weight of the model drug. Monitoring the release profile of model drugs illustrated that sodium salicylate loaded nanofibers had an initial fast release rate, which was slowed down over time. Finally, according to the large surface area provided by electrospun nanofibers, both rate and extent of release of the model drugs from electrospun fibers were significantly greater than those of as-cast films. Interestingly, Taepaiboon et al. showed that the application of a high electrical potential to the drug-containing solutions did not affect the chemical integrity of the drugs, which confirmed the applicability of electrospinning method for drug loading. During another study, Taepaiboon et al. (2007) investigated different properties and release profile of vitamin-loaded fibers. All-trans retinoic acid or vitamin A acid (Retin-A), a derivative of vitamin A or retinol, and a-tocopherol or vitamin E (Vit-E) were used as the model vitamins to load within the electrospun fibers based on cellulose acetate. The observed drug release pattern confirmed the initial burst release followed by enhancement in the rate of release to reach a plateau at the maximum release (Taepaiboon et al., 2007).

Targeting anticancer agents to the site of malignancy is one of the most important issues in cancer related therapies. Due to their high surfaces, nanofibers are capable of carrying a high amount of drug to the targeted site in order for the efficient treatment of malignant tissue avoiding destructive side effects of anticancer drugs. Xu et al. (2006) studied the antitumor activity of BCNU-loaded nanofibers with a polymeric base of poly (ethylene glycol)–poly (l-lactic acid) (PEG–PLLA); both of the polymers and also the drug were dissolved in the same organic solvent (chloroform) and nanofibers were fabricated via electrospinning. The release profile of drug showed a burst release at the beginning and, then, slowed down over time. The anticancer effect of drug-loaded fibers remained up to 72 h, while pure BCNU was degraded within 48 h. In addition, a relationship was found between the amount of loaded drug and rate of drug release. These findings allow researchers to control the rate of release by controlling the amount of embedded drug into the nanofibers. On the other hand, *in vivo* studies confirmed the anticancer effect of BCNU-loaded PEG-PLLA nanofibers on rat Glioma C6 cells, while unloaded nanofibers illustrate no effect (Xu et al., 2006). All of the mentioned studies confirmed the applicability of simple mixing followed by electrospinning method for loading a wide range of pharmaceutically active agents within the nanofibers. The nanofibers fabricated by this technique illustrate a burst release in few first hours or even minutes followed by a slow drug release rate. This pattern can be justified due to the initial simple diffusion of the drug particles dispersed on the very large surface of the nanofibers, and the subsequent slow release takes place because of the polymer degradation, which leads to a slow drug release rate. In conclusion, it can be said that many of the drug delivery systems made by means of simple mixing method could release the drug during several days (Yu et al., 2013).

6.2. Surface Immobilization on the Nanofiber

According to the literature, it is preferred to surface-immobilize bioactive molecules on the nanofibers by physical absorption or chemical conjugation. A dual electrospinning nozzle can be applied to create nanofiber sheet layers, which are stacked on top of one another. Therefore, the initial burst release is reduced compared with solid nanofibers because of these layers. The pharmaceutically active agent can be physically adsorbed on the surface of (or absorb into) the fabricated nanofibers; otherwise, it can chemically link to the surface of fibers (as shown in Figure 3). This purpose can be achieved by a simple deep coating method, which leads to the immobilization of the model drug on the surface of nanofibers by the formation of physical, chemical, or both types of forces, taking advantage of the very large surface to volume ratio of the nanofibers. The electrostatic interaction, hydrogen bonding, van der Waals interactions, and hydrophobic interactions are the most important bounding forces, which play a role in the physical absorption in order to incorporate either macromolecular or small molecular drugs onto the modified surface of the nanofiber. The ability of controlling the amount of loaded drug on the surface of fibers by controlling the proportional amount of fed drug is one of the unique advantages for this loading approach (Son, Kim, & Yoo, 2014; Yoo et al., 2009). Briefly, immobilization of the drug on the surface of fabricated nanofibers can be simply achieved by deep coating of fibers in a solution of drug. This method, similar to the simple mixing approach, is available for a variety of drugs (Son et al., 2014).

It is widely known that the most common and annoying problem after invasive surgeries is the infection of the site of surgery. One of the most disposed organs for postsurgical infection is the abdominal wall. Another difficulty after abdominal surgeries is the formation of fibrotic bands linking separate surfaces in the peritoneal cavity, known as "abdominal adhesion". In order to avoid the abdominal adhesion, a reliable way is to place a physical barrier between the injured site and other tissues close to it. Interpolation of an antibiotic agent to this physical barrier is a promising way to avoid the formation of abdominal adhesion as well as post-surgery infection. Nanofibers, due to the large surface area, which allows loading a high amount of the drug, and the high porous structure with pores in nanometer size

Figure 3. A simple view of nanofibers' surface modification

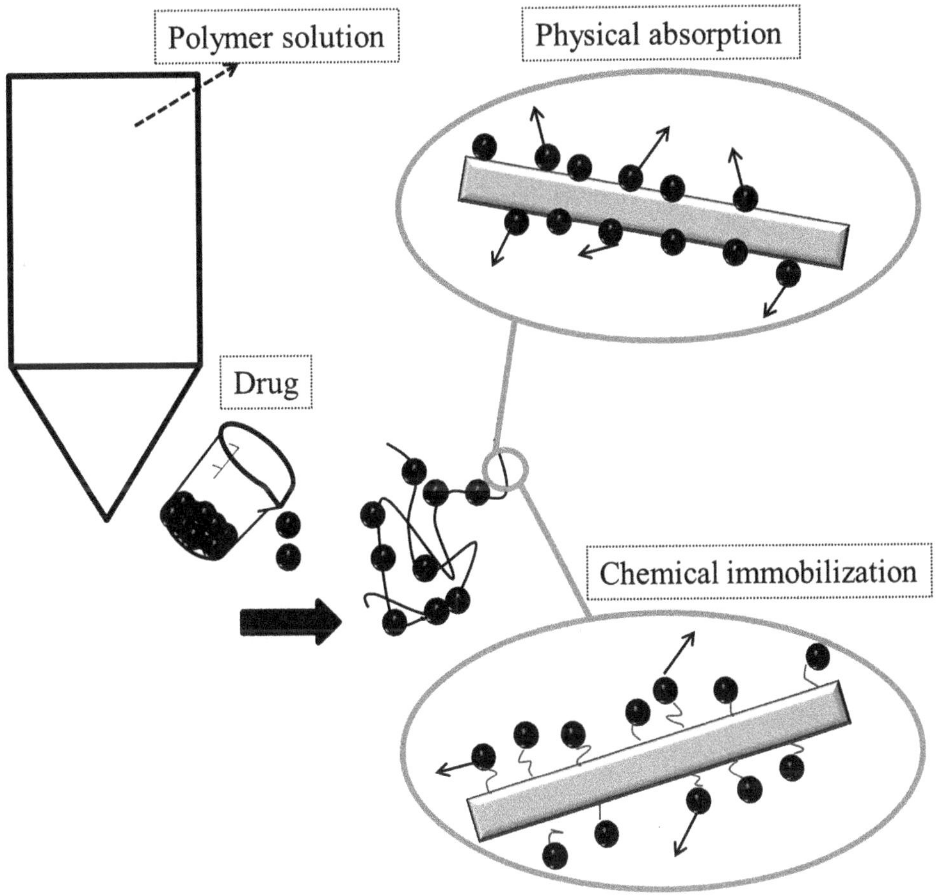

range that inhibits cell migration, seem to be the best choices to be applied as both physical barrier and antibiotic loaded carriers (Sill & von Recum, 2008). Bolgen et al. (2007) fabricated PCL based nanofibers via electrospinning and loaded ornidazole (Bitral@) on the surface of nanofibers by the absorption of drug solution into the fiber mat (Bölgen et al., 2007). In their study, the drug was dispersed on the surface of fibers and was not incorporated within them. *In vivo* investigations illustrated that, following the application of Bitral-loaded PCL nanofibers; both abdominal adhesion and infection were significantly reduced. In addition, studies showed that the rate of wound healing increased due to the application of drug-loaded nanofibers.

6.3. Core Shell Nanofibers

As mentioned above, simple mixing method, co-electrospinning, and surface immobilization have some limitations in the case of drug release that can be solved by designing sheath nanofibers via co-axial electrospinning method. A simple diagram describing drug encapsulation via co-axial electrospinning is represented in Figure 4. The simplest form of nanofibers produced by means of this method is the production of a sheath of polymer with a core of the drug dispersed in a matrix polymer. However, sometimes the core may contain drug itself. Other types for co-axial electrospinning include multiple drug loading within a single fiber and control of the release profile of each drug individually that can be achieved either by designing multilayer core consisting of different drugs or loading a drug in the core and dispersing the other one within the outer polymer solution. Multilayer stacked nanofibers may be produced via the application of pursuant electrospinning of two different solutions. It is also possible to provide a drug delivery system of a single drug with different release patterns. This purpose is achievable by dispersing a proportion of the drug into the polymer used to form the shell and loading the remaining drug within the core using another type of polymer. By means of this approach, the drug loaded within the shell will supply the initial dose, while the core will illustrate a prolonged release. It seems that there is no complication with electrospinning of two different solutions (consisting of drug and polymer), since it is simple electrospinning of two separate solutions using two separate, but concentric, capillaries (Huang et al., 2006; Jiang et al., 2005; Liao, Chew, & Leong, 2006; Sun, Zussman, Yarin, Wendorff, & Greiner, 2003; Wang et al., 2013; Zhang, Huang, Xu, Lim, & Ramakrishna, 2004). Drug loading efficiency of this method is high and the burst release effect observed by simple mixing method is eliminated due to the encapsulation of drug within the nanofiber. The release pattern of nanofibers fabricated by this method is more complicated than that of previous methods. After the diffusion of water to nanofiber system, dissolution of soluble parts and swelling of non-soluble swelling agents will be observed, which leads to the formation of a porous and perhaps swollen fiber system. The simple diffusion mechanism will be decreased significantly by hydrophobic shell, which acts as a barrier (Liao et al., 2006; Song, Yu, Markel, Shi, & Ren, 2013; Yu et al., 2013). This method is very common for encapsulating various drugs and more specially proteins within the nanofibers. As mentioned above, it is also possible to design

Figure 4. Schematic diagram of encapsulating drug particles within polymeric nanofiber via co-axial electrospinning

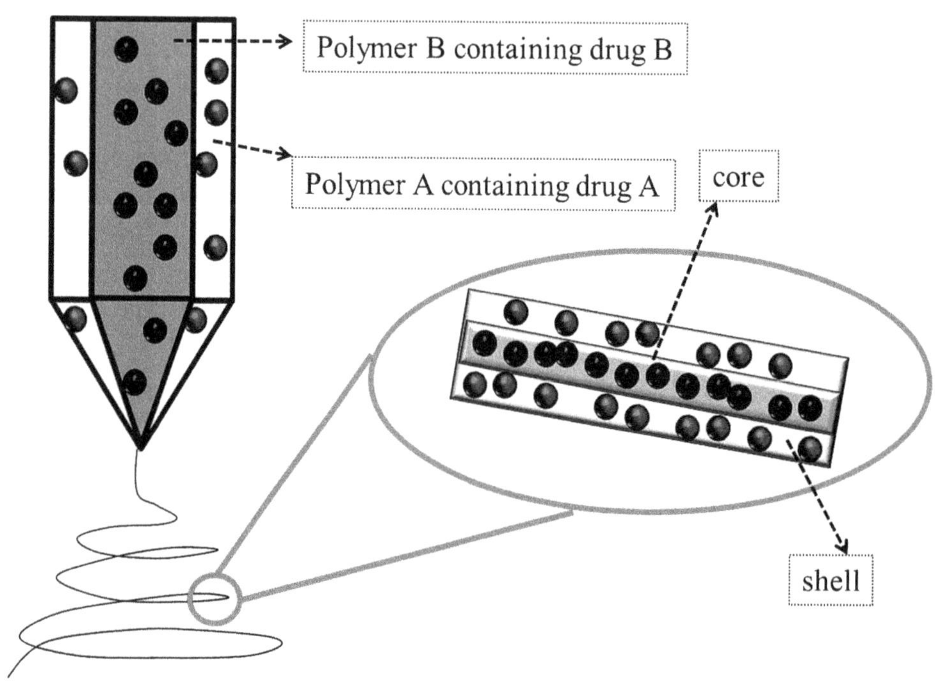

a multi-drug delivery system via two different loading methods, e.g. co-electrospinning of a simple mix and chemical surface modification. One drug can be loaded by electrospinning subsequent to dissolving in a solution (mostly aqueous) of polymer, which will form the core, and the other drug be incorporated on the shell by surface modification; the resulted nanofiber will illustrate a modified prolonged release (Cho, Choi, Jeong, & Yoo, 2010).

6.4. Layer-By-Layer Nanofibers

In order to obtain successful systemic drug delivery systems, layer-by-layer nanoparticles have shown promising potential due to the desirable capacity of this multidrug and multifunctional drug delivery system to control and modify the drug release pattern. Several investigations have illustrated the reduction of burst release effect by means of layer-by-layer devices. In addition, it is possible to control *in vivo* functionalities of these drug delivery systems via controlling (either aiding or avoiding) cell uptake. Furthermore, an effective targeted drug delivery to systemic tumors is achieved via layer-by-layer nanoparticles (Poon, Chang, Zhao, & Hammond, 2011).

The fabrication process of layer-by-layer nanofibers includes serial co-electrospinning of the several polymer solutions containing various drugs. As is obvious in Figure 5, the sequential electrospinning of solutions leads to the fabrication of several sheets of the drugs in polymeric matrices. In addition, polymer solutions with any drug dissolved will electrospun between two drug loaded sheets; therefore, each drug loaded polymer sheet (except the first layer) will be sandwiched between two polymeric sheet barriers (without drug) and the release profile will be controlled by means of these sheet barriers. As a result, although all of the sheets are produced via the same drug loading method, the first layer will release the drug earlier than the second drug loaded layer, which is due to the presence of controlling sheet barriers (Fathi-Azarbayjani & Chan, 2010; Okuda, Tominaga, & Kidoaki, 2010).

Figure 5. A schematic view of producing layer-by-layer nanofiber systems

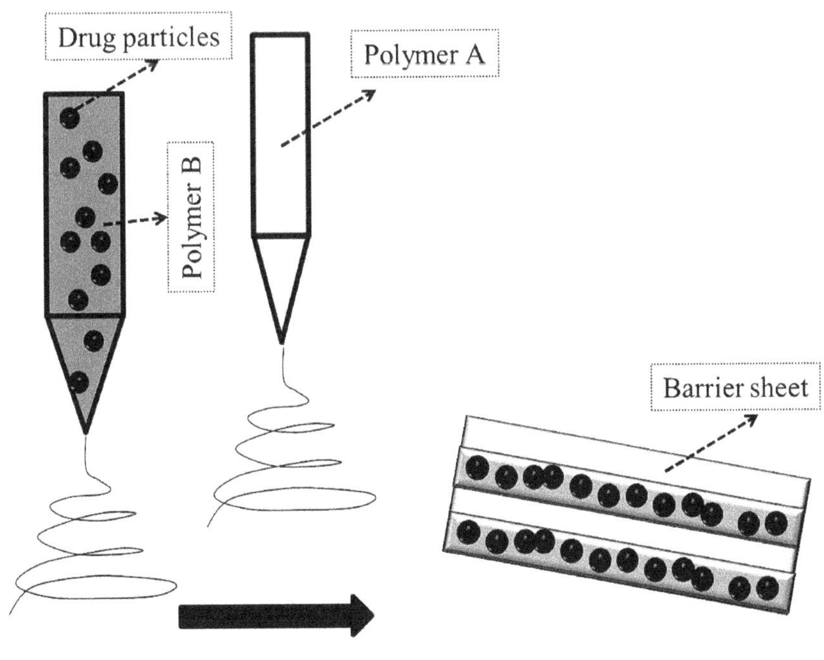

6.5. Hybrid Nanofiber Systems

Hybridization of two different drug delivery systems improves their advantages and it seems that the outstanding attributes of each system will increase synergistically by hybridization. Hybridization of nanofibers with other nano- or micro-drug delivery devices and hydrogels is discussed in this section. There are many investigations with a focus on the desirable efficiency and wide range applicability of hybridized systems in the case of drug delivery and other therapeutic goals. Drug loading efficiency, release profile, kinetic of release, and safety of designed drug delivery system are some of the most important factors, which can be modified via the hybridization of nanofibers with various types of drug delivery devices (Ionescu, Lee, Sennett, Burdick, & Mauck, 2010; Shao et al., 2011; Son & Yoo, 2012). Prolonged and well-controlled release patterns as well as the potency of these systems to embed the various drugs in a single fiber makes this approach a promising drug delivery system for multidrug loading in the case of resistant cancer therapies. Improving a multidrug delivery system looks easier and even more available by means of hybridization techniques, which use only a single nozzle to electrospun nanofibers in comparison with co-axial electrospinning method using two different concentricity nozzles. Two different types of drug delivery vehicles containing different drugs (a drug-loaded nano- or microparticles and a drug-loaded nanofibers produced by co-electrospinning or surface immobilization) will electrospun in the same polymer solution (Wang, Qiao, & Yin, 2010). Son and Yoo (2012) designed a drug delivery system by encapsulating dexamethasone micelles in the electrospun nanofibers based on PCL-PEG surface-modified using pluronic F127 (Son & Yoo, 2012).

Combination of nanofibers and hydrogels is another approach to design hybrid nanofiber based drug delivery devices. Hydrogels are well known for their high ability to water retention; so, they can be used in combination with nanofibers to modify the various properties of device. Moreover, they can form a delivery device with different release mechanisms. In order to improve effective nanofiber-based scaffolds in tissue engineering, hydrogels are very good candidates to use as a backbone device due to their hydrophilic nature which reduces the hydrophobicity of scaffolds and, therefore, significantly increases cell attachment (Lee, Park, & Koh, 2013; Loh, Peh, Liao, Sng, & Li, 2010). There is an initial burst release effect observed with most of the hydrogel nanofibers that can be modified via surface modification methods (He, Huang, & Han, 2009; Im, Yun, Lim, Kim, & Lee, 2010; Taepaiboon et al., 2006, 2007; Verreck et al., 2003; Zong et al., 2002)

CONCLUSION

Outstanding properties of the nanofibers including their desirable mechanical behavior and biological characteristics such as biocompatibility (and probably biodegradability) convert them into applicable materials in the medical and pharmaceutical areas. Furthermore, the physical and structural advantages such as their reduced size enhance the drugs solubility and dissolution rate. Additionally, high similarity of their structure to natural tissues ensures their ability to the promising mimesis of natural organs, especially extracellular matrix. Electrospinning is a very simple and applicable method for the production of nanofibers, especially polymer-based high functional and high performance nanofibers, with the ability of revolutionizing the world of structural materials. Electrospun nanofibers with diameters ranging from a few nanometers to several micrometers can be produced using an electrostatically driven jet of polymer solution or polymer melt and show enormous promise for developing different kinds of drug delivery systems due to their particular individuality. The current drug delivery systems based on electrospun nanofibers are composed of drug-loaded nanofibers including pharmaceuticals and biodegradable polymers. Drugs, proteins, genes, peptide, antibodies, as well as small molecule can be loaded within or on the surface of nanofibers according to their properties. Nanofibers can be also applied for scaffolds with high surface area and enhanced porosity. It has been demonstrated that these properties have a significant effect on cell adhesion, proliferation, and differentiation. The results of the recent studies have clearly indicated that nanofiber based scaffolds show excellent potential to be developed for a variety of tissue engineering applications. According to the related literature, the surface-immobilization of bioactive molecules on the nanofibers by physical absorption or chemical conjugation can stimulate cell differentiation and proliferation, especially in the case of chemically surface-immobilized proteins on a nanofiber mesh. A dual electrospinning nozzle can be used to produce nanofiber sheet layers, which are stacked on top of one another; therefore, the initial burst release is reduced compared with the solid nanofibers because of these layers.

Additionally, hybridization of electrospun nanofibers with other formulations such as nanoparticles and hydrogels is an efficient, indirect drug loading method into the nanofibers from the pharmaceutical point of view. It is also probable to produce multi-drug delivery systems with planned release profile using the hybridization of electrospun nanofibers. Hybridization of two different drug delivery systems can improve their benefits and it seems that the outstanding attributes of each system will increase synergistically by hybridization. Growing advancements in the nanotechnology (especially nanomedicine) have opened up some chances for application in a variety of medical areas. It seems that nanofibers in future would play a vital role in the treatment of human diseases.

REFERENCES

Adibkia, K. (2014). Preparation of Pharmaceutical Nanobeads and Nanofibers via Electrospinning Method. *J Mol Pharm Org Process Res*, *2*(01), e112. doi:10.4172/2329-9053.1000e112

Andrady, A. L. (2008). *Science and technology of polymer nanofibers*. John Wiley & Sons. doi:10.1002/9780470229842

Baker, S. C., Atkin, N., Gunning, P. A., Granville, N., Wilson, K., Wilson, D., & Southgate, J. (2006). Characterisation of electrospun polystyrene scaffolds for three-dimensional in vitro biological studies. *Biomaterials*, *27*(16), 3136–3146. doi:10.1016/j.biomaterials.2006.01.026 PMID:16473404

Barzegar-Jalali, M., Adibkia, K., Valizadeh, H., Shadbad, M. R. S., Nokhodchi, A., Omidi, Y., & Hasan, M. et al. (2008). Kinetic analysis of drug release from nanoparticles. *Journal of Pharmacy & Pharmaceutical Sciences*, *11*(1), 167–177. doi:10.18433/J3D59T PMID:18471378

Berry, C. C., & Curtis, A. S. G. (2003). Functionalisation of magnetic nanoparticles for applications in biomedicine. *Journal of Physics. D, Applied Physics*, *36*(13), R198–R206. doi:10.1088/0022-3727/36/13/203

Bölgen, N., Vargel, İ., Korkusuz, P., Menceloğlu, Y. Z., & Pişkin, E. (2007). In vivo performance of antibiotic embedded electrospun PCL membranes for prevention of abdominal adhesions. *Journal of Biomedical Materials Research. Part B, Applied Biomaterials*, *81*(2), 530–543. doi:10.1002/jbm.b.30694 PMID:17041925

Brannon-Peppas, L., & Blanchette, J. O. (2012). Nanoparticle and targeted systems for cancer therapy. *Advanced Drug Delivery Reviews*, *64*, 206–212. doi:10.1016/j.addr.2012.09.033 PMID:15350294

Burger, C., & Chu, B. (2007). Functional nanofibrous scaffolds for bone reconstruction. *Colloids and Surfaces. B, Biointerfaces*, *56*(1), 134–141. doi:10.1016/j.colsurfb.2006.09.023 PMID:17113762

Burgess, P., Hutt, P. B., Farokhzad, O. C., Langer, R., Minick, S., & Zale, S. (2010). On firm ground: IP protection of therapeutic nanoparticles. *Nature Biotechnology*, *28*(12), 1267–1270. doi:10.1038/nbt.1725 PMID:21139609

Chew, S. Y., Wen, J., Yim, E. K. F., & Leong, K. W. (2005). Sustained release of proteins from electrospun biodegradable fibers. *Biomacromolecules*, *6*(4), 2017–2024. doi:10.1021/bm0501149 PMID:16004440

Cho, K., Wang, X., Nie, S., Chen, Z., & Shin, D. M. (2008). Therapeutic nanoparticles for drug delivery in cancer. *Clinical Cancer Research*, *14*(5), 1310–1316. doi:10.1158/1078-0432.CCR-07-1441 PMID:18316549

Cho, Y. I., Choi, J. S., Jeong, S. Y., & Yoo, H. S. (2010). Nerve growth factor (NGF)-conjugated electrospun nanostructures with topographical cues for neuronal differentiation of mesenchymal stem cells. *Acta Biomaterialia*, *6*(12), 4725–4733. doi:10.1016/j.actbio.2010.06.019 PMID:20601229

Fang, , Niu, Lin, & Wang. (2008). Applications of electrospun nanofibers. *Chinese Science Bulletin*, *53*(15), 2265–2286.

Fathi-Azarbayjani, A., & Chan, S. Y. (2010). Single and multi-layered nanofibers for rapid and controlled drug delivery. *Chemical & Pharmaceutical Bulletin*, *58*(2), 143–146. doi:10.1248/cpb.58.143 PMID:20118570

Gelperina, S., Kisich, K., Iseman, M. D., & Heifets, L. (2005). The potential advantages of nanoparticle drug delivery systems in chemotherapy of tuberculosis. *American Journal of Respiratory and Critical Care Medicine*, *172*(12), 1487–1490. doi:10.1164/rccm.200504-613PP PMID:16151040

Goldberg, M., Langer, R., & Jia, X. (2007). Nanostructured materials for applications in drug delivery and tissue engineering. *Journal of Biomaterials Science. Polymer Edition*, *18*(3), 241–268. doi:10.1163/156856207779996931 PMID:17471764

Gopal, R., Kaur, S., Feng, C. Y., Chan, C., Ramakrishna, S., Tabe, S., & Matsuura, T. (2007). Electrospun nanofibrous polysulfone membranes as pre-filters: Particulate removal. *Journal of Membrane Science*, *289*(1), 210–219. doi:10.1016/j.memsci.2006.11.056

Hans, M. L., & Lowman, A. M. (2002). Biodegradable nanoparticles for drug delivery and targeting. *Current Opinion in Solid State and Materials Science*, *6*(4), 319–327. doi:10.1016/S1359-0286(02)00117-1

Hay, E. D. (2013). *Cell biology of extracellular matrix*. Springer Science & Business Media.

He, C.-L., Huang, Z.-M., & Han, X.-J. (2009). Fabrication of drug-loaded electrospun aligned fibrous threads for suture applications. *Journal of Biomedical Materials Research. Part A*, *89*(1), 80–95. doi:10.1002/jbm.a.32004 PMID:18428982

Henry, J. A., Simonet, M., Pandit, A., & Neuenschwander, P. (2007). Characterization of a slowly degrading biodegradable polyesterurethane for tissue engineering scaffolds. *Journal of Biomedical Materials Research. Part A*, *82*(3), 669–679. doi:10.1002/jbm.a.31094 PMID:17323319

Huang, Z.-M., He, C.-L., Yang, A., Zhang, Y., Han, X.-J., Yin, J., & Wu, Q. (2006). Encapsulating drugs in biodegradable ultrafine fibers through co-axial electrospinning. *Journal of Biomedical Materials Research. Part A*, *77*(1), 169–179. doi:10.1002/jbm.a.30564 PMID:16392131

Huang, Z.-M., Zhang, Y.-Z., Kotaki, M., & Ramakrishna, S. (2003). A review on polymer nanofibers by electrospinning and their applications in nanocomposites. *Composites Science and Technology*, *63*(15), 2223–2253. doi:10.1016/S0266-3538(03)00178-7

Im, J. S., Yun, J., Lim, Y.-M., Kim, H.-I., & Lee, Y.-S. (2010). Fluorination of electrospun hydrogel fibers for a controlled release drug delivery system. *Acta Biomaterialia*, *6*(1), 102–109. doi:10.1016/j.actbio.2009.06.017 PMID:19531386

Ionescu, L. C., Lee, G. C., Sennett, B. J., Burdick, J. A., & Mauck, R. L. (2010). An anisotropic nanofiber/microsphere composite with controlled release of biomolecules for fibrous tissue engineering. *Biomaterials*, *31*(14), 4113–4120. doi:10.1016/j.biomaterials.2010.01.098 PMID:20149432

Jafari-Aghdam, Adibkia, Payab, Barzegar-Jalali, Parvizpur, Mohammadi, & Sabzevari. (2014). Methylprednisolone acetate-Eudragit® RS100 electrospuns: Preparation and physicochemical characterization. *Artificial Cells, Nanomedicine, and Biotechnology*, 1-7.

Jahangiri, A., Davaran, S., Fayyazi, B., Tanhaei, A., Payab, S., & Adibkia, K. (2014). Application of electrospraying as a one-step method for the fabrication of triamcinolone acetonide-PLGA nanofibers and nanobeads. *Colloids and Surfaces. B, Biointerfaces*, *123*, 219–224. doi:10.1016/j.colsurfb.2014.09.019 PMID:25260224

Jiang, H., Hu, Y., Li, Y., Zhao, P., Zhu, K., & Chen, W. (2005). A facile technique to prepare biodegradable coaxial electrospun nanofibers for controlled release of bioactive agents. *Journal of Controlled Release*, *108*(2), 237–243. doi:10.1016/j.jconrel.2005.08.006 PMID:16153737

Jiang, H., Hu, Y., Zhao, P., Li, Y., & Zhu, K. (2006). Modulation of protein release from biodegradable core–shell structured fibers prepared by coaxial electrospinning. *Journal of Biomedical Materials Research. Part B, Applied Biomaterials*, *79*(1), 50–57. doi:10.1002/jbm.b.30510 PMID:16544305

Jiang, Y.-N., Mo, H.-Y., & Yu, D.-G. (2012). Electrospun drug-loaded core–sheath PVP/zein nanofibers for biphasic drug release. *International Journal of Pharmaceutics*, *438*(1), 232–239. doi:10.1016/j.ijpharm.2012.08.053 PMID:22981688

Jin, H.-J., Chen, J., Karageorgiou, V., Altman, G. H., & Kaplan, D. L. (2004). Human bone marrow stromal cell responses on electrospun silk fibroin mats. *Biomaterials*, *25*(6), 1039–1047. doi:10.1016/S0142-9612(03)00609-4 PMID:14615169

Kamaly, N., Xiao, Z., Valencia, P. M., Radovic-Moreno, A. F., & Farokhzad, O. C. (2012). Targeted polymeric therapeutic nanoparticles: Design, development and clinical translation. *Chemical Society Reviews*, *41*(7), 2971–3010. doi:10.1039/c2cs15344k PMID:22388185

Kenawy, E.-R., Bowlin, G. L., Mansfield, K., Layman, J., Simpson, D. G., Sanders, E. H., & Wnek, G. E. (2002). Release of tetracycline hydrochloride from electrospun poly (ethylene-co-vinylacetate), poly (lactic acid), and a blend. *Journal of Controlled Release*, *81*(1), 57–64. doi:10.1016/S0168-3659(02)00041-X PMID:11992678

Kenawy, E.-R., Layman, J. M., Watkins, J. R., Bowlin, G. L., Matthews, J. A., Simpson, D. G., & Wnek, G. E. (2003). Electrospinning of poly (ethylene-co-vinyl alcohol) fibers. *Biomaterials*, *24*(6), 907–913. doi:10.1016/S0142-9612(02)00422-2 PMID:12504511

Ki, C. S., Kim, J. W., Hyun, J. H., Lee, K. H., Hattori, M., Rah, D. K., & Park, Y. H. (2007). Electrospun three-dimensional silk fibroin nanofibrous scaffold. *Journal of Applied Polymer Science*, *106*(6), 3922–3928. doi:10.1002/app.26914

Kim, G. H. (2008). Electrospun PCL nanofibers with anisotropic mechanical properties as a biomedical scaffold. *Biomedical Materials (Bristol, England)*, *3*(2), 025010. doi:10.1088/1748-6041/3/2/025010 PMID:18458365

Kim, K., Luu, Y. K., Chang, C., Fang, D., Hsiao, B. S., Chu, B., & Hadjiargyrou, M. (2004). Incorporation and controlled release of a hydrophilic antibiotic using poly (lactide-co-glycolide)-based electrospun nanofibrous scaffolds. *Journal of Controlled Release*, *98*(1), 47–56. doi:10.1016/j.jconrel.2004.04.009 PMID:15245888

Kim, K.-H., Jeong, L., Park, H.-N., Shin, S.-Y., Park, W.-H., Lee, S.-C., & Lee, Y.-M. et al. (2005). Biological efficacy of silk fibroin nanofiber membranes for guided bone regeneration. *Journal of Biotechnology*, *120*(3), 327–339. doi:10.1016/j.jbiotec.2005.06.033 PMID:16150508

Kumar, M. N. V. R. (2000). Nano and microparticles as controlled drug delivery devices. *Journal of Pharmacy & Pharmaceutical Sciences*, *3*(2), 234–258. PMID:10994037

Kumari, A., Yadav, S. K., & Yadav, S. C. (2010). Biodegradable polymeric nanoparticles based drug delivery systems. *Colloids and Surfaces. B, Biointerfaces*, *75*(1), 1–18. doi:10.1016/j.colsurfb.2009.09.001 PMID:19782542

Labhasetwar, V., Song, C., & Levy, R. J. (1997). Nanoparticle drug delivery system for restenosis. *Advanced Drug Delivery Reviews*, *24*(1), 63–85. doi:10.1016/S0169-409X(96)00483-8

Lee, H. J., Park, Y. H., & Koh, W.-G. (2013). Fabrication of nanofiber microarchitectures localized within hydrogel microparticles and their application to protein delivery and cell encapsulation. *Advanced Functional Materials*, *23*(5), 591–597. doi:10.1002/adfm.201201501

Li, L., Bellan, L. M., Craighead, H. G., & Frey, M. W. (2006). Formation and properties of nylon-6 and nylon-6/montmorillonite composite nanofibers. *Polymer*, *47*(17), 6208–6217. doi:10.1016/j.polymer.2006.06.049

Li, S.-D., & Huang, L. (2008). Pharmacokinetics and biodistribution of nanoparticles. *Molecular Pharmaceutics*, *5*(4), 496–504. doi:10.1021/mp800049w PMID:18611037

Li, W.-J., Danielson, K. G., Alexander, P. G., & Tuan, R. S. (2003). Biological response of chondrocytes cultured in three-dimensional nanofibrous poly (ϵ-caprolactone) scaffolds. *Journal of Biomedical Materials Research. Part A*, *67*(4), 1105–1114. doi:10.1002/jbm.a.10101 PMID:14624495

Li, W.-J., Tuli, R., Okafor, C., Derfoul, A., Danielson, K. G., Hall, D. J., & Tuan, R. S. (2005). A three-dimensional nanofibrous scaffold for cartilage tissue engineering using human mesenchymal stem cells. *Biomaterials*, *26*(6), 599–609. doi:10.1016/j.biomaterials.2004.03.005 PMID:15282138

Lim, C. T., Tan, E. P. S., & Ng, S. Y. (2008). Effects of crystalline morphology on the tensile properties of electrospun polymer nanofibers. *Applied Physics Letters*, *92*(14), 141908. doi:10.1063/1.2857478

Loh, X. J., Peh, P., Liao, S., Sng, C., & Li, J. (2010). Controlled drug release from biodegradable thermo-responsive physical hydrogel nanofibers. *Journal of Controlled Release*, *143*(2), 175–182. doi:10.1016/j.jconrel.2009.12.030 PMID:20064568

Madduri, S., Papaloizos, M., & Gander, B. (2010). Trophically and topographically functionalized silk fibroin nerve conduits for guided peripheral nerve regeneration. *Biomaterials*, *31*(8), 2323–2334. doi:10.1016/j.biomaterials.2009.11.073 PMID:20004018

Mainardes, R. M., & Silva, L. P. (2004). Drug delivery systems: Past, present, and future. *Current Drug Targets*, *5*(5), 449–455. doi:10.2174/1389450043345407 PMID:15216911

Martins, A., Reis, R. L., & Neves, N. M. (2008). Electrospinning: Processing technique for tissue engineering scaffolding. *International Materials Reviews*, *53*(5), 257–274. doi:10.1179/174328008X353547

Matthews, J. A., Boland, E. D., Wnek, G. E., Simpson, D. G., & Bowlin, G. L. (2003). Electrospinning of collagen type II: A feasibility study. *Journal of Bioactive and Compatible Polymers*, *18*(2), 125–134. doi:10.1177/0883911503018002003

Matthews, J. A., Wnek, G. E., Simpson, D. G., & Bowlin, G. L. (2002). Electrospinning of collagen nanofibers. *Biomacromolecules*, *3*(2), 232–238. doi:10.1021/bm015533u PMID:11888306

Meinel, A. J., Germershaus, O., Luhmann, T., Merkle, H. P., & Meinel, L. (2012). Electrospun matrices for localized drug delivery: Current technologies and selected biomedical applications. *European Journal of Pharmaceutics and Biopharmaceutics*, *81*(1), 1–13. doi:10.1016/j.ejpb.2012.01.016 PMID:22342778

Melanko, J. B., Pearce, M. E., & Salem, A. K. (2009). *Nanotubes, nanorods, nanofibers, and fullerenes for nanoscale drug delivery. In Nanotechnology in Drug Delivery* (pp. 105–127). Springer.

Mickova, A., Buzgo, M., Benada, O., Rampichova, M., Fisar, Z., Filova, E., & Amler, E. et al. (2012). Core/shell nanofibers with embedded liposomes as a drug delivery system. *Biomacromolecules*, *13*(4), 952–962. doi:10.1021/bm2018118 PMID:22401557

Min, B.-M., Lee, G., Kim, S. H., Nam, Y. S., Lee, T. S., & Park, W. H. (2004). Electrospinning of silk fibroin nanofibers and its effect on the adhesion and spreading of normal human keratinocytes and fibroblasts in vitro. *Biomaterials*, *25*(7), 1289–1297. doi:10.1016/j.biomaterials.2003.08.045 PMID:14643603

Moghimi, S. (2005). Nanomedicine: Current status and future prospects. *The FASEB Journal*, *19*(3), 311–330. doi:10.1096/fj.04-2747rev PMID:15746175

Mohanraj, V. J., & Chen, Y. (2007). Nanoparticles-a review. *Tropical Journal of Pharmaceutical Research*, *5*(1), 561–573. doi:10.4314/tjpr.v5i1.14634

Nie, H., & Wang, C.-H. (2007). Fabrication and characterization of PLGA/HAp composite scaffolds for delivery of BMP-2 plasmid DNA. *Journal of Controlled Release*, *120*(1), 111–121. doi:10.1016/j.jconrel.2007.03.018 PMID:17512077

Okuda, T., Tominaga, K., & Kidoaki, S. (2010). Time-programmed dual release formulation by multilayered drug-loaded nanofiber meshes. *Journal of Controlled Release*, *143*(2), 258–264. doi:10.1016/j.jconrel.2009.12.029 PMID:20074599

Park, J.-Y., & Lee, I.-H. (2011). Controlled release of ketoprofen from electrospun porous polylactic acid (PLA) nanofibers. *Journal of Polymer Research*, *18*(6), 1287–1291. doi:10.1007/s10965-010-9531-0

Payab, Davaran, Tanhaei, Fayyazi, Jahangiri, Farzaneh, & Adibkia. (2014). Triamcinolone acetonide-Eudragit® RS100 nanofibers and nanobeads: Morphological and physicochemical characterization. *Artificial Cells, Nanomedicine, and Biotechnology*, 1-8.

Pham, Q. P., Sharma, U., & Mikos, A. G. (2006). Electrospinning of polymeric nanofibers for tissue engineering applications: A review. *Tissue Engineering*, *12*(5), 1197–1211. doi:10.1089/ten.2006.12.1197 PMID:16771634

Poon, Z., Chang, D., Zhao, X., & Hammond, P. T. (2011). Layer-by-layer nanoparticles with a pH-sheddable layer for in vivo targeting of tumor hypoxia. *ACS Nano*, *5*(6), 4284–4292. doi:10.1021/nn200876f PMID:21513353

Qian, X., Peng, X.-H., Ansari, D. O., Yin-Goen, Q., Chen, G. Z., Shin, D. M., & Nie, S. et al. (2008). In vivo tumor targeting and spectroscopic detection with surface-enhanced Raman nanoparticle tags. *Nature Biotechnology*, *26*(1), 83–90. doi:10.1038/nbt1377 PMID:18157119

Sakai, S., Yamada, Y., Yamaguchi, T., & Kawakami, K. (2006). Prospective use of electrospun ultrafine silicate fibers for bone tissue engineering. *Biotechnology Journal*, *1*(9), 958–962. doi:10.1002/biot.200600054 PMID:16941440

Schiffman, J. D., & Schauer, C. L. (2008). A review: Electrospinning of biopolymer nanofibers and their applications. *The Polish Review*, *48*(2), 317–352. doi:10.1080/15583720802022182

Shao, S., Li, L., Yang, G., Li, J., Luo, C., Gong, T., & Zhou, S. (2011). Controlled green tea polyphenols release from electrospun PCL/MWCNTs composite nanofibers. *International Journal of Pharmaceutics*, *421*(2), 310–320. doi:10.1016/j.ijpharm.2011.09.033 PMID:21983092

Shields, K. J., Beckman, M. J., Bowlin, G. L., & Wayne, J. S. (2004). Mechanical properties and cellular proliferation of electrospun collagen type II. *Tissue Engineering*, *10*(9-10), 1510–1517. doi:10.1089/ten.2004.10.1510 PMID:15588410

Sill, T. J., & von Recum, H. A. (2008). Electrospinning: Applications in drug delivery and tissue engineering. *Biomaterials*, *29*(13), 1989–2006. doi:10.1016/j.biomaterials.2008.01.011 PMID:18281090

Son, Y. J., Kim, W. J., & Yoo, H. S. (2014). Therapeutic applications of electrospun nanofibers for drug delivery systems. *Archives of Pharmacal Research, 37*(1), 69–78. doi:10.1007/s12272-013-0284-2 PMID:24234913

Son, Y. J., & Yoo, H. S. (2012). Dexamethasone-incorporated nanofibrous meshes for antiproliferation of smooth muscle cells: Thermally induced drug-loading strategy. *Journal of Biomedical Materials Research. Part A*, *100*(10), 2678–2685. doi:10.1002/jbm.a.34197 PMID:22619069

Song, W., Yu, X., Markel, D. C., Shi, T., & Ren, W. (2013). Coaxial PCL/PVA electrospun nanofibers: Osseointegration enhancer and controlled drug release device. *Biofabrication*, *5*(3), 035006. doi:10.1088/1758-5082/5/3/035006 PMID:23799653

Stankus, J. J., Guan, J., & Wagner, W. R. (2004). Fabrication of biodegradable elastomeric scaffolds with sub-micron morphologies. *Journal of Biomedical Materials Research. Part A*, *70*(4), 603–614. doi:10.1002/jbm.a.30122 PMID:15307165

Sun, Z., Zussman, E., Yarin, A. L., Wendorff, J. H., & Greiner, A. (2003). Compound core-shell polymer nanofibers by co-electrospinning. *Advanced Materials*, *15*(22), 1929–1932. doi:10.1002/adma.200305136

Taepaiboon, P., Rungsardthong, U., & Supaphol, P. (2006). Drug-loaded electrospun mats of poly (vinyl alcohol) fibres and their release characteristics of four model drugs. *Nanotechnology*, *17*(9), 2317–2329. doi:10.1088/0957-4484/17/9/041

Taepaiboon, P., Rungsardthong, U., & Supaphol, P. (2007). Vitamin-loaded electrospun cellulose acetate nanofiber mats as transdermal and dermal therapeutic agents of vitamin A acid and vitamin E. *European Journal of Pharmaceutics and Biopharmaceutics*, *67*(2), 387–397. doi:10.1016/j.ejpb.2007.03.018 PMID:17498935

Thandavamoorthy, S., Gopinath, N., & Ramkumar, S. S. (2006). Self-assembled honeycomb polyurethane nanofibers. *Journal of Applied Polymer Science*, *101*(5), 3121–3124. doi:10.1002/app.24333

Thassu, D., Deleers, M., & Pathak, Y. V. (2007). *Nanoparticulate drug delivery systems* (Vol. 166). CRC Press. doi:10.1201/9781420008449

Vasita, R., & Katti, D. S. (2006). Nanofibers and their applications in tissue engineering. *International Journal of Nanomedicine*, *1*(1), 15–30. doi:10.2147/nano.2006.1.1.15 PMID:17722259

Venugopal, J., Zhang, Y. Z., & Ramakrishna, S. (2005). Fabrication of modified and functionalized polycaprolactone nanofibre scaffolds for vascular tissue engineering. *Nanotechnology*, *16*(10), 2138–2142. doi:10.1088/0957-4484/16/10/028 PMID:20817986

Verreck, G., Chun, I., Rosenblatt, J., Peeters, J., Van Dijck, A., Mensch, J., & Brewster, M. E. et al. (2003). Incorporation of drugs in an amorphous state into electrospun nanofibers composed of a water-insoluble, nonbiodegradable polymer. *Journal of Controlled Release*, *92*(3), 349–360. doi:10.1016/S0168-3659(03)00342-0 PMID:14568415

Wang, Y., Qiao, W., & Yin, T. (2010). A novel controlled release drug delivery system for multiple drugs based on electrospun nanofibers containing nanoparticles. *Journal of Pharmaceutical Sciences*, *99*(12), 4805–4811. doi:10.1002/jps.22189 PMID:20821381

Wang, Y., Zhang, Y., Wang, B., Cao, Y., Yu, Q., & Yin, T. (2013). Fabrication of core–shell micro/nanoparticles for programmable dual drug release by emulsion electrospraying. *Journal of Nanoparticle Research, 15*(6), 1–12. doi:10.1007/s11051-013-1726-y

Xie, J., & Wang, C.-H. (2006). Electrospun micro-and nanofibers for sustained delivery of paclitaxel to treat C6 glioma in vitro. *Pharmaceutical Research, 23*(8), 1817–1826. doi:10.1007/s11095-006-9036-z PMID:16841195

Xu, X., Chen, X., Xu, X., Lu, T., Wang, X., Yang, L., & Jing, X. (2006). BCNU-loaded PEG–PLLA ultrafine fibers and their in vitro antitumor activity against Glioma C6 cells. *Journal of Controlled Release, 114*(3), 307–316. doi:10.1016/j.jconrel.2006.05.031 PMID:16891029

Xue, J., He, M., Liu, H., Niu, Y., Crawford, A., Coates, P. D., & Zhang, L. et al. (2014). Drug loaded homogeneous electrospun PCL/gelatin hybrid nanofiber structures for anti-infective tissue regeneration membranes. *Biomaterials, 35*(34), 9395–9405. doi:10.1016/j.biomaterials.2014.07.060 PMID:25134855

Yang, Y., Li, X., Qi, M., Zhou, S., & Weng, J. (2008). Release pattern and structural integrity of lysozyme encapsulated in core–sheath structured poly (DL-lactide) ultrafine fibers prepared by emulsion electrospinning. *European Journal of Pharmaceutics and Biopharmaceutics, 69*(1), 106–116. doi:10.1016/j.ejpb.2007.10.016 PMID:18078743

Yang, Chang, Yang, & Lin. (2010). Pharmacokinetics and physiologically-based pharmacokinetic modeling of nanoparticles. *Journal of Nanoscience and Nanotechnology, 10*(12), 8482-8490.

Yoo, H. S., Kim, T. G., & Park, T. G. (2009). Surface-functionalized electrospun nanofibers for tissue engineering and drug delivery. *Advanced Drug Delivery Reviews, 61*(12), 1033–1042. doi:10.1016/j.addr.2009.07.007 PMID:19643152

Yoshimoto, H., Shin, Y. M., Terai, H., & Vacanti, J. P. (2003). A biodegradable nanofiber scaffold by electrospinning and its potential for bone tissue engineering. *Biomaterials, 24*(12), 2077–2082. doi:10.1016/S0142-9612(02)00635-X PMID:12628828

Yu, D.-G., Li, X.-Y., Wang, X., Chian, W., Liao, Y.-Z., & Li, Y. (2013). Zero-order drug release cellulose acetate nanofibers prepared using coaxial electrospinning. *Cellulose (London, England), 20*(1), 379–389. doi:10.1007/s10570-012-9824-z

Yu, D. G., Wang, X., Li, X. Y., Chian, W., Li, Y., & Liao, Y. Z. (2013). Electrospun biphasic drug release polyvinylpyrrolidone/ethyl cellulose core/sheath nanofibers. *Acta Biomaterialia, 9*(3), 5665–5672. doi:10.1016/j.actbio.2012.10.021 PMID:23099302

Yu, H., Jia, Y., Yao, C., & Lu, Y. (2014). PCL/PEG core/sheath fibers with controlled drug release rate fabricated on the basis of a novel combined technique. *International Journal of Pharmaceutics, 469*(1), 17–22. doi:10.1016/j.ijpharm.2014.04.045 PMID:24751343

Zeng, J., Aigner, A., Czubayko, F., Kissel, T., Wendorff, J. H., & Greiner, A. (2005). Poly (vinyl alcohol) nanofibers by electrospinning as a protein delivery system and the retardation of enzyme release by additional polymer coatings. *Biomacromolecules, 6*(3), 1484–1488. doi:10.1021/bm0492576 PMID:15877368

Zhang, L., Gu, F. X., Chan, J. M., Wang, A. Z., Langer, R. S., & Farokhzad, O. C. (2008). Nanoparticles in medicine: Therapeutic applications and developments. *Clinical Pharmacology and Therapeutics*, *83*(5), 761–769. doi:10.1038/sj.clpt.6100400 PMID:17957183

Zhang, Y., Huang, Z.-M., Xu, X., Lim, C. T., & Ramakrishna, S. (2004). Preparation of core-shell structured PCL-r-gelatin bi-component nanofibers by coaxial electrospinning. *Chemistry of Materials*, *16*(18), 3406–3409. doi:10.1021/cm049580f

Zong, X., Kim, K., Fang, D., Ran, S., Hsiao, B. S., & Chu, B. (2002). Structure and process relationship of electrospun bioabsorbable nanofiber membranes. *Polymer*, *43*(16), 4403–4412. doi:10.1016/S0032-3861(02)00275-6

Chapter 14
Application of Nanoparticles as a Drug Delivery System

Vijay Kumar Singh
Bundelkhand University, India

Raj K. Keservani
Rajiv Gandhi Proudyogiki Vishawavidyalaya, India

ABSTRACT

Small colloidal particles having their diameter in the range of 50 to 500nm are defined as Nanoparticles. These are usually prepared either by using biodegradable or non-biodegradable polymers and are usually classified in two broad categories: (1) Nanocapsules: a type of reservoir system in which an oil or aqueous core is surrounded by a polymeric membrane. (2) Nanospheres: a type of matrix system. Preparation of nanoparticle as a drug delivery system is one of the most widely accepted approach since the prepration of nanoparticle were easy and convenient to scale up. Their high stability and conveniently easy to freeze-dried their preparations provide some additional advantages to choose Nanoparticles as a good drug delivery system. Inspite of them Nanoparticles were were able to achieve with success tissue targeting of many drugs (antibiotics, cytostatics, peptides and proteins, nucleic acids, etc.).

1. INTRODUCTION

In microcapsules drug is encapsulated as small particles or as a drug solution in a polymer fi lm or coat, whereas microspheres are solid polymeric spheres which entrap drug. Equivalent structures with particle diameters ranging from 50 to 500 nm are referred to as nanocapsules and nanoparticles. Nanoparticles (NPs) of different size and physicochemical properties have been introduced to many fields of life and biomedical sciences over the last decade (Oberdörster et al., 2005). It is worth noting that nanoparticles can be made from a fully variety of bulk materials and that they can explicate their actions depending on both the chemical composition and on the size and/or shape of the particles (Brunner et al., 2006). The literature on the ecotoxicity of nanoparticles and nanomaterials as well as the chemistry of both manufactured and natural NSPs is summarized in recent reports (Handy et al. 2008, Yu-Nam & Lead 2008). Medical therapies have become more tailored to specific diseases and patients in recent years.

DOI: 10.4018/978-1-5225-0751-2.ch014

Most pharmaceutical agents have primary targets within cells and tissues; ideally, these agents may be preferentially delivered to these sites of action within the cell. Selective subcellular delivery is likely to have greater therapeutic benefits. Cytosolic delivery, for instance, is desirable for drugs that undergo extensive exportation from the cell via efflux transporters such as multi-drug resistance proteins and P-glycoproteins (Faraji & Wipf, 2009).

2. PREPARATION OF NANOPARTICLES

Polymer nanoparticles including nanospheres and nanocapsules (Figure 1) can be prepared according to numerous methods that have been developed over the last 30 years. The development of these methods occurred in several steps. Historically, the first nanoparticles proposed as carriers for therapeutic applications were made of gelatin and cross-linked albumin (Scheffel et al., 1972; Marty et al., 1978). Then, to avoid the use of proteins that may stimulate the immune system and to limit the toxicity of the cross-linking agents, nanoparticles made from synthetic polymers were developed. At first, the nanoparticles were made by emulsion polymerization of acrylamide and by dispersion polymerization of methylmethacrylate (Birrenbach, Speiser 1976; Kreuter, 1976). These nanoparticles were proposed as adjuvants for vaccines. However, since they were made of non-biodegradable polymers, these nanoparticles were rapidly substituted by particles made of biodegradable synthetic polymers. Couvreur et al., proposed to make nanoparticles by polymerization of monomers from the family of alkylcyanoacrylates already used in vivo as surgical glue. They succeeded in making nanoparticles by polymerization of the monomers in oil-in-water type emulsions prepared with an acidified aqueous phase (Couvreur et al., 1979).

During the same period of time, Gurny et al., proposed a method based on the use of another biodegradable polymer consisting of poly(lactic acid) used as surgical sutures in humans (Gurny et al., 1981).

Figure 1. Schematic representation of a nanosphere (A) and of a nanocapsule (B). In nanospheres, the whole particle consists of a continuous polymer network. Nanocapsules present a core-shell structure with a liquid core surrounded by a polymer shell.

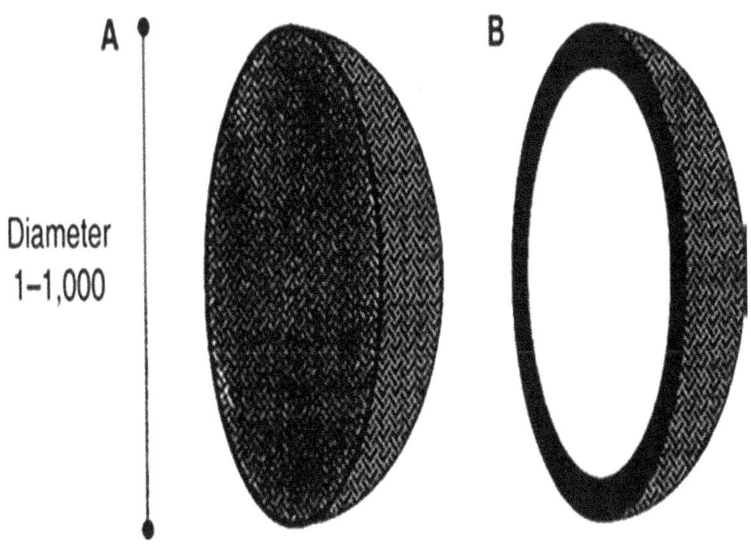

In this method, nanoparticles were formed directly from the polymer. Based on these initial investigations, several groups improved and modified the original processes mainly by reducing the amount of surfactant and organic solvents. At that time, the methods developed were only able to produce nanospheres (Figure 1) (Legrand et. al. 1999). A breakthrough in the development of nanoparticles occurred in 1986 with the development of methods allowing the preparation of nanocapsules corresponding to particles displaying a core-shell structure with a liquid core surrounded by a polymer shell. From 1986, there was also an acceleration in the development of new methodologies for the preparation of all types of nanoparticles.

The nanoprecipitation technique was proposed (Fessi et al., 1986) as well as the first method of interfacial polymerization in inverse microemulsion (Gasco & Trotta, 1986). In the following years, the methods based on salting-out, (Alle´man, 1992) emulsion–diffusion, (Quintanar & Guerrero, 1998) and double emulsion (Zambaux, 1998) were described. Finally, during the last decade, new approaches were considered to develop nanoparticles made from polysaccharides based on the gelation properties of these natural macromolecules (Vauthier & Couvreur, 2000a). These nanoparticles were developed for peptides and nucleic acid delivery. Another goal was the development of surface modified nanoparticles to produce long circulating particles able to avoid the capture by the macrophages of the mononuclear phagocyte system after intravenous administration (Gref, 1997).

All the methods can be classified into two groups depending on whether the nanoparticles are formed at the same time than the polymer itself requiring a polymerization reaction or are directly obtained from a polymer. There are numerous valuable reviews on the subject (Quintanar & Guerrero, 1998b). The general principles of the methods leading to nanoparticle preparation are described and details of the most representative over are given.

Preparation of Nanoparticles by Polymerization

Nanospheres (Kucuk & Edirisinghe 2014) are mostly prepared by emulsion polymerization whereas nanocapsules are obtained by interfacial polymerization performed in emulsion or in microemulsion. In emulsion polymerization, the monomer itself, if liquid, is dispersed under agitation in a continuous phase in which it is non-miscible.

The polymerization is usually initiated by the reaction of the initiators with the monomer molecules that are dissolved in the continuous phase of the emulsion.

The polymerization continues by further addition of monomer molecules that diffuse toward the growing polymer chain through the continuous phase. The growing polymer chain remains soluble until it reaches a certain molecular weight for which it becomes insoluble. Therefore, phase separation occurs leading to the nucleation of the polymer particles and the formation of the tyndall scattering effect. Further growth of the nucleated particles occurs according to a mechanism that depends on the stability conditions of the whole system. This includes capture of new growing polymer chains, fusion or collision between nucleated particles (Lowell, 1997). Throughout the polymerization, the monomer input in the continuous phase of the emulsion takes place by diffusion from the monomer droplets, which play the role of monomer reservoirs.

When the reaction is completed, the particles formed contains a large number of polymer chains (Lowell, 1997). Emulsion polymerization can be performed in emulsifier free systems and in both oil-in-water and waterin-oil emulsions. The poly(alkylcyanoacrylate) nanospheres, widely used as drug carriers, are prepared by emulsion polymerization according to a method initially introduced by Couvreur et al. The monomers (isobutylcyanoacrylate, isohexylcyanoacrylate, n-butylcyanoacrylate) are dispersed in a continuous acidified aqueous phase under magnetic agitation. The anionic polymerization of the alkylcyanoacrylate is rapidly and spontaneously initiated by the remaining OH_ ions of the acidified water and is completed within 3–4 h depending on the monomer type (Figure 2). The preparation is performed at low pH (pH _ 2.5) to slow down the anionic polymerization of the alkylcyanoacrylate, therefore allowing the polymer to arrange as colloidal particles. Dextran 70 or Pluronic_ F68 are usually dissolved in the aqueous phase to ensure the stability of the polymer particles. The size of the nanospheres can be controlled by the amount of Pluronic_ F68 from a diameter of 40–250nm for concentrations ranging from 3 to 0%, respectively. (Seijo, et. al. 1990) Numerous drugs have been associated with these nanospheres including doxorubicin, an anticancer agent, a peptide growth hormone, and several antibiotics. Antisense oligonucleotides were adsorbed on the nanosphere surface via the formation of an ion-pair with a cationic surfactant, cethyltrimethylammonium bromide. Finally, it should be mentioned that some drugs can lose their biological activity during the preparation of poly(alkylcyanoacrylate) nanospheres. Generally, these molecules contain chemical functions that are able to initiate the polymerization of alkylcyanoacrylates and be covalently attached to the polymer constituting the nanospheres. The mode of such an interaction has been elucidated for two molecules including phenylbutazone (an anti-inflammatory drug) and vidarabine (an antiviral molecule). In contrast, the side reactions can be used to achieve the covalent linkage of defined compounds to give specific properties to the nanospheres. This has been used with poly(ethylene glycol) that initiated the polymerization of isobutylcyanoacrylate to give poly(ethylene glycol)-coated nanospheres, therefore presenting a more hydrophilic surface than those prepared according to the original method (Seijo, 1990). Methylidene malonates are other monomers that give biodegradable polymers and polymerize according to a similar mechanism than alkylcyanoacrylates. These monomers were also used to make nanospheres by emulsion polymerization for drug delivery (De Keyser, 1991).

Nanocapsules can be prepared by interfacial polymerization of alkylcyanoacrylates. The main advantage of using these monomers is their very fast polymerization rate when they come into contact with water. Oil containing nanocapsules were prepared by the rapid dispersion of an ethanol phase including

Figure 2. Anionic polymerization of alkylcyanoacrylate initiated by the OH⁻ from the dissociation of the water molecule

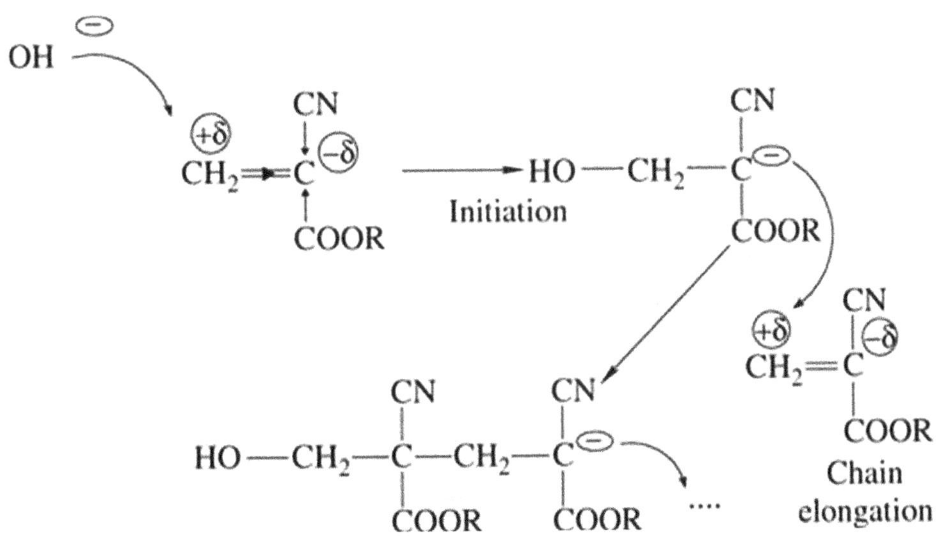

ethanol, the oil, the monomer, and the molecule to be encapsulated in an aqueous solution of surfactant. When the ethanol diffuses in the aqueous phase, tiny individual oil droplets form, and because of the contact with water at the oil/water interface, the polymerization of the alkylcyanoacrylate takes place on the droplet surface (Gallardo, 1993). This method is mainly adapted for the encapsulation of oily soluble substances. However, surprisingly, highly water-soluble molecules such as insulin could be entrapped in these nanocapsules with high encapsulation yields (up to 97%) (Aboubakar., 1999).

Water containing nanocapsules were prepared by interfacial polymerization of the alkylcyanoacrylate in water-in-oil microemulsions. In these systems, water swollen micelles of surfactants of small and uniform sizes are dispersed in an organic phase. To prepare nanocapsules, the monomer is added to the oily phase of the already prepared microemulsion.

The anionic polymerization of the alkylcyanoacrylate is initiated at the surface of the water swollen micelles and the polymer formed locally to make the shells of the nanocapsules. In the method first introduced by Gasco and Trotta, the microemulsions were prepared with hexane as the organic phase and Aerosol-OT as the surfactant. Both of these constituents are not compatible for the development of an acceptable drug carrier system. Thus, the method was recently adapted to microemulsions formulated with more biocompatible compounds, but still quite high concentrations of surfactant (up to 14 wt%) are required for their preparation (Watnasirichaikul, 2000). The nanocapsules obtained by this method are dispersed in an organic medium and can mainly be used for oral administration. Indeed, for intravenous administrations, it is necessary to transfer the nanocapsules into an aqueous continuous phase. Such a transfer still remained a problem until recently, since the total elimination of the organic phase and the redispersion of the nanocapsules, in water is a difficult task to achieve avoiding the aggregation of the nanocapsules. Recently, Lambert et al. proposed to perform this operation by ultracentrifugation of the nanocapsule dispersion over a layer of pure water. Using this simple approach, the nanocapsules transferred from the organic phase to the aqueous phase without any aggregation problem during the centrifugation. In addition, this technique allows the elimination of the excess surfactant, which remains in the organic phase. This nanoencapsulation method has special interest for the encapsulation of water soluble molecules such as peptides and nucleic acids including antisense oligonucleotides (Lambert et al., 1998).

Preparation of Nanoparticles Using a Polymer

In this group of methods, the nanoparticles are obtained from a polymer, which was prepared according to a totally independent method. This approach presents the major advantage that the polymers entering the composition of the nanoparticles are well characterized and their intrinsic physicochemical characteristics will not depend on the conditions encountered during the preparation of the nanoparticles as it can be the case with the previously described methods. Most methods starting from polymers have taken advantages of the physicochemical properties of the polymer used in terms of its solubility or its faculty to form a gel under certain conditions. Basically, two approaches are followed. One is based on the spontaneous formation of colloidal particles of the polymer that are then stabilized in a second step of the procedure. The second approach is based on the adaptation of methods initially developed to make microparticles. In this case, the goal is to reduce the size of the particles formed with these methods. A third approach leading to the formation of very specific particles named SupraMolecular BioVectors by their authors (De Miguel, 1995) is described separately. The different ways to produce nanoparticles from a polymer is summarized in Figure 3.

Figure 3. Summary of the different methods to prepare nanospheres and nanocapsules from a polymer
W/O: water-in-oil, O/W: oil-in-water, W/O/W: water-in-oil-in-water

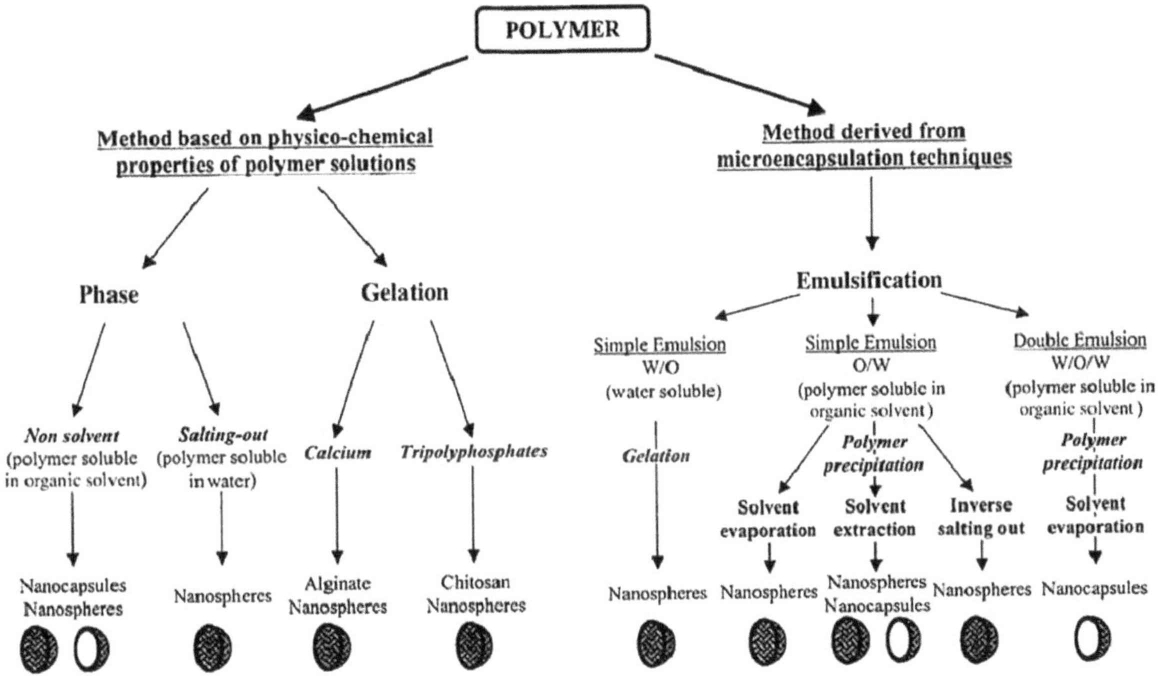

Methods Based on the Spontaneous Formation of the Nanoparticles

Spontaneous formation of nanoparticles can be achieved by taking advantage of the solubility and gelling properties of a dissolved polymer. Usually, the step allowing polymer colloidal particles to form is reversible, and it is necessary to complete the procedure by a second step required to stabilize the particles.

Based on the solubility properties of a polymer, the general principle is to prepare a solution of the polymer and to induce a phase separation by the addition of a non-solvent of the polymer or by a salting-out effect. The occurrence of the phase separation can be followed by turbidimetric measurements or investigated using ternary phase diagrams (Stainmesse, 1990). Phase separations leading to polymer colloid particles are usually obtained with diluted solutions of polymers. In a ternary phase diagram, it corresponds to a small domain.

Using higher polymer concentrations in the solvent, the colloidal particles formed at the limit of the phase separation as followed by turbidimetric measurements in the case of proteins. To facilitate the formation of colloidal dispersion of polymer particles, it is better to induce the phase separation in totally miscible solvent–non-solvent systems. At that stage, the particles form spontaneously and quasi-instantaneously.

Once the proper conditions to obtain the polymer colloidal nanoparticles are identified, the particles must be stabilized. This is usually achieved either by the elimination of the polymer solvent by evaporation or by chemical cross-linking of the polymer as it is the case with proteins (Weber, 2000).

This method, also known as the nanoprecipitation method, can be applied to numerous synthetic polymers. In general, the polymer is dissolved in acetone and the polymer solution is added into water.

The acetone is then evaporated to complete the formation of the particles. Surface active agents are usually added to water to ensure the stability of the polymer particles. This easy technique of nanoparticle preparation was scaled up for large batch production. It leads to the formation of nanospheres. Nanocapsules can easily be prepared by the same method just by adding a small amount of an organic oil in the polymer solution. When the polymer solution is poured into the water phase, the oil is dispersed as tiny droplets in the solvent–non-solvent mixture and the polymer precipitates on the oil droplet surface. This method leads to the preparation of oil-containing nanocapsules and can be valuably used for the encapsulation of liposoluble drugs. Techniques based on the use of proteins are much more adapted to the encapsulation of hydrosoluble compounds and were recently developed to produce gelatin nanospheres as carrier systems for gene delivery.

Based on the gelation properties displayed by certain polymers, nanoparticles are formed spontaneously by controlling the gelation process. This approach has been developed with alginate and chitosan that form highly water-swollen gels. The gelling agents for these two natural polysaccharides are respectively calcium and tripolyphosphate. Nanoparticles are formed in a certain domain of concentrations of the polysaccharide and of the gelling agent. With the alginate, it has been shown that nanoparticles can be prepared when the respective concentrations of alginate and calcium are comprised in the domain of the pregel stage of the alginate gelling process (alginate 0.6 wt%, calcium chloride 0.9 mM). At this composition, tiny particles of gels form resulting from inter and intramolecular aggregations of alginate molecules caused by the interaction with calcium. These aggregates are stabilized by the formation of a polyelectrolyte complex with polylysine. Alginate and chitosan nanoparticles are interested for nucleic acid and protein delivery as recently reviewed by (Vauthier & Couvreur, 2000).

Methods Derived from Microencapsulation Techniques

Methods derived from microencapsulation techniques require the formation of an emulsion as a first step of the procedure. To produce nanometer-scale-sized particles, the size of the emulsion droplets must be small enough. This can be achieved by the use of special equipments such as high pressure homogenizers and microfluidizers. The energy input produced by these apparatus is important and is mainly due to high turbulence and cavitation forces. It allows an efficient dispersion of the polymer solution in the continuous phase. Once the desired emulsion is prepared, the formation of the nanoparticles can be induced according to two routes including the gelation of the polymer and the precipitation of the polymer either by solvent displacement or by solvent evaporation. Gelation can be induced by increasing the pH, adding calcium, or decreasing the temperature of emulsions containing respectively, chitosan, alginate, and agarose. In the solvent displacement technique, the emulsion is formed with a solvent of the polymer, which is partially soluble in water and with an aqueous phase saturated with the solvent. Once the emulsion is formed with ethylacetate as an example, it is diluted by the further addition of water to displace the solvent from the dispersed phase inducing the polymer precipitation. This principle was also developed on the base of an inverse salting out method. In this procedure, a solution of polymer in acetone is dispersed in an aqueous phase containing a high concentration of salt to keep the acetone nonmiscible with water. Just by diluting the emulsion with a large amount of pure water, the acetone is then extracted from the dispersed phase inducing the polymer precipitation. The total elimination of the acetone can be achieved by evaporation. Finally, precipitation of the polymer solubilized in the dispersed phase can also be induced by the removal of the solvent by evaporation. In this method named emulsification solvent evaporation, the polymer solvent diffuses through the aqueous continuous phase and evaporates at the air/water interface. The emulsion should remain under agitation during the time required for the total evaporation of the solvent. These methods produce nanospheres. To make nanocapsules, small amounts of oil can be added in the dispersed phase of the emulsion that will form the nanocapsules by solvent displacement. Nanocapsules can also be prepared with the solvent evaporation technique from a double water-in-oil-in-water emulsion. The removal of the organic solvent of the intermediate phase of this double emulsion by evaporation causes the polymer to precipitate at the surface of the inner aqueous phase. Whereas nanocapsules made by the solvent displacement method is more adapted for the encapsulation of lipophilic compounds, this last method allows the encapsulation of hydrosoluble compounds.

Preparation of SupraMolecular BioVector

SupraMolecular BioVector consists of polysaccharide nanospheres surrounded by a bilayer of phospholipids (De Miguel, 1995). At the origin, these systems were developed to mimic the low density lipoproteins that are natural colloidal structures encountered in the blood circulation and designed for the transport of cholesterol and cholesterol esters in vivo. SupraMolecular Bio-Vector are prepared in several steps including the functionnalization and chemical cross-linking of a polysaccharide (starch or dextran), the purification and the drying of the modified polysaccharide followed by the fragmentation of the resulted powder under high pressure to produce small polysaccharide nanoparticles. Finally, a lipid bilayer is adsorbed on the surface of the nanoparticles. The chemical modification of the polysaccharide forming the core of the Supra Molecular BioVector lead to various possibilities in terms of the type of molecules that can be associated with such a carrier system. Indeed, the polysaccharide core can be either negatively or positively charged or even neutral opening large application potential.

Preparation of Surface Modified Nanoparticles

Once intravenously administered, the body distribution of the nanoparticles is controlled by their surface properties. Indeed, despite their small size, nanoparticles display an enormous specific surface area that makes the interaction with the surrounding medium very important especially for their fate in vivo. Thus, the preparation of surface modified nanoparticles received much attention during the last decade to produce nanoparticles that are able to circulate for a long period of time in the blood stream at first and, more recently, to achieve an effective targeting of the device or to improve their bioadhesivity to mucosae. Nanoparticles that are able to circulate for a long time in the blood stream should not be recognized by macrophages of the mononuclear phagocyte system. To achieve this goal, at least one of the two major known mechanisms involved in the recognition of foreign particles by macrophages should be avoided. These two mechanisms include the particle opsonisation and the complement activation, which consists in protein adsorption and subsequent recognition by macrophages. A barrier to protein adsorption could be achieved by creating an efficient barrier of steric hindrance, therefore, by coating or adsorbing hydrophilic polymers to nanoparticle surface.

Nanospheres coated with poly(ethylene glycol) were first obtained by the simple adsorption of triblock copolymers of poly(ethylene glycol)–poly(propyleneglycol)–poly(ethylene glycol) on the surface of already prepared nanospheres. To improve the stability of the poly(ethylene glycol) coating, nanospheres were prepared by nanoprecipitation or by emulsification solvent evaporation using copolymers of poly(lactic acid)–co-poly (ethylene glycol) or of poly(alkylcyanoacrylate)–co-poly(ethylene glycol). Finally, poly (ethylene glycol) can initiate the polymerization of alkylcyanoacrylate to produce poly(ethylene glycol)-coated poly-(alkylcyanoacrylate) nanoparticles by emulsion polymerization. To make nanoparticles able to escape complement activation, Passirani et al., proposed to coat nanospheres with heparin. This compound, which is a polysaccharide, is a physiological inhibitor of complement activation in vivo. Heparin-coated poly(methylmethacrylate) nanoparticles were prepared by emulsion polymerization. In the method, the radical polymerization of methylmethacrylate was initiated by heparin according to an original method involving cerium ions and allowing heparin to covalently attach to poly(methylmethacrylate) (Passirani, 1998; Passirani,1999).

The next step now is the development of targeted nanoparticles toward a specific cell type. This has recently been investigated by Stella et al., who prepared poly(alkylcyanoacrylate) nanoparticles showing residues of folic acid on their surface. These nanoparticles will be used to target cancer cells overexpressing a membrane receptor for the folic acid. The targeting moiety, consisting on the folic acid, was grafted on the surface of poly(aminopoly(ethylene glycol) cyanoco-hexadecylcyanoacrylate) nanoparticles that were obtained by nanoprecipitation (Stella et al., 2000). In another way, chitosan was used as a coating agent for nanoparticles to improve their bioadhesive properties after oral and nasal administration. Indeed, chitosan is known to have bioadhesive properties as well as an interesting absorption enhancing capacity.

3. CHARACTERIZATION OF NANOPARTICULATE DRUG CARRIERS

Nanoparticles can be characterized by all the different physico chemical techniques that apply for polymer colloids. Concerning the development procedure of nanoparticles as drug carriers, the main physico chemical parameters that are investigated are the shape, the size, the surface properties, the density, and the concentration of the particles. The size as well as the size distribution are important parameters to be determined to achieve safe intravenous administration. Surface properties are also important to consider as nanoparticles display considerable specific surface area responsible for the interactions with the surrounding medium. Finally, the density and the concentration are required to deduce the specific surface area of the particles together with the size.

Nanoparticles can be visualized using different microscopy techniques. Transmission electron microscopy is usually applied to nanoparticles after negative staining with phosphotungstate acid or with uranyl acetate after it has been checked that the staining agents do not modify the particles. Recent progress in transmission electron microscopy now allows direct observations of the nanoparticles without the use of any staining agent that may cause artefacts in some cases. In particular, direct observations of the nanoparticles after a sample of the nanoparticle dispersion has been freezing at very low temperature can be carried out by cryotransmission electron microscopy. Scanning electron microscopy is performed on samples coated with a thin layer of gold metal to produce the contrast. These techniques as well as those based on atomic force microscopy give useful images of the nanoparticles showing their shape. Measurements of the size and of the size distribution require determination of the diameters number of individual nanoparticles that may be assisted by the use of valuable image analysis softwares. The internal structure of the nanoparticles can be observed by freeze fracture and cryotransmission electron microscopy.

Generally, mean size and size distribution of nanoparticles are evaluated by quasi-elastic light scattering also named photocorrelation spectroscopy. This method is based on the evaluation of the translation diffusion coefficient, D, characterizing the Brownian motion of the nanoparticles. The nanoparticle hydrodynamic diameter, pH is then deduced from this parameter from the Stokes Einstein law. Other techniques can be used to determine the size and the size distribution of the nanoparticles. The field flow fractionation method is based on the separation of particles according to their size in a thin glass channel in which the flow carrying on the nanoparticles is submitted to an external perpendicular force produced either by a crossed flow or a sedimentation. This technique, which can be applied for particles in a wide range of size (10 nm to several hundred *m*m), will gain more attention in the future for size determination and also for nanoparticle surface analysis. Size and size distribution of nanoparticles can also be determined by size exclusion chromatography performed on appropriate gels. This approach, requiring less equipment than the previous methods, presents the main limitation that only particles having a diameter lower than 120nm can be characterized by this method. As mentioned earlier, surface characteristics of the nanoparticles are of primary importance for the interaction of the nanoparticles with the surrounding medium. The main nanoparticle surface characteristics that are considered are the charge, the hydrophilicity, the chemical composition and the capacity to absorb proteins and to induce complement activation.

The charge of the nanoparticle surface is usually evaluated by the measurement of their zeta potential, which gives information about the overall surface charge of the particles and how it is affected by changes in the environment. Zeta potential is affected by the surface composition of the nanoparticles, the presence or the absence of adsorbed compounds, and the composition of the dispersing phase, mainly the ionic strength and the pH. The hydrophilicity of the nanoparticle surface can be evaluated by hydrophobic interaction chromatography. This technique, based on affinity chromatography, allows a very rapid discrimination between hydrophilic and hydrophobic nanoparticles. The nanoparticles are passed through a column containing a hydrophobic interaction chromatography gel. The nanoparticles that are retained by the gel and only eluted after the addition of a surfactant are considered as hydrophobic, whereas the nanoparticles that do not interact with the gel and that are directly eluted from the column are considered as hydrophilic. Apart from the hydrophobic interaction chromatography, the field flow fractionation techniques recently appeared to present interesting potential for the characterization of nanoparticles with different surface characteristics.

X-ray photoelectron spectroscopy (ESCA) can be use to determine the chemical composition of the nanoparticle surface. This technique is a very useful tool for the development of surface modified nanoparticles providing a direct evidence of the presence of the components that are believed to be on the nanoparticle surface.

The capacity of the nanoparticles to adsorb proteins and to activate the complement in vivo after intravenous administration will influence the fate of the carrier and its body distribution. To approach this aspect, in vitro tests have been developed to investigate the profile of the type of serum proteins that adsorbed onto the nanoparticle surface after incubation in serum and to evaluate the capacity of the nanoparticles to induce complement activation. The analysis of the protein adsorbed onto the nanoparticle surface can be performed by 2D-polyacrylamide gel electrophoresis. This technique allows the identification of the proteins that adsorbed onto the nanoparticle surface. To evaluate modifications of the composition of the adsorbed protein with time, a faster method based on capillary electrophoresis can also be used. Finally, the activation of the complement produced by nanoparticles can be evaluated either by a global technique or by a specific method measuring the specific activation of the component C3. In the global technique, nanoparticles are incubated with serum and, after the incubation, the remaining non-activated complement in the serum is evaluated using a red blood cell lysis test. The concentration of nanoparticle in the dispersion can be deduced from gravimetric determination or by turbidimetric measurements based on the application of the Mie's law. Density of the nanoparticles is evaluated either by pycnometry or by isopycnic centrifugation (Quintanar-Guerrero, 1999).

4. PHARMACEUTICAL APPLICATIONS OF NANOPARTICLES

Nanoparticles were first developed in the mid-seventies by Birrenbach & Speiser. Later on, their application for the design of drug delivery systems was made available by the use of biodegradable polymers that were considered to be highly suitable for human applications. At that time, the research on colloidal carriers was mainly focusing on liposomes, but no one was able to produce stable lipid vesicles suitable for clinical applications. In some cases, nanoparticles have been shown to be more active than liposomes due to their better stability. This is the reason why in the last decades many drugs (e.g., antibiotics, antiviral and antiparasitic drugs, cytostatics, protein and peptides) were associated to nanoparticles (Birrenbach & Speiser, 1976).

Intravenous Administration

Fate of Nanoparticles and Their Content after Intravenous Administration

the main interest of nanoparticles is their ability to achieve tissue targeting and enhance the intracellular penetration of drugs. After intravenous administration, nanoparticules are taken up by the liver, spleen and to a lower extent the bone marrow. Within these tissues, nanoparticles are mainly taken up by cells of the mononuclear phagocyte system (MPS). The uptake occurs through an endocytosis process after which the particles end up in the lysosomal compartment where they are degraded producing low molecular weight soluble compounds that are eliminated from the body by renal excretion. As a result of the MPS site specific targeting, avoidance of some organs was made possible, thus reducing the side effects and toxicity of some active compounds. Due to their strong lysosomal localization, one could imagine that nanoparticles are not suitable to target to the cytoplasm. To avoid their trapping within the lysosomal compartment, several compounds able to destabilize the lysosomal membrane were added to the nanoparticulate systems (e.g., cationic surfactant) allowing some drugs to be delivered to the cytoplasm. Recently, to avoid MPS uptake, several groups have developed a strategy consisting of the linkage to the nanoparticles of poly(ethylene glycol) derivatives. (Peracchia, 1999) This linkage results in a lower uptake of nanoparticles by the MPS and in a longer circulation time. As a consequence, these so-called stealth_ nanoparticles would be able to extravasate across endothelium that becomes permeable due to the presence of solid tumors.

Application to the Treatment of Intracellular Infections

Intracellular infections were found to be a field of interest for drug delivery by means of nanospheres. Indeed, infected cells may constitute a ''reservoir'' for micro organisms, which are protected from antibiotics inside lysosomes. The resistance of intracellular infections to chemotherapy is often related to the low uptake of commonly used antibiotics or to their reduced activity at the acidic pH of lysosomes. To overcome these effects, the use of ampicillin, a β lactam antibiotic, bound to nanospheres was proposed as endocytozable formulation.(66) The effectiveness of polyisohexylcyanoacrylate (PIHCA) nanospheres was tested in the treatment of two experimental intracellular infections.

Firstly, ampicillin-loaded nanospheres were tested in the treatment of experimental Listeria monocytogenes infection in congenitally athymic nude mice, a model involving a chronic infection of both liver and spleen macrophages. After adsorption of ampicillin onto nanospheres, the therapeutic activity of ampicillin was found to increase dramatically over that of the free drug. Bacterial counts in the liver were at least 20-fold reduced after linkage of ampicillin to PIHCA nanospheres. In addition, nanoparticulate ampicillin was capable of ensuring liver sterilization after two injections of 0.8 mg of nanospheres bound drug, whereas no such sterilization was ever observed with any of other regimens tested. Reappearance of living bacteria in the liver after the end of the treatment was probably due to a secondary infection derived from other organs such as the spleen, which was not completely sterilized by the treatment. Secondly, nanosphere-bound ampicillin was tested in the treatment of experimental salmonellosis in C57/BL6 mice, a model involving an acute fatal infection. All mice treated with a single injection of nanoparticle-bound ampicillin survived, whereas all control mice and all those treated with unloaded nanospheres died within 10 days post infection. With free ampicillin, an effective-curative effect required three doses of 32mg each. Lower doses (3 _ 0.8mg and 3 _ 16 mg) delayed but did not reduce mortality. Thus, the therapeutic index of ampicillin, calculated on the basis of mice mortality, was increased by 120-fold when the drug was bound to nanospheres.

In order to clarify the mechanism by which nanospheres improved the antimicrobial efficacy of ampicillin, Forestier et al., have compared in vitro the efficacy of ampicillin bound to poly(isobutylcyanoacrylate) (PIBCA) nanospheres with that of free ampicillin in terms of survival of L. monocytogenes in mouse peritoneal macrophages. After 30 h of incubation, nanospheres-bound ampicillin decreased the number of viable bacteria by 99% as compared to the controls whereas with free ampicillin, the number of bacteria was slightly lower than in the controls (Forestier et al., 1992). Nanoparticle-ampicillin thus appeared to bemuchmore effective than free ampicillin for inhibiting intracellular growth of L. monocytogenes. With in vitro Salmonella typhimurium infected macrophages, the situation was a little bit more complicated since the bactericidal effect of ampicillin-bound PIHCA nanospheres was poor although the intracellular capture of ampicillin was dramatically increased and its efflux in the extracellular medium reduced. In another study, confocal microscopy and transmission electron microscopy were used to establish the intracellular traffic of ampicillin bound-PIHCA nanospheres and its relation with the bacteria within the subcellular compartments. The data obtained clearly demonstrated the active uptake by phagocytosis of ampicillin-bound PIHCA nanospheres by murine macrophages and their localization in the same vacuoles as the infecting bacteria, but in a restrictive way. Thus, it was difficult to understand the limited bactericidal effect of ampicillin-bound nanospheres. The most probable explanation is to be found in the resistance mechanism of S. typhimurium involving the inhibition of the phagosome–lysosome fusion, which lets some bacteria in phagosomes free of nanospheres. If this proposed hypothesis (inhibition of phagosome–lysosome fusion) is correct, the dramatic efficiency observed in vivo should rather be due to the specific targeting of the infected tissues (rich in reticuloendothelial cells), than to an efficient intracellular targeting as it could be supposed.

In order to eliminate both dividing and non-dividing bacteria, a fluoroquinolone antibiotic, ciprofloxacin, has been associated with PIBCA and PIHCA nanospheres. In an animal model of persisting Salmonella infection, although an effect on the early phase of the infection was observed, neither free nor nanospherebound ciprofloxacin was able to eradicate truly persisting bacteria. Since they accumulate in the MPS, nanospheres hold promise as drug carriers for the treatment of visceral leishmaniosis. Thus, it has been shown that PIHCA nanospheres can be used as a carrier of primaquine whose activity was increased 21-fold against intracellular Leishmania donovani when associated with nanospheres. A part of the activity was attributed to the fact that phagocytosis of nanospheres led to the induction of a respiratory burst, which was more pronounced in infected than in non-infected macrophages. Dehydroemetine is also one of the drug candidates for this treatment but has some side effects involving the heart, which were reduced after linkage with nanospheres.

Application to the Treatment of Cancer

When given intravenously, anticancer drugs are distributed throughout the body as a function of the physicochemical properties of the molecule. A pharmacologically active concentration is reached in the tumor tissue at the expense of massive contamination of the rest of the body. For cytostatic compounds, this poor specificity raises a toxicological problem, which presents a serious obstacle to effective therapy. The use of colloidal drug carriers could represent a more rational approach to specific cancer therapy. In addition, the possibility of overcoming multidrug resistance might be achieved by using cytostatics-loaded nanospheres. The antitumor efficacy of doxorubicin-loaded nanospheres was first tested using the lymphoid leukemia L-1210 as a tumor model. In this study, one intravenous injection of doxorubicin-loaded PIBCA nanospheres was found to be more effective against L1210 leukemia than when the drug was administered in its free form following the same dosing schedule. Although the increased life span (ILS %) of mice injected with doxorubicin-loaded PIBCA nanospheres was twice as high as the ILS % for free doxorubicin, there were no long-term survivors.

The effectiveness of doxorubicin-loaded PIHCA nanospheres against L1210 leukemia was even more pronounced than that of doxorubicin loaded onto PIBCA nanospheres. The drug toxicity was markedly decreased when it was bound to this sort of nanospheres, so that impressive results were obtained with this formulation at doses for which the therapeutic efficiency of free doxorubicin was completely masked by the overpowering toxicity of the drug. Furthermore, preliminary experiments suggested that one i.v. bolus injection of doxorubicin-loaded nanospheres was more active, in L1210-bearing mice, than perfusion of the free drug for 24 h.

The superiority of doxorubicin targeted with the aid of poly(alkylcyanoacrylate) nanospheres was later confirmed in a murine hepatic metastases model (M5076 reticulosarcoma). Irrespective of the dose and the administration schedule, the reduction in the number of metastases was much greater with doxorubicin-loaded nanospheres than with free doxorubicin, particularly if treatment was given only when the metastases were well established. The improved efficacy of the targeted drug, as clearly confirmed by histological examinations, shows that both the number and the size of the tumor nodules were lower when doxorubicin was administered in its nanoparticulate form. Furthermore, liver biopsies of animals treated with the nanosphere-targeted drug showed a lower cancer cell density inside tumor tissue. Necrosis was often less widespread with the nanosphere-associated drug than in the control group and the group treated with free doxorubicin.

Studies performed on total homogenates of livers from both healthy and metastases-bearing mice showed extensive capture of nanoparticulate doxorubicin by the liver; no difference in hepatic concentrations was noted between healthy and tumor-bearing animals. In order to elucidate the mechanism behind the enhanced efficiency of doxorubicin-loaded nanospheres, doxorubicin measurements were made in both metastatic nodules and neighboring healthy hepatic tissue. This provided quantitative information concerning the drug distribution within these tissues. During the first 6 h after administration, the exposure of the liver to doxorubicin was 18 times greater for nanosphere-associated doxorubicin. However, no special affinity for the tumor tissue was detected and the nanospheres were seen by electron microscopy to be located within Kupffer cells (macrophages). However, at later time-points, the amount of drug in the tumor tissue increased in nanosphere-treated animals to 2.5 times the level found in animals given free doxorubicin. Since uptake of nanospheres by neoplastic tissue is unlikely, this increase in the doxorubicin concentration in tumor tissue probably resulted from doxorubicin released from healthy tissue, in particular Kupffer cells. Hepatic tissue could play the role of drug reservoir from which prolonged diffusion of the free drug (from nanospheres entrapped in Ku¨ pffer cell lysosomes) toward the neighboring malignant cells occurs.

This hypothesis raises the question of the long-term effect of an 18-fold increase of doxorubicin concentration in the liver. Although toxicological data have shown that doxorubicin-loaded nanospheres were not significantly or unexpectedly toxic to the liver in terms of survival rate at high doses, body weight loss, and histological appearance, this possibility should be borne in mind, especially since a temporary depletion in the number of Kupffer cells, and hence the ability to clear bacteria, was observed in rats treated with doxorubicin-loaded liposomes. A systematic study using unloaded poly(alkylcyanoacrylate) nanoparticles confirmed a reversible decline in the phagocytic capacity of the liver after repeated dosing, as well as a slightinflammatory response. Nanoparticle-associated doxorubicin also accumulated in bone marrow, leading to a myelosuppressive effect. However, this tropism of carriers might be useful to deliver myelostimulating compounds such as granulocyte colony stimulating factor to reverse the suppressive effects of intense chemotherapy. Nanospheres are also captured by splenic macrophages. In this study, the spleen architecture was shown to play a role in the localization of the nanospheres: in mice, uptake was mainly observed in metallophilic macrophages of the marginal zone whereas in rats, which have sinusoidal spleens similar to that of humans, particles were found in the red pulp macrophages.

On the other hand, alteration of the drug distribution profile by linkage to nanospheres can, in some cases, considerably reduce the toxicity of a drug because of reduced accumulation in organs where the most acute toxic effects are exerted. This concept was indeed illustrated with doxorubicin, which displays severe acute and chronic cardiomyopathy. After intravenous administration to mice, plasma levels of doxorubicin were higher when the drug was adsorbed onto nanospheres and at the same time the cardiac concentration of the drug was dramatically reduced. In accordance with the observed distribution profile, doxorubicin associated with nanospheres was found to be less toxic than free doxorubicin. The ability of tumor cells to develop simultaneous resistance to multiple lipophilic compounds represents a major problem in cancer chemotherapy. Cellular resistance to anthracyclines has been attributed to an active drug efflux from resistant cells linked to the presence of transmembrane P-glycoprotein, which was not detectable in the parental drug-sensitive cellline. Drugs, such as doxorubicin, appear to enter the cell by passive diffusion through the lipid bilayer. Upon entering the cell, these drugs bind to P-glycoprotein, which forms transmembrane channels and uses energy from ATP hydrolysis to pump these compounds out of the cell. To solve this problem, many authors have proposed the use of competitive P-glycoprotein inhibitors, such as the calcium channel blocker verapamil, which are able to bind to P-glycoprotein and to overcome pleiotropic resistance. However, since the adverse effects of verapamil are serious, its clinical use to overcome multidrug resistance is limited.

During the past few years, many studies have been devoted to evaluating the antitumor potential of carrier-drug complexes (Brasseur, et. al., 1980). The effect of nanospheres loaded with doxorubicin, resistance to which is known to be related to the presence of P-glycoprotein, was evaluated. The cytotoxicity of free-doxorubicin, doxorubicin- loaded PIHCA nanospheres (NP-Doxorubicin) (mean diameter 300 nm), and nanospheres without drug (NP), against sensitive (MCF7) and multidrug resistant (Doxorubicin R MCF7) human breast cancer cell lines was compared. MCF7 cells were more sensitive to free-doxorubicin than Doxorubicin R MCF7 cells with a 150-fold difference in the IC50. No significant difference was observed in the survival rate of MCF7 treated with free-Doxorubicin or NPdoxorubicin. In contrast, for doxorubicin R MCF7, the IC50 for doxorubicin was 130-fold lower when NPdoxorubicin were used instead of free-doxorubicin. These results indicated that nanospheres provided an effective carrier for introducing a cytotoxic dose of doxorubicin into the pleiotropic resistant human cancer cell line Doxorubicin R MCF7.

Complementary experiments, conducted with other sensitive and resistant cell lines, have confirmed this efficacy of nanospheres. Doxorubicin resistance was circumvented in the majority of the cell lines tested, and some encouraging results were obtained in vivo in a P388 model growing as ascites. Further studies were undertaken to elucidate the mechanism of action of polyalkylcyanoacrylate nanospheres. The incubation time and number of particles per cell were important factors and, when PIBCA nanospheres were used, doxorubicin accumulation within P388/ADR resistant leukemic cells was increased compared with free drug, although no endocytosis of nanospheres occurred. On the other hand, when the less rapidly degradable PIHCA nanospheres were used, reversion was observed in the absence of increased intracellular drug. The degradation products of poly (alkylcyanoacrylate) nanospheres (mainly poly(cyanoacrylic acid)) were also able to increase both accumulation and cytotoxicity of doxorubicin, although they were soluble in the culture medium. Hence, the reversion of resistance seems to be due both to the adsorption of nanospheres on the cell surface and to theformation of a doxorubicin-poly(cyanoacrylic acid) ion pair, which facilitates the transport of the drug across the cell membrane.

In the light of the results obtained with doxorubicinloaded nanospheres in the liver metastases model described earlier, (Chiannilkulchai, 1989) the role of macrophages as a reservoir for doxorubicin was tested in a two-compartment coculture system in vitro with both resistant and sensitive P388 cells. Even after prior uptake by macrophages, doxorubicin-loaded PIBCA nanospheres were able to overcome resistance. However, this reversion was only partial. It was decided to take advantage of the particulate drug carrier offers to associate an anticancer drug and a compound capable of inhibiting the P-glycoprotein. This approach was tested with doxorubicin and cyclosporin A bound to the same nanospheres and was found to be extremely effective in

reversing P388 resistance (Soma, 1999). The association of cyclosporine A with nanospheres would ensure that it reaches the same sites as the anticancer drug at the same time and would also reduce its toxic side effects.

As early as 1986, researcher observed that other colloidal carriers, like nanocapsules, administered by the IV route in rabbits, were taken up rapidly by organs of the mononuclear phagocyte system (Khouri et al., 1986). One application that takes advantage of this uptake concerns nanocapsules of (muramyl tripeptide cholesterol) (MTP-Chol). This immunostimulating agent is able to activate macrophages and induce toxicity toward tumor cells, and would therefore be a useful agent to treat metastatic cancer. The mechanisms by which activated macrophages arrest tumor proliferation include production of nitric oxide and TNF-*a*. It was showed in in vitro models of rat alveolar macrophages and RAW 264.7 mouse monocyte macrophage line that nanocapsules based on poly(D,L-lactide) containing MTP-Chol are more efficient activators than the free drug. This action could be due to an intracellular delivery of the immunomodulator encapsulated in nanocapsules after phagocytosis and to an intermediate transfer of the drug to serum proteins (Seyler, 1999). This system has also demonstrated its efficiency in vivo; in fact (Barratt et al. 1994), reported that antimetastatic effects of nanocapsules contained MTP-Chol in a model of liver metastases. Some antimetastatic activity was also seen after oral administration.

Nanospheres for Oligonucleotide Delivery

Oligodeoxynucleotides are potentially powerful new drugs because of their selectivity for particular gene products in both sense and antisense strategies. However, using antisense oligonucleotides in therapeutics is a challenge to pharmaceutical technology because of their susceptibility to enzymatic degradation and their poor penetration across biological membranes. Nanoparticulate preparations might be an interesting alternative because of better stability in the presence of biological fluids. In the case of nanospheres made of synthetic polymers (poly(alkylcyanoacrylate), poly (lactic acid)), since oligonucleotides have no affinity for the polymeric matrix, association with nanoparticles has been achieved by ion pairing with a cationic surfactant, cetyltimethylammonium bromide (CTAB) adsorbed onto the nanoparticle surface (Fattal, 1998). Oligonucleotides bound to poly(alkylcyanoacrylate) nanospheres in this way were protected from nucleases in vitro and their intracellular uptake was increased (Chavany, 1994). In addition, nanospheres were able to concentrate intact oligonucleotides in the liver and in the spleen (Nakada, et. al. 1996). Antisense oligonucleotides formulated in this way were able to specifically inhibit mutated Ha-ras-mediated cell proliferation and tumorigenicity in nude mice (Schwab, 1994).

This approach has recently been applied to the association of a phosphodiester antisense oligonucleotide directed against the 30 non-translated region of the PKC*a* gene with nanospheres prepared from PIBCA. These nanospheres were able to inhibit PKC*a* neoexpression in cultured Hep G6 cells. Nanospheres containing oligonucleotides have also been formulated from a naturally occurring polysaccharide, alginate, which forms a gel in the presence of calcium ions. In this case, the oligonucleotides penetrate into the gel matrix by reptation, thus providing a high loading yield and good protection against nuclease (Aynie, 1999).

Subcutaneous/Intramuscular Administration

Subcutaneous administration of nanoparticles was achieved mainly for the delivery of peptides and vaccines. It allows slow release of the entrapped drugs therefore reducing the number of administrations, increasing blood half-life of the active drug, and finally, in some cases, reducing side effects.

PIBCA nanospheres were injected subcutaneously to rats. Autoradiographic pictures obtained after using radiolabelled polymer have shown a progressive staining reduction in the muscular tissue suggesting that nanospheres were slowly biodegraded. In the same study, nanospheres were found to release a peptide (GRF) in a sustained manner. Comparison of the

AUC of free GRF and GRF-loaded nanospheres showed that in addition to the slow release process nanospheres were able to improve the bioavailability of the peptide. This improvement could be attributed to the fact that free administered GRF is very quickly metabolized at the injection site, whereas it is partly protected from massive enzymatic degradation when it is administered associated with nanospheres (Gautier, 1992).

A few examples of the use of nanospheres as adjuvant for antigens/allergens delivery were described in the literature. The main advantage of this approach is to design single shot vaccine. In this case the drug carrier has to remain at the site of administration and deliver either continuously or pulsatively the antigen. The use of slowly degradable polymers (PLA, PMMA) is suitable for this application, since peptide or protein release is more adequate. Poly(methyl methacrylate) were first investigated as adjuvants for injectable vaccines. These nanospheres were claimed to be biodegradable after subcutaneous or intramuscular injection and shown to exhibit very powerful adjuvant properties for a number of antigens. However, the adjuvant properties were shown to be better when the antigen was incorporated during the polymerization process than when adsorbed onto nanospheres (Mahmoudi et al., 2010). When comparing the effect of PMMA with other polymers (polystyrene and 2-hydroxyethyl methacrylate/methyl methacrylate copolymer, HEMA: MMA), it was also demonstrated that a decrease in particle size and an increase in the hydrophobicity of nanospheres increased the antibody response after immunization against influenza whole and split virus, bovine serum albumin, and HIV2 split virus (Kreuter, 1978).

Oral Route

There are numerous reports showing that uptake and translocation of nanoparticles and microparticles take place after oral administration to animals (Jani, 1989). Different mechanisms have been proposed to explain the translocation of particulate material across the intestine: i) uptake via Peyer's patches or isolated lymphoid follicles; ii) intracellular uptake; and iii) intracellular/paracellular passage. The uptake of poly(alkylcyanoacrylate) nanocapsules by Peyer's patches has been shown by Damge´ et al., (Damge et al., 1988) When administered in the lumen of an isolated ileal segment of the rat, polylalkylcyanoacrylate nanocapsules were found preferentially over Peyer's patches through which they passed massively and rapidly.Nanocapsules were clearly visible in M-cells and in intercellular spaces around the lymph cells. Intracellular uptake of nanospheres has been proposed by Kreuter, Muller and Munz (Kreuter, 1989; Muller & Munz, 2000) based on electron-microscopic autoradiographic investigations showing radioactivity into epithelial and goblet cells after oral administration of poly(hexylcyanoacrylate) (PHCA) nanospheres labeled with 14C. The translocation of particles by a paracellular pathway has been evidenced in a study done by Aprahamian et al., using PIBCA nanocapsules. Nanocapsules were filled with an iodinized oil (lipiodol) in order to render them detectable using a scanning electron microscope equipped with an energy-dispersive X-ray spectrometer (Aprahamian et al., 1987). When they were administered in an isolated segment of a dog jejunum, they appeared as vesicles associated with intraluminal mucus. Subsequently, they were observed in intravillus capillaries in close contact with red cells or adsorbed to the inner wall of endothelial cells. Among these three mechanisms and according to many studies involving nanoparticles made of other biodegradable and nondegradable polymers, translocation via the uptake in Peyer's patches seems to be the major pathway for a rapid and substantial passage after oral administration of nanoparticles. Although it might exist in certain situations, the passage of particles between the absorptive cells is rather less likely if the barrier of tight junctions has not been disrupted. Although there are abundant reports from various independent workers showing evidence of absorption of particulate systems by the gastrointestinal tract, the oral absorption of nanoparticles remains a controversial issue. However, even if a more clear estimation of the quantity of absorbed particles is needed as well as a better understanding of the factors affecting particles uptake, it must be concluded that translocation of small sized particles like poly(alkylcyanoacrylate) nanoparticles is possible. The question remains if the extent of particle translocation is compatible with a strategy of drug administration with therapeutic perspectives. This will be discussed below.

Oral Delivery of Peptides and Proteins and Vaccines

Poly(isobutylcyanoacrylate) nanocapsules were shown 10 years ago to be able to encapsulate insulin and to increase its activity as assessed by a reduction of glycemia. Several aspects of this phenomenon are surprising: encapsulation of a hydrophilic drug in the oily core of nanocapsules; reduction of glycemia was only obtained with diabetic animals; hypoglycaemia appeared two days after a single administration and was maintained for up to 20 days depending on the insulin doses, although the amplitude of the pharmacological effect (minimum level of blood glucose) did not depend on the insulin dose. Damge´ et al. (Damge et al., 1990) and Lowe and Temple (Lowe and Temple, 1994) suggested that nanocapsules could protect insulin from proteolytic degradation in intestinal fluids, based on the protection of encapsulated insulin, observed in the presence of different enzymes in vitro. Later studies showed that insulin did not react with the alkylcyanoacrylate monomer during the formation of nanocapsules and was located within the oily core rather than adsorbed on their surface.

The capacity of insulin nanocapsules to reduce glycemia could be explained by their translocation through the intestinal barrier, as suggested by Damge´ et al., (Damge et al. 1997) for example by paracellular pathway or via M cells in Peyer's patches (Michel, 1991). Recently, the use of Texas Red_-labeled insulin allowed this translocation to be visualized more readily (Aboubakar, 2000). One hour after oral administration, nanocapsules reached the ileum. The presence of fluorescent areas within the mucosa and even in the lamina propria suggested that insulin-loaded nanocapsules could cross the intestinal epithelium. Although this passage is certainly an important factor, it does not explain the duration of the hypoglycemia. This prolonged action could be due to the retention of a part of the colloidal system in the gastrointestinal tract. Interestingly, a prolonged hypoglycemic effect was also observed with insulin entrapped in poly(alkylcyanoacrylate) nanospheres when these were dispersed in an oily phase containing surfactant. This suggests that some components of nanocapsules could act as promoters of absorption. Recently, Damge´ et al. showed that the incorporation of octreotide, a somatostatin analogue, in poly(alkylcyanoacrylate) nanocapsules also improved and prolonged the therapeutic effect of this peptide, after administration by the oral route (Damge et al., 1997).

Even if the main limitation to oral administration of poly(alkylcyanoacrylate) nanoparticles is that their passage through the intestinal barrier is probably restricted and sometimes erratic, they represent an interesting tool for oral delivery of antigens. Indeed, M-cells appear to be the main site for the uptake of poly(alkylcyanoacrylate) nanoparticles after oral administration (Damge et al., 1997).and, furthermore, it is generally accepted that limited doses of antigen are sufficient for a mucous immunization. In fact, oral delivery of antigens may be considered as the most convenient means of producing an IgA antibody response. However, it is importantly limited by enzymatic degradation of antigens in the GI tract and, additionally by their poor absorption (Yildirimera et al., 2011). Thus, it has been postulated that the use of micro- or nanoparticles for the oral delivery of antigens should be efficient if those systems are able to achieve the protection of the antigenic molecule. Poly(alkylcyanoacrylate) nanoparticles have been shown to enhance the secretory immune response after their oral administration in association with ovalbumin (O'Hagan, 1989). This result was not fully reproduced in the case of poly(acrylamide) nanoparticles loaded with the same antigen. It was postulated that in the case of poly(acrylamide) nanospheres, much of the antigen was located at the surface of the polymer and could have been degraded during its passage through the gut. The relatively high surface concentration of ovalbumin adsorbed onto poly(butylcyanoacrylate) nanospheres may have reduced the ability of the proteolytic enzymes in the gut to gain access to and to degrade the antigen, resulting in a greater antigen availability.

Ocular Delivery

The anatomical structure and the protective physiological process of the eye exert a strong defense against ocular drug delivery. This is the reason why conventional ocular dosage forms exhibit extremely low bioavailability. Limited absorption of the drug through the lipophilic corneal barrier is mainly because of short precorneal residence time due to the tear turn-over, rapid nasolacrimal drainage of instilled drug from the tear fluid, and non-productive absorption through the conjonctiva. Only a small proportion (1–3%) of the applied drug penetrates the cornea and reaches intraocular tissues. For these reasons, it is necessary to develop efficient and more acceptable ocular therapeutic systems.

Different strategies can be carried out to improve the precorneal residence time and/or penetration ability of the active ingredient. Among them, one approach consists of using colloidal drug delivery systems such as nanoparticles. Initial studies carried out with nanocapsules, as ocular drug carriers, attempted to increase the penetration of lipophilic drugs into the eye by prolonging the precorneal residence time, as observed with other colloidal systems, liposomes and nanospheres. These studies, which concerned antiglaucomatous agents, such as betaxolol, carteolol, and metipranolol encapsulated in nanocapsules, only showed a reduction of the non-corneal absorption (systemic circulation) leading to reduced side-effects as compared with the free drug (Losa, 1993). These systemic side-effects are due to a poor ocular retention of drugs that are directly absorbed into the systemic circulation by conjunctival and nasal blood vessels. In two cases (carteolol and betaxolol), encapsulation in nanocapsules produced an improved pharmacological effect (reduction of intraocular pressure) than produced by free drug and nanospheres (although the penetration of nanocapsules was not tested) and reduced cardiovascular systemic side-effects. Metipranolol showed the same activity alone and associated with nanocapsules but, as in the case of carteolol and betaxolol, its side-effects were reduced. When betaxolol was used, the nature of the polymer making up the nanocapsule wall was found to be important, and poly (*e*-caprolactone) was more efficient than PIBCA or poly(lactic-co-glycolic acid) (Marchal-Heussler, 1993).

Calvo et al., explored the mechanisms of interaction of nanocapsules with ocular tissues to better understand the pharmacological responses obtained with antiglaucomatous agents. By confocal microscopy, they showed that poly(*e*-caprolactone) nanocapsules could specifically penetrate the corneal epithelium by an endocytic process without causing any damage to the cells, in contrast with PIBCA nanoparticles, the uptake of which was associated with cellular lysis (Calvo et al., 2001). These results explained the improved therapeutic effect and the reduction of systemic side-effects as a result of drug loss through the conjunctiva provided by poly(*e*-caprolactone) nanocapsules by increasing corneal epithelium penetration of lipophilic drugs. Calvo et al., also excluded the influence of the oily inner structure in the activity of the nanocapsules, in the light of the absence of differences in penetration between nanospheres and nanocapsules (Park et al. 2015; Afrooz et al., 2015), in contrast with Marchal-Heussler et al., who observed a better therapeutic effect with nanocapsules than with nanospheres (Marchal-Heussler et al. 1992). Moreover, Calvo et al. demonstrated with indomethacin-loaded nanocapsules that the colloidal nature of the carrier was the main factor influencing its ocular bioavailability. The same authors were also interested in the influence of the nature and the charge of the surface of nanocapsules on their physical stability and on their ocular bioavailability. They found that coating the negatively charged surface of poly(*e*-caprolactone) nanocapsules with cationic polymers could prevent their degradation caused by the adsorption of lysozyme, a positively charged enzyme found in tear fluid (Calvo et al. 1997). Moreover, they noticed that a cationic polymer, chitosan, adsorbed on the surface of nanocapsules was able to provide the best corneal drug penetration without any local intolerance as compared to another positively charged polymer. This was achieved by a combination of effects: Penetration of particles into the corneal epithelial cells, mucoadhesion of positively charged particles onto negatively charged membranes, and a specific effect on the tight junctions (Calvo et al. 1997).

This effect of improvement of ocular absorption was also reported by Calvo et al. 1996 with the immunosuppressive peptide cyclosporin A. The corneal level of the drug was increased fivefold as compared with an oily solution of the drug owing to a highly loaded nanocapsule preparation, also containing poly (*e*-caprolactone). The efficacy of this topical formulation has also been observed on a penetrating keratoplasty rejection model in the rat (Holzwarth et al., 2014) and also proposed an alternative preparation of cyclosporin nanocapsules based on poly(alkylcyanoacrylate) dispersed in poly(acrylic acid) gel able to drastically reduce toxicity of poly(alkylcyanocrylates) on the cornea and to promote absorption of the drug (Harper et al., 2015).

REFERENCES

Aboubakar, M., Couvreur, P., Pinto-Alphandary, H., Gouritin, B., Lacour, B., Farinotti, R., & Vauthier, C. et al. (2000). Insulin-loaded nanocapsules for oral administration: In vitro and in vivo investigation. *Drug Development Research*, *49*(2), 109–117. doi:10.1002/(SICI)1098-2299(200002)49:2<109::AID-DDR4>3.0.CO;2-#

Aboubakar, M., Puisieux, F., Couvreur, P., Deyme, M., & Vauthier, C. (1999). Study of the mechanism of insulin encapsulation in poly(isobutylcyanoacrylate) nanocapsules obtained by interfacial polymerization. *Journal of Biomedical Materials Research*, *47*(4), 568–576. doi:10.1002/(SICI)1097-4636(19991215)47:4<568::AID-JBM14>3.0.CO;2-X PMID:10497293

Afrooz, A. R. M. N., Hussain, S. M., & Saleh, N. B. (2015). Erratum to: Aggregate size and structure determination of nanomaterials in physiological media: importance of dynamic evolution. *Journal of Nanoparticle Research*, *17*(5), 232–243. doi:10.1007/s11051-015-2933-5

Alle'man, E., Doelker, E., & Gurny, R. (1992). Preparation of aqueous polymeric nanodispersions by a reversible salting-out process, influence of process parameters on particle size. *International Journal of Pharmaceutics*, *87*(1-3), 247–253. doi:10.1016/0378-5173(92)90249-2

Aprahamian, M., Michel, C., Humbert, W., Devissaguet, J. P., & Damge, C. (1987). Transmucosal passage of polyalkylcyanoacrylate nanocapsules as a new drug carrier in the small intestine. *Biology of the Cell*, *61*(1-2), 69–76. doi:10.1111/j.1768-322X.1987.tb00571.x PMID:2833966

Aynie, I., Vauthier, C., Chacun, H., Fattal, E., & Couvreur, P. (1999). Spongelike alginate nanoparticles as a new potential system for the delivery of antisense oligonucleotides. antisense. *Nucleic Acid Drug Dev*, *9*(3), 301–312. doi:10.1089/oli.1.1999.9.301 PMID:10435755

Barratt, G., Puisieux, F., Yu, W. P., Foucher, C., Fessi, H., & Devissaguet, J. P. (1994). Anti-metastatic activity of MDPL- alanyl-cholesterol incorporated into various types of nanocapsules. *International Journal of Immunopharmacology*, *16*(5-6), 457–461. doi:10.1016/0192-0561(94)90036-1 PMID:7927993

Birrenbach, G., & Speiser, P. (1976). Polymerized micelles and their use as adjuvants in immunology. *Journal of Pharmaceutical Sciences*, *65*(12), 1763–1766. doi:10.1002/jps.2600651217 PMID:1036442

Brasseur, F., Couvreur, P., Kante, B., Deckers-Passau, L., Roland, M., Deckers, C., & Speisers, P. (1980). Actinomycin D absorbed on polymethylcyanoacrylate nanoparticles: Increased efficiency against an experimental tumor. *European Journal of Cancer*, *16*(11), 1441–1445. doi:10.1016/0014-2964(80)90053-5 PMID:7227421

Brunner, T. I., Wick, P., Manser, P., Spohn, P., Grass, R. N., Limbach, L. K., & Stark, W. J. et al. (2006). In vitro cytotoxicity of oxide nanoparticles: Comparison to asbestos, silica, and effect of particle solubility. *Environmental Science & Technology*, *40*(14), 4374–4381. doi:10.1021/es052069i PMID:16903273

Calvo, P., Alonso, M. J., Vila-Jato, J. L., & Robinson, J. R. (1996). Improved ocular bioavailability of indomethacin by novel ocular drug carriers. *The Journal of Pharmacy and Pharmacology*, *48*(11), 1147–1152. doi:10.1111/j.2042-7158.1996.tb03911.x PMID:8961163

Calvo, P., Gouritin, B., & Chacunm, H. et al.. (2001). Long-circulating PEGylated polycyanoacrylate nanoparticles as new drug carrier for brain delivery. *Pharmaceutical Research*, *18*(8), 1157–1166. doi:10.1023/A:1010931127745 PMID:11587488

Calvo, P., Gouritin, B., Villarroya, H., Eclancher, F., Giannavola, C., Klein, C., & Couvreur, P. et al. (2002). Quantification and localization of PEGylated polycyanoacrylate nanoparticles in brain and spinal cord during experimental allergic encephalomyelitis in the rat. *The European Journal of Neuroscience*, *15*(8), 1317–1326. doi:10.1046/j.1460-9568.2002.01967.x PMID:11994126

Calvo, P., Vila-Jato, J. L., & Alonso, M. J. (1997). Effect of lysozyme on the stability of polyester nanocapsules and nanoparticles: Stabilization approaches. *Biomaterials*, *18*(19), 1305–1310. doi:10.1016/S0142-9612(97)00061-6 PMID:9307220

Chavany, C., Saison-Behmoaras, T., Le Doan, T., Puisieux, F., Couvreur, P., & Helene, C. (1994). Adsorption of oligonucleotides onto polyisohexylcyanoacrylate nanoparticles protects them against nucleases and increases their cellular uptake. *Pharmaceutical Research*, *11*(9), 1370–1378. doi:10.1023/A:1018923301967 PMID:7816773

Chiannilkulchai, N., Driouich, Z., Benoit, J. P., Parodi, A. L., & Couvreur, P. (1989). Doxorubicin-loaded nanoparticles: Increased efficiency in murine hepatic metastases. *Selective Cancer Therapeutics*, *5*(1), 1–11. doi:10.1089/sct.1989.5.1 PMID:2756244

Couvreur, P., Kante, B., Roland, M., Guiot, P., Baudhuin, P., & Speiser, P. (1979). Poly(cyanoacrylate) nanoparticles as potential lysosomotropic carriers: Preparation, morphological and sorptive properties. *The Journal of Pharmacy and Pharmacology*, *31*(1), 331–332. doi:10.1111/j.2042-7158.1979.tb13510.x PMID:37304

Damge, C., Michel, C., Aprahamian, M., & Couvreur, P. (1988). New approach for oral administration of insulin with polyalkylcyanoacrylate nanocapsules as drug carrier. *Diabetes*, *37*(2), 246–251. doi:10.2337/diab.37.2.246 PMID:3292320

Damge, C., Michel, C., Aprahamian, M., Couvreur, P., & Devissaguet, J. P. (1990). Nanocapsules as carriers for oral peptide delivery. *Journal of Controlled Release*, *13*(2-3), 233–239. doi:10.1016/0168-3659(90)90013-J

Damge, C., Vonderscher, J., Marbach, P., & Pinget, M. (1997). Poly(alkyl cyanoacrylate) nanocapsules as a delivery system in the rat for octreotide, a long-acting somatostatin analogue. *The Journal of Pharmacy and Pharmacology*, *49*(10), 949–954. doi:10.1111/j.2042-7158.1997.tb06022.x PMID:9364401

DeKeyser, J. L., Poupaert, J. H., & Dumont, P. (1991). Poly(diethylmethylidenemalonate) nanoparticles as a potential drugcarrier: Preparation, distribution and elimination after intravenous and peroral administration to mice. *Journal of Pharmaceutical Sciences*, *80*(1), 67–70. doi:10.1002/jps.2600800117 PMID:2013853

DeMiguel, I., Ioualalen, K., Bonnefous, M., Peyrot, M., Nguyen, F., & Cervilla, M. et al.. (1995). Synthesis and characterization of supramolecular biovector (SMBV) specifically designed for the entrapment of ionic molecules. *Biochimica et Biophysica Acta*, *1237*(1), 49–58. doi:10.1016/0005-2736(95)00079-I PMID:7619842

Faraji, A. H., & Wipf, P. (2009). Nanoparticles in cellular drug delivery. *Bioorganic & Medicinal Chemistry*, *17*(8), 2950–2962. doi:10.1016/j.bmc.2009.02.043 PMID:19299149

Fattal, E., Vauthier, C., Aynie, I., Nakada, Y., Lambert, G., Malvy, C., & Couvreur, P. (1998). Biodegradable polyalkylcyanoacrylate nanoparticles for the delivery of oligonucleotides. *Journal of Controlled Release*, *53*(1-3), 137–143. doi:10.1016/S0168-3659(97)00246-0 PMID:9741921

Forestier, F., Gerrier, P., Chaumard, C., Quero, A. M., Couvreur, P., & Labarre, C. (1992). Effect of nanoparticle-bound ampicillin on the survival of listeria monocytogenes in mouse peritoneal macrophages. *The Journal of Antimicrobial Chemotherapy*, *30*(2), 173–179. doi:10.1093/jac/30.2.173 PMID:1399927

Gallardo, M. M., Couarraze, G., Denizot, B., Treupel, L., Couvreur, P., & Puisieux, F. (1993). Preparation and purification of isohexylcyanoacrylate nanocapsules. *International Journal of Pharmaceutics*, *100*, 55–64. doi:10.1016/0378-5173(93)90075-Q

Gasco, M., & Trotta, M. (1986). Nanoparticles from microemulsions. *International Journal of Pharmaceutics*, *29*(2-3), 267–268. doi:10.1016/0378-5173(86)90125-0

Gautier, J. C., Grangier, J. L., Barbier, A., Dupont, P., Dussosoy, D., Pastor, G., & Couvreur, P. (1992). Biodegradable nanoparticles for subcutaneous administration of growth hormone releasing factor (hGRF). *Journal of Controlled Release*, *3*, 205–210.

Gref, R., Minamitake, Y., Peracchia, M. T., Domb, A., Trubetskoy, V., Torchilin, V., & Langer, R. (1997). Poly(ethylene Glycol)-coated nanospheres: Potential carriers for intravenous drug administration. *Pharmaceutical Biotechnology*, *10*, 167–198. doi:10.1007/0-306-46803-4_6 PMID:9160372

Gurny, R., Peppas, N. A., Harrington, D. D., & Banker, G. S. (1981). Development of biodegradable and injectable lattices for controlled release potent drugs. *Drug Development and Industrial Pharmacy*, *7*(1), 1–25. doi:10.3109/03639048109055684

Handy, R. D., Owen, R., & Valsami-Jones, E. (2008). The ecotoxicology of nanoparticles and nanomaterials: Current status, knowledge gaps, challenges and future nedds. *Ecotoxicology (London, England)*, *17*(5), 315–325. doi:10.1007/s10646-008-0206-0 PMID:18408994

Harper, B., Thomas, D., Chikkagoudar, S., Baker, N., Tang, K., Heredia-Langner, A., & Harper, S. et al. (2015). Comparative hazard analysis and toxicological modeling of diverse nanomaterials using the embryonic zebrafish (EZ) metric of toxicity. *Journal of Nanoparticle Research*, *17*(6), 250–255. doi:10.1007/s11051-015-3051-0 PMID:26069453

Holzwarth, U., Bellido, E., Dalmiglio, M., Kozempel, J., Cotogno, G., & Gibson, N. (2014). Be-recoil radiolabelling of industrially manufactured silica nanoparticles. *Journal of Nanoparticle Research*, *16*(9), 2574–2589. doi:10.1007/s11051-014-2574-0 PMID:25285032

Jani, P., Halbert, G. W., Langridge, J., & Florence, A. T. (1989). The uptake and translocation of latex nanospheres and microspheres after oral administration to rats. *The Journal of Pharmacy and Pharmacology*, *41*(12), 809–812. doi:10.1111/j.2042-7158.1989.tb06377.x PMID:2576440

Kreuter, J., & Haenzel, I. (1978). Mode of action of immunological adjuvants: Some physicochemical factors influencing the effectivity of polyacrylic adjuvants. *Infection and Immunity*, *19*, 667–675. PMID:631894

Kreuter, J., Muller, V., & Munz, K. (1989). Quantitative and microautoradiographic study on mouse intestinal distribution of polycyanoacrylate nanoparticles. *International Journal of Pharmaceutics*, *55*(1), 39–45. doi:10.1016/0378-5173(89)90274-3

Kreuter, J., & Speiser, P. P. (1976). In vitro studies of poly(methyl methacrylate) adjuvants. *Journal of Pharmaceutical Sciences*, *65*(11), 1624–1627. doi:10.1002/jps.2600651115 PMID:993993

Kucuk, I., & Edirisinghe, M. (2014). Microfluidic preparation of polymer nanospheres. *Journal of Nanoparticle Research*, *16*(12), 2626–2638. doi:10.1007/s11051-014-2626-5 PMID:25484617

Lambert, G., Fattal, E., Pinto-Alphandary, H., Gulik, A., & Couvreur, P. (1998). Polyisobutylcyanoacrylate nanocapsules containing an aqueous core as a novel colloidal carrier for the delivery of oligonucleotides. *Biochimie*, *80*, 969–976. doi:10.1016/S0300-9084(99)80002-9 PMID:9924975

LeBourlais, C. A., Chevanne, F., Turlin, B., Acar, L., Zia, H., Sado, P. A., & Leverge, R. et al. (1997). Effect of cyclosporine a formulations on bovine corneal absorption: Ex-vivo study. *Journal of Microencapsulation*, *14*(4), 457–467. doi:10.3109/02652049709033830 PMID:9229345

Losa, C., Marchal-Heussler, L., Orallo, F., Vila Jato, J. L., & Alonso, M. J. (1993). Design of new formulations for topical ocular administration: Polymeric nanocapsules containing metipranolol. *Pharmaceutical Research*, *10*(1), 80–87. doi:10.1023/A:1018977130559 PMID:8094245

Lowe, P. J., & Temple, C. S. (1994). Calcitonin and Insulin in Isobutylcyanoacrylate nanocapsules: Protection against proteases and effect on intestinal absorption in rats. *The Journal of Pharmacy and Pharmacology*, *46*(7), 547–552. doi:10.1111/j.2042-7158.1994.tb03854.x PMID:7996380

Lowell, P. A., & El-Aasser, M. S. (1997). *Emulsion Polymerization and Emulsion Polymers* (p. 801). New York: Wiley.

Mahmoudi, M., Simchi, A., Imani, M., Shokrgozar, M. A., Milani, A. S., Häfeli, U. O., & Stroeve, P. (2010). A new approach for the in vitro identification of the cytotoxicity of superparamagnetic iron oxide nanoparticles. *Colloids and Surfaces. B, Biointerfaces*, *75*(1), 300–309. doi:10.1016/j.colsurfb.2009.08.044 PMID:19781921

Marchal-Heussler, L., Fessi, H., Devissaguet, J. P., Hoffman, M., & Maincent, P. (1992). Colloidal drug delivery systems for the eye. A comparison of the efficacy of three different polymers: Polyisobutylcyanoacrylate, poly (lactic-co-glycolic Acid, poly-epsilon caprolactone. *S.T.P. Pharma*, *2*, 98–104.

Marchal-Heussler, L., Sirbat, D., Hoffman, M., & Maincent, P. (1993). Poly(epsilon-caprolactone) nanocapsules in carteolol ophthalmic delivery. *Pharmaceutical Research*, *10*(3), 386–390. doi:10.1023/A:1018936205485 PMID:8464811

Marty, J. J., Oppenheim, R. C., & Speiser, P. (1978). Nanoparticles: A new colloidal drug delivery systems. *Pharmaceutica Acta Helvetiae*, *53*, 17–23. PMID:643885

Michel, C., Aprahamian, M., Defontaine, L., Couvreur, P., & Damge, C. (1991). The effect of site of administration in the gastrointestinal tract on the absorption of insulin from nanocapsules in diabetic rats. *The Journal of Pharmacy and Pharmacology*, *43*(1), 1–5. doi:10.1111/j.2042-7158.1991.tb05437.x PMID:1676051

Muller, R. H., Mader, K., & Gohla, S. (2000). Solid lipid nanoparticles (SLN) for controlled drug delivery – a review of the state of the art. *European Journal of Pharmaceutics and Biopharmaceutics*, *50*, 161–177. doi:10.1016/S0939-6411(00)00087-4 PMID:10840199

Nakada, Y., Fattal, E., Foulquier, M., & Couvreur, P. (1996). Pharmacokinetics and biodistribution of oligonucleotide adsorbed onto poly(isobutylcyanoacrylate) nanoparticles after intravenous administration in mice. *Pharmaceutical Research*, *13*(1), 38–43. doi:10.1023/A:1016017014573 PMID:8668676

O'Hagan, D. T., Palin, K., & Davis, S. S. (1989). Poly(butyl2cyanoacrylate) particles as adjuvant for oral immunization. *Vaccine*, *7*(3), 213–216. doi:10.1016/0264-410X(89)90231-4 PMID:2781856

Oberdörster, G., Oberdörster, E., & Oberdörster, J. (2005). Nanotoxicology: An emerging discipline evolving from studies of ultrafine particles. *Environmental Health Perspectives*, *113*(7), 823–839. doi:10.1289/ehp.7339 PMID:16002369

Park, H. J., Sohn, J. H., Kim, Y.-J., Park, Y. H., Han, H., Park, K. H., & Lee, J.-H. et al. (2015). Acute exposure to silica nanoparticles aggravate airway inflammation: Different effects according to surface characteristics. *Experimental & Molecular Medicine*, *47*(7), e173. doi:10.1038/emm.2015.50 PMID:26183169

Passirani, C., Barratt, G., Devissaguet, J. P., & Labarre, D. (1998). Interactions of nanoparticles bearing heparin or dextran covalently bound to poly(methylmethacrylate) with the complement system. *Life Sciences*, *62*(8), 775–785. doi:10.1016/S0024-3205(97)01175-2 PMID:9489513

Passirani, C., Ferrarini, L., Barratt, G., Devissaguet, J. P., & Labarre, D. (1999). Preparation and characterization of nanoparticles bearing heparin or dextran covalently-linked to poly(methylmethacrylate). *J. Biomater. Sci. Polym*, *10*(1), 47–62. doi:10.1163/156856299X00270 PMID:10091922

Peracchia, M. T., Fattal, E., Desmaële, D., Besnard, M., Noël, J. P., Gomis, J. M., & Couvreur, P. et al. (1999). Stealth (R) PEGylated polycyanoacrylate nanoparticles for intravenous administration and splenic targeting. *Journal of Controlled Release*, *60*(1), 121–128. doi:10.1016/S0168-3659(99)00063-2 PMID:10370176

Quintanar-Guerrero, D., Alle'man, E., Doelker, E., & Fessi, H. (1998a). Preparation and characterization of nanocapsules from preformed polymers by a new process based on emulsification–diffusion technique. *Pharmaceutical Research*, *15*(7), 1056–1062. doi:10.1023/A:1011934328471 PMID:9688060

Quintanar-Guerrero, D., Alle'man, E., Fessi, H., & Doelker, E. (1998b). Preparation techniques and mechanisms of formation of biodegradable nanoparticles from preformed polymers. *Drug Development and Industrial Pharmacy*, *24*(12), 1113–1128. doi:10.3109/03639049809108571 PMID:9876569

Quintanar-Guerrero, D., Alle'man, E., Fessi, H., & Doelker, E. (1999). Pseudolatex preparation using a novel emulsion– diffusion process involving direct displacement of partially water-miscible solvents by distillation. *International Journal of Pharmaceutics*, *188*(2), 155–164. doi:10.1016/S0378-5173(99)00216-1 PMID:10518671

Scheffel, U., Rhodes, B. A., Natarajan, T. K., & Wagner, H. N. (1972). Albumin microspheres for the study of the reticulo-endothelial system. *Journal of Nuclear Medicine*, *13*, 498–503. PMID:5033902

Schwab, G., Duroux, I., Chavany, C., Helene, C., & Saison-Behmoaras, E. (1994). An approach for new anticancer drugs: Oncogene-targeted antisense DNA. *Annals of Oncology*, *5*(suppl 4), 55–58. doi:10.1093/annonc/5.suppl_4.S55 PMID:8060898

Seijo, B., Fattal, E., Roblot-Treupel, L., & Couvreur, P. (1990). Design of nanoparticles of less than 50nm in diameter. Preparation, characterization and drug loading. *International Journal of Pharmaceutics*, *62*(1), 1–7. doi:10.1016/0378-5173(90)90024-X

Seyler, I., Appel, M., Devissaguet, J. P., Legrand, P., & Barratt, G. (1999). Macrophage activation by a lipophilic derivative of muramyldipeptide. *Journal of Nanoparticle Research*, *1*(1), 91–97. doi:10.1023/A:1010016128378

Soma, C. E., Dubernet, C., Barratt, G., Nemati, F., Appel, M., Benita, S., & Couvreur, P. (1999). Ability of doxorubicin-loaded nanoparticles to overcome multidrug resistance of tumor cells after their capture by macrophages. *Pharmaceutical Research*, *16*(11), 1710–1716. doi:10.1023/A:1018902031370 PMID:10571276

Stainmesse, S. (1990). *Etude gale'nique D'un Nouveau Proce'de´ D'obtention De Vecteurs Colloı¨daux Submicroniques a` Partir D'une Prote'ine Ou D'un Polyme`re Synthe'tique.* (Thesis). Universite´ De Paris Sud.

Stella, B., Arpicco, S., & Peracchia, M. T. (2000). Characterization of Folic Acid-Nanoparticles Conjugates for Tumoral Targeting. *Proceedings of the 27th International Symposium on Controlled Release of Bioactive Materials of the Controlled Release Society, Inc.*

Vauthier, C., & Couvreur, P. (2000). Development of polysaccharide nanoparticles as novel drug carrier systems. In C. Trantolo & S. Inyang (Eds.), *Handbook of Pharmaceutical Controlled Release Technology; Wise* (pp. 413–429). New York: Marcel Dekker, Inc.

Watnasirichaikul, S., Rades, R., Tucker, I. G., & Davies, N. M. (2000). Manipulating the Release of Insulin from Nanocapsules Prepared by Interfacial Polymerization of Microemulsions. *Proceedings of the 27th International Symposium on Controlled Release of Bioactive Materials of the Controlled Release Society, Inc.*

Weber, C., Coester, C., Kreuter, J., & Langer, K. (2000). Dessolvation process and surface characterization of protein nanoparticles. *International Journal of Pharmaceutics*, *194*(1), 94–102. doi:10.1016/S0378-5173(99)00370-1

Yildirimera, L., Thanhb, N. T. K., Loizidoua, M., & Seifaliana, A. M. (2011). Toxicology and clinical potential of nanoparticles. *Nano Today*, *6*(6), 585–607. doi:10.1016/j.nantod.2011.10.001 PMID:23293661

Yu-Nam, Y., & Lead, R. (2008). Manufactured nanoparticles: An overview of their chemistry, interactions and potential environmental implications. *The Science of the Total Environment*, *400*(1-3), 396–414. doi:10.1016/j.scitotenv.2008.06.042 PMID:18715626

Zambaux, M. F., Bonneauz, F., Gref, R., Maincent, P., Dellacherie, E., Alonso, M. J., & Vigneron, C. et al. (1998). Influence of experimental parameters on the characteristics of poly(lactic acid) nanoparticles prepared by a double emulsion method. *Journal of Controlled Release*, *50*(1-3), 31–40. doi:10.1016/S0168-3659(97)00106-5 PMID:9685870

Chapter 15
Therapeutic Applications of Nanobiomaterials

Anuj Garg
National Institute of Pharmaceutical Education and Research (NIPER), Raebareli, India

ABSTRACT

The most exciting advancement in the fields of biomaterial science is its ability to engineer new materials at the nanoscale level for various biological applications particularly drug and gene delivery for therapeutic applications. The main focus of this chapter is to review the therapeutic applications of different nanobiomaterials. Thus, it is proposed to discuss type of nanobiomaterials, general biological barriers for therapeutics, surface functionalization of nanobiomaterials and their therapeutics application in the present chapter. The therapeutic applications are explained on the basis of type of nanobiomaterials. The biocompatibility and toxicological response towards nanobiomaterials is an important issue that requires investigation for clinical development and their commercialization. The commercial prospects and future challenges in development of nanobiomaterials particularly for drug delivery are also discussed in the present chapter.

1. INTRODUCTION

The most exciting advancement in the fields of biomaterial science is its ability to engineer new materials at the nanoscale level for various biological applications particularly drug and gene delivery for therapeutic applications. Nanotechnology-based approaches are being explored for many applications such as for drug delivery, diagnosis, tissue engineering, and biosensors. Most of these approaches employ nanobiomaterials for developing unique functionalities required by these biomedical systems. The main focus of this chapter is to provide perspective of therapeutic application of nanobiomaterials. The application of nanobiomaterials to tumor delivery and targeting of therapeutics for cancer treatment have received significant attention in the last decade (Golla et al., 2013; Luo et al., 2010; Heister et al., 2009; Maeda et al., 2000). A wide range of nanobiomaterials materials have been used to construct nanoparticles for encapsulation of chemotherapeutics to increase the capability of delivery or to provide unique optical, magnetic, electrical and structural properties for therapy as well as imaging.

DOI: 10.4018/978-1-5225-0751-2.ch015

Nanobiomaterials are used as reservoir of the drugs for prolonged or extended delivery. Therapeutics-drug and gene delivery systems include metallic, inorganic, organic/carbon, protein/peptide, polymeric and lipid, polymeric-lipid hybrid and biologically directed (virus) nanobiomaterials. These nanobiomaterials can be capable to provide a unique solution to overcome the limitations of existing conventional drug delivery systems, which include low bioavailability, non- targeting and potential toxicity. General biological barriers for therapeutics are also explained in this chapter for better understanding of the limitations of nanobiomaterials. The understanding of these limitations provides help in development of the nanobiomaterials based drug delivery systems to overcome the biological barriers.

Further, surface properties of these nanobiomaterials can be manipulated to enhance their therapeutic efficacy by increasing their targeting potential and immunocompatibility. Surface modification of nanobiomaterials can also influence their stability in *in-vivo*. The surface modification/functionalization of nanobiomaterials received significant attention in the treatment of cancers. Surface functionalization of nanobiomaterials includes conjugation with antibodies and receptor targeting ligands for active targeting of nanobiomaterials (Yu et al., 2013).

In the present chapter, therapeutic applications of nanobiomaterials are discussed with relevant examples on the basis of type of nanobiomaterials as shown in outline of the chapter. Metallic nanobiomaterials like gold nanoparticles are used for the drug delivery and photo thermal therapy in treatment of tumours. Inorganic based nanobiomaterials like hydroxyapatite possess a potential therapeutic application in the management of osteoporosis, a bone disease (Linovitz & Peppas, 2002). Carbon based nanobiomaterials like *carbon nanotubes* and *fullerenes* have various applications in the field of therapeutics like used as photsensitizers in photodynamic therapy (Zhou et al., 2009; Carlson & Krauss, 2008). The peptide based nanobiomaterials can incorporate the small hydrophobic molecules like lipophilic drugs and to be easily functionalized with targeting moeity. Also some peptide based nanobiomaterials exhibited strong antimicrobial properties. The application of peptide nanobiomaterials in gene delivery is also to be summarized in the present chapter. The polymeric and lipid based nanobiomaterials are widely used as drug delivery platform to overcome the stability, bioavailability and toxicity related issues for various type of drug molecules like anticancer agents, antimicrobial agents, anti diabetic agents etc. The main focus of this chapter is to review the therapeutic applications of different nanobiomaterials.

Thus, it is proposed to discuss type of nanobiomaterials, general biological barriers for therapeutics, surface functionalization of nanobiomaterials and their therapeutics application in the present chapter. The therapeutic applications are explained on the basis of type of nanobiomaterials. The biocompatibility and toxicological response towards nanobiomaterials is an important issue that requires investigation for clinical development and their commercialization. The commercial prospects and future challenges in development of nanobiomaterials particularly for drug delivery are also discussed in the present chapter.

2. TYPE OF NANOBIOMATERIALS

Nanobiomaterials can be classified based on the dimensions, which are not confined to the nanoscale range. The classification is as follows:

1. **Zero Dimensional (0-D):** All dimensions are at nanoscale like drug loaded nanoparticles
2. **One dimensional (1-D):** Two dimensions are at nanoscale, other dimension is not at nanoscale like nanowires, nanrods and nanotubes (carbon nanotubes)

3. **Two Dimensional (2-D):** One dimension at nanoscale other two dimensions are not at nanoscale like nanofilms, nanocoatings and nanoplates like graphene.
4. **Three Dimensional (3-D):** All three dimensions are not at nanoscale range. For example bulk nanobiomaterials composed of a multiple arrangement of nanoscale crystals, most typically in different orientations.

In addition to their size, nanobiomaterials can also be classified based on their composition as shown in Figure 1.

3. GENERAL BIOLOGICAL BARRIERS FOR THERAPEUTICS

Biological barriers must be overcome to achieve the successful delivery of the drug from the nanobiomaterials. The initial barriers encountered depend on the desired mode of administration which include oral, pulmonary, parenteral (intravenous route) etc. For example, drug loaded nanobiomaterials given by oral route must address stability of nanobiomaterials during the harsh condition in gastrointestinal tract and simultaneously target a specific site for entry whereas intravenous injections must overcome

Figure 1. Classification of nanobiomaterials based on their composition

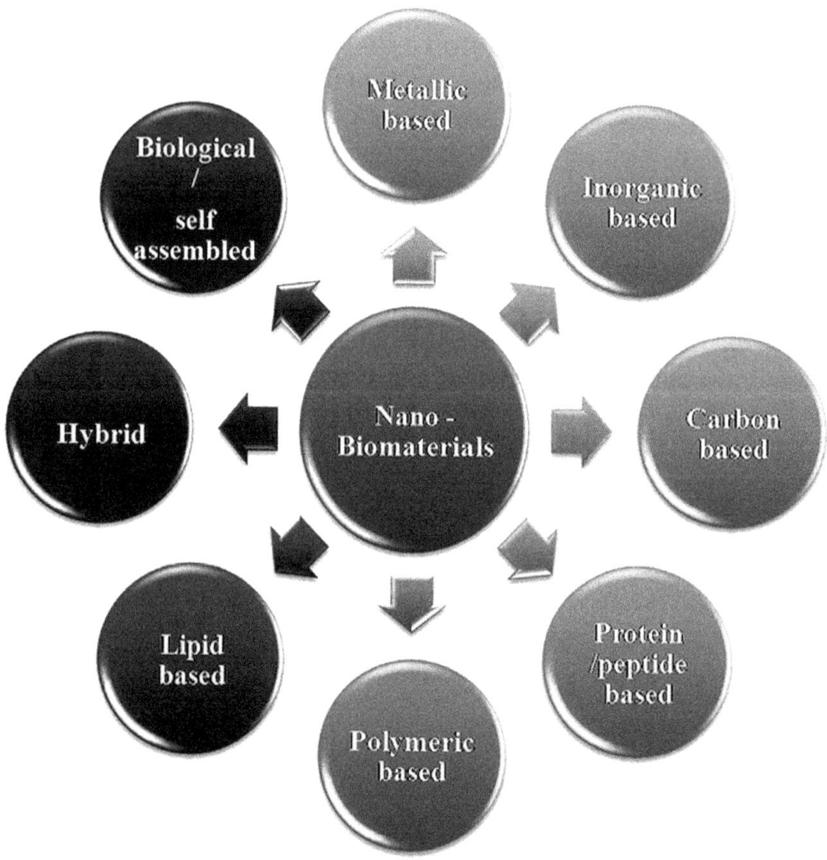

the reticular-endothelial system if prolonged circulation is to be achieved (Roger et al., 2010; Petros & DeSimone, 2010). Further to achieve specific site targeting like intracellular drug delivery, various biological barriers from system level, to the organ level, to the cellular level must be overcome. The biological barriers at system level are initial barrier and depend on the mode of administration as explained above. The multiple organ level clearance mechanisms such as occurring in the liver and spleen must be overcome if the carrier or drug loaded nanobiomaterials is to reach its intended target. There are several strategies to overcome these barriers first, altering the hydrophilicity of the carrier surface to reduce the rate of protein opsonization, which ultimately marks carriers for sequestration and removal (Torchilin & Trubetskoy, 1995; Adams et al., 2003; Owens and Peppas, 2006; Howard et al., 2008). There are many biological barriers at the cellular level that a nanobiomaterial must overcome to achieve successful intracellular drug delivery. The biological barrier includes cell membrane, which blocks diffusion of complexes larger than 1000 Dalton. Several endocytic mechanisms can be engaged to facilitate the internalization of nanobiomaterials (Table 1).

The route of endocytosis determines the path of trafficking through various possible subcellular compartments. Nanobiomaterials internalized through clathrin mediated endocytosis are reached for a lysosomal compartment, whereas those internalized through caveolin mediated process are not reached to lysosomal compartment (Bareford & Swan, 2007). Ligands conjugated to the surface of nanobiomaterials can influence the endocytic route of cellular internalization. Ligands for glycoreceptors promote clathrin mediated endocytosis whereas ligands such as folic acid, albumin and cholesterol facilitate the uptake through caveolin mediated endocytosis (Bareford & Swan, 2007).

4. SURFACE FUNCTIONALIZATION OF NANOBIOMATERIALS

Surface of the nanobiomaterial is the primary medium by which it interacts with its environment. The surface properties/characteristics of nano size range biomaterials are of greater importance as their large surface to volume ratio. The interaction between the surface of the nanobiomaterials and its environment *in vivo* ultimately influence the colloidal stability of the particles, and may yield to a controlled assembly or to the delivery of nanoparticles to a target, e.g. by appropriate functional molecules or attaching ligand on the particle surface. The following desirable characteristics for successful drug delivery from nanobiomaterials can be achieved as a result of the surface modification of nanobiomaterials.

Table 1. Endocytic routes for cellular internalization of nanobiomaterials

S.No.	Endocytic Route	Characteristics
1.	Phagocytosis	For internalization of larger particles
2.	Macropinocytosis	For internalization of smaller particles
3.	Caveolar mediated endocytosis	For nanobiomaterials (-60 nm) and ligand such as folic acid facilitate the uptake through this route
4.	Clathrin mediated endocytosis	For nanobiomaterials (120 nm) and ligands for glycoreceptors like mannose promote this endocytosis
5.	Clathrin and caveolin independent endocytosis	Internalization of many virus like simian virus 40 into host cell example of this type of endocytosis

1. Longevity: to increase half life of nanobiomaterials in the circulation
2. Targeting: active or passive targeting
3. Desirable bio-distribution
4. Stabilization against aggregation

There are many approaches for the surface modifications of nanobiomaterials to achieve successful delivery of drugs which lead to enhance the therapeutic activity of drug molecules. The different approaches of surface modifications are shown in Figure 2.

In the active targeting different targeting ligands like antibodies, peptides, sugar moieties and other functional group listed in Table 2 can be attach to the surface of the nanoparticles as shown in Figure 3.

Surface functionalization of nanobiomaterial can be used to control their *in-vivo* or biological properties and make them to simultaneously perform various therapeutically or diagnostically important functions. It has a significant role in controlling longevity, and biodistribution and targeting property of nanobiomaterials.

5. THERAPEUTIC APPLICATIONS OF NANOBIOMATERIALS

a. Metallic Nanobiomaterials

Many metal and metalloid elements like silver, gold, galdolinium, titanium, iron oxide etc. are able to form nano-scale structures. Some of the better known nanoparticles currently being investigated include those based on silver and gold.

Figure 2. Different approaches for surface modifications of nanobiomaterials

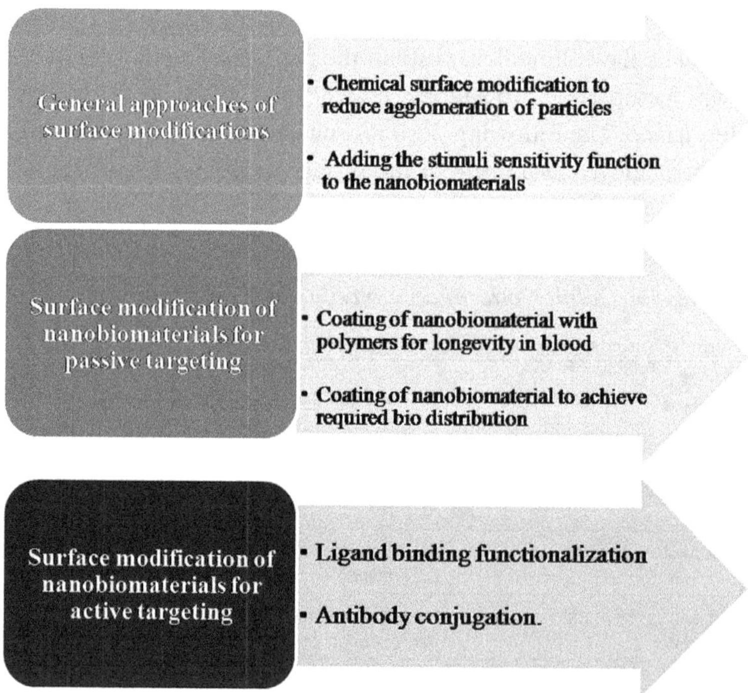

Table 2. Different ligands used to modify surface of nanobiomaterials for active targeting

Protein and Peptides Based	Carbohydrate Based	Miscellaneous
Antibodies	Galactose	Folic acid
Immunotoxins	Mannose	Lectins
Modified albumin	Heparin	
Lipoproteins	Chitosan	
Vasoactive intestinal peptide (VIP)		
Cyclic RGD		

Figure 3. Surface modification of the carrier by different targeting ligands for active targeting

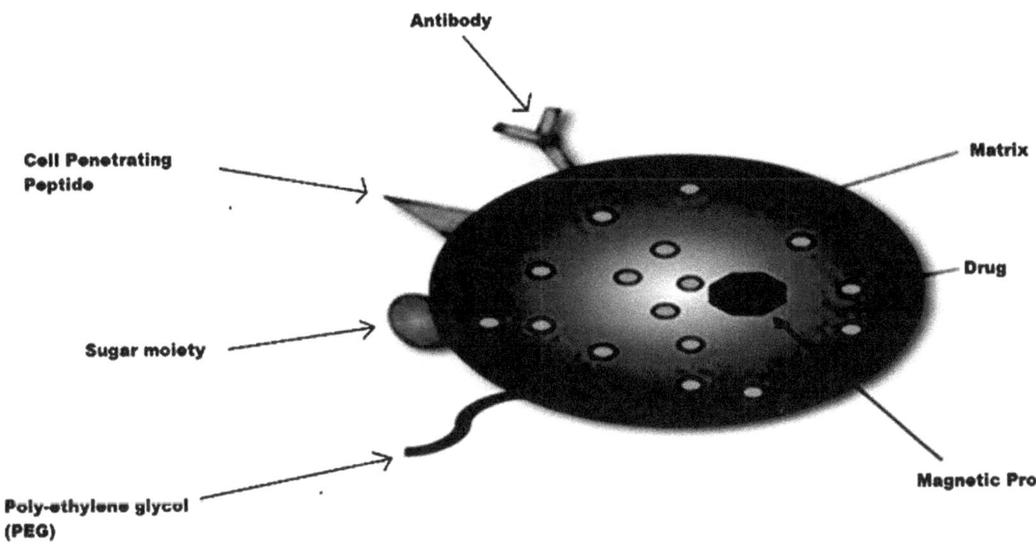

Silver Nanoparticles

Silver nanoparticles are known for their anti-microbial and anti-inflammatory properties (Chaloupka et al., 2010). Silver has long been known for its ability to combat infection, being able to inhibit various aspects of respiration; silver nanoparticles have larger surface area, increasing the area available for interactions, making them even more effective anti-microbial agents (Chen & Schluesener, 2008; Rai et al., 2009). In addition to antimicrobial activity, applications of silver nanoparticles have been expanded to drug delivery and other therapeutic applications like as antiviral agent, photosensitizer/radiosensitizer and anticancer agents. Therapeutic application of different surface modified silver nanoparticles has been investigated and found to be effective in the treatment of leukaemia, breast cancer, lung cancer, skin and oral carcinoma. Recently, therapeutic applications of silver nanoparticles are reviewed by Wei et al., (2015). Wei et al., (2015) reviewed the synthesis; properties and therapeutic application of silver nanoparticle and also discuss the toxicity of silver nanoparticles.

Gold Nanoparticles

Gold nanoparticles are widely used in drug delivery, photothermal therapy, cell tracking and sensing applications (Giljohnan et al., 2010). Colloidal gold nanoparticles can be easily prepared and bind with range of organic molecules and due to their tunable physical and chemical properties so they can be used as therapeutic agent or vaccine carriers in to specific cells. The gold nanoparticles has extensive applications in drug delivery because of the compatibility, conjugation of these particles to the biomolecules and their tunable optical properties which are due to the shape, size and surface area of the gold nanoparticles. Due to the small size and large surface, shape and crystallinity, nanoparticles are proved to be excellent therapeutic agents because they can easily travel into the target cells and can bear high drug load (Guo et al., 2014; Lan et al., 2013)

Gold nanocages coated with temperature-sensitive polymer were used as drug carrier which releases their effectors with interaction of near-infrared irradiations (Guo et al., 2010). Singh et al., (2014) explored the potential antitumour activity of biologically synthesized gold nanoparticles in lung and liver tumour system in vitro by activation of molecular mechanism of cell death. The main objective of development of targeted drug delivery systems is to differentiate between malignant and non-malignant cells, making them a promising alternative to existing drugs. This type of targeting efficiency of gold nanoparticles can be accomplished in future therapies using peptide conjugation, which directly targets tumor cells without affecting normal cells. Thus, a study of the exact mechanism by which gold nanoparticles inhibit signalling cascades responsible for the development and progression of the disease would be a tremendous breakthrough in the field of nanomedicine and make these agents an effective alternative in tumor and angiogenesis related diseases (Singh et al., 2014).

Iron Oxide Nanoparticles

Iron oxide nanoparticles are the only type of magnetic nanoparticles (MNPs) approved for clinical use by Food Drug Administration. Iron oxide- magnetite (Fe_3O_4) or maghemite (Fe_2O_3) occurs naturally in human heart, spleen, and liver, which indicates their biocompatibility and non toxic at physiological concentration (Grassi et al., 1997). Magnetite or maghemite are the most frequently used for biomedical application. These two compounds fulfil the prerequisites of chemical stability under physiological conditions, low toxicity and sufficiently high magnetic moments (Filippousi et al., 2014). However, it is essential to determine a safe upper limit of iron oxide nanoparticles for biomedical use.

Iron oxide nanoparticles are highly promising carriers for drug delivery because of their easy handling with the aid of external applied magnetic field, the ability of visualization, the possibility of using passive and active drug delivery strategies and enhanced uptake by the target tissue which results in improving efficacy of the treatment at same therapeutically optimal dose (Arruebo, 2007). The process of drug localization is based on the competing forces exerted on the particles in the blood compartment using the magnetic force generated by the external magnetic field. Moreover, the administration route of the MNPs seems to be crucial for the successful of the therapy. Intra artery delivery avoids or at least minimizes the particle clearance by the mononuclear phagocyte system in liver and spleen in comparison to intravenously applied particles.

The magnetically-guided nanoparticle has allowed the usual accumulation of nanoparticles observed in particular pathologies, such as tumors, inflammatory and infectious sites, to be enhanced. Those pathologies are characterized by structural abnormalities in the vasculature.

This phenomenon, known as the enhanced permeability and retention (EPR) effect (Maeda, 2007), is a consequence of the affected tissues possessing "leaky" vasculature, which allows macromolecules and nanoparticles to extravasate and accumulate more readily. Iron oxide nanoparticles exhibit potential in cancer treatment by magnetic hyperthermia (Liu et al., 2005; Balivada et al., 2010).

Surface modification or coating of Iron oxide particles further improve the targeting of the MNPs to the brain. Chertok et al.(2010) used iron oxide nanoparticles coated with starch or gum arabic modified with polyethyleneimine (PEI) as a potential vascular drug/gene carrier for delivery to brain tumors. The MNPs were injected into rats harboring orthotopic gliosarcoma. The intra-carotid administration route was shown to be optimal. The study showed that the surface modification with polycationic PEI resulted in 5.2-fold higher tumor accumulation of PEI-MNPs compared to uncoated MNPs.

Iron oxide magnetic nanoparticles have also been used to transfect the vector DNA and antisense oligonucleotides in vitro for effective gene therapy using a process called magnetofection. PEI-coated magnetic particles were first reported by Scherer *et al.* (2002) and provided the first example of *in vitro* MNP-mediated non-viral gene delivery. This process increases the efficiency of conventional transfection methods and decreases the toxicity (Chen et al. 2009; Namgung et al. 2010).

b. Inorganic Based Nanobiomaterials

Mesoporous Silica Nanoparticles

Among inorganic nanoparticles, silica based nanobiomaterials are most often selected for drug delivery and other biological applications. The advantages of silica based nanobiomaterials as drug delivery systems include their biocompatibility, highly porous framework and an ease in terms of functionalization (Amato, 2010; Slowing et al., 2007). There are different types of silica-based nanoparticles which include monoliths, rod like particles, fibers, hollow and solid nanospheres, silica nanotubes, and mesoporous silica nanoparticles (MSNs) (Jafelicci et al. 1999; Miyaji et al. 1999; Fan et al. 2003; Miyazaki et al. 2004; Blasi et al. 2005; Deng et al. 2006; Han et al. 2006). Among them mesoporous silica nanoparticles are widely used for development of drug delivery systems. Mesoporous silica nanoparticles (MSN), due to honeycomb-like porous structures, permit incorporation of both small and large drug molecules (Slowing et al. 2007). The mechanism of drug loading into mesoporous silica material is a chemical or physical adsorption (Di Pasqua et al., 2009). Silica nanoparticles can also act as magnetic hyperthermia agents after complexed with super paramagnetic iron oxide (Matín-Saavedra et al. 2010).

MSNs exhibit several characteristics that could be beneficial for gene-delivery. First characteristic is a narrow pore size distribution of MSNs which can provide efficient protection of the cargo until the point of release if the plasmid is present inside the mesopore system, and second, easy modification of the surfaces lead to optimize plasmid adsorption and release characteristics. However, the loading of DNA or RNAs into the mesopore of MSNs is not straightforward, and in many reports on MSNs for gene delivery DNA was primarily only adsorbed to the outer surface of the particles of cationically modified MSNs (Xia et al., 2009; Meng et al., 2010). Many research works focusing on adsorption of plasmids into and onto MSNs have been reported which indicated the potential of MSNs to serve as efficient carriers for plasmids (Mamaeva et al., 2013).

In addition to cancer therapy, MSNs can be served as drug delivery systems for the treatment of other diseases. For example, formulations of bone cement based on MSNs as antibiotic carrier and novel filler is developed to prevent inflammation and osteomyelitis in hip and joint replacement surgery (Shen et al., 2011). The formulation provides extended drug release and also increased drug release efficiency.

MSNs can also be used to treat intracellular pathogens like *Mycobacterium tuberculosis* infected macrophages. MSNs are taken up by the components of reticuloendothelial system (RES). Clemens, et al (2012) reported a successful *in-vitro* study on targeted intracellular delivery of antituberculosis drugs rifampin and Isoniazid to *Mycobacterium tuberculosis*-infected macrophages which exploits the accumulation of MSNs by components of RES, a phenomenon, which otherwise nanomedicine is trying to avoid (Clemens et al., 2012).

Hydroxyapatite Based Nanobiomaterials

Hydroxyapatite is the inorganic component of bones and teeth. Hydroxyapatite based nanobiomaterials like dental restoratives and bone defect repair platforms are now commercially available (Linovitz & Peppas, 2002). Hydroxyapatite based systems with and without collagen or elastin nanofibers may be formulated to match the size and shape of the diseased bone tissue of the specific patient. Furthermore, these systems may be loaded with an antibacterial drug or with growth factor to enhance bone tissue regeneration (Laffargue et al., 2000; Shinto et al., 1992). Hydroxyapatite nanoparticles containing Docetaxel, an anticancer agent, were prepared which found to possess more cytotoxicity against prostate cancer cell line (PC3 and DU145) as compared to Docetaxel alone (Luo et al., 2010).

Carbon Based Nanobiomaterials

Carbon nanotubes (CNT) and fullerenes are well known carbon based nanobiomaterials used in drug delivery and other biomedical application. Surface modifications of these hydrophobic nanobiomaterials are required to make them water solubilise for biological applications. Many surface modifications methods are reported in the literature (Liu et al., 2009; Wu et al., 2008).

Carbon Nanotubes

The carbon nanotube (CNT), an allotrope of carbon with a cylindrical structure, was first discovered by Iijima in 1991 (Iijima, 1991). Depending of the number of cylindrical grapheme layers, CNTs can be mainly categorized into two groups: single-walled carbon nanotubes (SWNTs) and multi-walled carbon nanotubes (MWNTs). Carbon nanotubes have been investigated as novel drug delivery systems for treatment of the cancer (Heister et al., 2009; Chen et al., 2008; Dhar et al., 2008).

Various drug molecules with aromatic ring structures and biomolecules like oligonucleotides and small interference RNAs (siRNAs) can easily be immobilized onto CNTs by physical adsorption. The presence of high density of carboxyl group on the sidewalls of CNTs due to acid-mediated oxidation of CNTs make them accessible to attach ligands or drug molecules with amino groups. The amino group can be attached to carboxyl group of CNTs via the conventional 1-ethyl-3-(3-dimethylaminopropyl) carbodiimide/N-hydroxysuccinimide (EDC/NHS) crosslinking method to enhance the targeting selectivity (Heister et al., 2009). CNTs because of their unique small size and shape (needle like structure of nanotubes) and functionalized by oxidations, coated by surfactants or polymers are able to cross the cell membrane by endocytosis pathways which further implies their potential to serve as multifunctional drug delivery system (Liu et al., 2009; Kam et al., 2004; Kam et al., 2006; Jin et al., 2008; Wu et al., 2008; Chen et al., 2006).

Moreover, carbon nanotubes also demonstrate strong optical absorption in the near-infrared region, thus making them promising nanobiomaterial for use in the photothermal ablation of tumors (Zhou et al., 2009; Carlson & Krauss, 2008).

CNTs have been identified as a potential alternative for the gene therapy or transfection because of their simple-functionalized surface, great membrane penetration and low immunogenicity (Yu et al., 2013).

Fullerenes

The "buckyball" was the first fullerene ever discovered and has the molecular formula of C60. Fullerene or buckyball is a molecule composed entirely of carbon, in form of a hollow geodesic structure. Fullerene is a nanoscale carbon material having unique photo, electrochemical, physical properties with low systemic toxicity.

Photoirradiation of fullerenes in the presence of molecular oxygen generated singlet oxygen making them suitable as photosensitizers for photodynamic therapy (Iwamoto and Yamakoshi, 2006). Moreover, Fullerene based photodynamic therapy nanocomposites can be served as both photosensitizer and its carrier to improve photodynamic efficacy (Shi et al., 2013).

c. Polymer Based Nanobiomaterials

Polymer based nanobiomaterials are extensively used in the field of drug delivery systems. Polymeric nanoparticles are widely used because of their increased stability and the unique ability to create extended release. The polymers used in the development of drug delivery systems are either of natural or synthetic in origin as given in Table 3.

The advantage of using natural polymer for the development of nanobiomaterials is their biocompatibility, which assists in cell adhesion and tissue regeneration. However, these polymers have poor mechanical properties and failed to provide stability and extended drug release from the delivery systems. On the other hand, synthetic polymers possess better mechanical strength than natural polymers. Further, these can be synthetically manipulated to allow biodegradation. However, these show lower biocompatibility compared to natural polymers.

Table 3. List of widely used polymers for development of nanoparticulate based drug delivery systems

Natural Polymers	Synthetic Polymers
Starch	Poly (lactic acid) (PLA)
Sodium alginate	Poly (lactic-glycolic acid) (PLGA
Chitin/Chitosan	Poly (hydroxyl butyrate) (PHB)
Hyaluronic acid & derivatives	Poly (ε-caprolactone)
Dextran	Polyacrylamide
Albumin	Polyanhydride
Gelatin	

Drugs can be encapsulated in polymeric nanoparticles after a polymerization reaction or can be encapsulated in polymeric nanoparticles during a polymerization step (Luo et al., 2010; Mora-Huertas et al., 2010). Drugs may be released by desorption, diffusion, or nanoparticle erosion in target tissue (Torchilin, 2008). Polymeric nanoparticles are usually coated with nonionic surfactants in order to reduce immunological interactions such as opsonization. Further, surface of polymeric nanoparticles can also be modified with ligands to develop active targeted drug delivery systems as discussed earlier in this chapter. Some examples of polymeric nanobiomaterial as drug delivery systems are given in Table 4 which showed their extensive application in therapeutics.

d. Protein/Peptide Based Nanobiomaterials

Protein and polypeptides are promising biomaterial for constructing the nanocarrier systems. Application of protein/peptide based nanobiomaterials as drug delivery systems are rapidly growing due to their amphiphilic nature which allow them to interact well with both drug and solvent (Locharoenkal et al., 2014). Moreover, they are biodegradable and easily amenable to surface modifications to allow attachment of drugs and ligands for active targeting. Proteins/peptides including gelatin, albumin, gliadin, legumin, elastin, soy protein and milk protein (casein) can be utilized to prepare nanobiomaterials for drug delivery. There are many review articles which discuss the preparation, characterization and application of nanoparticles derived from protein and peptides (Locharoenkal et al., 2014; Wang and Uludag, 2008; Chen et al., 2006). Gelatin and albumin are most widely used for development of nanoparticulate based drug delivery systems, while plant proteins and milk proteins have just begun to be explored for drug delivery applications, and they represent highly promising protein based nanobiomaterials. Zhen et al. (2013) demonstrated the ability of cisplatin loaded casein nanoparticles to penetrate cell membranes, target tumors, and inhibit tumor growth in hepatic tumor bearing mice (Zhen et al., 2013). Nanoparticles prepared from cow milk-derived lactoferrin have been evaluated as an oral delivery system for doxorubicin to treat hepatocellular carcinoma (HCC). Hepatocellular carcinoma cell are highly metabolically active and express a high level of lactoferrin receptors, thus are a potential target of lactoferrin nanoparticles (Schneider et al., 1984). Doxorubicin-loaded lactoferrin nanoparticles were found to exhibit improved efficacy, bioavailability, and safety as compared to free doxorubicin. This nanoparticle formulation was shown to reduce the number of liver nodules by >93% without affecting the body weight (Golla et al., 2013)

Table 4. Polymeric nanobiomaterial as drug delivery system

Drug	Polymer Used	Therapeutic Activity	Reference
Gemcitabine	Chitosan	Antitumour activity	
Campothecin	PLGA	Intracranial glioma	Householder et al., 2015
Rapamycin	Chitosan/PLA	Immunosuppression in corneal transplantation	Yuan et al., 2008
Quinine	Corn Starch	Anti malarial activity	Heikham et al., 2015
Ursolic acid	Polyethylene glycol (PEG)-Poly Caprolactone (PCL)	Treatment of Gastric Cancer	Zhang et al., 2013
Plasmid DNA	Hyaluronic acid/Chitosan	Gene delivery targeting Osteoarthiritis	Lu et al., 2011
Rifampicin	Gelatin	Antituberculosis	Saraogi et al., 2010

e. Lipid Based Nanobiomaterials

Lipid based nanobiomaterials have been extensively exploited for the dermal, peroral, ocular, pulmonary and rectal route (Garg & Singh, 2014; Hu et al., 2010; Souto & Muller, 2010; Liu et al., 2008; Hippalgaonkar et al., 2013). Lipid based nanobiomaterials include solid lipid nanoparticles (SLN), nanostructured lipid carriers (NLC) and lipid drug conjugates (LDC). SLN are particles made of solid lipids such as purified triglycerides, fatty acids like stearic acid etc. The lipids used in the preparation of solid lipid nanoparticles (SLN) are included in the category of GRAS (Generally Recognized as Safe) substances (Muller et al., 2000) and therefore, they encounter less regulatory hurdles for the FDA approvals. The other interesting characteristics of SLN include a good physical stability, protection of incorporated drugs from degradation, controlled drug release, and good tolerability. Solid lipid nanoparticles possess some disadvantages like low loading capacity, drug expulsion after crystallization during storage (Muller et al., 2002). NLC and LDC have been developed to overcome the problems associated with SLN. NLC are prepared by using mixture of solid and liquid lipid. The presence of liquid lipid such as oleic acid produces the imperfect structure in crystalline solid lipid and prevents the expulsion of drug from the solid lipid nanoparticles (Üner & Yener, 2007). LDC was developed to overcome the limited drug loading of hydrophilic drugs in SLN. The hydrophilic drug -lipid conjugates can be prepared by salt formation or by covalent linking followed by homogenization (Muller and Keck, 2004). Lipid based nanoparticles are mainly exploited for their dermal application. SLNs can provide benefits of accumulation of drug in the skin strata to treat various skin diseases such as acne, eczema and fungal infections (Garg & Singh, 2011). Garg & Singh (2014), evaluate the skin targeting ability of lipid based nanoparticles to increase the concentration of eugenol at epidermis, site of fungal infection and decrease the systemic absorption of eugenol. However, solid lipid nanoparticles are less viscous and not suitable for dermal application as such. Garg and Singh (2014), incorporate the eugenol loaded SLN into carbopol hydrogel and makes them suitable for dermal application. The carbopol hydrogel accommodates EG-SLN in the empty spaces inside its three dimensional structure. Although eugenol has high diffusion coefficient but developed EG-SLN enriched hydrogel can effectively localize eugenol in the epidermis with less penetration into deep skin layers (Garg and Singh, 2014). Hydration of epidermal layer of skin results in penetration of EG-SLN and forms depot in the epidermis where eugenol is released slowly. They also demonstrated the effect of shape of particles of SLN on their interaction with skin surface which could affect the density of film and thus, hydration of skin. The hydrogel containing SLN can be promising nanobiomaterials for targeting drug molecules to the epidermis and hence improve the efficacy against the fungal and other skin related infections.

Lipid based nanobiomaterials draw lot of attention for developing topical products for medicinal as well as cosmetic purposes. In past years, many topical products based on lipid nanoparticles were launched in market (Table 5).

f. Hybrid Nanobiomaterials

Nanobiomaterial has been extensively explored in last decade and evolved toward more complex nanoscopic core–shell architecture. A new type of nanobiomaterial platform, named polymer-lipid hybrid nanoparticles has been developed that combines the positive attributes of both lipid based nanoparticles and polymeric nanoparticles while excluding some of their disadvantages.

Table 5. List of marketed topical products based on lipid nanobiomaterials

Product Name	Producer/Distributor	Main Active Ingredients
Nano Lipid Restore	Chemisches Laboratorium Dr. Kurt Richter, CLR Berlin	Coenzyme Q-10 and omega unsaturated fatty acids
NLC Deep effect	Beate Johnen	Cocunut oil, tamanu tree extract,
Intensive Serum Nanorepair Q-10	Dr. Rimpler Gmbh	Q-10, Polypeptide, Mafane extract (Anti-wrinkle effect)

The lipid-polymer hybrid nanobiomaterials consist of a hydrophobic polymeric core, a lipid shell surrounding the polymeric core, and a hydrophilic polymer stealth layer outside the lipid shell as schematic representation shown in Figure 4.

The poorly water soluble drug are incorporated with high loading yields whereas a lipid layer surrounding the core acts as a highly biocompatible shell and as a molecular fence to promote drug retention inside the polymeric core. The presence of hydrophilic polymer stealth layer outside the lipid shell lead to enhance stability and systemic circulation lifetime of hybrid nanoparticles. The hydrophobic interactions, van der Waals forces, electrostatic interactions or other non-covalent forces are involved in polymeric core and the lipid shell association while hydrophilic polymer stealth layer is often conjugated to the lipid shell through covalent bonds.

In general, lipid polymer hybrid nanoparticles can be prepared by using two distinct approaches. One approach involves the two step process while second approach involves a single step process. In two step process, polymer core and lipid shell are prepared separately and then merged together. In single step process, the hybrid nanoparticles are prepared through a one pot nanoprecipitation and self assembly method.

Hybrid nanoparticles are used to deliver a wide variety of therapeutic agents. The drugs can be loaded inside the nanoparticle alone or in combination with more drugs. Hybrid nanoparticles possess great potential for combinatorial drug delivery.

Figure 4. Schematic representation of hybrid nanobiomaterial

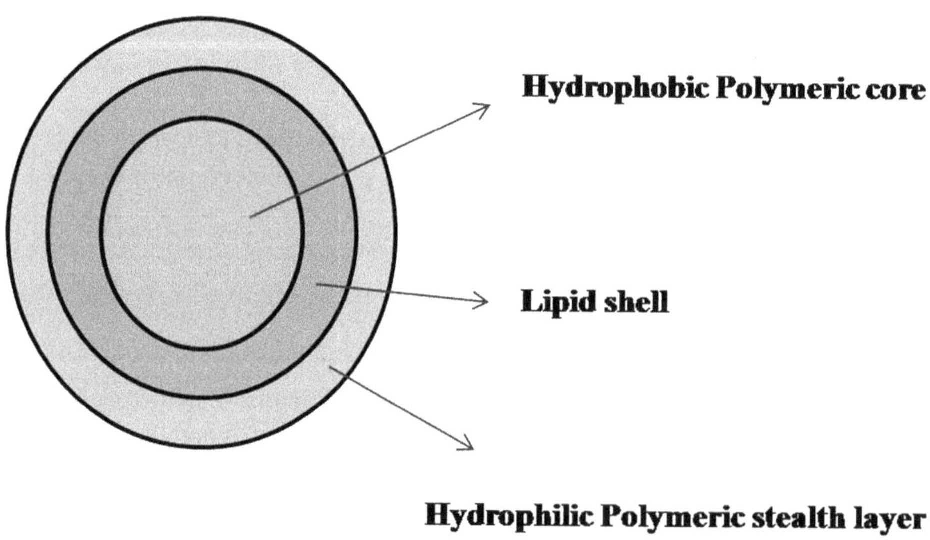

Wang et al.,2010 prepared a targeted hybrid nanoparticle system in which an anticancer drug, docetaxel, was first encapsulated inside the polymer core during the nanoprecipitation process, and then a radioisotope, In^{111}, was chelated onto the particle surface to concurrently deliver chemotherapy and radiotherapy agents for the treatment of prostate cancer. The resulting dual-drug-loaded nanoparticles showed distinct release profiles for both drugs and enhanced killing of tumor cells.

g. Biologically/Self-Assembled Nanobiomaterials

Virus Based Nanocarriers

Virus based nanocarriers are an emerging platform which offer great advantages of morphological uniformity, biocompatibility and easy functionalization. Different viruses which have been studied in the field of nanotechnology for drug delivery are cowpea mosaic virus (CPMV), cowpea chlorotic mottle virus (CCMV), red clover necrotic mosaic virus (RCNMV), Tobacco mosaic virus (TMV), M13 bacteriophage and MS2.

CPMV is an icosahedral plant virus belonging to the Comoviridae family. CPMV is stable at a rather wide range of temperatures (up to 60 °C), in the pH range of 3–9, and in the presence of certain organic solvents. The outstanding stability of CPMV made it a very-well studied virus for nanotechnology and drug delivery (Singh et al., 2006).

The cowpea chlorotic mottle virus (CCMV) is a member of the bromovirus group of Bromoviridae, a family of plant viruses. One of the most attractive characteristics of CCMV lies in the fact that it has a dynamic structure and it undergoes a reversible pH dependent swelling, resulting in the formation of 60 separate openings with diameters of 2 nm at the quasi-threefold axes (Speir et al., 1995). The 180 coat protein subunits are able to self assemble and dissemble in-vitro depending upon changing the pH and ionic strength. Thus, by using this feature, the viral RNA could be removed from the virus and be replaced with functional species. The inner cavity of this virus is of 18 nm (twice the diameter of ferritin) and carries high positive charge density due to presence of arginine and lysine residues. Because of the positive charge cavity, it is particularly useful for encapsulating negatively charged species.

Virus based nanobiomaterials are useful in their specificity, but causes problems upon using them as drug delivery carriers. Viruses are made of proteins and therefore, the human immune system will attack the viral nanoparticles, even though the viruses are non-human viruses. Thus, the viral nanoparticles cannot have repeated use.

6. COMMERCIAL PROSPECTS AND FUTURE CHALLENGES

According to a study by Grand View Research, Inc., the global market for healthcare nanotechnology is expected to reach USD 196.02 billion by 2020 growing at a CAGR of 12.1%. A number of well known drugs based on nanobiomaterial delivery platform have already been in the market. The industry and the scientific community hold a greater responsibility toward ethical and regulatory issues regarding use of nanobiomaterials upon increasing their commercial applications. The successful translation of nanobiomaterials from research lab to the clinic requires the development of simple, safe, reproducible, eco friendly and cost-effective methods for synthesis of nanobiomaterials, and in depth understanding of the safety control mechanisms as well as the biodistribution and pharmacokinetics of nanobiomaterials in clinical applications.

Thus, the main challenges for the nanobiomaterials to be used more effectively in drug delivery include in depth understanding of their biological interactions, safety concerns, manufacturing issues and economic and financial barriers.

In order to use nanobiomaterials as drug delivery systems in human, it is essential to have in depth understanding of the mechanisms underlying intracellular uptake, trafficking and the fate of nanomaterials in complex biological networks. Nanobiomaterial based drug delivery systems suffer from some major hindrances like rapid clearance by the macrophages, low targeting efficiency and difficulty in crossing biological barriers. A full understanding of the mechanism of transport will result in achieving the ability to control and manipulate drug delivery by using nanobiomaterials. Although, attempt has been made in this regard but more research studies are being required to explore the mechanisms of intracellular uptake and fate of nanobiomaterials in human body.

The most important concern to use nanobiomaterials is their toxic effects on human body. Because of their submicron size, nanobiomaterials can be inhaled, ingested or absorbed through the skin, and they can penetrate cells, even into the cell nucleus, where, if sufficiently small, they can come into close contact with genetic material. Therefore, nanobiomaterial toxicity should be considered in the patients as well as in the individuals exposed during the entire manufacturing and disposal processes. A new field known as "Nanotoxicology" has emerged with the development of nanobiomaterials. This refers to the study of the potential deleterious or harmful effects on the biological systems upon interaction with nanoparticles. Preliminary nanotoxicological studies showed that nanobiomaterials may contribute to the formation of free radicals, damage of brain cells and undesirable penetration through the epidermis or other physiological barriers into areas of the body that are more susceptible to toxic effects. Several mechanisms have been proposed to affect the toxicity of nanomaterials, depending on multiple factors derived from physiochemical properties, physical characteristics and environmental conditions. For example, it was reported that most cationic NPs can cause hemolysis and blood clotting, while neutral and anionic NPs are quite nontoxic. Based on safety concerns, the establishment of robust regulations and specific guidelines outlining the limitations on human exposure levels, environmental leakage issues, and waste disposal for each nanobiomaterial is essential rather than issuing general outlines.

The large-scale production of nanobiomaterials in terms of scaling up laboratory or pilot technologies for consistent and reproducible production and commercialization is another major limitation to use nanobiomaterials in drug delivery systems. A number of nanobiomaterial delivery technologies may not be compatible with large-scale production owing to the nature of the preparation method and high cost of materials employed. It is much easier to modify or maintain the size or composition of nanobiomaterials at the laboratory scale for improved performance than at a large scale.

Despite the number of patents for nanobiomaterials in drug delivery technologies, commercialization is still in its nascent stage due to above mentioned limitations. High development costs and lack of expertise required to achieve regulatory and commercial success are other additional obstacles to bring nanobiomaterial based drug delivery systems to the market.

7. CONCLUSION

The nanobiomaterials exhibit unique properties different from the bulk biomaterials and thus, can serve as a novel platform to deliver the drugs. The nanobiomaterials based platform can be utilized to deliver the drugs in better way and increase the potential of their existing and also provide the new therapeutic applications. Although, the development of nanobiomaterials based drug delivery systems are challenging, but provide potentially rewarding opportunity to develop the next generation drug delivery and biomedical products. In particular, these nanobiomaterials could revolutionize the treatment of cancer and multiple resistant microbial infections which lead to improve the life several patients suffering from these diseases.

ACKNOWLEDGMENT

Author would like to acknowledge the support and facilities provided by National Institute of Pharmaceutical Education and Research (NIPER), Raebareli.

REFERENCES

Adams, M. L., Lavasanifar, A., & Kwon, G. S. (2003). Amphiphilic block copolymers for drug delivery. *Journal of Pharmaceutical Sciences*, *92*(7), 1343–1355. doi:10.1002/jps.10397 PMID:12820139

Amato, G. (2010). Silica-encapsulated efficient and stable siquantum dots with high biocompatibility. *Nanoscale Research Letters*, *5*(7), 1156–1160. doi:10.1007/s11671-010-9619-9 PMID:20596494

Arruebo, M., Fernández-Pacheco, R., Ibarra, M. R., & Santamaría, J. (2007). Magnetic nanoparticles for drug delivery. *Nano Today*, *2*(3), 22–32. doi:10.1016/S1748-0132(07)70084-1

Balivada, S., Rachakatla, R. S., Wang, H., Samarakoon, T. N., Dani, R. K., Pyle, M., & Troyer, D. L. et al. (2010). A/C magnetic hyperthermia of melanoma mediated by iron(0)/iron oxide core/shell magnetic nanoparticles: A mouse study. *BMC Cancer*, *10*(1), 119. doi:10.1186/1471-2407-10-119 PMID:20350328

Bareford, L. M., & Swaan, P. W. (2007). Endocytic mechanisms for targeted drug delivery. *Advanced Drug Delivery Reviews*, *59*(8), 748–758. doi:10.1016/j.addr.2007.06.008 PMID:17659804

Blasi, L., Longo, L., Vasapollo, G., Cingolani, R., Rinaldi, R., Rizzello, T., & Maffia, M. et al. (2005). Characterization of glutamate dehydrogenase immobilization on silica surface by atomic force microscopy and kinetic analyses. *Enzyme and Microbial Technology*, *36*(5-6), 818–823. doi:10.1016/j.enzmictec.2005.01.014

Carlson, L. J., & Krauss, T. D. (2008). Photo physics of individual single-walled carbon nanotubes. *Accounts of Chemical Research*, *41*(2), 235–243. doi:10.1021/ar700136v PMID:18281946

Chaloupka, K., Malam, Y., & Seifalian, A. M. (2010). Nanosilver as a new generation of nano product in biomedical applications. *Trends in Biotechnology*, *28*(11), 580–588. doi:10.1016/j.tibtech.2010.07.006 PMID:20724010

Chen, C. B., Chen, J. Y., & Lee, W. C. (2009). Fast transfection of mammalian cells using super paramagnetic nanoparticles under strong magnetic field. *Journal of Nanoscience and Nanotechnology*, *9*(4), 2651–2659. doi:10.1166/jnn.2009.449 PMID:19438016

Chen, J., Chen, S., Zhao, X., Kuznetsova, L. V., Wong, S. S., & Ojima, L. (2008). Functionalized single-walled carbon nanotubes as rationally designed vehicles for tumor-targeted drug delivery. *Journal of the American Chemical Society*, *130*(49), 16778–16785. doi:10.1021/ja805570f PMID:19554734

Chen, L., Remondetto, G. E., & Subirade, M. (2006). Food protein based materials as nutraceutical delivery systems. *Trends in Food Science & Technology*, *17*(5), 272–283. doi:10.1016/j.tifs.2005.12.011

Chen, X., & Schluesener, H. J. (2008). Nanosilver: A nanoproduct in medical application. *Toxicology Letters*, *176*(1), 1–12. doi:10.1016/j.toxlet.2007.10.004 PMID:18022772

Chen, X., Tam, U. C., Czlapinski, J. L., Lee, G. S., Rabuka, D., Zettl, A., & Bertozzi, C. R. (2006). Interfacing Carbon Nanotubes with Living Cells. *Journal of the American Chemical Society*, *128*(19), 6292–6293. doi:10.1021/ja060276s PMID:16683774

Chertok, B., David, A. E., & Yang, V. C. (2010). Polyethyleneimine-modified iron oxide nanoparticles for brain tumor drug delivery using magnetic targeting and intracarotid administration. *Biomaterials*, *31*(24), 6317–6324. doi:10.1016/j.biomaterials.2010.04.043 PMID:20494439

Clemens, D. L., Lee, B.-Y., Xue, M., Thomas, C. R., Meng, H., Ferris, D., & Horwitz, M. A. et al. (2012). Targeted intracellular delivery of antituberculosis drugs to Mycobacterium tuberculosis-infected macrophages via functionalized mesoporous silica nanoparticles. *Antimicrobial Agents and Chemotherapy*, *56*(5), 2535–2545. doi:10.1128/AAC.06049-11 PMID:22354311

Damm, E. M., Pelkmans, L., Kartenbeck, J., Mezzacasa, A., Kurzchalia, T., & Helenius, A. (2005). Clathrin- and caveolin-1-independent endocytosis: Entry of simian virus 40 into cells devoid of caveolae. *The Journal of Cell Biology*, *168*(3), 477–488. doi:10.1083/jcb.200407113 PMID:15668298

Deng, A. D., Chen, M., Zhou, S. X., You, B., & Wu, L. M. (2006). A novel method for the fabrication ofmonodisperse hollow silica spheres. *Langmuir*, *22*(14), 6403–6407. doi:10.1021/la060944n PMID:16800706

Dhar, S., Liu, Z., Thomale, J., Dai, H., & Lippard, S. J. (2008). Targeted single-wall carbon nanotube-mediated Pt (IV) prodrug delivery using folate as a homing device. *Journal of the American Chemical Society*, *130*(34), 11467–11476. doi:10.1021/ja803036e PMID:18661990

Fan, J., Lei, J., Wang, L. M., Yu, C. Z., Tu, B., & Zhao, D. Y. (2003). Rapid and high capacity immobilization of enzymes based on mesoporous silica with controlled morphologies. *Chemical Communications (Cambridge)*, *17*, 2140–2141. doi:10.1039/b304391f PMID:13678170

Filippousi, M., Angelakeris, M., Katsikini, M., Paloura, E., Efthimiopoulos, I., Wang, Y., & van Tendeloo, G. et al. (2014). Surfactant effects on the structural and magnetic properties of iron oxide nanoparticles. *J. Phys. Chem. C Nanomater. Interfaces*, *118*, 16209–16217.

Garg, A., & Singh, S. (2011). Enhancement in antifungal activity of eugenol in immunosuppressed rats through lipid nanocarriers. *Colloids and Surfaces. B, Biointerfaces*, *87*(2), 280–288. doi:10.1016/j.colsurfb.2011.05.030 PMID:21689909

Garg, A., & Singh, S. (2014). Targeting of eugenol loaded solid lipid nanoparticles to the epidermal layer of human skin. *Nanomedicine (London)*, *9*(8), 1223–1238. doi:10.2217/nnm.13.33 PMID:23987096

Giljohann, D. A., Seferos, D. S., Daniel, W. L., Massich, M. D., Patel, P. C., & Mirkin, C. A. (2010). Gold nanoparticles for biology and medicine. *Angewandte Chemie International Edition in English*, *49*(19), 3280–3294. doi:10.1002/anie.200904359 PMID:20401880

Golla, K., Bhaskar, C., Ahmed, F., & Kondapi, A. K. (2013). A target specific oral formulation of doxorubicin-protein nanoparticles: Efficacy and safety in hepatocellular cancer. *Journal of Cancer*, *4*(8), 644–652. doi:10.7150/jca.7093 PMID:24155776

Gou, X. C., Liu, J., & Zhang, H. L. (2010). Monitoring human telomere DNA hybridization and G-quadruplex formation using gold nanorods. *Analytica Chimica Acta*, *668*(2), 208–214. doi:10.1016/j.aca.2010.04.027 PMID:20493300

Grassi-Schultheiss, P. P., Heller, F., & Dobson, J. (1997). Analysis ofmagnetic material in the human heart, spleen and liver. *Biometals*, *10*(4), 351–355. doi:10.1023/A:1018340920329 PMID:9353885

Guo, Q., Yuan, J., & Zeng, J. (2014). Biosynthesis of gold nanoparticles using a kind of flavonol:Dihydromyricetin. *Colloids and Surfaces. A, Physicochemical and Engineering Aspects*, *441*, 127–132. doi:10.1016/j.colsurfa.2013.08.067

Han, Y., Lee, S. S., & Ying, J. Y. (2006). Pressure-driven enzyme entrapment in siliceous mesocellular foam. *Chemistry of Materials*, *18*(3), 643–649. doi:10.1021/cm0520618

Heikham, K. D., Gupta, A., Kumar, A., Singh, C., Saxena, J., Srivastava, K., & Misra, A. et al. (2015). Preferential targeting of human erythrocytes infected with the malaria parasite Plasmodium falciparum via hexose transporter surface proteins. *International Journal of Pharmaceutics*, *483*(1-2), 57–62. doi:10.1016/j.ijpharm.2015.02.011 PMID:25666024

Heister, E., Neves, V., T^ılmaciu, C., Lipert, K., Beltr'an, V. S., Coley, H. M., & McFadden, J. et al. (2009). Triple functionalisation of single-walled carbon nanotubes with doxorubicin, a monoclonal antibody, and a fluorescent marker for targeted cancer therapy. *Carbon*, *47*(9), 2152–2160. doi:10.1016/j.carbon.2009.03.057

Hippalgaonkar, K., Adelli, G. R., Hippalgaonkar, K., Repka, M. A., & Majumdar, S. (2013). Indomethacin-Loaded Solid Lipid Nanoparticles for Ocular Delivery: Development, Characterization, and *In Vitro* Evaluation. *Journal of Ocular Pharmacology and Therapeutics*, *29*(2), 216–228. doi:10.1089/jop.2012.0069 PMID:23421502

Householder, K. T., DiPerna, D. M., Chung, E. P., Wohlleb, G. M., Dhruv, H. D., Berens, M. E., & Sirianni, R. W. (2015). Intravenous delivery of camptothecin-loaded PLGA nanoparticles for the treatment of intracranial glioma. *International Journal of Pharmaceutics*, *479*(2), 374–380. doi:10.1016/j.ijpharm.2015.01.002 PMID:25562639

Howard, M. D., Jay, M., Dziublal, T. D., & Lu, X. L. (2008). PEGylation of nanocarrier drug delivery systems: State of the art. *J. Biomed. Nanotechnol.*, *4*(2), 133–148. doi:10.1166/jbn.2008.021

Hu, L., Xing, Q., Meng, J., & Shang, C. (2010). Preparation and enhanced oral bioavailability of cryptotanshinone loaded solid lipid nanoparticles. *AAPS PharmSciTech*, *11*(2), 582–587. doi:10.1208/s12249-010-9410-3 PMID:20352534

Iijima, S. (1991). HELICAL Microtubules of graphitic carbon. *Nature*, *354*(6348), 56–58. doi:10.1038/354056a0

Iwamoto, Y., & Yamakoshi, Y. (2006). A highly water-soluble C60-NVP copolymer: A potential material for photodynamic therapy. *Chemical Communications (Cambridge)*, *46*(46), 4805–4807. doi:10.1039/B614305A PMID:17345735

Jafelicci, M. Jr, Davolos, M. R., Santos, F. J., & Andrade, S. J. (1999). Hollow silica particles from microemulsion. *Journal of Non-Crystalline Solids*, *247*(1-3), 98–102. doi:10.1016/S0022-3093(99)00040-X

Jin, H., Heller, D. A., & Strano, M. S. (2008). Single-Particle Tracking of Endocytosis and Exocytosis of Single-Walled Carbon Nanotubes in NIH-3T3 Cells. *Nano Letters*, *8*(6), 1577–1585. doi:10.1021/nl072969s PMID:18491944

Kam, N. W. S., Jessop, T. C., Wender, P. A., & Dai, H. (2004). Nanotube Molecular Transporters: Internalization of Carbon Nanotube–Protein Conjugates into Mammalian Cells. *Journal of the American Chemical Society*, *126*(22), 6850–6851. doi:10.1021/ja0486059 PMID:15174838

Kam, N. W. S., Liu, Z., & Dai, H. (2006). Carbon Nanotubes as Intracellular Transporters for Proteins and DNA: An Investigation of the Uptake Mechanism and Pathway. *Angewandte Chemie International Edition*, *45*(4), 577–581. doi:10.1002/anie.200503389 PMID:16345107

Laffargue, P., Fialdes, P., Frayssinet, P., Rtaimate, M., Hildebrand, H. F., & Marchandise, X. (2000). Adsorption and release of insulin-like growth factor-I on porous tricalcium phosphate Implant. *Journal of Biomedical Materials Research*, *49*(3), 415–421. doi:10.1002/(SICI)1097-4636(20000305)49:3<415::AID-JBM15>3.0.CO;2-Z PMID:10602075

Lan, M. Y., Hsu, Y. B., Hsu, C. H., Ho, C. Y., Lin, J. C., & Lee, S. W. (2013). Induction of apoptosis by high-dose gold nanoparticles in nasopharyngeal carcinoma cells. *Auris, Nasus, Larynx*, *40*(6), 563–568. doi:10.1016/j.anl.2013.04.011 PMID:23722198

Linovitz, R. J., & Peppers, T. A. (2002). Use of an advanced formulation of beta-tricalcium phosphate as a bone extender in inter body lumbar fusion. *Orthopedics*, *25*, S585–S589. PMID:12038846

Liu, J., Gong, T., Fu, H., Wang, C., Wang, X., Chen, Q., & Zhang, Z. et al. (2008). Solid lipid nanoparticles for pulmonary delivery of insulin. *International Journal of Pharmaceutics*, *356*(1-2), 333–344. doi:10.1016/j.ijpharm.2008.01.008 PMID:18281169

Liu, X., Xu, B., Xia, Q. S., Zhao, T. D., & Tang, T. P. (2005). A method of showing thermal effect of iron oxide nanoparticles in alternating magnetic field. *Ai Zheng*, *24*(9), 1148–1150. PMID:16159444

Liu, Z., Tabakman, S., Welsher, K., & Dai, H. (2009). Carbon nanotubes in biology and medicine: *In vitro* and *in vivo* detection, imaging and drug delivery. *Nano Res.*, *2*(2), 85–120. doi:10.1007/s12274-009-9009-8 PMID:20174481

Lohcharoenkal, W., Wang, L., Chen, Y. C., & Rojanasakul, Y. (2014). Protein nanoparticles as drug delivery carriers for cancer therapy.BioMed Research International.

Lu, H. D., Zhao, H. Q., Wang, K., & Lu-Lu, L. (2011). Novel hyaluronic acid–chitosan nanoparticles as non-viral gene delivery vectors targeting osteoarthritis. *International Journal of Pharmaceutics*, *420*(2), 358–365. doi:10.1016/j.ijpharm.2011.08.046 PMID:21911044

Luo, G., Yu, X., Jin, C., Yang, F., Fu, D., Long, J., & Lu, W. et al. (2010). LyP-1-conjugated nanoparticles for targeting drug delivery to lymphatic metastatic tumors. *International Journal of Pharmaceutics*, *385*(1-2), 150–156. doi:10.1016/j.ijpharm.2009.10.014 PMID:19825404

Luo, Y., Ling, Y., Guo, W., Pang, J., Liu, W., Fang, Y., & Gao, X. et al. (2010). Docetaxel loaded oleic acid-coated hydroxyapatite nanoparticles enhance the docetaxel-induced apoptosis through activation of caspase-2 in androgenindependent prostate cancer cells. *Journal of Controlled Release*, *147*(2), 278–288. doi:10.1016/j.jconrel.2010.07.108 PMID:20655966

Maeda, H., Wu, J., Sawa, T., Matsumura, Y., & Hori, K. (2000). Tumor vascular permeability and the EPR effect in macromolecular therapeutics: A review. *Journal of Controlled Release*, *65*(1-2), 271–284. doi:10.1016/S0168-3659(99)00248-5 PMID:10699287

Mamaeva, V., Sahlgren, C., & Lindén, M. (2013). Mesoporous silica nanoparticles in medicine- Recent advances. *Advanced Drug Delivery Reviews*, *65*(5), 689–702. doi:10.1016/j.addr.2012.07.018 PMID:22921598

Martín-Saavedra, F. M., Ruíz-Hernández, E., Boré, A., Arcos, D., Vallet-Regí, M., & Vilaboa, N. (2010). Magneticmesoporous silica spheres for hyperthermia therapy. *Acta Biomaterialia*, *6*(12), 4522–4531. doi:10.1016/j.actbio.2010.06.030 PMID:20601238

Meng, H. A., Liong, M., Xia, T., Li, Z., Ji, Z., Zink, J. I., & Nel, A. E. (2010). Engineered design of mesoporous silica nanoparticles to deliver doxorubicin & P-glycoprotein siRNA to overcome drug resistance in a cancer cell line. *ACS Nano*, *4*(8), 4539–4550. doi:10.1021/nn100690m PMID:20731437

Miyaji, F., Davis, S. A., Charmant, J. P. H., & Mann, S. (1999). Organic crystal templating of hollow silica fibers. *Chemistry of Materials*, *11*(11), 3021–3024. doi:10.1021/cm990449v

Miyazaki, M., Kaneno, J., Kohama, R., Uehara, M., Kanno, K., Fujii, M., & Maeda, H. et al. (2004). Preparation of functionalized nanostructures on micro channel surface and their use for enzyme micro reactors. *Chemical Engineering Journal*, *101*(1-3), 277–284. doi:10.1016/j.cej.2003.11.010

Mora-Huertas, C. E., Fessi, H., & Elaissari, A. (2010). Polymer-based nanocapsules for drug delivery. *International Journal of Pharmaceutics*, *385*(1-2), 113–142. doi:10.1016/j.ijpharm.2009.10.018 PMID:19825408

Müller, R. H., & Keck, C. M. (2004). Challenges and solutions for the delivery of biotech drugs – a review of drug nanocrystals technology and lipid nanoparticles. *Journal of Biotechnology, 113*(1-3), 151–170. doi:10.1016/j.jbiotec.2004.06.007 PMID:15380654

Müller, R. H., Radtke, M., & Wissing, S. A. (2002). Nanostructured lipid matrices for improved microencapsulation of drugs. *International Journal of Pharmaceutics, 242*(1-2), 121–128. doi:10.1016/S0378-5173(02)00180-1 PMID:12176234

Namgung, R., Singh, K., Yu, M. K., Jon, S., Kim, Y. S., Ahn, Y., & Kim, W. J. et al. (2010). Hybrid superparamagneticiron oxide nanoparticle-branched polyethyleniminemagnetoplexes for gene transfection of vascular endothelial cells. *Biomaterials, 31*(14), 4204–4213. doi:10.1016/j.biomaterials.2010.01.123 PMID:20170956

Owens, D. E. III, & Peppas, N. A. (2006). Opsonization, biodistribution, & pharmacokinetics of polymeric nanoparticles. *International Journal of Pharmaceutics, 307*(1), 93–102. doi:10.1016/j.ijpharm.2005.10.010 PMID:16303268

Pasqua, D. A. J., Wallner, S., Kerwood, D. J., & Dabrowiak, J. C. (2009). Adsorption of the Pt(II) anticancer drug carboplatin bymesoporous silica. *Chemistry & Biodiversity, 6*(9), 1343–1349. doi:10.1002/cbdv.200900021 PMID:19774597

Petros, R. A., & DeSimone, J. M. (2010). Strategies in the design of nanoparticles for therapeutic applications. *Nature Reviews. Drug Discovery, 9*(8), 615–627. doi:10.1038/nrd2591 PMID:20616808

Rai, M., Yadav, A., & Gade, A. (2009). Silver nanoparticles as a new generation of antimicrobials. *Biotechnology Advances, 27*(1), 76–83. doi:10.1016/j.biotechadv.2008.09.002 PMID:18854209

Roger, E., Lagarce, F., Garcion, E., & Benoit, J. P. (2010). Biopharmaceutical parameters to consider in orderto alter the fate of nanocarriers after oral delivery. *Nanomedicine, 5,* 287–306.

Saraogia, G. K., Gupta, P., Gupta, U. D., Jain, N. K., & Agrawala, G. P. (2010). Gelatin nanocarriers as potential vectors for effective management of tuberculosis. *International Journal of Pharmaceutics, 385*(1-2), 143–149. doi:10.1016/j.ijpharm.2009.10.004 PMID:19819315

Scherer, F., Anton, M., Schillinger, U., Henke, J., Bergemann, C., Kruger, A., & Plank, C. et al. (2002). Magnetofection: Enhancing and targeting gene delivery by magnetic force *in vitro* and *in vivo. Gene Therapy, 9*(2), 102–109. doi:10.1038/sj.gt.3301624 PMID:11857068

Schneider, Y., Abarca, J., Pirak, A. E., Baurain, R., Ceulemans, F., Campeneere, D. D., . . . Trouet, A. (1984). Drug targeting in human cancer chemotherapy. In Receptor-Mediated Targeting of Drugs. Springer. doi:10.1007/978-1-4684-4862-7_1

Shen, S. C., Ng, W. K., Shi, Z., Chia, L., Neoh, K. G., & Tan, R. B. H. (2011). Mesoporous silica nanoparticle-functionalized poly (methylmethacrylate)-based bone cement for effective antibiotics delivery. *Journal of Materials Science. Materials in Medicine, 22*(10), 2283–2292. doi:10.1007/s10856-011-4397-1 PMID:21786132

Shinto, Y., Uchida, A., Korkusuz, F., Araki, N., & Ono, K. (1992). Calcium hydroxyapatite ceramic used as a delivery system for antibiotics. *The Journal of Bone and Joint Surgery. British Volume*, *74*, 600–604. PMID:1320622

Singh, M., Kumar, M., Manikandan, S., Chandrasekaran, N., & Mukherjee, A. (2014). Drug delivery system for controlled cancer therapy using physico-chemically stabilized bioconjugated gold nanoparticles synthesized from marine macroalgae, *PadinaGymnospora*. *J. Nanomed Nanotechol.*, *5*, 9.

Singh, P., Gonzalez, M. J., & Manchester, M. (2006). Viruses & their uses in nanotechnology. *Drug Development Research*, *6*(1), 23–41. doi:10.1002/ddr.20064

Slowing, I., Trewyn, B. G., Giri, S., & Lin, V. S.-Y. (2007). Mesoporous silica nanoparticles for drug delivery and biosensing gapplications. *Advanced Functional Materials*, *17*(8), 1225–1236. doi:10.1002/adfm.200601191

Souto, E. B., & Muller, R. H. (2010). Lipid nanoparticles: Effect on bioavailability and pharmacokinetic changes. *Handbook of Experimental Pharmacology*, *197*, 115–141. doi:10.1007/978-3-642-00477-3_4 PMID:20217528

Speir, J.A., Munshi, S., Wang, G.J., Baker, T.S., & Johnson, J.E. (1995). Structures of the native &swollen forms of cowpea chlorotic mottle virus determined by X-ray crystallography & cryoelectron microscopy. *Structure, 3*, 63–78.

Torchilin, V. (2008). *Multifunctional Pharmaceutical Nanocarriers*. Springer Science + Business Media, LLC.

Torchilin, V. P., & Trubetskoy, V. S. (1995). Which polymers can make nanoparticulate drug carriers long-circulating. *Advanced Drug Delivery Reviews*, *16*(2-3), 141–155. doi:10.1016/0169-409X(95)00022-Y

Üner, M., & Yener, G. (2007). Importance of solid lipid nanoparticles (SLN) in various administration routes and future perspectives. *International Journal of Nanomedicine*, *2*, 289–300. PMID:18019829

Wang, A. Z., Yuet, K., Zhang, L., Gu, F. X., Huynh-Le, M., Radovic-Moreno, A. F., & Farokhzad, O. C. et al. (2010). Chemo Rad nanoparticles: A novel multifunctional nanoparticle platform for targeted delivery of concurrent chemo radiation. *Nanomedicine (London)*, *5*(3), 361–368. doi:10.2217/nnm.10.6 PMID:20394530

Wang, G., & Uludag, H. (2008). Recent developments in nanoparticle-based drug delivery and targeting systems with emphasis on protein-based nanoparticles. *Expert Opinion on Drug Delivery*, *5*(5), 499–515. doi:10.1517/17425247.5.5.499 PMID:18491978

Wei, L., Lu, J., Xu, H., Patel, A., Chen, Z., & Chen, G. (2015, May). Silver nanoparticles: Synthesis, properties, & therapeutic applications. *Drug Discovery Today*, *20*(5), 595–601. doi:10.1016/j.drudis.2014.11.014 PMID:25543008

Wu, P., Chen, X., Hu, N., Tam, U. C., Blixt, O., Zettl, A., & Bertozzi, C. R. (2008). Biocompatible Carbon Nanotubes Generated by Functionalization with Glycodendrimers. *Angewandte Chemie International Edition in English*, *47*(27), 5022–5025. doi:10.1002/anie.200705363 PMID:18509843

Xia, T. A., Kovochich, M., Liong, M., Meng, H., Kabehie, S., George, S., & Nel, A. E. et al. (2009). Polyethyleneimine coating enhances the cellular uptake of mesoporous silica nanoparticles and allows safe delivery of siRNA and DNA constructs. *ACS Nano*, *3*(10), 3273–3286. doi:10.1021/nn900918w PMID:19739605

Yu, C. C. (2013). Non-metallic nanomaterials in cancer theranostics: A review of silica- and carbon-based drug delivery systems. *Science and Technology of Advanced Materials*, *14*(4), 044407. doi:10.1088/1468-6996/14/4/044407

Yuan, X. B., Yuan, Y., Jiang, W., Liu, J., Tian, E., Shun, H., & Sheng, J. et al. (2008). Preparation of rapamycin-loaded chitosan/PLA nanoparticles for immunosuppression in corneal transplantation. *International Journal of Pharmaceutics*, *349*(1-2), 241–248. doi:10.1016/j.ijpharm.2007.07.045 PMID:17919859

Zhanga, H., Xiaolin, L. A., Jing, D., Xu, H., & Daid, X. (2013). Delivery of ursolic acid in polymeric nanoparticles effectively promotesthe apoptosis of gastric cancer cells through enhanced inhibition of cyclooxygenase 2. *International Journal of Pharmaceutics*, *441*(1-2), 261–268. doi:10.1016/j.ijpharm.2012.11.034 PMID:23194884

Zhen, X., Wang, X., Xie, C., Wu, W., & Jiang, X. (2013). Cellular uptake,antitumor response and tumor penetration of cisplatin-loaded milk protein nanoparticles. *Biomaterials*, *34*(4), 1372–1382. doi:10.1016/j.biomaterials.2012.10.061 PMID:23158934

Zhou, F., Xing, D., Ou, Z., Wu, B., Resasco, D. E., & Chen, W. R. (2009). Cancer photothermal therapy in the near-infra red region by using single-walled carbon nanotubes. *Journal of Biomedical Optics*, *14*(2), 021009. doi:10.1117/1.3078803 PMID:19405722

Compilation of References

Aagaard, L., & Rossi, J. J. (2007). RNAi therapeutics: Principles, prospects and challenges. *Advanced Drug Delivery Reviews*, *59*(2), 75–86. doi:10.1016/j.addr.2007.03.005 PMID:17449137

Aathimanikandan, S. V., Savariar, E. N., & Thayumanavan, S. (2005). Temperature-sensitive dendritic micelles. *Journal of the American Chemical Society*, *127*(42), 14922–14929. doi:10.1021/ja054542y PMID:16231948

Abdallah, M. H., Omaima, A., Sammour, H., Ghamry, E., & Mohammed, E. (2013). Design and development of piroxicam-entrapped niosomes as an oral drug delivery system. *International Journal of Advances in Pharmaceutical Research*, *4*(6), 205–215.

Abdelaziz, A. A., Elbanna, T. E., Sonbol, F. I., Gamaleldin, N. M., & El Maghraby, G. M. (2015). Optimization of niosomes for enhanced antibacterial activity and reduced bacterial resistance: in vitro and in vivo evaluation. *Expert Opinion on Drug Delivery*, *12*(2).163-180.

Abdelbary, G., & El-gendy, N. (2008). Niosome-encapsulated gentamicin for ophthalmic controlled delivery. *AAPS PharmSciTech*, *9*(3), 740–747. doi:10.1208/s12249-008-9105-1 PMID:18563578

Abdelkader, H., Ismail, S., Hussein, A., Wu, Z., Al-Kassas, R., & Alany, R. G. (2012). Conjunctival and corneal tolerability assessment of ocular naltrexone niosomes and their ingredients on the hen's egg chorioallantoic membrane and excised bovine cornea models. *International Journal of Pharmaceutics*, *432*(1-2), 1–10. doi:10.1016/j.ijpharm.2012.04.063 PMID:22575752

Abdelkader, H., Ismail, S., Kamal, A., & Alany, R. G. (2010). Preparation of niosomes as an ocular delivery system for naltrexone hydrochloride: Physicochemical characterization. *Die Pharmazie-An International Journal of Pharmaceutical Sciences*, *65*(11), 811–817. PMID:21155387

Abdelkader, H., Ismail, S., Kamal, A., & Alany, R. G. (2011). Design and evaluation of controlled-release niosomes and discomes for naltrexone hydrochloride ocular delivery. *Journal of Pharmaceutical Sciences*, *100*(5), 1833–1846. doi:10.1002/jps.22422 PMID:21246556

Abdel-Mottaleb, M. M., Neumann, D., & Lamprecht, A. (2011). Lipid nanocapsules for dermal application: A comparative study of lipid-based versus polymer-based nanocarriers. *European Journal of Pharmaceutics and Biopharmaceutics*, *79*(1), 36–42. doi:10.1016/j.ejpb.2011.04.009 PMID:21558002

Abdul-Fatta, A., Zhang, J., Bennett, D. B., & Ballesteros Lechuga, D. (2003). Characterization of spray-dried powders in the liquid crystalline state. *Journal of Pharmaceutical Sciences*, *4*, 1286–1289.

Aboubakar, M., Couvreur, P., Pinto-Alphandary, H., Gouritin, B., Lacour, B., Farinotti, R., & Vauthier, C. et al. (2000). Insulin-loaded nanocapsules for oral administration: In vitro and in vivo investigation. *Drug Development Research*, *49*(2), 109–117. doi:10.1002/(SICI)1098-2299(200002)49:2<109::AID-DDR4>3.0.CO;2-#

Aboubakar, M., Puisieux, F., Couvreur, P., Deyme, M., & Vauthier, C. (1999). Study of the mechanism of insulin encapsulation in poly(isobutylcyanoacrylate) nanocapsules obtained by interfacial polymerization. *Journal of Biomedical Materials Research*, *47*(4), 568–576. doi:10.1002/(SICI)1097-4636(19991215)47:4<568::AID-JBM14>3.0.CO;2-X PMID:10497293

Abraham, S. A., Waterhouse, D. N., Mayer, L. D., Cullis, P. R., Madden, T. D., & Bally, M. B. (2005). The liposomal formulation of doxorubicin. *Methods in Enzymology*, *391*, 71–97. doi:10.1016/S0076-6879(05)91004-5 PMID:15721375

Abu Hashim, I. I., El-dahan, M. S., Yusif, R. M., Abd-ElGawad, A. E. H., & Arima, H. (2014). Potential use of niosomal hydrogel as an ocular delivery system for atenolol. *Biological & Pharmaceutical Bulletin*, *37*(4), 541–551. doi:10.1248/bpb.b13-00724 PMID:24694602

Adams, M. L., Lavasanifar, A., & Kwon, G. S. (2003). Amphiphilic block copolymers for drug delivery. *Journal of Pharmaceutical Sciences*, *92*(7), 1343–1355. doi:10.1002/jps.10397 PMID:12820139

Adhikari, T., Kundu, S., & Rao, A. S. (2013). Impact of SiO2 and Mo Nano Particles on Seed Germination of Rice (Oryza Sativa L.). *Int J Agric Food Sci Tec*, *4*, 809–816.

Adibkia, K. (2014). Preparation of Pharmaceutical Nanobeads and Nanofibers via Electrospinning Method. *J Mol Pharm Org Process Res*, *2*(01), e112. doi:10.4172/2329-9053.1000e112

Afrooz, A. R. M. N., Hussain, S. M., & Saleh, N. B. (2015). Erratum to: Aggregate size and structure determination of nanomaterials in physiological media: importance of dynamic evolution. *Journal of Nanoparticle Research*, *17*(5), 232–243. doi:10.1007/s11051-015-2933-5

Afroze, F., Nies, E., & Berghmans, H. (2000). Phase transitions in the system poly (*N*-isopropylacrylamide)/water and swelling behaviour of the corresponding networks. *Journal of Molecular Structure*, *554*(1), 55–68. doi:10.1016/S0022-2860(00)00559-7

Aggarwal, D., Garg, A., & Kaur, I. P. (2004). Development of a topical niosomal preparation of acetazolamide: Preparation and evaluation. *The Journal of Pharmacy and Pharmacology*, *56*(12), 1509–1517. doi:10.1211/0022357044896 PMID:15563757

Aggarwal, D., Pal, D., Mitra, A. K., & Kaur, I. P. (2007). Study of the extent of ocular absorption of acetazolamide from a developed niosomal formulation, by microdialysis sampling of aqueous humor. *International Journal of Pharmaceutics*, *338*(1), 21–26. doi:10.1016/j.ijpharm.2007.01.019 PMID:17300885

Aguilar, M. R., Elvira, C., Gallardo, A., Vázquez, B., & Román, J. S. (2007). Smart polymers and their applications as biomaterials. Topics in Tissue Engineering, 3(6).

Ahmad, H., Nurunnabi, M., Rahman, M. M., Kumar, K., Tauer, K., Minami, H., & Gafur, M. A. (2014). Magnetically doped multi stimuli-responsive hydrogel microspheres with IPN structure and application in dye removal. *Colloids and Surfaces. A, Physicochemical and Engineering Aspects*, *459*, 39–47. doi:10.1016/j.colsurfa.2014.06.038

Ahmed, A. M., Ghourab, M. M., Shedid, S. G., & Qushawy, M. K. (2013). Optimization of piroxicam niosomes using central composite design. *International Journal of Pharmacy and Pharmaceutical Sciences*, *5*(3), 229–236.

Ahmed, A., Barry, B. W., Williams, A. C., & Davis, A. F. (2004). Pencyclovir solubility in Eudragit films: A comparison of x-ray, thermal, microscopic and release rate techniques. *Journal of Pharmaceutical and Biomedical Analysis*, *34*(5), 945–956. doi:10.1016/j.jpba.2003.11.018 PMID:15019028

Ahola, M. S., Säilynoja, E. S., Raitavuo, M. H., Vaahtio, M. M., Salonen, J. I., & Yli-Urpo, A. U. (2001). In vitro release of heparin from silica xerogels. *Biomaterials*, *22*(15), 2163–2170. doi:10.1016/S0142-9612(00)00407-5 PMID:11432596

Aiello, C., Andreozzi, P., La Mesa, C., & Risuleo, G. (2010). Biological activity of SDS-CTAB cat-anionic vesicles in cultured cells and assessment of their cytotoxicity ending in apoptosis. *Colloids and Surfaces. B, Biointerfaces*, *78*(2), 149–154. doi:10.1016/j.colsurfb.2010.02.013 PMID:20347276

Akbari, V., Abedi, D., Pardakhty, A., & Sadeghi-Aliabadi, H. (2013). Ciprofloxacin nano-niosomes for targeting intracellular infections: An in vitro evaluation. *Journal of Nanoparticle Research*, *15*(4), 1–14. doi:10.1007/s11051-013-1556-y

Akbari, V., Abedi, D., Pardakhty, A., & Sadeghi-Aliabadi, H. (2015). Release Studies on Ciprofloxacin Loaded Non-ionic Surfactant Vesicles. *Avicenna Journal of Medical Biotechnology*, *7*(2), 69–75. PMID:26140184

Akbarzadeh, A., Rezaei-Sadabady, R., Davaran, S., Joo, S. W., Zarghami, N., Hanifehpour, Y., & Nejati-Koshki, K. (2013). Liposome: Classification, preparation, and applications. *Nanoscale Research Letters*, *8*(1), 102. PMID:23432972

Akhter, S., Kushwaha, S., Warsi, M. H., Anwar, M., Ahmad, M. Z., Ahmad, I., & Ahmad, F. J. et al. (2012). Development and evaluation of nanosized niosomal dispersion for oral delivery of Ganciclovir. *Drug Development and Industrial Pharmacy*, *38*(1), 84–92. doi:10.3109/03639045.2011.592529 PMID:21726136

Alami, N., Banerjee, K., Page, V., Hayashi, T., Igarashi, E., & Leyland-Jones, B. (2005). Long term survival with no apparent toxicity observed with a novel cisplatin-incorporated polymeric micelle, NC-6004, in the MCF-7 breast cancer model. *Breast Cancer Research and Treatment*, *94*, S64–S65.

Alam, M. M., Oka, T., Ohta, N., & Yamazaki, M. (2011). Kinetics of low pH-induced lamellar to bicontinuous cubic phase transition in dioleoyl phosphatidyl serine/monoolein. *The Journal of Chemical Physics*, *134*(14), 145102. doi:10.1063/1.3575240 PMID:21495771

Alexandridis, P., Zhou, D., & Khan, A. (1996). *Lyotropic liquid crystallinity in amphiphilic block copolymers: temperature effect on phase behavior and structure copolymers of different composition*. Academic Press.

Alexis, F., Rhee, J. W., Richie, J. P., Radovic-Moreno, A. F., Langer, R., & Farokhzad, O. (2008). New frontiers in nanotechnology for cancer treatment. *Urologic Oncology*, *26*(1), 74–85. doi:10.1016/j.urolonc.2007.03.017 PMID:18190835

Al-Jamal, W. T., & Kostarelos, K. (2011). Liposomes: From a clinically established drug delivery system to a nanoparticle platform for theranostic nanomedicine. *Accounts of Chemical Research*, *44*(10), 1094–1104. doi:10.1021/ar200105p PMID:21812415

Alle'man, E., Doelker, E., & Gurny, R. (1992). Preparation of aqueous polymeric nanodispersions by a reversible salting-out process, influence of process parameters on particle size. *International Journal of Pharmaceutics*, *87*(1-3), 247–253. doi:10.1016/0378-5173(92)90249-2

Allen, T. M., & Cullis, P. R. (2013). Liposomal drug delivery systems: From concept to clinical applications. *Advanced Drug Delivery Reviews*, *65*(1), 36–48. doi:10.1016/j.addr.2012.09.037 PMID:23036225

Allen, T. M., Hansen, C. B., & de Menezes, D. E. L. (1995). Pharmacokinetics of long-circulating liposomes. *Advanced Drug Delivery Reviews*, *16*(2), 267–284. doi:10.1016/0169-409X(95)00029-7

Allen, T. M., Hansen, C., & Rutledge, J. (1989). Liposomes with prolonged circulation times: Factors affecting uptake by reticuloendothelial and other tissues. *Biochimica et Biophysica Acta (BBA)-. Biomembranes*, *981*(1), 27–35. doi:10.1016/0005-2736(89)90078-3

Almutairi, A., Rossin, R., Shokeen, M., Hagooly, A., Ananth, A., Capoccia, B., & Fréchet, J. M. J. et al. (2009). Biodegradable dendritic positron-emitting nanoprobes for the noninvasive imaging of angiogenesis. *Proceedings of the National Academy of Sciences of the United States of America*, *106*(3), 685–690. doi:10.1073/pnas.0811757106 PMID:19129498

Alomrani, A. H., Al-Agamy, M. H., & Badran, M. M. (2015). In vitro skin penetration and antimycotic activity of itraconazole loaded niosomes: Various non-ionic surfactants. *Journal of Drug Delivery Science and Technology*, *28*, 37–45. doi:10.1016/j.jddst.2015.04.009

Alsarra, I. A., Bosela, A., Ahmed, S., & Mahrous, G. (2005). Proniosomes as a drug carrier for transdermal delivery of ketorolac. *European Journal of Pharmaceutics and Biopharmaceutics*, *59*(3), 485–490. doi:10.1016/j.ejpb.2004.09.006 PMID:15760729

Alvarez-Lorenzo, C., Bromberg, L., & Concheiro, A. (2009). Light-sensitive intelligent drug delivery systems. *Photochemistry and Photobiology*, *85*(4), 848–860. doi:10.1111/j.1751-1097.2008.00530.x PMID:19222790

Alvi, I. A., Madan, J., Kaushik, D., Sardana, S., Pandey, R. S., & Ali, A. (2011). Comparative study of transfersomes, liposomes, and niosomes for topical delivery of 5-fluorouracil to skin cancer cells: Preparation, characterization, in-vitro release, and cytotoxicity analysis. *Anti-Cancer Drugs*, *22*(8), 774–782. doi:10.1097/CAD.0b013e328346c7d6 PMID:21799471

Amanatfard, A., Khazaeli, P., Pardakhty, A., Najafi, M. L., & Mohammadi, A. (2015). Preparation and characterization of physicochemical properties of N, N-diethyl-meta-toluamide niosomes. *International Journal of Pharmaceutical Investigation*, *5*(4), 259–265. doi:10.4103/2230-973X.167691 PMID:26682196

Amar Yuli, I., & Garti, N. (2005). Transitions induced by solubilized fat into reverse hexagonal mesophases. *Colloids and Surfaces. B, Biointerfaces*, *43*(2), 72–82. doi:10.1016/j.colsurfb.2005.03.011 PMID:15921902

Amato, G. (2010). Silica-encapsulated efficient and stable Si quantum dots with high biocompatibility. *Nanoscale Research Letters*, *5*(7), 1156–1160. doi:10.1007/s11671-010-9619-9 PMID:20596494

Amselem, S., Gabizon, A., & Barenholz, Y. (1993). A large-scale method for the preparation of sterile and non-pyrogenic liposomal formulations of defined size distributions for clinical use. *Liposome Technology, 1*, 501-525.

Anderson, D., & Schindler, J. (2014). *U.S. Patent Application 14/213,808*. Washington, DC: U.S. Patent and Trademark Office.

Andolina, C. M., Klemm, P. J., Floyd, W. C. III, Fréchet, J. M., & Raymond, K. N. (2012). Analysis of lanthanide complex dendrimer conjugates for bimodal NIR and MRI imaging. *Macromolecules*, *45*(22), 8982–8990. doi:10.1021/ma302206g PMID:23226878

Andrady, A. L. (2008). *Science and technology of polymer nanofibers*. John Wiley & Sons. doi:10.1002/9780470229842

Ansel, H. C., Allen, L. V., & Popovich, N. G. (1999). Pharmaceutical dosage forms and drug delivery systems. Philadelphia: Lippincott Williams and Wilkins.

Antonietti, M., & Förster, S. (2003). Vesicles and liposomes: A self-assembly principle beyond lipids. *Advanced Materials*, *15*(16), 1323–1333. doi:10.1002/adma.200300010

APG. (2011). *Procurement and prescribing practices for biologics in the UK*. APG.

Aprahamian, M., Michel, C., Humbert, W., Devissaguet, J. P., & Damge, C. (1987). Transmucosal passage of polyalkylcyanoacrylate nanocapsules as a new drug carrier in the small intestine. *Biology of the Cell*, *61*(1-2), 69–76. doi:10.1111/j.1768-322X.1987.tb00571.x PMID:2833966

Araújo, F., Kelmann, R., Araujo, B., Finatto, R., Teixeira, H., & Koester, L. (2011). Development and characterization of parenteral nanoemulsions containing thalidomide. *European Journal of Pharmaceutical Sciences*, *42*(3), 238–245. doi:10.1016/j.ejps.2010.11.014 PMID:21130164

Armes, S. P., Madsen, P. J., Vo, C.-D., & Li, C. (2007). *WO Patent Application 07/063320.*

Arnardottir, H. B., Sveinsson, S. L., & Kristmundsdottir, T. (1995). The use of a high intensity ultrasonic processor equipped with a flow cell in the production of reverse-phase liposomes. *International Journal of Pharmaceutics*, *117*(2), 237–241. doi:10.1016/0378-5173(94)00356-A

Aronoff, D. M., & Neilson, E. G. (2001). Antipyretics: Mechanisms of action and clinical use in fever suppression. *The American Journal of Medicine*, *111*(4), 304–315. doi:10.1016/S0002-9343(01)00834-8 PMID:11566461

Arruebo, M., Fernández-Pacheco, R., Ibarra, M. R., & Santamaría, J. (2007). Magnetic nanoparticles for drug delivery. *Nano Today*, *2*(3), 22–32. doi:10.1016/S1748-0132(07)70084-1

Arunothayanun, P., Bernard, M. S., Craig, D., Uchegbu, I., & Florence, A. (2000). The effect of processing variables on the physical characteristics of non-ionic surfactant vesicles (niosomes) formed from a hexadecyl diglycerol ether. *International Journal of Pharmaceutics*, *201*(1), 7–14. doi:10.1016/S0378-5173(00)00362-8 PMID:10867260

Arunothayanun, P., Turton, J. A., Uchegbu, I. F., & Florence, A. T. (1999). Preparation and in vitro/in vivo evaluation of luteinizing hormone releasing hormone (LHRH)-loaded polyhedral and spherical/tubular niosomes. *Journal of Pharmaceutical Sciences*, *88*(1), 34–38. doi:10.1021/js980286u PMID:9874699

Arzani, G., Haeri, A., Daeihamed, M., Bakhtiari-Kaboutaraki, H., & Dadashzadeh, S. (2015). Niosomal carriers enhance oral bioavailability of carvedilol: Effects of bile salt-enriched vesicles and carrier surface charge. *International Journal of Nanomedicine*, *10*, 4797. PMID:26251598

Asadi, A. P., Moshafi, M., & Sharifi, M. I. (2012). Preparation and in vivo administration of paromomycin niosomes in balb/c mice. *Research in Pharmaceutical Sciences*, *7*(5), S373.

Ashley, G. W., Santi, D. V., & Henise, J. C. (2012). *U.S. Patent Application 14/343,819*. Washington, DC: U.S. Patent and Trademark Office.

Astruc, D., Boisselier, E., & Ornelas, C. (2010). Dendrimers Designed for Functions: From Physical, Photophysical, and Supramolecular Properties to Applications in Sensing, Catalysis, Molecular Electronics, Photonics, and Nanomedicine. *Chemical Reviews*, *110*(4), 1857–1959. doi:10.1021/cr900327d PMID:20356105

Attama, A., Schicke, B., Paepenmüller, T., & Müller-Goymann, C. (2007). Solid lipid nanodispersions containing mixed lipid core and a polar heterolipid: Characterization. *European Journal of Pharmaceutics and Biopharmaceutics*, *67*(1), 48–57. doi:10.1016/j.ejpb.2006.12.004 PMID:17276663

Attia, I. A., El-Gizawy, S. A., Fouda, M. A., & Donia, A. M. (2007). Influence of a niosomal formulation on the oral bioavailability of acyclovir in rabbits. *AAPS PharmSciTech*, *8*(4), 206–212. doi:10.1208/pt0804106 PMID:18181527

Atyabi, F., Khodaverdi, E., & Dinarvand, R. (2007). Temeperature modulated drug permeation through liquid crystal embedded cellulose membranes. *International Journal of Pharmaceutics*, *339*(1-2), 213–221. doi:10.1016/j.ijpharm.2007.03.004 PMID:17448615

Awad, T. S., Okamoto, Y., Masum, S. M., & Yamazaki, M. (2005). Formation of cubic phases from large unilamellar vesicles of dioleoylphosphatidylglycerol/monoolein membranes induced by low concentrations of Ca^{2+}. *Langmuir*, *21*(25), 11556–11561. doi:10.1021/la051782i PMID:16316079

Aynie, I., Vauthier, C., Chacun, H., Fattal, E., & Couvreur, P. (1999). Spongelike alginate nanoparticles as a new potential system for the delivery of antisense oligonucleotides. antisense. *Nucleic Acid Drug Dev*, *9*(3), 301–312. doi:10.1089/oli.1.1999.9.301 PMID:10435755

Azagarsamy, M. A., Yesilyurt, V., & Thayumanavan, S. (2010). Disassembly of dendritic micellar containers due to protein binding. *Journal of the American Chemical Society*, *132*(13), 4550–4551. doi:10.1021/ja100746d PMID:20232866

Babu, S., Fan, C., Stepanskiy, L., Uitto, J., & Papazoglou, E. (2009). Effect of size at the nanoscale and bilayer rigidity on skin diffusion of liposomes. *Journal of Biomedical Materials Research. Part A*, *91*(1), 140–148. doi:10.1002/jbm.a.32197 PMID:18770522

Bae, Y. H., & Kim, S. W. (1993). *U.S. Patent No. 5,262,055*. Washington, DC: U.S. Patent and Trademark Office.

Bae, Y. H., & Park, S. Y. (2000). *U.S. Patent No. 6,103,865*. Washington, DC: U.S. Patent and Trademark Office.

Baillie, A., Florence, A., Hume, L., Muirhead, G., & Rogerson, A. (1985). The preparation and properties of niosomes--non-ionic surfactant vesicles. *The Journal of Pharmacy and Pharmacology*, *37*(12), 863–868. doi:10.1111/j.2042-7158.1985.tb04990.x PMID:2868092

Bajpai, S. K., & Saxena, S. (2004). Enzymatically degradable and pH-sensitive hydrogels for colon-targeted oral drug delivery. I. Synthesis and characterization. *Journal of Applied Polymer Science*, *92*(6), 3630–3643. doi:10.1002/app.20283

Baker, S. C., Atkin, N., Gunning, P. A., Granville, N., Wilson, K., Wilson, D., & Southgate, J. (2006). Characterisation of electrospun polystyrene scaffolds for three-dimensional in vitro biological studies. *Biomaterials*, *27*(16), 3136–3146. doi:10.1016/j.biomaterials.2006.01.026 PMID:16473404

Balakrishnan, P., Shanmugam, S., Lee, W. S., Lee, W. M., Kim, J. O., Oh, D. H., & Choi, H. G. et al. (2009). Formulation and in vitro assessment of minoxidil niosomes for enhanced skin delivery. *International Journal of Pharmaceutics*, *377*(1), 1–8. doi:10.1016/j.ijpharm.2009.04.020 PMID:19394413

Balivada, S., Rachakatla, R. S., Wang, H., Samarakoon, T. N., Dani, R. K., Pyle, M., & Troyer, D. L. et al. (2010). A/C magnetic hyperthermia of melanoma mediated by iron(0)/iron oxide core/shell magnetic nanoparticles:A mouse study. *BMC Cancer*, *10*(1), 119. doi:10.1186/1471-2407-10-119 PMID:20350328

Ballatori, N., Krance, S. M., Notenboom, S., Shi, S., Tieu, K., & Hammond, C. L. (2009). Glutathione dysregulation and the etiology and progression of human diseases. *Biological Chemistry*, *390*(3), 191–214. doi:10.1515/BC.2009.033 PMID:19166318

Bally, M. B., Mayer, L. D., Loughrey, H., Redelmeier, T., Madden, T. D., Wong, K., & Cullis, P. R. et al. (1988). Dopamine accumulation in large unilamellar vesicle systems induced by transmembrane ion gradients. *Chemistry and Physics of Lipids*, *47*(2), 97–107. doi:10.1016/0009-3084(88)90078-3 PMID:2457454

Bal, T., Murthy, P. N., & Sengupta, S. (2012). Preparation and evaluation of mucoadhesive simvastatin microcapsules using orifice gelation technique. *Asian Journal of Pharmaceutics*, *6*(1), 74. doi:10.4103/0973-8398.100152

Bangham, A. (1982). Techniques in the Life Science, B4/11. *Lipid and Membrane Biochemistry B*, *420*, 1–25.

Bangham, A. D., Hill, M. V., & Miller, N. G. (1974). Methods in cell biology. *The Journal of Membrane Biology*, *1*, 1–68.

Bangham, A. D., & Horne, R. (1964). Negative staining of phospholipids and their structural modification by surface-active agents as observed in the electron microscope. *Journal of Molecular Biology*, *8*(5), 660–IN610. doi:10.1016/S0022-2836(64)80115-7 PMID:14187392

Bangham, A. D., Standish, M. M., & Watkins, J. C. (1965). Diffusion of univalent ions across the lamellae of swollen phospholipids. *Journal of Molecular Biology*, *13*(1), 238–252. doi:10.1016/S0022-2836(65)80093-6 PMID:5859039

Bangham, A., Standish, M., & Weissmann, G. (1965). The action of steroids and streptolysin S on the permeability of phospholipid structures to cations. *Journal of Molecular Biology*, *13*(1), 253–IN228. doi:10.1016/S0022-2836(65)80094-8 PMID:5859040

Ban, J. F., Lu, S. R., & Zhang, C. X. (2010). Synthesis and characterization of biphenylnate liquid crystalline polyurethanes. *Key Engineering Materials*, *428-429*, 158–161. doi:10.4028/www.scientific.net/KEM.428-429.158

Banker, G. S., Siepmann, J., & Rhodes, C. (2002). *Modern pharmaceutics*. CRC Press. doi:10.1201/9780824744694

Bansal,S.(n.d.) A Comparative Review On Vesicular Drug Delivery System and Stability Issues. *International Journal of Research in Pharmacy and Chemistry*, *4*, 704.

Barata, T. S., Shaunak, S., Teo, I., Zloh, M., & Brocchini, S. (2011). Structural studies of biologically active glycosylated polyamidoamine (PAMAM) dendrimers. *Journal of Molecular Modeling*, *17*(8), 2051–2060. doi:10.1007/s00894-010-0907-1 PMID:21161557

Barauskas, J., Johnsson, M., & Tiberg, F. (2005). Self-assembled lipid superstructures: Beyond vesicles and liposome. *Nano Letters*, *5*(8), 1615–1619. doi:10.1021/nl050678i PMID:16089498

Barauskas, J., & Landh, T. (2003). Phase behavior of the phytantriol/water system. *Langmuir*, *19*(23), 9562–9565. doi:10.1021/la0350812

Bardajee, G. R., Hooshyar, Z., Asli, M. J., Shahidi, F. E., & Dianatnejad, N. (2014). Synthesis of a novel supermagnetic iron oxide nanocomposite hydrogel based on graft copolymerization of poly((2-dimethylamino)ethyl methacrylate) onto salep for controlled release of drug. *Materials Science and Engineering C*, *36*, 277–286. doi:10.1016/j.msec.2013.11.022 PMID:24433913

Bareford, L. M., & Swaan, P. W. (2007). Endocytic mechanisms for targeted drug delivery. *Advanced Drug Delivery Reviews*, *59*(8), 748–758. doi:10.1016/j.addr.2007.06.008 PMID:17659804

Barenholz, Y. (2001). Liposome application: Problems and prospects. *Current Opinion in Colloid & Interface Science*, *6*(1), 66–77. doi:10.1016/S1359-0294(00)00090-X

Barenholz, Y. C. (2012). Doxil®—the first FDA-approved nano-drug: Lessons learned. *Journal of Controlled Release*, *160*(2), 117–134. doi:10.1016/j.jconrel.2012.03.020 PMID:22484195

Barratt, G., Puisieux, F., Yu, W. P., Foucher, C., Fessi, H., & Devissaguet, J. P. (1994). Anti-metastatic activity of MDPL-alanyl-cholesterol incorporated into various types of nanocapsules. *International Journal of Immunopharmacology*, *16*(5-6), 457–461. doi:10.1016/0192-0561(94)90036-1 PMID:7927993

Barraud, L., Merle, P., Soma, E., Lefrançois, L., Guerret, S., Chevallier, M., & Vitvitski, L. et al. (2005). Increase of doxorubicin sensitivity by doxorubicin-loading into nanoparticles for hepatocellular carcinoma cells in vitro and in vivo. *Journal of Hepatology*, *42*(5), 736–743. doi:10.1016/j.jhep.2004.12.035 PMID:15826724

Barreto, J. A., O'Malley, W., Kubeil, M., Graham, B., Stephan, H., & Spiccia, L. (2011). Nanomaterials: Applications in cancer imaging and therapy. *Advanced Materials*, *23*(12), H18–H40. doi:10.1002/adma.201100140 PMID:21433100

Barrett, C. J., Mamiya, J. I., Yager, K. G., & Ikeda, T. (2007). Photo-mechanical effects in azobenzene-containing soft materials. *Soft Matter*, *3*(10), 1249–1261. doi:10.1039/b705619b

Bartlett, G. R. J. (1959). Purification of polysaccharide-protein conjugate vaccines by ultrafiltration with ammonium sulfate solutions. *The Journal of Biological Chemistry*, *234*, 466. PMID:13641241

Barua, S., Ramos, J., Potta, T., Taylor, D., Huang, H.-C., Montanez, G., & Rege, K. (2011). Discovery of cationic polymers for non-viral gene delivery using combinatorial approaches. *Combinatorial Chemistry & High Throughput Screening*, *14*(10), 908–924. doi:10.2174/138620711797537076 PMID:21843141

Barzegar-Jalali, M., Adibkia, K., Valizadeh, H., Shadbad, M. R. S., Nokhodchi, A., Omidi, Y., & Hasan, M. et al. (2008). Kinetic analysis of drug release from nanoparticles. *Journal of Pharmacy & Pharmaceutical Sciences*, *11*(1), 167–177. doi:10.18433/J3D59T PMID:18471378

Batzre, S., & Korn, E. D. (1973). Single bilayer liposomes prepared without sonication. *Biochimica et Biophysica Acta*, *298*(4), 1015–1019. doi:10.1016/0005-2736(73)90408-2 PMID:4738145

Bawa, P., Pillay, V., Choonara, Y. E., & Du Toit, L. C. (2009). Stimuli-responsive polymers and their applications in drug delivery. *Biomedical Materials (Bristol, England)*, *4*(2), 022001. doi:10.1088/1748-6041/4/2/022001 PMID:19261988

Bayindir, Z. S., & Yuksel, N. (2010). Characterization of niosomes prepared with various nonionic surfactants for paclitaxel oral delivery. *Journal of Pharmaceutical Sciences*, *99*(4), 2049–2060. doi:10.1002/jps.21944 PMID:19780133

Beg, S., Rizwan, M., Sheikh, A. M., Hasnain, M. S., Anwer, K., & Kohli, K. (2011). Advancement in carbon nanotubes: Basics, biomedical applications and toxicity. *The Journal of Pharmacy and Pharmacology*, *63*(2), 141–163. doi:10.1111/j.2042-7158.2010.01167.x PMID:21235578

Bendas, E. R., Abdullah, H., El-Komy, M. H., & Kassem, M. A. (2013). Hydroxychloroquine niosomes: A new trend in topical management of oral lichen planus. *International Journal of Pharmaceutics*, *458*(2), 287–295. doi:10.1016/j.ijpharm.2013.10.042 PMID:24184035

Bender, J., Ericson, M. B., Merclin, N., Iani, V., Rosén, A., Engström, S., & Moan, J. (2005). Lipid cubic phases for improved topical drug delivery in photodynamic therapy. *Journal of Controlled Release*, *106*(3), 350–360. doi:10.1016/j.jconrel.2005.05.010 PMID:15967535

Bender, J., Simonsson, C., Smedh, M., Engstrom, S., & Ericson, M. B. (2008). Lipid cubic phases in topical drug delivery: Visualization of skin distribution using two-photon microscopy. *Journal of Controlled Release*, *129*(3), 163–169. doi:10.1016/j.jconrel.2008.04.020 PMID:18538886

Bennett, D., Cabot, K., Foster, L., Lechuga-Ballesteros, D., & Tan, T. (1999). *Liquid crystal forms of cyclosporin.* US Patent Application 990352, WO 99/42124.

Benson, H. A. (2006). Transfersomes for transdermal drug delivery. *Expert Opinion on Drug Delivery*, *3*(6), 727–737. doi:10.1517/17425247.3.6.727 PMID:17076595

Benvegnu, T., Lemiègre, L., & Cammas-Marion, S. (2009). New generation of liposomes called archaeosomes based on natural or synthetic archaeal lipids as innovative formulations for drug delivery. *Recent Patents on Drug Delivery & Formulation*, *3*(3), 206–220. doi:10.2174/187221109789105630 PMID:19534669

Berry, C. C., & Curtis, A. S. G. (2003). Functionalisation of magnetic nanoparticles for applications in biomedicine. *Journal of Physics. D, Applied Physics*, *36*(13), R198–R206. doi:10.1088/0022-3727/36/13/203

Bertrand, N., & Leroux, J. C. (2011). The journey of a drug carrier in the body: An anatomo-physiological perspective. *Journal of Controlled Release*, *161*(2), 152–163. doi:10.1016/j.jconrel.2011.09.098 PMID:22001607

Bhadra, D., Bhadra, S., Jain, S., & Jain, N. (2003). A PEGylated dendritic nanoparticulate carrier of fluorouracil. *International Journal of Pharmaceutics*, *257*(1), 111–124. doi:10.1016/S0378-5173(03)00132-7 PMID:12711167

Bhandari, U., Jain, N., & Pillai, K. K. (2007). Further studies on antioxidant potential and protection of pancreatic beta-cells by Embelia ribes in experimental diabetes. *Experimental Diabetes Research*, 15803–15808. PMID:17641739

Bhatia, A., & Kumar, R. (2004). Tamoxifen in topical liposomes: Development, characterization and in-vitro evaluation. *Journal of Pharmaceutical Sciences*, *7*(2), 252–259. PMID:15367383

Bhirde, A. A., Patel, V., Gavard, J., Zhang, G., Sousa, A. A., Masedunskas, A., & Rusling, J. F. et al. (2009). Targeted killing of cancer cells in vivo and in vitro with EGF-directed carbon nanotube-based drug delivery. *ACS Nano*, *3*(2), 307–316. doi:10.1021/nn800551s PMID:19236065

Bhise, S. D. (2011). Ternary solid dispersions of fenofibrate with Poloxamer 188 and TPGS for enhancement of solubility and bioavailability. *Int J Res Pharm Biomed Sci*, *2*(2), 583–595.

Bhowmik, D., Chiranjib, C. R., & Jayakar, B. (2009). Role of nanotechnology in novel drug delivery system. *Journal of Pharmaceutical Science and Technology*, *1*(1), 20–35.

Biju, S. S., Taleganokar, S., Misra, P. R., & Khar, R. K. (2006). Vesicular systems: An overview. *Indian Journal of Pharmaceutical Sciences*, *68*(2), 141–153. doi:10.4103/0250-474X.25707

Biju, S.S., Talegaonkar, S., & Mishra, P.R., Khar & K.R. (2009). Vesicular System: An overveiw. *Indian Journal of Pharmaceutical Sciences*, *71*(4), 421–427. PMID:20502548

Biosimilars Market Product (BMP) [Recombinant Non-Glycosylated Proteins (Insulin, Filgrastim, Somatropin), Glycosylated (Monoclonal Antibodies, Erythropoietin), Peptides (Glucagon, Calcitonin)] & Application (Oncology, Blood Disorders) - Global Forecast to 2018. (n.d.). Retrieved from http://www.marketsandmarkets.com/Market-Reports/biosimilars-40.html

Biosimilarsnews.com. (2012). *Ranbaxy will boost biosimilar business*. Retrieved from www.biosimilarnews.com/ranbaxy-will-boost-biosimilar-business

Birrenbach, G., & Speiser, P. (1976). Polymerized micelles and their use as adjuvants in immunology. *Journal of Pharmaceutical Sciences*, *65*(12), 1763–1766. doi:10.1002/jps.2600651217 PMID:1036442

Bladé, J., Sonneveld, P., San Miguel, J. F., Sutherland, H. J., Hajek, R., Nagler, A., & Zhuang, S. H. et al. (2011). Efficacy and safety of pegylated liposomal doxorubicin in combination with bortezomib for multiple myeloma: Effects of adverse prognostic factors on outcome. *Clinical Lymphoma Myeloma and Leukemia*, *11*(1), 44–49. doi:10.3816/CLML.2011.n.005 PMID:21454189

Blasi, L., Longo, L., Vasapollo, G., Cingolani, R., Rinaldi, R., Rizzello, T., & Maffia, M. et al. (2005). Characterization of glutamate dehydrogenase immobilization on silica surface by atomic force microscopy and kinetic analyses. *Enzyme and Microbial Technology*, *36*(5-6), 818–823. doi:10.1016/j.enzmictec.2005.01.014

Bogardus, J. B. (1982). Phase equilibria of nafcillin sodium–water. *Journal of Pharmaceutical Sciences*, *71*(1), 105–109. doi:10.1002/jps.2600710125 PMID:7057360

Bölgen, N., Vargel, İ., Korkusuz, P., Menceloğlu, Y. Z., & Pişkin, E. (2007). In vivo performance of antibiotic embedded electrospun PCL membranes for prevention of abdominal adhesions. *Journal of Biomedical Materials Research. Part B, Applied Biomaterials*, *81*(2), 530–543. doi:10.1002/jbm.b.30694 PMID:17041925

Bonig, H., Becker, P. S., Schwebig, A., & Turner, M. (2015). Biosimilar granulocyte–colony-stimulating factor for healthy donor stem cell mobilization: Need we be afraid. *Transfusion*, *55*(2), 430–539. doi:10.1111/trf.12770 PMID:24965197

Boni, L. T., & Hui, S. W. (1983). Polymorphic phase behaviour of dilinoleoyl phosphatidyl ethanolamine and palmitoyl oleoyl phosphatidyl choline mixtures. Structural changes between hexagonal, cubic and bilayer phases. *Biochimica et Biophysical Acta Biomembranes*, *731*(2), 177–185. doi:10.1016/0005-2736(83)90007-X PMID:6849915

Bordi, F., Cametti, C., & Sennato, S. (2006). Electrical properties of aqueous liposome suspensions. *Advances in Planar Lipid Bilayers and Liposomes*, *4*, 281–320. doi:10.1016/S1554-4516(06)04009-9

Bosman, A. W., Janssen, H. M., & Meijer, E. W. (1999). About Dendrimers: Structure, Physical Properties, and Applications. *Chemical Reviews*, *99*(7), 1665–1688. doi:10.1021/cr970069y PMID:11849007

Bosworth, M. E., Hunt, C. A., & Pratt, D. (1982). Liposome dialysis for improved size distributions. *Journal of Pharmaceutical Sciences*, *71*(7), 806–812. doi:10.1002/jps.2600710722 PMID:7120068

Boulikas, T. (2009). Clinical overview on Lipoplatin™: A successful liposomal formulation of cisplatin. *Expert Opinion on Investigational Drugs*, *18*(8), 1–22. doi:10.1517/13543780903114168 PMID:19053877

Bouwstra, J. A., van Hal, D. A., Hofl, H. E., & Junginger, H. E. (1997). Preparation and characterization of nonionic surfactant vesicles. *Colloids and Surfaces. A, Physicochemical and Engineering Aspects*, *123*, 71–80. doi:10.1016/S0927-7757(96)03800-9

Boyd, B. J., Davey, G., & Drummond, C. J. (2004). *Surfactants and lyotropic phases formed there from.* International patent WO, 2004/022530.

Boyd, B. J., Davey, G., Khoo, S. M., & Whittaker, D. V. (2005). *Compositions and methods of delivery of biologically active agents.* International patent WO2005021046.

Boyd, B. J., Khoob, S., Whittaker, D. V., & Davey, S. M. (2006). Lyotropic liquid crystalline phases formed from glycerate surfactants as sustained release drug delivery systems. *International Journal of Pharmaceutics*, *309*(1-2), 218–226. doi:10.1016/j.ijpharm.2005.11.033 PMID:16413980

Boyd, B. J., Khoo, S. M., Whittaker, D. V., Davey, G., & Porter, C. J. H. (2007). A lipid-based liquid crystalline matrix that provides sustained release and enhanced oral bioavailability for a model poorly water soluble drug in rats. *International Journal of Pharmaceutics*, *340*(1), 52–60. doi:10.1016/j.ijpharm.2007.03.020 PMID:17467935

Boyd, B. J., Whittaker, D. V., Khoob, S., & Davey, S. M. (2006). Hexosome formed from glycerate surfactants-Formulation as a colloidal carrier for irinotecan. *International Journal of Pharmaceutics*, *318*(1-2), 154–162. doi:10.1016/j.ijpharm.2006.03.010 PMID:16621358

Bragagni, M., Mennini, N., Furlanetto, S., Orlandini, S., Ghelardini, C., & Mura, P. (2014). Development and characterization of functionalized niosomes for brain targeting of dynorphin-B. *European Journal of Pharmaceutics and Biopharmaceutics*, *87*(1), 73–79. doi:10.1016/j.ejpb.2014.01.006 PMID:24462793

Bragagni, M., Mennini, N., Ghelardini, C., & Mura, P. (2012). Development and characterization of niosomal formulations of doxorubicin aimed at brain targeting. *Journal of Pharmacy & Pharmaceutical Sciences*, *15*(1), 184–196. doi:10.18433/J3230M PMID:22365096

Bramlett, K., Onel, E., Viscusi, E. R., & Jones, K. (2012). A randomized, double-blind, dose-ranging study comparing wound infiltration of DepoFoam bupivacaine, an extended-release liposomal bupivacaine, to bupivacaine HCl for postsurgical analgesia in total knee arthroplasty. *The Knee*, *19*(5), 530–536. doi:10.1016/j.knee.2011.12.004 PMID:22285545

Brandl, M., Bachmann, D., Drechsler, M., & Bauer, K. (1990). Liposome preparation by a new high pressure homogenizer Gaulin Micron Lab 40. *Drug Development and Industrial Pharmacy*, *16*(14), 2167–2191. doi:10.3109/03639049009023648

Brannon-Peppas, L., & Blanchette, J. O. (2012). Nanoparticle and targeted systems for cancer therapy. *Advanced Drug Delivery Reviews*, *64*, 206–212. doi:10.1016/j.addr.2012.09.033 PMID:15350294

Brasseur, F., Couvreur, P., Kante, B., Deckers-Passau, L., Roland, M., Deckers, C., & Speisers, P. (1980). Actinomycin D absorbed on polymethylcyanoacrylate nanoparticles: Increased efficiency against an experimental tumor. *European Journal of Cancer, 16*(11), 1441–1445. doi:10.1016/0014-2964(80)90053-5 PMID:7227421

Bressler, N. M., & Bressler, S. B. (2000). Photodynamic therapy with verteporfin (Visudyne): Impact on ophthalmology and visual sciences. *Investigative Ophthalmology & Visual Science, 41*(3), 624–628. PMID:10711673

Brewer, J., & Alexander, J. (1992). The adjuvant activity of non-ionic surfactant vesicles (niosomes) on the BALB/c humoral response to bovine serum albumin. *Immunology, 75*(4), 570. PMID:1592432

Brooks, C. J. W., Machachlan, J., Cole, W. J., & Lawric, T. D. V. (1984). Vesicular system.*International Symposium, 349*.

Brown, G. H., & Shaw, W. G. (1957). The mesomorphic state: Liquid crystals. *Chemical Reviews, 57*(6), 1049–1157. doi:10.1021/cr50018a002

Brunner, T. I., Wick, P., Manser, P., Spohn, P., Grass, R. N., Limbach, L. K., & Stark, W. J. et al. (2006). In vitro cytotoxicity of oxide nanoparticles: Comparison to asbestos, silica, and effect of particle solubility. *Environmental Science & Technology, 40*(14), 4374–4381. doi:10.1021/es052069i PMID:16903273

Bunjes, H., & Rades, T. (2005). Thermotropic liquid crystalline drugs. *The Journal of Pharmacy and Pharmacology, 57*(7), 807–816. doi:10.1211/0022357056208 PMID:15969938

Burger, C., & Chu, B. (2007). Functional nanofibrous scaffolds for bone reconstruction. *Colloids and Surfaces. B, Biointerfaces, 56*(1), 134–141. doi:10.1016/j.colsurfb.2006.09.023 PMID:17113762

Burgess, P., Hutt, P. B., Farokhzad, O. C., Langer, R., Minick, S., & Zale, S. (2010). On firm ground: IP protection of therapeutic nanoparticles. *Nature Biotechnology, 28*(12), 1267–1270. doi:10.1038/nbt.1725 PMID:21139609

Burrows, R., Collett, J. H., & Attwood, D. (1994). The release of drugs from monoglyceride-water liquid crystalline phases. *International Journal of Pharmaceutics, 111*(3), 283–293. doi:10.1016/0378-5173(94)90351-4

Business Monitor International. (2008). First Biosimilar Submitted for Approval. In BMI Industry Insights—Pharma and Healthcare, Asia.

Cain, C. C., Sipe, D. M., & Murphy, R. F. (1989). Regulation of endocytic pH by the Na+/K+-ATPase in living cells. *Proceedings of the National Academy of Sciences of the United States of America, 86*(2), 544–548. doi:10.1073/pnas.86.2.544 PMID:2536168

Cai, W., Anderson, E. C., & Gupta, R. B. (2001). Separation of lignin from aqueous mixtures by ionic and nonionic temperature-sensitive hydrogels. *Industrial & Engineering Chemistry Research, 40*(10), 2283–2288. doi:10.1021/ie0009435

Calvo, P., Alonso, M. J., Vila-Jato, J. L., & Robinson, J. R. (1996). Improved ocular bioavailability of indomethacin by novel ocular drug carriers. *The Journal of Pharmacy and Pharmacology, 48*(11), 1147–1152. doi:10.1111/j.2042-7158.1996.tb03911.x PMID:8961163

Calvo, P., Gouritin, B., & Chacunm, H. et al.. (2001). Long-circulating PEGylated polycyanoacrylate nanoparticles as new drug carrier for brain delivery. *Pharmaceutical Research, 18*(8), 1157–1166. doi:10.1023/A:1010931127745 PMID:11587488

Calvo, P., Gouritin, B., Villarroya, H., Eclancher, F., Giannavola, C., Klein, C., & Couvreur, P. et al. (2002). Quantification and localization of PEGylated polycyanoacrylate nanoparticles in brain and spinal cord during experimental allergic encephalomyelitis in the rat. *The European Journal of Neuroscience, 15*(8), 1317–1326. doi:10.1046/j.1460-9568.2002.01967.x PMID:11994126

Calvo, P., Vila-Jato, J. L., & Alonso, M. J. (1997). Effect of lysozyme on the stability of polyester nanocapsules and nanoparticles: Stabilization approaches. *Biomaterials*, *18*(19), 1305–1310. doi:10.1016/S0142-9612(97)00061-6 PMID:9307220

Caminade, A.-M., & Turrin, C.-O. (2014). Dendrimers for drug delivery. *Journal of Materials Chemistry B*, *2*(26), 4055–4066. doi:10.1039/c4tb00171k

Cantor, A. S. (1999). Drug and excipient diffusion and solubility in acrylate adhesives measured by infrared-attenuated total reflectance (IR-ATR) spectroscopy. *Journal of Controlled Release*, *61*(1-2), 219–231. doi:10.1016/S0168-3659(99)00119-4 PMID:10469917

Cao, Y., He, Y., Liu, H., Luo, Y., Shen, M., Xia, J., & Shi, X. (2015). Targeted CT imaging of human hepatocellular carcinoma using low-generation dendrimer-entrapped gold nanoparticles modified with lactobionic acid. *Journal of Materials Chemistry B*, *3*(2), 286–295. doi:10.1039/C4TB01542H

Caracciolo, G., Pozzi, D., Caminiti, R., Marianecci, C., Moglioni, S., Carafa, M., & Amenitsch, H. (2008). Effect of hydration on the structure of solid-supported Niosomal membranes investigated by in situ energy dispersive X-ray diffraction. *Chemical Physics Letters*, *462*(4-6), 307–312. doi:10.1016/j.cplett.2008.07.094

Carafa, M. L., Marzio, D., Marianecci, C., Cinque, B., Lucania, G., Kajiwara, K., & Santucci, E. et al. (2006). Designing novel pH-sensitive non-phospholipid vesicle: Characterization and cell interaction. *European Journal of Pharmaceutical Sciences*, *28*(5), 385–393. doi:10.1016/j.ejps.2006.04.009 PMID:16797946

Carafa, M., Santucci, E., Alhaique, F., Coviello, T., Murtas, E., Riccieri, F., & Torrisi, M. et al. (1998). Preparation and properties of new unilamellar non-ionic/ionic surfactant vesicles. *International Journal of Pharmaceutics*, *160*(1), 51–59. doi:10.1016/S0378-5173(97)00294-9

Carlson, L. J., & Krauss, T. D. (2008). Photo physics of individual single-walled carbon nanotubes. *Accounts of Chemical Research*, *41*(2), 235–243. doi:10.1021/ar700136v PMID:18281946

Castor, T. P. (2005). Phospholipid nanosomes. *Current Drug Delivery*, *2*(4), 329–340. doi:10.2174/156720105774370195 PMID:16305436

Cervin, C., Vandoolaeghe, P., Nistor, C., Tiberg, F., & Johnssona, M. (2009). A combined in vitro and in vivo study on the interactions between somatostatin and lipid-based liquid crystalline drug carriers and bilayers. *European Journal of Pharmaceutical Sciences*, *36*(4-5), 377–385. doi:10.1016/j.ejps.2008.11.001 PMID:19041716

Cevc, G. (1996). Transfersomes, liposomes and other lipid suspensions on the skin: permeation enhancement, vesicle penetration, and transdermal drug delivery. *Critical Reviews™ in Therapeutic Drug Carrier Systems, 13*(3-4).

Cevc, G. (1987). How membrane chain melting properties are regulated by the polar surface of the lipid bilayer. *Biochemistry*, *26*(20), 6305–6310. doi:10.1021/bi00394a002 PMID:3427005

Cevc, G. (1991). How membrane chain-melting phase-transition temperature is affected by the lipid chain asymmetry and degree of unsaturation: An effective chain-length model. *Biochemistry*, *30*(29), 7186–7193. doi:10.1021/bi00243a021 PMID:1854729

Cevc, G. (1991). Isothermal lipid phase. *Transitions Chemistry and Physics of Lipids*, *57*(2-3), 293–299. doi:10.1016/0009-3084(91)90082-M PMID:2054910

Cevc, G. (1993). *Phospholipids handbook*. CRC Press.

Cevc, G. (2004). Lipid vesicles and other colloids as drug carriers on the skin. *Advanced Drug Delivery Reviews*, *56*(5), 675–711. doi:10.1016/j.addr.2003.10.028 PMID:15019752

Cevc, G., Blume, G., & Schatzlein, A. (1997). Transfersomes-mediated transepidermal delivery improves the regio-specificity and biological activity of corticosteroids in vivo. *Journal of Controlled Release*, *45*, 211–226. doi:10.1016/S0168-3659(96)01566-0

Cevc, G., Blume, G., Sehatzlein, A., Gebauer, D., & Paul, A. (1996). The skin- a pathway for systemic treatment with patches and lipid-based agent carriers. *Advanced Drug Delivery Reviews*, *18*(3), 349–378. doi:10.1016/0169-409X(95)00091-K

Chahar, P., & Cummings, K. C. III. (2012). Liposomal bupivacaine: A review of a new bupivacaine formulation. *Journal of Plant Research*, *5*, 257–264. PMID:23049275

Chalker-Scott, L. (2013). The Myth of Polyacrylamide Hydrogels. In *The informed gardener*. Washington, DC: University of Washington Press.

Chaloupka, K., Malam, Y., & Seifalian, A. M. (2010). Nanosilver as a new generation of nano product in biomedical applications. *Trends in Biotechnology*, *28*(11), 580–588. doi:10.1016/j.tibtech.2010.07.006 PMID:20724010

Chandra, A. & Sharma, P. (2008). Proniosome based drug delivery system of piroxicam. *African Journal of Pharmacy and Pharmacology*, *2*(9),184-190.

Chandraprakash, K., Udupa, N., Umadevi, P., & Pillai, G. (1990). Pharmacokinetic evaluation of surfactant vesicle-entrapped methotrexate in tumor-bearing mice. *International Journal of Pharmaceutics*, *61*(1-2), R1–R4. doi:10.1016/0378-5173(90)90056-A

Chandraprakash, K., Udupa, N., Umadevi, P., & Pillai, G. (1992). Formulation and evaluation of Methotrexate niosomes. *Indian Journal of Pharmaceutical Sciences*, *54*, 197–197.

Chandrasekhar, S. (1993). *Liquid Crystals* (2nd ed.). Cambridge Univ Pr Published.

Chang, C. M., & Bodmeier, R. (1997). Swelling of and drug release from monoglyceride-based drug delivery systems. *Journal of Pharmaceutical Sciences*, *86*(6), 747–752. doi:10.1021/js960256w PMID:9188059

Chan, H. K., & Gonda, I. (1991). Methotrexate: Existence of different types of solid. *International Journal of Pharmaceutics*, *68*(1-3), 179–190. doi:10.1016/0378-5173(91)90140-J

Chan, K. W., Yu, T., Qiao, Y., Liu, Q., Yang, M., Patel, H., & Bulte, J. W. et al. (2014). A diaCEST MRI approach for monitoring liposomal accumulation in tumors. *Journal of Controlled Release*, *180*, 51–59. doi:10.1016/j.jconrel.2014.02.005 PMID:24548481

Chan, Y. N., Bulmus, V., Zareie, M. H., Byrne, F. L., Barner, L., & Kavallaris, M. (2006). Acid-cleavable polymeric core–shell particles for delivery of hydrophobic drugs. *Journal of Controlled Release*, *115*(2), 197–207. doi:10.1016/j.jconrel.2006.07.025 PMID:16996635

Chan, Y. N., Wong, T., Byrne, F., Kavallaris, M., & Bulmus, V. (2008). Acid-labile core cross-linked micelles for pH-triggered release of antitumor drugs. *Biomacromolecules*, *9*(7), 1826–1836. doi:10.1021/bm800043n PMID:18564874

Chapman, S. J., & Walsh, A. (1990). Desmosomes and desquamation: An ultrastructural study of adult pig epidermis. *Archives of Dermatological Research*, *282*(5), 304–310. doi:10.1007/BF00375724 PMID:2221982

Chaterji, S., Kwon, I. K., & Park, K. (2007). Smart polymeric gels: Redefining the limits of biomedical devices. *Progress in Polymer Science*, *32*(8), 1083–1122. doi:10.1016/j.progpolymsci.2007.05.018 PMID:18670584

Chaturvedi, M., Kumar, M., Sinhal, A., & Saifi, A. (2011). Recent development in novel drug delivery systems of herbal drugs. *International Journal of Green Pharmacy*, *5*(2), 87. doi:10.4103/0973-8258.85155

Chavany, C., Saison-Behmoaras, T., Le Doan, T., Puisieux, F., Couvreur, P., & Helene, C. (1994). Adsorption of oligonucleotides onto polyisohexylcyanoacrylate nanoparticles protects them against nucleases and increases their cellular uptake. *Pharmaceutical Research*, *11*(9), 1370–1378. doi:10.1023/A:1018923301967 PMID:7816773

Chen, C. B., Chen, J. Y., & Lee, W. C. (2009). Fast transfection of mammalian cells using super paramagnetic nanoparticles under strong magnetic field. *Journal of Nanoscience and Nanotechnology*, *9*(4), 2651–2659. doi:10.1166/jnn.2009.449 PMID:19438016

Cheng, Y., Zhao, L., Li, Y., & Xu, T. (2011). Design of biocompatible dendrimers for cancer diagnosis and therapy: Current status and future perspectives. *Chemical Society Reviews*, *40*(5), 2673–2703. doi:10.1039/c0cs00097c PMID:21286593

Chen, J. P., Tsai, M. J., & Liao, H. T. (2013). Incorporation of biphasic calcium phosphate microparticles in injectable thermoresponsive hydrogel modulates bone cell proliferation and differentiation. *Colloids and Surfaces. B, Biointerfaces*, *110*, 120–129. PMID:23711782

Chen, J., Chen, S., Zhao, X., Kuznetsova, L. V., Wong, S. S., & Ojima, L. (2008). Functionalized single-walled carbon nanotubes as rationally designed vehicles for tumor-targeted drug delivery. *Journal of the American Chemical Society*, *130*(49), 16778–16785. doi:10.1021/ja805570f PMID:19554734

Chen, J., Qiu, X. Z., Ouyang, J., Kong, J. M., Zhong, W., & Xing, M. M. Q. (2011). pH and reduction dual-sensitive copolymeric micelles for intracellular doxorubicin delivery. *Biomacromolecules*, *12*(10), 3601–3611. doi:10.1021/bm200804j PMID:21853982

Chen, L., Remondetto, G. E., & Subirade, M. (2006). Food protein based materials as nutraceutical delivery systems. *Trends in Food Science & Technology*, *17*(5), 272–283. doi:10.1016/j.tifs.2005.12.011

Chen, M., Zhong, Z., Tan, W., Wang, S., & Wang, Y. (2011). Recent advances in nanoparticle formulation of oleanolic acid. *Chinese Medicine*, *6*(1), 20. doi:10.1186/1749-8546-6-20 PMID:21619582

Chen, Q., Li, K., Wen, S., Liu, H., Peng, C., Cai, H., & Shi, X. et al. (2013). Targeted CT/MR dual mode imaging of tumors using multifunctional dendrimer-entrapped gold nanoparticles. *Biomaterials*, *34*(21), 5200–5209. doi:10.1016/j.biomaterials.2013.03.009 PMID:23583039

Chen, Q., Wang, H., Liu, H., Wen, S., Peng, C., Shen, M., & Shi, X. et al. (2015). Multifunctional Dendrimer-Entrapped Gold Nanoparticles Modified with RGD Peptide for Targeted Computed Tomography/Magnetic Resonance Dual-Modal Imaging of Tumors. *Analytical Chemistry*, *87*(7), 3949–3956. doi:10.1021/acs.analchem.5b00135 PMID:25768040

Chen, W., Meng, F. H., Li, F., Ji, S. J., & Zhong, Z. Y. (2009). pH-responsive biodegradable micelles based on acid-labile polycarbonate hydrophobe: Synthesis and triggered drug release. *Biomacromolecules*, *10*(7), 1727–1735. doi:10.1021/bm900074d PMID:19469499

Chen, X., & Schluesener, H. J. (2008). Nanosilver: A nanoproduct in medical application. *Toxicology Letters*, *176*(1), 1–12. doi:10.1016/j.toxlet.2007.10.004 PMID:18022772

Chen, X., Tam, U. C., Czlapinski, J. L., Lee, G. S., Rabuka, D., Zettl, A., & Bertozzi, C. R. (2006). Interfacing Carbon Nanotubes with Living Cells. *Journal of the American Chemical Society*, *128*(19), 6292–6293. doi:10.1021/ja060276s PMID:16683774

Chen, Y., & Liu, L. (2012). Modern methods for delivery of drugs across the blood–brain barrier. *Advanced Drug Delivery Reviews*, *64*(7), 640–665. doi:10.1016/j.addr.2011.11.010 PMID:22154620

Chen, Y., Lu, Y., Zhong, Y., Wang, Q., Wu, W., & Gao, S. (2012). Ocular delivery of cyclosporine A based on glyceryl monooleate/poloxamer 407 liquid crystalline nanoparticles: Preparation, characterization, in vitro corneal penetration and ocular irritation. *Journal of Drug Targeting*, *20*(10), 856–863. doi:10.3109/1061186X.2012.723214 PMID:23050903

Chen, Z., & Rand, R. (1997). The influence of cholesterol on phospholipid membrane curvature and bending elasticity. *Biophysical Journal*, *73*(1), 267–276. doi:10.1016/S0006-3495(97)78067-6 PMID:9199791

Chertok, B., David, A. E., & Yang, V. C. (2010). Polyethyleneimine-modified iron oxide nanoparticles for brain tumor drug delivery using magnetic targeting and intracarotid administration. *Biomaterials*, *31*(24), 6317–6324. doi:10.1016/j.biomaterials.2010.04.043 PMID:20494439

Chew, S. Y., Wen, J., Yim, E. K. F., & Leong, K. W. (2005). Sustained release of proteins from electrospun biodegradable fibers. *Biomacromolecules*, *6*(4), 2017–2024. doi:10.1021/bm0501149 PMID:16004440

Chiannilkulchai, N., Driouich, Z., Benoit, J. P., Parodi, A. L., & Couvreur, P. (1989). Doxorubicin-loaded nanoparticles: Increased efficiency in murine hepatic metastases. *Selective Cancer Therapeutics*, *5*(1), 1–11. doi:10.1089/sct.1989.5.1 PMID:2756244

Chime, S., Kenechukwu, F., & Attama, A. (2014). Nanoemulsions—Advances in Formulation, Characterization and applications in drug delivery. In Application of nanotechnology in drug delivery. Croatia: In Tech.

Chiranjeevi, G., Muthukumaran, M., & Krishnamoorthy, B. (2013). A review on potency of vesicular systems in targeting drug delivery. *Research Journal of Pharmaceutical Biological Chemical Sciences*, *4*(2), 156–170.

Chirino, A. J., & Mire-Sluis, A. (2004). Characterizing biological products and assessing comparability following manufacturing changes. *Nature Biotechnology*, *22*(11), 1383–1391. doi:10.1038/nbt1030 PMID:15529163

Chitra, M., Sukumar, E., Suja, V., & Devi, C. S. (1994). Antitumor, anti-inflammatory and analgesic property of embelin, aplant product. *Chemotherapy*, *40*(2), 109–113. doi:10.1159/000239181 PMID:7510605

Cho, Z. K., & Hong, S. K. (2014). *Patent Application KR 2014/0115542*. Lead Biotech Co Ltd.

Cho, K., Wang, X., Nie, S., Chen, Z., & Shin, D. M. (2008). Therapeutic nanoparticles for drug delivery in cancer. *Clinical Cancer Research*, *14*(5), 1310–1316. doi:10.1158/1078-0432.CCR-07-1441 PMID:18316549

Chomoucka, J., Drbohlavova, J., Huska, D., Adam, V., Kizek, R., & Hubalek, J. (2010). Magnetic nanoparticles and targeted drug delivering. *Pharmacological Research*, *62*(2), 144–149. doi:10.1016/j.phrs.2010.01.014 PMID:20149874

Chong, J. Y. T., Mulet, X., Waddington, L. J., Boyd, B. J., & Drummond, C. J. (2011). Steric stabilisation of self-assembled cubic lyotropic liquid crystalline nanoparticles: High throughput evaluation of triblock polyethylene oxide-polypropylene oxidepolyethylene oxide copolymers. *Soft Matter*, *7*(10), 4768–4777. doi:10.1039/c1sm05181d

Chong, J. Y. T., Mulet, X., Waddington, L. J., Boyd, B. J., & Drummond, C. J. (2012). High-throughput discovery of novel steric stabilizers for cubic lyotropic liquid crystal nanoparticle dispersions. *Langmuir*, *28*(25), 9223–9232. doi:10.1021/la301874v PMID:22630595

Chong, P. L.-G., Ayesa, U., Prakash Daswani, V., & Hur, E. C. (2012). On physical properties of tetraether lipid membranes: Effects of cyclopentane rings. *Archaea (Vancouver, B.C.)*, 2012. PMID:23028246

Choudhary, N., & Sekhon, B. S. (2012). An overview of advances in the standardization of herbal drugs. *Journal of Pharmaceutical Education and Research*, *2*, 2.

Chowhan, Z. T., & Pritchard, R. (1975). Release of corticoids from oleaginous ointment bases containing drug in suspension. *Journal of Pharmaceutical Sciences*, *64*(5), 754–759. doi:10.1002/jps.2600640505 PMID:1151642

Cho, Y. I., Choi, J. S., Jeong, S. Y., & Yoo, H. S. (2010). Nerve growth factor (NGF)-conjugated electrospun nanostructures with topographical cues for neuronal differentiation of mesenchymal stem cells. *Acta Biomaterialia*, *6*(12), 4725–4733. doi:10.1016/j.actbio.2010.06.019 PMID:20601229

Chujo, Y., Sada, K., & Saegusa, T. (1990). Polyoxazoline having a coumarin moiety as a pendant group. Synthesis and photogelation. *Macromolecules*, *23*(10), 2693–2697. doi:10.1021/ma00212a017

Chung, H., & Caffrey, M. (1995). Polymorphism, mesomorphism, and metastability of monoelaidin in excess water. *Biophysical Journal*, *69*(5), 1951–1963. doi:10.1016/S0006-3495(95)80065-2 PMID:8580338

Ciolino, J. B., Hoare, T. R., & Kohane, D. S. (2014). *Patent Application AU 2014/215997*, Massachusetts Inst. Technology.

Clark, M. A., Jepson, M. A., & Hirst, B. H. (2001). Exploiting M cells for drug and vaccine delivery. *Advanced Drug Delivery Reviews*, *50*(1), 81–106. doi:10.1016/S0169-409X(01)00149-1 PMID:11489335

Clemens, D. L., Lee, B.-Y., Xue, M., Thomas, C. R., Meng, H., Ferris, D., & Horwitz, M. A. et al. (2012). Targeted intracellular delivery of antituberculosis drugs to Mycobacterium tuberculosis-infected macrophages via functionalized mesoporous silica nanoparticles. *Antimicrobial Agents and Chemotherapy*, *56*(5), 2535–2545. doi:10.1128/AAC.06049-11 PMID:22354311

Clogston, J., & Caffrey, M. (2005). Controlling release from the lipidic cubic phase. Amino acids, peptides, proteins and nucleic acids. *Journal of Controlled Release*, *107*(1), 97–111. doi:10.1016/j.jconrel.2005.05.015 PMID:15990192

Cohen Avrahami, M., Aserin, A., & Garti, N. (2010). HII mesophase and peptide cell-penetrating enhancers for improved transdermal delivery of sodium diclofenac. *Colloids and Surfaces. B, Biointerfaces*, *77*(2), 131–138. doi:10.1016/j.colsurfb.2010.01.013 PMID:20189781

Cohen-Avrahami, M., Libster, D., Aserin, A., & Garti, N. (2012). Penetratin-induced transdermal delivery from H *II* mesophases of sodium diclofenac. J*ournal of Controlled Release,* 15*9(3)*, 419–428. doi:10.1016/j.jconrel.2012.01.025 PMID:22306174

Cole, A. J., Yang, V. C., & David, A. E. (2011). Cancer theranostics: The rise of targeted magnetic nanoparticles. T*rends in Biotechnology,* 2*9(*7), 323–332. doi:10.1016/j.tibtech.2011.03.001 PMID:21489647

Coles-Harry, J., & Mikhail, N. (2005). Liquid crystal 'blue phases' with a wide temperature range. *Nature Materials*, *436*(7053), 997–1000. doi:10.1038/nature03932

Collings, P. J., & Hird, M. (1997). *Introduction to Liquid Crystals*. Bristol, PA: Taylor & Francis. doi:10.4324/9780203211199

Conacher, M., Alexander, J., & Brewer, J. M. (2001). Oral immunisation with peptide and protein antigens by formulation in lipid vesicles incorporating bile salts (bilosomes). *Vaccine*, *19*(20), 2965–2974. doi:10.1016/S0264-410X(00)00537-5 PMID:11282208

Consensus Information Paper (CIP). (2013). *What you need to know about Biosimilar Medicinal Products*. CIP.

Correia, J. C. D. S., de Oliveira, J. M. A., De Oliveira, J. M. T., De Sousa, R. P. A. R., & Dos Reis, R. L. G. (2015). *U.S. Patent No. 9,012,415*. Washington, DC: U.S. Patent and Trademark Office.

Cortesi, R., Esposito, E., Corradini, F., Sivieri, E., Drechsler, M., Rossi, A., & Menegatti, E. et al. (2007). Non-phospholipid vesicles as carriers for peptides and proteins: Production, characterization and stability studies. *International Journal of Pharmaceutics*, *339*(1), 52–60. doi:10.1016/j.ijpharm.2007.02.024 PMID:17395411

Cosco, D., Paolino, D., Muzzalupo, R., Celia, C., Citraro, R., Caponio, D., & Fresta, M. et al. (2009). Novel PEG-coated niosomes based on bola-surfactant as drug carriers for 5-fluorouracil. *Biomedical Microdevices*, *11*(5), 1115–1125. doi:10.1007/s10544-009-9328-2 PMID:19507033

Costa Balogh, F. O., Sparr, E., Sousa, J. J. S., & Pais, A. C. (2010). Drug release from lipid liquid crystalline phases: Relation with phase behavior. *Drug Development and Industrial Pharmacy*, *36*(4), 470–481. doi:10.3109/03639040903261997 PMID:19848561

Couvreur, P., Kante, B., Roland, M., Guiot, P., Baudhuin, P., & Speiser, P. (1979). Poly(cyanoacrylate) nanoparticles as potential lysosomotropic carriers: Preparation, morphological and sorptive properties. *The Journal of Pharmacy and Pharmacology*, *31*(1), 331–332. doi:10.1111/j.2042-7158.1979.tb13510.x PMID:37304

Couvreur, P., & Vauthier, C. (2006). Nanotechnology: Intelligent Design to Treat Complex Disease. *Pharmaceutical Research*, *23*(7), 1417–1450. doi:10.1007/s11095-006-0284-8 PMID:16779701

Cowan-Lincoln, M. (n.d.). *FORMULATION-Solubility| Improve the Bioavailability of Poorly Soluble Drugs*. Academic Press.

Cox, J. S. G., Woodard, G. D., & McCrone, W. C. (1971). Solid state chemistry of cromolyn sodium (disodium cromoglycate). *Journal of Pharmaceutical Sciences*, *60*(10), 1453–1465. doi:10.1002/jps.2600601003 PMID:5001963

Crommelin, D. J., Bermejo, T., Bissig, M., Damiaans, J., Krämer, I., Rambourg, P., & Tredree, R. (2005). Pharmaceutical evaluation of biosimilars: Important differences from generic low-molecular weight pharm. *Eur J Hosp Pharm Sci*, *1*, 11–17.

Cui, Z.-K., & Lafleur, M. (2014). Lamellar self-assemblies of single-chain amphiphiles and sterols and their derived liposomes: Distinct compositions and distinct properties. *Colloids and Surfaces. B, Biointerfaces*, *114*, 177–185. doi:10.1016/j.colsurfb.2013.09.042 PMID:24184913

Cullins, P. R., & Hope, M. J. (1986). Biochemistry of lipid and membrane. Benzain/Cumning.

Cullis, P., Mayer, L., Bally, M., Madden, T., & Hope, M. (1989). Generating and loading of liposomal systems for drug-delivery applications. *Advanced Drug Delivery Reviews*, *3*(3), 267–282. doi:10.1016/0169-409X(89)90024-0

Czarnobaj, K. (2008). Preparation and characterization of silica xerogels as carriers for drugs. *Drug Delivery*, *15*(8), 485–492. doi:10.1080/10717540802321495 PMID:18798086

Czarnobaj, K., & Czarnobaj, J. (2008). Sol–gel processed porous silica carriers for the controlled release of diclofenac diethylamine. *Journal of Biomedical Materials Research. Part B, Applied Biomaterials*, *87*(1), 114–120. doi:10.1002/jbm.b.31076 PMID:18437709

Czarnobaj, K., & Łukasiak, J. (2007). In vitro release of cisplatin from sol–gel processed organically modified silica xerogels. *Journal of Materials Science. Materials in Medicine*, *18*(10), 2041–2044. doi:10.1007/s10856-007-3139-x PMID:17558477

Czarnobaj, K., & Sawicki, W. (2012). The sol-gel prepared SiO2-CaO-P2O5 composites doped with Metronidazole for application in local delivery systems. *Pharmaceutical Development and Technology*, *17*(6), 697–704. doi:10.3109/10837450.2011.572894 PMID:21480825

Czeslik, C., Winter, R., Rapp, G., & Bartels, K. (1995). Temperature and pressure-dependent phase behavior of monoacylglycerides monoolein and monoelaidin. *Biophysical Journal*, *68*(4), 1423–1429. doi:10.1016/S0006-3495(95)80315-2 PMID:7787028

Damge, C., Michel, C., Aprahamian, M., & Couvreur, P. (1988). New approach for oral administration of insulin with polyalkylcyanoacrylate nanocapsules as drug carrier. *Diabetes*, *37*(2), 246–251. doi:10.2337/diab.37.2.246 PMID:3292320

Damge, C., Michel, C., Aprahamian, M., Couvreur, P., & Devissaguet, J. P. (1990). Nanocapsules as carriers for oral peptide delivery. *Journal of Controlled Release*, *13*(2-3), 233–239. doi:10.1016/0168-3659(90)90013-J

Damge, C., Vonderscher, J., Marbach, P., & Pinget, M. (1997). Poly(alkyl cyanoacrylate) nanocapsules as a delivery system in the rat for octreotide, a long-acting somatostatin analogue. *The Journal of Pharmacy and Pharmacology*, *49*(10), 949–954. doi:10.1111/j.2042-7158.1997.tb06022.x PMID:9364401

Damm, E. M., Pelkmans, L., Kartenbeck, J., Mezzacasa, A., Kurzchalia, T., & Helenius, A. (2005). Clathrin- and caveolin-1-independent endocytosis: Entry of simian virus 40 into cells devoid of caveolae. *The Journal of Cell Biology*, *168*(3), 477–488. doi:10.1083/jcb.200407113 PMID:15668298

Danhier, F., Feron, O., & Préat, V. (2010). To exploit the tumor microenvironment: Passive and active tumor targeting of nanocarriers for anti-cancer drug delivery. *Journal of Controlled Release*, *148*(2), 135–146. doi:10.1016/j.jconrel.2010.08.027 PMID:20797419

Dapergolas, G., & Gregoriadis, G. (1976). Hypoglycaemic effect of liposome-entrapped insulin administered intragastrically into rats. *Lancet, 2*(7990), 824-827.

Darwish, I. A., & Uchegbu, I. F. (1997). The evaluation of crown ether based niosomes as cation containing and cation sensitive drug delivery systems. *International Journal of Pharmaceutics*, *159*(2), 207–213. doi:10.1016/S0378-5173(97)00289-5

Davis, M. E., Chen, Z., & Shin, D. M. (2008). Nanoparticle therapeutics: An emerging treatment modality for cancer. *Nature Reviews. Drug Discovery*, *7*(9), 771–782. doi:10.1038/nrd2614 PMID:18758474

Dayan, N., & Touitou, E. (2000). Carriers for skin delivery of trihexyphenidyl HCl: Ethosomes vs. liposomes. *Biomaterials*, *21*(18), 1879–1885. doi:10.1016/S0142-9612(00)00063-6 PMID:10919691

De La Rica, R., Aili, D., & Stevens, M. M. (2012). Enzyme-responsive nanoparticles for drug release and diagnostics. *Advanced Drug Delivery Reviews*, *64*(11), 967–978. doi:10.1016/j.addr.2012.01.002 PMID:22266127

De Villiers, M. M., Aramwit, P., & Kwon, G. S. (Eds.). (2009). *Nanotechnology in drug delivery*. New York, NY: Springer. doi:10.1007/978-0-387-77667-5

Deamer, D. W., & Ann, N. Y. (1978). Preparation and properties of ether-injection liposomes. National Academy of Sciences, 308, 250.

Deamer, D. W. (2010). From "Banghasomes" to liposomes: A memoir of Alec Bangham, 1921–2010. *The FASEB Journal*, *24*(5), 1308–1310. doi:10.1096/fj.10-0503 PMID:20430797

Deamer, D. W., & Bangham, A. D. (1976). large voume liposomes by anether vaporisation method. *Biochimica et Biophysica Acta*, *443*, 629. PMID:963074

Declerck, P. J. (2012). Biologicals and biosimilars: A review of the science and its implications. *Generics and Biosimilars Initiative Journal*, *1*(1), 13–16. doi:10.5639/gabij.2012.0101.005

DeForest, C. A., & Anseth, K. S. (2011). Cytocompatible click-based hydrogels with dynamically tunable properties through orthogonal photoconjugation and photocleavage reactions. *Nature Chemistry*, *3*(12), 925–931. doi:10.1038/nchem.1174 PMID:22109271

DeKeyser, J. L., Poupaert, J. H., & Dumont, P. (1991). Poly(diethylmethylidenemalonate) nanoparticles as a potential drugcarrier: Preparation, distribution and elimination after intravenous and peroral administration to mice. *Journal of Pharmaceutical Sciences*, *80*(1), 67–70. doi:10.1002/jps.2600800117 PMID:2013853

D'Emanuele, A., & Attwood, D. (2005). Dendrimer–drug interactions. *Advanced Drug Delivery Reviews*, *57*(15), 2147–2162. doi:10.1016/j.addr.2005.09.012 PMID:16310283

D'Emanuele, A., Kost, J., Hill, J. L., & Langer, R. (1992). An investigation of the effects of ultrasound on degradable polyanhydride matrices. *Macromolecules*, *25*(2), 511–515. doi:10.1021/ma00028a002

DeMiguel, I., Ioualalen, K., Bonnefous, M., Peyrot, M., Nguyen, F., & Cervilla, M. et al.. (1995). Synthesis and characterization of supramolecular biovector (SMBV) specifically designed for the entrapment of ionic molecules. *Biochimica et Biophysica Acta*, *1237*(1), 49–58. doi:10.1016/0005-2736(95)00079-I PMID:7619842

Deng, A. D., Chen, M., Zhou, S. X., You, B., & Wu, L. M. (2006). A novel method for the fabrication ofmonodisperse hollow silica spheres. *Langmuir*, *22*(14), 6403–6407. doi:10.1021/la060944n PMID:16800706

Deng, C., Jiang, Y., Cheng, R., Meng, F., & Zhong, Z. (2012). Biodegradable polymeric micelles for targeted and controlled anticancer drug delivery: Promises, progress and prospects. *Nano Today*, *7*(5), 467–480. doi:10.1016/j.nantod.2012.08.005

Derwent, J. J. K., & Mieler, W. F. (2008). Thermoresponsive hydrogels as a new ocular drug delivery platform to the posterior segment of the eye. *Transactions of the American Ophthalmological Society*, *106*, 206. PMID:19277236

des Rieux, A., Fievez, V., Garinot, M., Schneider, Y.-J., & Préat, V. (2006). Nanoparticles as potential oral delivery systems of proteins and vaccines: A mechanistic approach. *Journal of Controlled Release*, *116*(1), 1–27. doi:10.1016/j.jconrel.2006.08.013 PMID:17050027

Desai, T., & Finlay, W. (2002). Nebulization of niosomal all-trans-retinoic acid: An inexpensive alternative to conventional liposomes. *International Journal of Pharmaceutics*, *241*(2), 311–317. doi:10.1016/S0378-5173(02)00245-4 PMID:12100858

Devaraj, G., Parakh, S., Devraj, R., Apte, S., Rao, B., & Rambhau, D. (2002). Release studies on niosomes containing fatty alcohols as bilayer stabilizers instead of cholesterol. *Journal of Colloid and Interface Science*, *251*(2), 360–365. doi:10.1006/jcis.2002.8399 PMID:16290741

Dew, N., Edwards, K., Eriksson, J., Edsman, K., & Björk, E. (2012). Gel formulations containing catanionic vesicles composed of alprenolol and SDS: Effects of drug release and skin penetration on aggregate structure. *Colloids and Surfaces. B, Biointerfaces*, *89*(10), 53–60. doi:10.1016/j.colsurfb.2011.08.022 PMID:21958537

Dhanikula, R. S., Argaw, A., Bouchard, J.-F., & Hildgen, P. (2008). Methotrexate loaded polyether-copolyester dendrimers for the treatment of gliomas: Enhanced efficacy and intratumoral transport capability. *Molecular Pharmaceutics*, *5*(1), 105–116. doi:10.1021/mp700086j PMID:18171013

Dhar, S., Liu, Z., Thomale, J., Dai, H., & Lippard, S. J. (2008). Targeted single-wall carbon nanotube-mediated Pt (IV) prodrug delivery using folate as a homing device. *Journal of the American Chemical Society*, *130*(34), 11467–11476. doi:10.1021/ja803036e PMID:18661990

Dhawan, V. V., Joshi, G. V., Jain, A. S., Nikam, Y. P., Gude, R. P., Mulherkar, R., & Nagarsenker, M. S. (2014). Apoptosis induction and anti-cancer activity of LeciPlex formulations. *Cellular Oncology*, *37*(5), 339–351. doi:10.1007/s13402-014-0183-7 PMID:25204961

Di Marzio, L., Esposito, S., Rinaldi, F., Marianecci, C., & Carafa, M. (2012). Polysorbate 20 vesicles as oral delivery system: In-vitro characterization. *Colloids and Surfaces. B, Biointerfaces*, *104*, 200–206. doi:10.1016/j.colsurfb.2012.10.036 PMID:23314494

Di Marzio, L., Marianecci, C., Petrone, M., Rinaldi, F., & Carafa, M. (2011). Novel pH-sensitive non-ionic surfactant vesicles: Comparison between Tween 21 and Tween 20. *Colloids and Surfaces. B, Biointerfaces*, *82*(1), 18–24. doi:10.1016/j.colsurfb.2010.08.004 PMID:20832262

Di Pasqua, A. J., Wallner, S., Kerwood, D. J., & Dabrowiak, J. C. (2009). Adsorption of the PtII anticancer drug carboplatin by mesoporous silica. *Chemistry & Biodiversity*, *6*(9), 1343–1349. doi:10.1002/cbdv.200900021 PMID:19774597

Dierking, I. (2003). *Textures of Liquid Crystals*. Weinheim: Wiley-VCH. doi:10.1002/3527602054

Dinarvand, R., Khodaverdi, E., Atyabi, F., & Erfan, M. (2006). Thermoresponsive drug delivery using liquid crystal-embedded cellulose nitrate membranes. *Drug Delivery*, *13*(5), 345–350. doi:10.1080/10717540500394729 PMID:16877309

Ding, C. X., Gu, J. X., Qu, X. Z., & Yang, Z. Z. (2009). Preparation of multifunctional drug carrier for tumor-specific uptake and enhanced intracellular delivery through the conjugation of weak acid labile linker. *Bioconjugate Chemistry*, *20*(6), 1163–1170. doi:10.1021/bc800563g PMID:19472997

Dixit, R., & Nagarsenker, M. (2008). Self-nanoemulsifying granules of ezetimibe: Design, optimization and evaluation. *European Journal of Pharmaceutical Sciences*, *35*(3), 183–192. doi:10.1016/j.ejps.2008.06.013 PMID:18652892

Djekic, L., Krajisnik, D., Martinovic, M., Djordjevic, D., Primorac, M. (2015). Characterization of gelation process and drug release profile of thermosensitive liquid lecithin/poloxamer 407 based gels as carriers for percutaneous delivery of ibuprofen. *International Journal of Pharmaceutics, 490*(1-2), 180-189.

Djekic, L., Krajisnik, D., & Micic, Y. (2015). Polyphenolics-Phospholipid Complexes as Natural Cosmetic Ingredients: Properties and Application. Tenside, Surfactants. *Detergents*, *52*(3), 186–192.

Dobrovolskaia, M. A., & McNeil, S. E. (2007). Immunological properties of engineered nanomaterials. *Nature Nanotechnology*, *2*(8), 469–478. doi:10.1038/nnano.2007.223 PMID:18654343

Doijad, R. C., Bhambere, D. S., Fakirappa, M. V., & Deshmukh, N. V. (2009). Formulation and characterization of vesicular drug delivery system for Anti-HIV drug. *Journal of Global Pharma Technology*, *1*, 94–100.

Dong, Y. D., Larson, I., Hanley, T., & Boyd, B. J. (2006). Bulk and dispersed aqueous phase behavior of phytantriol: Effect of vitamin E acetate and F127 polymer on liquid crystal nanostructure. *Langmuir*, *22*(23), 9512–9518. doi:10.1021/la061706v PMID:17073473

Drummond, C. J., & Fong, C. (1999). Surfactant self-assembly objects as novel drug delivery vehicles. *Current Opinion in Colloid & Interface Science*, *4*(6), 449–456. doi:10.1016/S1359-0294(00)00020-0

Dubey, V., Mishra, D., Asthana, A., & Jain, N. K. (2006). Transdermal delivery of a pineal hormone: Melatonin via elastic liposomes. *Biomaterials*, *27*(18), 3491–3496. doi:10.1016/j.biomaterials.2006.01.060 PMID:16513163

Dubey, V., Mishra, D., Nahar, M., & Jain, N. K. (2007). Vesicles as tools for the modulation of skin permeability. *Expert Opinion on Drug Delivery*, *4*(6), 579–593. doi:10.1517/17425247.4.6.579 PMID:17970662

Dufes, C., Gaillard, F., Uchegbu, I. F., Schatzlein, A. G., Olivier, J. C., & Muller, J. M. (2004). Glucose-targeted niosomes deliver vasoactive intestinal peptide (VIP) to the brain. *International Journal of Pharmaceutics*, *285*(1-2), 77–85. doi:10.1016/j.ijpharm.2004.07.020 PMID:15488681

Dufes, C., Schätzlein, A., Tetley, L., Gray, A., Watson, D., Olivier, J., & Uchegbu, I. et al. (2000). Niosomes and polymeric chitosan based vesicles bearing transferrin and glucose ligands for drug targeting. *Pharmaceutical Research*, *17*(10), 1250–1258. doi:10.1023/A:1026422915326 PMID:11145231

Du, J.-Z., Du, X.-J., Mao, C.-Q., & Wang, J. (2011). Tailor-Made Dual pH-Sensitive Polymer-Doxorubicin Nanoparticles for Efficient Anticancer Drug Delivery. *Journal of the American Chemical Society*, *133*(44), 17560–17563. doi:10.1021/ja207150n PMID:21985458

Duncan, R., & Sat, Y. N. (1998). Tumour targeting by enhanced permeability and retention (EPR) effect. *Annals of Oncology*, *9*(Suppl.2), 39–44. doi:10.1023/A:1008418325819

Dušek, K., & Prins, W. (1969). *Structure and elasticity of non-crystalline polymer networks*. Springer Berlin Heidelberg.

Ebato, Y., Kato, Y., Onishi, H., Nagai, T., & Machida, Y. (2003). In vivo efficacy of a novel double liposome as an oral dosage form of salmon calcitonin. *Drug Development Research*, *58*(3), 253–257. doi:10.1002/ddr.10162

EBE-EFPIA. (2006). *Position Paper: Inapplicability of automatic substitution rules to biotechnology products, including biosimilar medicinal products: recommendation for addressing unique safety concerns*. Author.

Eccleston, G. M., & Beattie, L. (1988). Micro structural changes during the storage of system containing cetostearyl alcohol/polyxyethylene alkyl ether surfactant. *Drug Development and Industrial Pharmacy*, *14*(15-17), 2499–2518. doi:10.3109/03639048809152029

Echegoyen, L. E., Hernandez, J. C., Kaifer, A. E., Gokel, G. W., & Echegoyen, L. (1988). Aggregation of steroidal lariat ethers: The first example of nonionic liposomes (niosomes) formed from neutral crown ether compounds. *Journal of the Chemical Society. Chemical Communications*, *12*(12), 836–837. doi:10.1039/c39880000836

Echeverria, C., López, D., & Mijangos, C. (2009). UCST responsive microgels of poly (acrylamide–acrylic acid) copolymers: Structure and viscoelastic properties. *Macromolecules*, *42*(22), 9118–9123. doi:10.1021/ma901316k

Eddington, D. T., & Beebe, D. J. (2004). A valved responsive hydrogel microdispensing device with integrated pressure source. *Journal of Microelectromechanical Systems*, *13*(4), 586–593. doi:10.1109/JMEMS.2004.832190

Egbaria, K., & Weiner, N. D. (1990). Liposomes as a topical drug delivery system. *Advanced Drug Delivery Reviews*, *5*(3), 287–300. doi:10.1016/0169-409X(90)90021-J

Elbashir, S. M., Lendeckel, W., & Tuschl, T. (2001). RNA interference is mediated by 21-and 22-nucleotide RNAs. *Genes & Development*, *15*(2), 188–200. doi:10.1101/gad.862301 PMID:11157775

ElBayoumi, T. A., & Torchilin, V. P. (2009). Tumor-targeted nanomedicines: Enhanced antitumor efficacy in vivo of doxorubicin-loaded, long-circulating liposomes modified with cancer-specific monoclonal antibody. *Clinical Cancer Research*, *15*(6), 1973–1980. doi:10.1158/1078-0432.CCR-08-2392 PMID:19276264

Elliott, S., Egrie, J., Browne, J., Lorenzini, T., Busse, L., Rogers, N., & Ponting, I. (2004). Control of rHuEPO biological activity: The role of carbohydrate. *Experimental Hematology*, *32*(12), 1146–1155. doi:10.1016/j.exphem.2004.08.004 PMID:15588939

Elliott, S., Lorenzini, T., Chang, D., Barzilay, J., Delorme, E., Giffin, J., & Hesterberg, L. (1996). Fine structure epitope mapping of antierythropoietin monoclonal antibodies reveals a model of recombinant human erythropoietin structure. *Blood*, *87*, 2702–2713. PMID:8639886

El-Menshawe, S. F., & Hussein, A. K. (2013). Formulation and evaluation of meloxicam niosomes as vesicular carriers for enhanced skin delivery. *Pharmaceutical Development and Technology*, *18*(4), 779–786. doi:10.3109/10837450.2011.598166 PMID:21913880

Elnaggar, Y. S., El-Refaie, W. M., El-Massik, M. A., & Abdallah, O. Y. (2014). Lecithin based nanostructured gels for skin delivery: An update on state of art and recent applications. *Journal of Controlled Release*, *180*, 10–24. doi:10.1016/j.jconrel.2014.02.004 PMID:24531009

El-Ridy, M. S., Abdelbary, A., Nasr, E. A., Khalil, R. M., Mostafa, D. M., El-Batal, A. I., & Abd El-Alim, H. S. (2011). Niosomal encapsulation of the antitubercular drug, pyrazinamide. *Drug Development and Industrial Pharmacy*, *37*(9), 1110–1118. doi:10.3109/03639045.2011.560605 PMID:21417612

El-Ridy, M. S., Yehia, S. A., Kassem, M. A. E. M., Mostafa, D. M., Nasr, E. A., & Asfour, M. H. (2015). Niosomal encapsulation of ethambutol hydrochloride for increasing its efficacy and safety. *Drug Delivery*, *22*(1), 21–36. doi:10.3109/10717544.2013.868556 PMID:24359403

Elsabahy, M., & Wooley, K. L. (2012). Design of polymeric nanoparticles for biomedical delivery applications. *Chemical Society Reviews*, *41*(7), 2545–2561. doi:10.1039/c2cs15327k PMID:22334259

Elsayed, M. M. A., Abdallah, O. Y., Naggar, V. F., & Khalafallah, N. M. (2007). Lipid vesicles for skin delivery of drugs: Reviewing three decades of research. *International Journal of Pharmaceutics*, *332*(1-2), 1–16. doi:10.1016/j.ijpharm.2006.12.005 PMID:17222523

Elsayed, M. M., Abdallah, O. Y., & Nagar, V. F. (2006). Deformable liposomes and ethosomes: Mechanism of enhanced skin delivery. *International Journal of Pharmaceutics*, *322*(1-2), 60–66. doi:10.1016/j.ijpharm.2006.05.027 PMID:16806755

EMEA. (2009). *Scientific Guidelines for Human Medicines*. Retrieved from http://www.emea.Europa .eu/ htms /human/humanguidelines/multidiscipline.htm

Engstrom, S., Larsson, K., & Lindman, B. (1984). *Method of preparing controlled-release preparations for biologically active materials.* European Patent EP0126751 A1.

Ercan, M. T. (1992). Rapid determination of hydrolyzed-reduced technetium-99m in particulate radiopharmaceuticals. *International Journal of Radiation Applications and Instrumentation. Part A, Applied Radiation and Isotopes*, *43*(9), 1175–1177. doi:10.1016/0883-2889(92)90065-M

Eriksson, P. O., & Lindblom, G. (1993). Lipid and water diffusion in bicontinuous cubic phases measured by NMR. *Biophysical Journal*, *64*(1), 129–136. doi:10.1016/S0006-3495(93)81347-X PMID:8431537

Esposito, E., Carotta, V., Scabbia, A., Trombelli, L., D'Antona, P., Menegatti, E., & Nastruzzi, C. (1996). Comparative analysis of tetracycline-containing dental gels: Poloxamer- and monoglyceride-based formulations. *International Journal of Pharmaceutics*, *142*(1), 9–23. doi:10.1016/0378-5173(96)04649-2

Esposito, E., Cortesi, R., Drechsler, M., Paccamiccio, L., Mariani, P., Contado, C., & Puglia, C. et al. (2005). Cubosome dispersions as delivery systems for percutaneous administration of indomethacin. *Pharmaceutical Research*, *22*(12), 2163–2173. doi:10.1007/s11095-005-8176-x PMID:16267633

Estrela, J. M., Ortega, A., & Obrador, E. (2006). Glutathione in cancer biology and therapy. *Critical Reviews in Clinical Laboratory Sciences*, *43*(2), 143–181. doi:10.1080/10408360500523878 PMID:16517421

Etheridge, M. L., Campbell, S. A., Erdman, A. G., Haynes, C. L., Wolf, S. M., & McCullough, J. (2013). The big picture on nanomedicine: The state of investigational and approved nanomedicine products. *Nanomedicine; Nanotechnology, Biology, and Medicine*, *9*(1), 1–14. doi:10.1016/j.nano.2012.05.013 PMID:22684017

European Biopharmaceutical Enterprises (EBE). (n.d.). *Biosimilars*. EBE.

European Medicines Agency (EMA). (2012). *Questions and Answers on biosimilar medicines (similar medicinal products).* European Medicines Agency. Retrieved from http://www.ema.europa.eu/ema/index.jsp?curl=pages/special_topics/document_listing/document_listing_000318.jsp

European Medicines Agency (EMA). (n.d.). *Guideline on similar biological medicinal products containing biotechnology-derived proteins as active substance: quality issues (revision 1).* European Medicines Agency - Europa.

Evans, J. R., Fildes, F. J., & Oliver, J. E. (1983). *U.S. Patent No. 4,370,349.* Washington, DC: U.S. Patent and Trademark Office.

Fang, , Niu, Lin, & Wang. (2008). Applications of electrospun nanofibers. *Chinese Science Bulletin, 53*(15), 2265–2286.

Fang, J. Y., Hong, C. T., Chiu, W. T., & Wang, Y. Y. (2001). Effect of liposomes and niosomes on skin permeation of enoxacin. *International Journal of Pharmaceutics, 219*(1-2), 61–72. doi:10.1016/S0378-5173(01)00627-5 PMID:11337166

Fan, H. L., Huang, J., Li, Y. P., Yu, J. H., & Chen, J. H. (2010). Fabrication of reduction-degradable micelle based on disulfide-linked graft copolymer–camptothecin conjugate for enhancing solubility and stability of camptothecin. *Polymer, 51*(22), 5107–5114. doi:10.1016/j.polymer.2010.09.004

Fan, J., Lei, J., Wang, L. M., Yu, C. Z., Tu, B., & Zhao, D. Y. (2003). Rapid and high capacity immobilization of enzymes based on mesoporous silica with controlled morphologies. *Chemical Communications (Cambridge), 17*, 2140–2141. doi:10.1039/b304391f PMID:13678170

Faraji, A. H., & Wipf, P. (2009). Nanoparticles in cellular drug delivery. *Bioorganic & Medicinal Chemistry, 17*(8), 2950–2962. doi:10.1016/j.bmc.2009.02.043 PMID:19299149

Fariya, M., Jain, A., Dhawan, V., Shah, S., & Nagarsenker, M. S. (2014). Bolaamphiphiles: A Pharmaceutical Review. *Advanced Pharmaceutical Bulletin, 4*(Suppl 2), 483.

Farkas, E., Kiss, D., & Zelk, O. R. (2007). Study on the release of chlorhexidine base and salts from different liquid crystalline structures. *International Journal of Pharmaceutics, 340*(1-2), 71–75. doi:10.1016/j.ijpharm.2007.03.038 PMID:17467206

Farkas, E., Zelko, R., Nemeth, Z., Palinkas, J., Marton, S., & Racz, I. (2000). The effect of liquid crystalline structure on chlorhexidine diacetate release. *International Journal of Pharmaceutics, 193*(2), 239–245. doi:10.1016/S0378-5173(99)00346-1 PMID:10606788

Farokhzad, O. C., & Langer, R. (2009). Impact of nanotechnology on drug delivery. *ACS Nano, 3*(1), 16–20. doi:10.1021/nn900002m PMID:19206243

Farooq, S. A., Saini, V., Singh, R., & Kaur, K. (2013). Application of novel drug delivery system in the pharmacotherapy of Hyperlipidemia. *Journal Of Chemical and Pharmaceutical Sciences, 6*(3), 138–144.

Farraj, N., Johansen, B., Davis, S., & Illum, L. (1990). Nasal administration of insulin using bioadhesive microspheres as a delivery system. *Journal of Controlled Release, 13*(2), 253–261. doi:10.1016/0168-3659(90)90016-M

Fasol, U., Frost, A., Büchert, M., Arends, J., Fiedler, U., Scharr, D., & Mross, K. et al. (2012). Vascular and pharmacokinetic effects of EndoTAG-1 in patients with advanced cancer and liver metastasis. *Annals of Oncology, 23*(4), 1030–1036. doi:10.1093/annonc/mdr300 PMID:21693769

Fathi-Azarbayjani, A., & Chan, S. Y. (2010). Single and multi-layered nanofibers for rapid and controlled drug delivery. *Chemical & Pharmaceutical Bulletin, 58*(2), 143–146. doi:10.1248/cpb.58.143 PMID:20118570

Fattal, E., Vauthier, C., Aynie, I., Nakada, Y., Lambert, G., Malvy, C., & Couvreur, P. (1998). Biodegradable polyalkylcyanoacrylate nanoparticles for the delivery of oligonucleotides. *Journal of Controlled Release*, *53*(1-3), 137–143. doi:10.1016/S0168-3659(97)00246-0 PMID:9741921

Fedorchak, M. V., Little, S. R., Schuman, J. S., & Cugini, A. (2014). *WO Patent Application 14/138085*.

Feher, A., Urban, E., Eros, I., Szabove, P., & Csanyi, E. (2008). Lyotropic liquid crystal perconcentrates for the treatment of periodontal disease. *International Journal of Pharmaceutics*, *358*(1-2), 23–26. doi:10.1016/j.ijpharm.2008.02.025 PMID:18403142

Felgner, P. L., Gadek, T. R., Holm, M., Roman, R., Chan, H. W., Wenz, M., & Danielsen, M. et al. (1987). Lipofection: A highly efficient, lipid-mediated DNA-transfection procedure. *Proceedings of the National Academy of Sciences of the United States of America*, *84*(21), 7413–7417. doi:10.1073/pnas.84.21.7413 PMID:2823261

Ferry, J. D. (1980). *Viscoelastic Properties of Polymers*. New York, NY: Wiley.

Fidalgo, A., Lopez, T. M., & Ilharco, L. M. (2009). Wet sol–gel silica matrices as delivery devices for phenytoin. *Journal of Sol-Gel Science and Technology*, *49*(3), 320–328. doi:10.1007/s10971-008-1880-3

Filippousi, M., Angelakeris, M., Katsikini, M., Paloura, E., Efthimiopoulos, I., Wang, Y., & van Tendeloo, G. et al. (2014). Surfactant effects on the structural and magnetic properties of iron oxide nanoparticles. *J. Phys. Chem. C Nanomater. Interfaces*, *118*, 16209–16217.

Fire, A., Xu, S., Montgomery, M. K., Kostas, S. A., Driver, S. E., & Mello, C. C. (1998). Potent and specific genetic interference by double-stranded RNA in Caenorhabditis elegans. *Nature, 391*(6669), 806-811.

Florence, A. (1993). Nonionic surfactant vesicles: preparation and characterization. *Liposome technology 2*,157-176.

Flory, P. J., & Rehner, J. Jr. (1943). Statistical mechanics of cross-linked polymer networks II. Swelling. *The Journal of Chemical Physics*, *11*(11), 521–526. doi:10.1063/1.1723792

Fomina, N., McFearin, C., Sermsakdi, M., Edigin, O., & Almutairi, A. (2010). UV and near-IR triggered release from polymeric nanoparticles. *Journal of the American Chemical Society*, *132*(28), 9540–9542. doi:10.1021/ja102595j PMID:20568765

Fong, C., Wells, D., Krodkiewska, I., Booth, J., & Hartley, P. G. (2007). Synthesis and mesophases of glycerate surfactants. *The Journal of Physical Chemistry B*, *111*(6), 1384–1392. doi:10.1021/jp0659655 PMID:17286353

Fong, W. K., Hanley, T., & Boyd, B. J. (2009). Stimuli responsive liquid crystals provide 'on-demand' drug delivery *in vitro* and *in vivo*. *Journal of Controlled Release*, *135*(3), 218–226. doi:10.1016/j.jconrel.2009.01.009 PMID:19331865

Forestier, F., Gerrier, P., Chaumard, C., Quero, A. M., Couvreur, P., & Labarre, C. (1992). Effect of nanoparticle-bound ampicillin on the survival of listeria monocytogenes in mouse peritoneal macrophages. *The Journal of Antimicrobial Chemotherapy*, *30*(2), 173–179. doi:10.1093/jac/30.2.173 PMID:1399927

Foster, T., Dorfman, K. D., & Davis, H. T. (2010). Giant biocompatible and biodegradable PEG–PMCL vesicles and microcapsules by solvent evaporation from double emulsion droplets. *Journal of Colloid and Interface Science*, *351*(1), 140–150. doi:10.1016/j.jcis.2010.05.020 PMID:20627256

Fox, G. F., & Sothinathan, U. (2005). The choice of surfactant for treatment of respiratory distress syndrome in preterm infants: A review of the evidence. *Infant*, *1*, 8–12.

Fraley, R., Wyatt, J. P., & Papahadjopoulus, D. (1981). Liposomes: From Physical Structues to Therapeutics Applications. Elsevier.

Franco, R., & Cidlowski, J. A. (2009). Apoptosis and glutathione: Beyond an antioxidant. *Cell Death and Differentiation*, *16*(10), 1303–1314. doi:10.1038/cdd.2009.107 PMID:19662025

Franco, R., Schoneveld, O. J., Pappa, A., & Panayiotidis, M. I. (2007). The central role of glutathione in the pathophysiology of human diseases. *Archives of Physiology and Biochemistry*, *113*(4-5), 234–258. doi:10.1080/13813450701661198 PMID:18158646

Frank, D., Tyagi, C., Tomar, L., Echoonara, Y., du Toit, L. C., Kumar, P., & Pillay, V. et al. (2014). Overview of the role of nanotechnological innovations in the detection and treatment of solid tumors. *International Journal of Nanomedicine*, *9*, 589–613. PMID:24489467

Freiberg, S., & Zhu, X. (2004). Polymer microspheres for controlled drug release. *International Journal of Pharmaceutics*, *282*(1), 1–18. doi:10.1016/j.ijpharm.2004.04.013 PMID:15336378

Fry, D. W., White, J. C., & Goldman, I. D. (1978). Rapid separation of low molecular weight solutes from liposomes without dilution. *Journal of Analytical Biochemistry*, *90*(2), 809–815. doi:10.1016/0003-2697(78)90172-0 PMID:727510

Fuchs, S., Otto, H., Jehle, S., Henklein, P., & Schlüter, A. D. (2005). Fluorescent dendrimers with a peptide cathepsin B cleavage site for drug delivery applications. *Chemical Communications*, (14): 1830–1832. doi:10.1039/B415651J PMID:15795757

Fuller, J. M., Raghupathi, K. R., Ramireddy, R. R., Subrahmanyam, A. V., Yesilyurt, V., & Thayumanavan, S. (2013). Temperature-Sensitive Transitions below LCST in Amphiphilic Dendritic Assemblies: Host–Guest Implications. *Journal of the American Chemical Society*, *135*(24), 8947–8954. doi:10.1021/ja402019c PMID:23692369

Gaafar, P. M., Abdallah, O. Y., Farid, R. M., & Abdelkader, H. (2014). Preparation, characterization and evaluation of novel elastic nano-sized niosomes (ethoniosomes) for ocular delivery of prednisolone. *Journal of Liposome Research*, *24*(3), 204–215. doi:10.3109/08982104.2014.881850 PMID:24484536

Gabizon, A., & Papahadjopoulos, D. (1988). Liposome formulations with prolonged circulation time in blood and enhanced uptake by tumors. *Proceedings of the National Academy of Sciences of the United States of America*, *85*(18), 6949–6953. doi:10.1073/pnas.85.18.6949 PMID:3413128

Gallardo, M. M., Couarraze, G., Denizot, B., Treupel, L., Couvreur, P., & Puisieux, F. (1993). Preparation and purification of isohexylcyanoacrylate nanocapsules. *International Journal of Pharmaceutics*, *100*, 55–64. doi:10.1016/0378-5173(93)90075-Q

Gamal, M., Maghraby, M., Williams, A. C., & Barry, B. W. (1999). Skin delivery of oestradiol from deformable and traditional liposomes- Mechanistic studies. *The Journal of Pharmacy and Pharmacology*, *51*(10), 1123–1134. doi:10.1211/0022357991776813 PMID:10579683

Gambling, D., Hughes, T., Martin, G., Horton, W., & Manvelian, G. (2005). A comparison of Depodur, a novel, single-dose extended-release epidural morphine, with standard epidural morphine for pain relief after lower abdominal surgery. *Anesthesia and Analgesia*, *100*(4), 1065–1074. doi:10.1213/01.ANE.0000145009.03574.78 PMID:15781524

Gana-Weisz, M., Halaschek-Wiener, J., Jansen, B., Elad, G., Haklai, R., & Kloog, Y. (2002). The Ras inhibitor S-trans, trans-farnesylthiosalicylic acid chemosensitizes human tumor cells without causing resistance. *Clinical Cancer Research*, *8*(2), 555–565. PMID:11839677

Ganem-Quintanar, A., Quintanar-Guerrero, D., & Buri, P. (2000). Monoolein: A review of the pharmaceutical applications. *Drug Development and Industrial Pharmacy*, *26*(8), 809–820. doi:10.1081/DDC-100101304 PMID:10900537

Ganesan, M. G., Weiner, N. D., Flynn, G. I., & Ho, N. F. H. (1984). Influence of liposomal drug entrapment on percutaneous absorption. *International Journal of Pharmaceutics*, *20*(1-2), 139–154. doi:10.1016/0378-5173(84)90225-4

Gangwar, M., Singh, R., Goel, R. K., & Nath, G. (2011). Recent Advances In Various Emerging Vescicular Systems: An Overview. *Asian Pacific Journal of Tropical Biomedicine*, *33*, 848.

Ganta, S., Devalapally, H., Shahiwala, A., & Amiji, M. (2008). A review of stimuli-responsive nanocarriers for drug and gene delivery. *Journal of Controlled Release*, *126*(3), 187–204. doi:10.1016/j.jconrel.2007.12.017 PMID:18261822

Gao, Y., Kuang, Y., & Xu, B. (2014). *U.S. Patent No. 8,658,600*. Washington, DC: U.S. Patent and Trademark Office.

Gao, X., Huang, Y., Makhov, A. M., Epperly, M., Lu, J., Grab, S., & Li, S. et al. (2013). Nanoassembly of surfactants with interfacial drug-interactive motifs as tailor-designed drug carriers. *Molecular Pharmaceutics*, *10*(1), 187–198. doi:10.1021/mp300319m PMID:23244299

Garg, A., & Singh, S. (2011). Enhancement in antifungal activity of eugenol in immunosuppressed rats through lipid nanocarriers. *Colloids and Surfaces. B, Biointerfaces*, *87*(2), 280–288. doi:10.1016/j.colsurfb.2011.05.030 PMID:21689909

Garg, A., & Singh, S. (2014). Targeting of eugenol loaded solid lipid nanoparticles to the epidermal layer of human skin. *Nanomedicine (London)*, *9*(8), 1223–1238. doi:10.2217/nnm.13.33 PMID:23987096

Garg, T., Rath, G., Murthy, R. R., Gupta, U. D., Vatsala, P. G., & Goyal, A. K. (2015). Current nanotechnological approaches for an effective delivery of bioactive drug molecules to overcome drug resistance tuberculosis. *Current Pharmaceutical Design*, *21*(22), 3076–3089. doi:10.2174/1381612821666150531163254 PMID:26027577

GarimaChawla, P. G., Koradia, V., & Bansal, A. K. (2013). *Gastroretention, a means to address regional variability in intestinal drug absorption*. Academic Press.

Gasco, M., & Trotta, M. (1986). Nanoparticles from microemulsions. *International Journal of Pharmaceutics*, *29*(2-3), 267–268. doi:10.1016/0378-5173(86)90125-0

Gautier, J. C., Grangier, J. L., Barbier, A., Dupont, P., Dussosoy, D., Pastor, G., & Couvreur, P. (1992). Biodegradable nanoparticles for subcutaneous administration of growth hormone releasing factor (hGRF). *Journal of Controlled Release*, *3*, 205–210.

Gayathri Devi, S., & Udupa, N. (2000). Niosomal Sumartriptan Succinate For Nasal Administration. *Indian Journal of Pharmaceutical Sciences*, *62*(6), 479–486.

Geary, R. S., & Schlameus, H. W. (1993). Vancomycin and insulin used as models for oral delivery of peptides. *Journal of Controlled Release*, *23*(1), 65–74. doi:10.1016/0168-3659(93)90071-C

Gebicki, J., & Hicks, M. (1973). Ufasomes are stable particles surrounded by unsaturated fatty acid membranes. *Nature*, *243*(5404), 232–234. doi:10.1038/243232a0 PMID:4706295

Gelperina, S., Kisich, K., Iseman, M. D., & Heifets, L. (2005). The potential advantages of nanoparticle drug delivery systems in chemotherapy of tuberculosis. *American Journal of Respiratory and Critical Care Medicine*, *172*(12), 1487–1490. doi:10.1164/rccm.200504-613PP PMID:16151040

Generics and Biosimilars Initiative. (2012). *India releases draft similar biologic guidelines*. Retrieved from www.gabionline.net/layout/set/print/guidelines/india-releases-draft-similar-biologic-guidelines

Gennes, P. G., & Prost, J. (1993). *The Physics of Liquid Crystals*. Oxford, UK: Clarendon Press.

George, P. M., LaVan, D. A., Burdick, J. A., Chen, C. Y., Liang, E., & Langer, R. (2006). Electrically Controlled Drug Delivery from Biotin-Doped Conductive Polypyrrole. *Advanced Materials*, *18*(5), 577–581. doi:10.1002/adma.200501242

Geraghty, P. B., Attwood, D., Collett, J. H., & Dandiker, Y. (1996). The in vitro release of some antimuscarinic drugs from monoolein/water lyotropic liquid crystalline gels. *Pharmaceutical Research*, *13*(8), 1265–1271. doi:10.1023/A:1016036908947 PMID:8865324

Ghannoum, M., Isham, N., Henry, W., Kroon, H.-A., & Yurdakul, S. (2012). Evaluation of the Morphological Effects of TDT 067 (Terbinafi ne in Transfersome) and Conventional Terbinafi ne on Dermatophyte Hyphae In Vitro and In Vivo. *Antimicrobial Agents and Chemotherapy*, *56*(5), 2530–2534. doi:10.1128/AAC.05998-11 PMID:22354309

Ghizal, R., Fatima, G. R., & Srivastava, S. (2014). Smart Polymers and Their Applications. *International Journal of Engineering Technology. Management and Applied Sciences*, *2*(4), 104–115.

Giljohann, D. A., Seferos, D. S., Daniel, W. L., Massich, M. D., Patel, P. C., & Mirkin, C. A. (2010). Gold nanoparticles for biology and medicine. *Angewandte Chemie International Edition in English*, *49*(19), 3280–3294. doi:10.1002/anie.200904359 PMID:20401880

Gillies, E. R., & Fréchet, J. M. J. (2003). A new approach towards acid sensitive copolymer micelles for drug delivery. *Chemical Communications*, *14*(14), 1640–1641. doi:10.1039/B304251K PMID:12877480

Gillies, E. R., Jonsson, T. B., & Fréchet, J. M. J. (2004). Stimuli-responsive supramolecular assemblies of linear-dendritic copolymers. *Journal of the American Chemical Society*, *126*(38), 11936–11943. doi:10.1021/ja0463738 PMID:15382929

Ginsburg, G. S., Atkinson, D., & Small, D. M. (1984). Physical properties of cholesteric esters. *Progress in Lipid Research*, *23*(3), 135–167. doi:10.1016/0163-7827(84)90002-X PMID:6399750

Giorgione, J. R., Huang, Z., & Epand, R. M. (1998). Increased activation of protein kinase C with cubic phase lipid compared with liposomes. *Biochemistry*, *37*(8), 2384–2392. doi:10.1021/bi970873e PMID:9485386

Glangchai, L. C., Caldorera-Moore, M., Shi, L., & Roy, K. (2008). Nanoimprint lithography based fabrication of shape-specific, enzymatically-triggered smart nanoparticles. *Journal of Controlled Release*, *125*(3), 263–272. doi:10.1016/j.jconrel.2007.10.021 PMID:18053607

Glantz, M. J., LaFollette, S., Jaeckle, K. A., Shapiro, W., Swinnen, L., Royental, J. R., & Howell, S. B. et al. (1999). Randomized trial of a slow-release versus a standard formulation of cytarabine for the intrathecal treatment of lymphomatous meningitis. *Journal of Clinical Oncology*, *17*, 3110–3116. PMID:10506606

Global Industry Analysts Inc. (GIAI). (2012). *Biosimilars – a global strategic business report.* GIAI.

Glück, R. (1999). Adjuvant activity of immunopotentiating reconstituted influenza virosomes (IRIVs). *Vaccine*, *17*(13-14), 1782–1787. doi:10.1016/S0264-410X(98)00440-X PMID:10194840

Goeddel, D. V., Heyneker, H. L., Hozumi, T., Arentzen, R., Itakura, K., Yansura, D. G., & Seeburg, P. H. (1979). Direct expression in *Escherichia coli* of a DNA sequence coding for human growth hormone. *Nature*, *281*(5732), 544–548. doi:10.1038/281544a0 PMID:386136

Goldberg, E. P. (1983). *Local chemo- and immunotherapy by intratumor drug injection: opportunities for polymer-drug compositions. In Targeted Drugs* (p. 312). New York: Wiley.

Goldberg, M., Langer, R., & Jia, X. (2007). Nanostructured materials for applications in drug delivery and tissue engineering. *Journal of Biomaterials Science. Polymer Edition*, *18*(3), 241–268. doi:10.1163/156856207779996931 PMID:17471764

Golla, K., Bhaskar, C., Ahmed, F., & Kondapi, A. K. (2013). A target specific oral formulation of doxorubicin-protein nanoparticles: Efficacy and safety in hepatocellular cancer. *Journal of Cancer*, *4*(8), 644–652. doi:10.7150/jca.7093 PMID:24155776

Gompper, G., & Kroll, D. M. (1995). Driven transport of fluid vesicles through narrow pores. *Physical Review E: Statistical Physics, Plasmas, Fluids, and Related Interdisciplinary Topics*, *52*(4), 4198–4211. doi:10.1103/PhysRevE.52.4198 PMID:9963891

Gopalakrishnan, A. M., Kundu, A. K., Mandal, T. K., & Kumar, N. (2013). Novel nanosomes for gene delivery to Plasmodium falciparum-infected red blood cells. *Scientific Reports*, *3*, 1534. doi:10.1038/srep01534 PMID:23525038

Gopal, R., Kaur, S., Feng, C. Y., Chan, C., Ramakrishna, S., Tabe, S., & Matsuura, T. (2007). Electrospun nanofibrous polysulfone membranes as pre-filters: Particulate removal. *Journal of Membrane Science*, *289*(1), 210–219. doi:10.1016/j.memsci.2006.11.056

Gopferich, A., & Lee, G. (1992). Determining the solubility and crystal form of clenbuterol in thin films of Eudragit NE30D. *Drug Development and Industrial Pharmacy*, *18*(3), 319–331. doi:10.3109/03639049209043702

Gopinath, D., Ravi, D., Rao, B., Apte, S., Renuka, D., & Rambhau, D. (2004). Ascorbyl palmitate vesicles (Aspasomes): Formation, characterization and applications. *International Journal of Pharmaceutics*, *271*(1), 95–113. doi:10.1016/j.ijpharm.2003.10.032 PMID:15129977

Górski, G., Szopiński, P., Michalak, J., Marianowska, A., Borkowski, M., Geremek, M., & Noszczyk, W. et al. (2005). Liposomal heparin spray: A new formula in adjunctive treatment of superficial venous thrombosis. *Angiology*, *56*(1), 9–17. doi:10.1177/000331970505600102 PMID:15678251

Gou, X. C., Liu, J., & Zhang, H. L. (2010). Monitoring human telomere DNA hybridization and G-quadruplex formation using gold nanorods. *Analytica Chimica Acta*, *668*(2), 208–214. doi:10.1016/j.aca.2010.04.027 PMID:20493300

Goyal, P., & Goyal, K., Kumar, S. G. V., Singh, A., Katare, O. P., & Mishra, D. N. (2005). Liposomal drug delivery systems-clinical applications. *Acta Pharmaceutica (Zagreb, Croatia)*, *55*(1), 1–25. PMID:15907221

Goyal, P., Goyal, K., Kumar, S. G., Singh, A., Katare, O. P., & Mishra, D. N. (2005). Liposomal drug delivery systems: Clincal applications. *Acta Pharmaceutica (Zagreb, Croatia)*, *55*, 1–25. PMID:15907221

Graham, N. B. (1992). Poly(ethylene glycol) chemistry. In J. M. Harris (Ed.), *Biotechnical and biomedical application* (pp. 1–13). New York, NY: Plenum Press.

Graham, T. (1861). On liquid transpiration in relation to chemical composition. *Philosophical Transactions of the Royal Society*, *151*, 183–224. doi:10.1098/rstl.1861.0011

Graham, T. (1864). On the properties of silicic acid and other analogous colloidal substances. *Journal of the Chemical Society of London*, *17*, 318–327.

Gramaglia, D., Conway, B. R., Kett, V. L., Malcolm, R. K., & Batchelor, H. K. (2005). High speed DSC (HyperDSC) as a tool to measure the solubility of a drug within a solid or semi-solid matrix. *International Journal of Pharmaceutics*, *301*(1-2), 1–5. doi:10.1016/j.ijpharm.2005.04.038 PMID:16061335

Grant, R., & Grant, C. (Eds.). (1987). *Grant & Hackh's Chemical Dictionary* (5th ed.). New York, NY: McGraw-Hill.

Grassi-Schultheiss, P. P., Heller, F., & Dobson, J. (1997). Analysis ofmagnetic material in the human heart, spleen and liver. *Biometals*, *10*(4), 351–355. doi:10.1023/A:1018340920329 PMID:9353885

Greenberger, J. S., Sakakeeny, M. A., Humphries, R. K., Eaves, C. J., & Eckner, R. J. (1983). Demonstration of permanent factor-dependent multipotential (erythroid/neutrophil/basophil) hematopoietic progenitor cell lines. *Proceedings of the National Academy of Sciences of the United States of America*, *80*(10), 2931–2935. doi:10.1073/pnas.80.10.2931 PMID:6574462

Gref, R., Domb, A., Quellec, P., Blunk, T., Müller, R., Verbavatz, J., & Langer, R. (2012). The controlled intravenous delivery of drugs using PEG-coated sterically stabilized nanospheres. *Advanced Drug Delivery Reviews*, *64*, 316–326. doi:10.1016/j.addr.2012.09.008 PMID:25170183

Gref, R., Minamitake, Y., Peracchia, M. T., Domb, A., Trubetskoy, V., Torchilin, V., & Langer, R. (1997). Poly(ethylene Glycol)-coated nanospheres: Potential carriers for intravenous drug administration. *Pharmaceutical Biotechnology*, *10*, 167–198. doi:10.1007/0-306-46803-4_6 PMID:9160372

Gregoriadis, G. (Ed.). (2007). Liposome Technology. New York, NY: Informa Healthcare.

Gregoriadis, G. (1976a). The carrier potential of liposomes in biology and medicine. *The New England Journal of Medicine*, *295*(13), 704–710. doi:10.1056/NEJM197609232951305 PMID:958245

Gregoriadis, G. (1976b). The carrier potential of liposomes in biology and medicine (second of two parts). *The New England Journal of Medicine*, *295*(14), 765–770. doi:10.1056/NEJM197609302951406 PMID:785256

Gregoriadis, G. (1977). Targeting of drugs. *Controlled drug delivery. Nature*, *265*(5593), 407–411. doi:10.1038/265407a0 PMID:834290

Gregoriadis, G. (1995). Engineering liposomes for drug delivery: Progress and problems. *Trends in Biotechnology*, *13*(12), 527–537. doi:10.1016/S0167-7799(00)89017-4 PMID:8595139

Gubernator, J., Lipka, D., Korycińska, M., Kempińska, K., Milczarek, M., Wietrzyk, J., & Kozubek, A. et al. (2014). Efficient Human Breast Cancer Xenograft Regression after a Single Treatment with a Novel Liposomal Formulation of Epirubicin Prepared Using the EDTA Ion Gradient Method. *PLoS ONE*, *9*(3), e91487. doi:10.1371/journal.pone.0091487 PMID:24621591

Gude, R., Jadhav, M., Rao, S., & Jagtap, A. (2002). Effects of niosomal cisplatin and combination of the same with theophylline and with activated macrophages in murine B16F10 melanoma model. *Cancer Biotherapy & Radiopharmaceuticals*, *17*(2), 183–192. doi:10.1089/108497802753773801 PMID:12030112

Guedj, C., Pucci, B., Zarif, L., Coulomb, C., Riess, J., & Pavia, A. (1994). Vesicles and other supramolecular systems from biocompatible synthetic glycolipids with hydrocarbon and/or fluorocarbon chains. *Chemistry and Physics of Lipids*, *72*(2), 153–173. doi:10.1016/0009-3084(94)90099-X PMID:7954977

Guinedi, A. S., Mortada, N. D., Mansour, S., & Hathout, R. M. (2005). Preparation and evaluation of reverse-phase evaporation and multilamellar niosomes as ophthalmic carriers of acetazolamide. *International Journal of Pharmaceutics*, *306*(1-2), 71–82. doi:10.1016/j.ijpharm.2005.09.023 PMID:16263229

Gunter, K. K., Gunter, T. E., Jarkowski, A., & Rosier, R. N. (1982). evidence for more than one calcium ion transport mechanism in mitochondria. *Analytical Biochemistry*, *110*, 123.

Guo, C., Wang, J., Cao, F., Lee, R. J., & Zhai, G. (2010). Lyotropic liquid crystal systems in drug delivery. *Drug Discovery Today*, *15*(23-24), 1032–1040. doi:10.1016/j.drudis.2010.09.006 PMID:20934534

Guo, J., Zhuang, J., Wang, F., Raghupathi, K. R., & Thayumanavan, S. (2014). Protein AND enzyme gated supramolecular disassembly. *Journal of the American Chemical Society*, *136*(6), 2220–2223. doi:10.1021/ja4108676 PMID:24447098

Guo, Q., Yuan, J., & Zeng, J. (2014). Biosynthesis of gold nanoparticles using a kind of flavonol:Dihydromyricetin. *Colloids and Surfaces. A, Physicochemical and Engineering Aspects*, *441*, 127–132. doi:10.1016/j.colsurfa.2013.08.067

Guo, S., & Huang, L. (2011). Nanoparticles escaping RES and endosome: Challenges for siRNA delivery for cancer therapy. *Journal of Nanomaterials*, *2011*, 11. doi:10.1155/2011/742895

Gupta, N., Srivastava, V., Saxena, S., & Pandey, A. (2010). Formulation and evaluation of non-ionic surfactant vesicles for ocular delivery of ofloxacin, *International Journal of Life Science and Pharma Reviews*, (7), 413-418.

Gupta, A., Stait-Gardner, T., de Campo, L., Waddington, L. J., Kirby, N., Price, W. S., & Moghaddam, M. J. (2014). Nano assemblies of Gd-DTPA-monooleyl and glycerol monooleate amphiphiles as potential MRI contrast agents. *Journal of Materials Chemistry B*, *2*(9), 1225–1233. doi:10.1039/c3tb21069c

Gupta, P. N., Mishra, V., Singh, P., Rawat, A., Dubey, P., Mahor, S., & Vyas, S. P. (2005). Tetanus toxoid-loaded transfersomes for topical immunization. *The Journal of Pharmacy and Pharmacology*, *57*(3), 295–301. doi:10.1211/0022357055515 PMID:15807984

Gupta, P., Vermani, K., & Garg, S. (2002). Hydrogels: From controlled release to pH-responsive drug delivery. *Drug Discovery Today*, *7*(10), 569–579. doi:10.1016/S1359-6446(02)02255-9 PMID:12047857

Gupta, S., Singh, R. P., Lokwani, P., Yadav, S., & Gupta, S. K. (2011). Vesicular system as targeted drug delivery system: An overview. *International Journal of Pharmacy and Technology*, *3*(2), 987–1021.

Gupta, V., Agrawal, R., & Triwedi, P. (2011). Reduction in cisplatin genotoxity in non-target cells of mice by protrasfersome gel formulation used for management of cutaneous squamous cell carcinoma. *Acta Pharmaceutica (Zagreb, Croatia)*, *61*, 63–71. doi:10.2478/v10007-011-0004-8 PMID:21406344

Gurny, R., Peppas, N. A., Harrington, D. D., & Banker, G. S. (1981). Development of biodegradable and injectable lattices for controlled release potent drugs. *Drug Development and Industrial Pharmacy*, *7*(1), 1–25. doi:10.3109/03639048109055684

Gustafsson, J., Ljusberg Wahren, H., Almgren, M., & Larsson, K. (1997). Submicron particles of reversed lipid phases in water stabilized by a nonionic amphiphilic polymer. *Langmuir*, *13*(26), 6964–6971. doi:10.1021/la970566+

H.R. 1548 (112th Congress), Title I (a)(4)(A)(i)(II).

Haba, Y., Harada, A., Takagishi, T., & Kono, K. (2004). Rendering poly (amidoamine) or poly (propylenimine) dendrimers temperature sensitive. *Journal of the American Chemical Society*, *126*(40), 12760–12761. doi:10.1021/ja047755g PMID:15469255

Haba, Y., Kojima, C., Harada, A., & Kono, K. (2006). Control of temperature-sensitive properties of poly (amidoamine) dendrimers using peripheral modification with various alkylamide groups. *Macromolecules*, *39*(21), 7451–7453. doi:10.1021/ma061019a

Haefeli, U., Atcher, R., Morris, C., & Beresford, B. (1992). Polymeric radiopharmaceutical delivery systems. *Radioactivity and Radiochemistry*, *3*, 11–11.

Hafer, C., Goble, R., Deering, P., Lehmer, A., & Breut, J. (1999). Formulation of interleukin-2 and Interferon-a containing ultradeformable carriers for potential transdermal application. *Journal of Anticancer Research*, *19*(2c), 1505–1512. PMID:10365133

Hamaguchi, T., Kato, K., Yasui, H., Morizane, C., Ikeda, M., Ueno, H., & Matsumura, Y. et al. (2007). A phase I and pharmacokinetic study of NK105, a paclitaxel-incorporating micellar nanoparticle formulation. *British Journal of Cancer*, *97*(2), 170–176. doi:10.1038/sj.bjc.6603855 PMID:17595665

Hamilton, A., Biganzoli, L., Coleman, R., Mauriac, L., Hennebert, P., Awada, A., & de Valeriola, D. et al. (2002). A phase I clinical and pharmacokinetic study of polyethylene glycol liposomal doxorubicin (Caelyx, Doxil) at a 6-week interval in patients with metastatic breast cancer. *Annals of Oncology*, *13*(6), 910–918. doi:10.1093/annonc/mdf157 PMID:12123337

Hamishehkar, H., Rahimpour, Y., & Kouhsoltani, M. (2013). Niosomes as a propitious carrier for topical drug delivery. *Expert Opinion on Drug Delivery*, *10*(2), 261–272. doi:10.1517/17425247.2013.746310 PMID:23252629

Han, I. S., Lew, S., & Han, M. H. (2004). *U.S. Patent No. 6,835,553*. Washington, DC: U.S. Patent and Trademark Office.

Handjani-Vila, R. M., Ribier, A., Rondot, B., & Vanlerberghie, G. (1979). Dispersions of lamellar phases of non-ionic lipids in cosmetic products. *International Journal of Cosmetic Science*, *1*(5), 303–314. doi:10.1111/j.1467-2494.1979.tb00224.x PMID:19467076

Handy, R. D., Owen, R., & Valsami-Jones, E. (2008). The ecotoxicology of nanoparticles and nanomaterials: Current status, knowledge gaps, challenges and future nedds. *Ecotoxicology (London, England)*, *17*(5), 315–325. doi:10.1007/s10646-008-0206-0 PMID:18408994

Han, K., Pan, X., Chen, M., Wang, R., Xu, Y., Feng, M., & Wu, C. (2010). Phytantriol-based inverted type bicontinuous cubic phase for vascular embolization and drug sustained release. *European Journal of Pharmaceutical Sciences*, *41*(5), 692–699. doi:10.1016/j.ejps.2010.09.012 PMID:20883779

Hann, I. M., & Prentice, H. G. (2001). Lipid-based amphotericin B: A review of the last 10 years of use. *International Journal of Antimicrobial Agents*, *17*(3), 161–169. doi:10.1016/S0924-8579(00)00341-1 PMID:11282260

Hans, M. L., & Lowman, A. M. (2002). Biodegradable nanoparticles for drug delivery and targeting. *Current Opinion in Solid State and Materials Science*, *6*(4), 319–327. doi:10.1016/S1359-0286(02)00117-1

Han, Y., Lee, S. S., & Ying, J. Y. (2006). Pressure-driven enzyme entrapment in siliceous mesocellular foam. *Chemistry of Materials*, *18*(3), 643–649. doi:10.1021/cm0520618

Hao, Y., & Li, K. (2010). Entrapment and release difference resulting from hydrogen bonding interactions in niosome. *International Journal of Pharmaceutics*, *403*(1-2), 245–253. doi:10.1016/j.ijpharm.2010.10.027 PMID:20971171

Hao, Y., Zhao, F., Li, N., Yang, Y., & Li, K. (2002). Studies on a high encapsulation of colchicine by a niosome system. *International Journal of Pharmaceutics*, *244*(1-2), 73–80. doi:10.1016/S0378-5173(02)00301-0 PMID:12204566

Hargreaves, W. R., & Deamer, D. W. (1978). Evidence against the partially and cost effectiveness of gram positive culture. *Biochemistry*, *17*, 3759. doi:10.1021/bi00611a014 PMID:698196

Harnoy, A. J., Rosenbaum, I., Tirosh, E., Ebenstein, Y., Shaharabani, R., Beck, R., & Amir, R. J. (2014). Enzyme-Responsive Amphiphilic PEG-Dendron Hybrids and Their Assembly into Smart Micellar Nanocarriers. *Journal of the American Chemical Society*, *136*(21), 7531–7534. doi:10.1021/ja413036q PMID:24568366

Harper, B., Thomas, D., Chikkagoudar, S., Baker, N., Tang, K., Heredia-Langner, A., & Harper, S. et al. (2015). Comparative hazard analysis and toxicological modeling of diverse nanomaterials using the embryonic zebrafish (EZ) metric of toxicity. *Journal of Nanoparticle Research*, *17*(6), 250–255. doi:10.1007/s11051-015-3051-0 PMID:26069453

Hartshorne, N. H., & Woodard, G. D. (1973). Mesomorphism in the system disodium chromoglycate-water. *Molecular Crystals & Liquid Crystals*, *23*(3-4), 343–368. doi:10.1080/15421407308083381

Hato, M., & Minamikawa, H. (1996). The effects of oligosaccharide stereochemistry on the physical properties of aqueous synthetic glycolipids. *Langmuir*, *12*(6), 1658–1665. doi:10.1021/la950326z

Hauser, C., & Seow, W. Y. (2014). *WO Patent Application 2014/116187*. Agency For Science, Technology and Research, SG.

Hauser, H., & Gains, N. (1982). Spontaneous vesiculation of phospholipids: A simple and quick method of forming unilamellar vesicles. *Proceedings of the National Academy of Sciences of the United States of America*, *79*(6), 1683–1687. doi:10.1073/pnas.79.6.1683 PMID:6952221

Hay, E. D. (2013). *Cell biology of extracellular matrix*. Springer Science & Business Media.

Heather, A., & Benson, E. (2005). Transdermal drug delivery: Penetration enhancement techniques. *Current Drug Delivery*, *2*(1), 23–33. doi:10.2174/1567201052772915 PMID:16305405

Heavner, G. A., Arakawa, T., Philo, J. S., & Labrenz, S. (2007). Protein isolation from biopharmaceutical formulations cannot be used for comparative studies: Follow-up to ''A case study using Epoetin Alfa fromEpogen and EPREX. *Journal of Pharmaceutical Sciences*, *96*(12), 3214–3225. doi:10.1002/jps.20993 PMID:17721976

He, C.-L., Huang, Z.-M., & Han, X.-J. (2009). Fabrication of drug-loaded electrospun aligned fibrous threads for suture applications. *Journal of Biomedical Materials Research. Part A*, *89*(1), 80–95. doi:10.1002/jbm.a.32004 PMID:18428982

Heffernan, M. J., & Murthy, N. J. (2005). Polyketal nanoparticles: A new pHsensitive biodegradable drug delivery vehicle. *Bioconjugate Chemistry*, *16*(6), 1340–1342. doi:10.1021/bc050176w PMID:16287226

He, H., Cao, X., & Lee, L. J. (2004). Design of a novel hydrogel-based intelligent system for controlled drug release. *Journal of Controlled Release*, *95*(3), 391–402. doi:10.1016/j.jconrel.2003.12.004 PMID:15023451

Heikham, K. D., Gupta, A., Kumar, A., Singh, C., Saxena, J., Srivastava, K., & Misra, A. et al. (2015). Preferential targeting of human erythrocytes infected with the malaria parasite Plasmodium falciparum via hexose transporter surface proteins. *International Journal of Pharmaceutics*, *483*(1-2), 57–62. doi:10.1016/j.ijpharm.2015.02.011 PMID:25666024

Heister, E., Neves, V., T^ılmaciu, C., Lipert, K., Beltr'an, V. S., Coley, H. M., & McFadden, J. et al. (2009). Triple functionalisation of single-walled carbon nanotubes with doxorubicin, a monoclonal antibody, and a fluorescent marker for targeted cancer therapy. *Carbon*, *47*(9), 2152–2160. doi:10.1016/j.carbon.2009.03.057

Helledi, L. S., & Schubert, L. (2001). Release kinetics of acyclovir from a suspension of acyclovir incorporated in a cubic phase delivery system. *Drug Development and Industrial Pharmacy*, *27*(10), 1073–1081. doi:10.1081/DDC-100108370 PMID:11794810

Heller, J., & Hoffman, A. (1996). Drug delivery systems. *Biomaterials science: An introduction to materials in medicine*, 346-356.

Henry, J. A., Simonet, M., Pandit, A., & Neuenschwander, P. (2007). Characterization of a slowly degrading biodegradable polyesterurethane for tissue engineering scaffolds. *Journal of Biomedical Materials Research. Part A*, *82*(3), 669–679. doi:10.1002/jbm.a.31094 PMID:17323319

He, Q., Gao, Y., Zhang, L., Zhang, Z., Gao, F., Ji, X., & Shi, J. et al. (2011). A pH-responsive mesoporous silica nanoparticles-based multi-drug delivery system for overcoming multi-drug resistance. *Biomaterials*, *32*(30), 7711–7720. doi:10.1016/j.biomaterials.2011.06.066 PMID:21816467

Herber, S., Bomer, J., Olthuis, W., Bergveld, P., & Van Den Berg, A. (2005). A miniaturized carbon dioxide gas sensor based on sensing of pH-sensitive hydrogel swelling with a pressure sensor. *Biomedical Microdevices*, *7*(3), 197–204. doi:10.1007/s10544-005-3026-5 PMID:16133807

Herzog, C., Hartmann, K., Künzi, V., Kürsteiner, O., Mischler, R., Lazar, H., & Glück, R. (2009). Eleven years of Inflexal® V-a virosomal adjuvanted influenza vaccine. *Vaccine*, *27*(33), 4381–4387. doi:10.1016/j.vaccine.2009.05.029 PMID:19450630

Heskins, M., & Guillet, J. E. (1968). Solution properties of poly (*N*-isopropylacrylamide). *Journal of Macromolecular Science. Chemistry*, *2*(8), 1441–1455. doi:10.1080/10601326808051910

He, X., Alves, C. S., Oliveira, N., Rodrigues, J., Zhu, J., Bányai, I., & Shi, X. et al. (2015). RGD peptide-modified multifunctional dendrimer platform for drug encapsulation and targeted inhibition of cancer cells. *Colloids and Surfaces. B, Biointerfaces*, *125*(0), 82–89. doi:10.1016/j.colsurfb.2014.11.004 PMID:25437067

Hippalgaonkar, K., Adelli, G. R., Hippalgaonkar, K., Repka, M. A., & Majumdar, S. (2013). Indomethacin-Loaded Solid Lipid Nanoparticles for Ocular Delivery: Development, Characterization, and *In Vitro* Evaluation. *Journal of Ocular Pharmacology and Therapeutics*, *29*(2), 216–228. doi:10.1089/jop.2012.0069 PMID:23421502

Hirlekar, R., Jain, S., Patel, M., Garse, H., & Kadam, V. (2010). Hexosomes: A novel drug delivery system. *Current Drug Delivery*, *7*(1), 28–35. doi:10.2174/156720110790396526 PMID:20044910

Hodgson, J. (2009). WHO guidelines presage US biosimilars legislation? *Nature Biotechnology*, *27*(11), 963–965. doi:10.1038/nbt1109-963a PMID:19898430

Hoffman, A. S. (2012). Hydrogels for biomedical applications. *Advanced Drug Delivery Reviews*, *64*, 18–23. doi:10.1016/j.addr.2012.09.010 PMID:11755703

Hofland, H. E. J., Bouwstra, J. A., Gooris, G. S., Spies, F., Talsma, H., & Junginger, H. E. (1993). Nonionic surfactant vesicles: A study of vesicle formation, characterization, and stability. *Journal of Colloid and Interface Science*, *161*(2), 366–376. doi:10.1006/jcis.1993.1479

Hofland, H. E., van der Geest, R., Bodde, H. E., Junginger, H. E., & Bouwstra, J. A. (1994). Estradiol permeation from nonionic surfactant vesicles through human stratum corneum in vitro. *Pharmaceutical Research*, *11*(5), 659–664. doi:10.1023/A:1018963910260 PMID:8058633

Hofland, H., Bootstrap, J. A., Spies, F., Gooris, G., & Nagelkerke, J. F. (1994). Liposomes as carriers for topical and transdermal delivery. *Journal of Pharmaceutical Sciences*, *83*(9), 1189–1203. doi:10.1002/jps.2600830902 PMID:7830230

Hofland, H., Bouwstra, J., Verhoef, J., Buckton, G., Chowdry, B., Ponec, M., & Junginger, H. (1992). Safety Aspects of Non-ionic Surfactant Vesicles: A Toxicity Study Related to the Physicochemical Characteristics of Non-ionic Surfactants. *The Journal of Pharmacy and Pharmacology*, *44*(4), 287–294. doi:10.1111/j.2042-7158.1992.tb03608.x PMID:1355538

Holzer, B. R., Hatz, C., Schmid-Sissolak, D., Glück, R., Althaus, B., & Egger, M. (1996). Immunogenicity and adverse effects of inactivated virosome versus alum-adsorbed hepatitis A vaccine: A randomized controlled trial. *Vaccine*, *14*(10), 982–986. doi:10.1016/0264-410X(96)00042-4 PMID:8873392

Holzwarth, U., Bellido, E., Dalmiglio, M., Kozempel, J., Cotogno, G., & Gibson, N. (2014). Be-recoil radiolabelling of industrially manufactured silica nanoparticles. *Journal of Nanoparticle Research*, *16*(9), 2574–2589. doi:10.1007/s11051-014-2574-0 PMID:25285032

Honeywell-Nguyen, P. L., & Bouwstra, J. A. (2005). Vesicles as a tool for transdermal and dermal delivery. *Drug Discovery Today. Technologies*, *2*(1), 67–74. doi:10.1016/j.ddtec.2005.05.003 PMID:24981757

Hong, M., Zhu, S., Jiang, Y., Tang, G., & Pei, Y. (2009). Efficient tumor targeting of hydroxycamptothecin loaded PEGylated niosomes modified with transferrin. *Journal of Controlled Release*, *133*(2), 96–102. doi:10.1016/j.jconrel.2008.09.005 PMID:18840485

Hope, M. J., Bally, M. B., Webb, G., & Cullis, P. R. (1985). Production of large unilamellar vesicles by a rapid extrusion procedure. *Biochimica et Biophysica Acta*, *812*(1), 55–65. doi:10.1016/0005-2736(85)90521-8 PMID:23008845

Hoshi, K. (1996). Approved indications of lipo-PGE 1 in Japan. *Advanced Drug Delivery Reviews*, *20*(2), 171–176. doi:10.1016/0169-409X(95)00120-V

Hospira Symp on Assessing Biosimilars. (2015). Retrieved from http://www.corporatecitizenship.novartis.com/downloads/businessconduct/Novartis_Perspective_Pharmacovigilance_for_Biosimilars. pdf

Householder, K. T., DiPerna, D. M., Chung, E. P., Wohlleb, G. M., Dhruv, H. D., Berens, M. E., & Sirianni, R. W. (2015). Intravenous delivery of camptothecin-loaded PLGA nanoparticles for the treatment of intracranial glioma. *International Journal of Pharmaceutics*, *479*(2), 374–380. doi:10.1016/j.ijpharm.2015.01.002 PMID:25562639

Howard, M. D., Jay, M., Dziublal, T. D., & Lu, X. L. (2008). PEGylation of nanocarrier drug delivery systems: State of the art. *J. Biomed. Nanotechnol.*, *4*(2), 133–148. doi:10.1166/jbn.2008.021

Hrubý, M., Koňák, Č., & Ulbrich, K. (2005). Polymeric micellar pH-sensitive drug delivery system for doxorubicin. *Journal of Controlled Release*, *103*(1), 137–148. doi:10.1016/j.jconrel.2004.11.017 PMID:15710507

Huang, C. H. (1969). Studies on phosphatidylcholine vesicles. Formation and physical characteristics. *Biochemistry*, *8*(1), 344–352. doi:10.1021/bi00829a048 PMID:5777332

Huang, C.-H., Nwe, K., Al Zaki, A., Brechbiel, M. W., & Tsourkas, A. (2012). Biodegradable Polydisulfide Dendrimer Nanoclusters as MRI Contrast Agents. *ACS Nano*, *6*(11), 9416–9424. doi:10.1021/nn304160p PMID:23098069

Huang, Y. C., Yang, Y. S., Lai, T. Y., & Jan, J. S. (2012). Lysine-block-tyrosine block copolypeptides: Self-assembly, cross-linking, and conjugation of targeted ligand for drug encapsulation. *Polymer*, *53*(4), 913–922. doi:10.1016/j.polymer.2012.01.010

Huang, Y., Lu, J., Gao, X., Li, J., Zhao, W., Sun, M., & Li, S. et al. (2012). PEGderivatized embelin as a dual functional carrier for the delivery of paclitaxel. *Bioconjugate Chemistry*, *23*(7), 1443–1451. doi:10.1021/bc3000468 PMID:22681537

Huang, Z., Li, X., Zhang, T., Song, Y., She, Z., Li, J., & Deng, Y. (2014). Progress involving new techniques for liposome preparation. *Asian Journal of Pharmaceutical Sciences*, *9*(4), 176–182. doi:10.1016/j.ajps.2014.06.001

Huang, Z.-M., He, C.-L., Yang, A., Zhang, Y., Han, X.-J., Yin, J., & Wu, Q. (2006). Encapsulating drugs in biodegradable ultrafine fibers through co-axial electrospinning. *Journal of Biomedical Materials Research. Part A*, *77*(1), 169–179. doi:10.1002/jbm.a.30564 PMID:16392131

Huang, Z.-M., Zhang, Y.-Z., Kotaki, M., & Ramakrishna, S. (2003). A review on polymer nanofibers by electrospinning and their applications in nanocomposites. *Composites Science and Technology*, *63*(15), 2223–2253. doi:10.1016/S0266-3538(03)00178-7

Hua, W., & Liu, T. (2007). Preparation and properties of highly stable innocuous niosome in Span 80/PEG 400/H 2 O system. *Colloids and Surfaces. A, Physicochemical and Engineering Aspects*, *302*(1), 377–382. doi:10.1016/j.colsurfa.2007.02.068

Huh, K. M., Lee, S. C., Ch, Y. W., Lee, J., Jeong, J. H., & Park, K. (2005). Hydrotropic polymer micelle system for delivery of paclitaxel. *Journal of Controlled Release*, *101*(1–3), 59–68. doi:10.1016/j.jconrel.2004.07.003 PMID:15588894

Hu, L., Xing, Q., Meng, J., & Shang, C. (2010). Preparation and enhanced oral bioavailability of cryptotanshinone loaded solid lipid nanoparticles. *AAPS PharmSciTech*, *11*(2), 582–587. doi:10.1208/s12249-010-9410-3 PMID:20352534

Hu, W., Cheng, L., Cheng, L., Zheng, M., Lei, Q., Hu, Z., & Chen, D. et al. (2014). Redox and pH-responsive poly (amidoamine) dendrimer–poly (ethylene glycol) conjugates with disulfide linkages for efficient intracellular drug release. *Colloids and Surfaces. B, Biointerfaces*, *123*, 254–263. doi:10.1016/j.colsurfb.2014.09.024 PMID:25277289

Ibrahim, H. G., Sallam, E., Takieddin, M., & Habboub, M. (1993). Effects of solute characteristics and concentration on a lyotropic liquid crystal: Solute induced phase change. *Pharmaceutical Research*, *10*(5), 5–12. doi:10.1023/A:1018920118631 PMID:8321840

ICH Q6B Note for guidance on specifications: test procedures and acceptance criteria for biotechnological/biological products (CPMP/ICH/365/96).

Igarashi, R., Takenaga, M., Takeuchi, J., Kitagawa, A., Matsumoto, K., & Mizushima, Y. (2001). Marked hypotensive and blood flow-increasing effects of a new lipo-PGE 1 (lipo-AS013) due to vascular wall targeting. *Journal of Controlled Release*, *71*(2), 157–164. doi:10.1016/S0168-3659(00)00373-4 PMID:11274747

Ihre, H. R., Padilla De Jesús, O. L., Szoka, F. C., & Fréchet, J. M. J. (2002). Polyester Dendritic Systems for Drug Delivery Applications: Design, Synthesis, and Characterization. *Bioconjugate Chemistry*, *13*(3), 443–452. doi:10.1021/bc010102u PMID:12009932

Iijima, S. (1991). HELICAL Microtubules of graphitic carbon. *Nature*, *354*(6348), 56–58. doi:10.1038/354056a0

Ilić-Stojanović, S., Mladenović-Ranisavljević, I., Nikolić, V., Takić, L., Stojiljković, D., Stojiljković, S., & Nikolić, L. (2011). Thermo-responsive hydrogels for controlled release of paracetamol, In *Proceedings of 43rd International October Conference on Mining and Metallurgy* (pp. 707-710). Kladovo, Republic of Serbia: University of Belgrade Technical Faculty in Bor.

Ilić-Stojanović, S., Nikolić, L., Nikolić, V., Petrović, S. D., & Stanković, M. (2014). *RS Patent No. 53220 B*. The Intellectual Property Office of the Republic of Serbia.

Ilić-Stojanović, S. (2015). *Synthesis and characterization of negatively thermosensitive hydrogels*. Saarbrücken, Germany: LAP Lambert Academic Publishing, Akademikeverlag GmbH & Co. KG.

Ilić-Stojanović, S. S., Nikolić, L. B., Nikolić, V. D., Milić, J. R., Petrović, S. D., Nikolić, G. M., & Kapor, A. J. (2012). Potential application of thermo-sensitive hydrogels for controlled release of phenacetin. *Hem. Ind.*, *66*(6), 831–839. doi:10.2298/HEMIND120222089I

Ilić-Stojanović, S. S., Nikolić, L. B., Nikolić, V. D., Milić, J. R., Stamenković, J., Nikolić, G. M., & Petrović, S. D. (2013). Synthesis and characterization of thermosensitive hydrogels and the investigation of modified release of ibuprofen. *Hem. Ind.*, *67*(6), 901–912. doi:10.2298/HEMIND130119038I

Ilić-Stojanović, S. S., Nikolić, L. B., Nikolić, V. D., Petrović, S. D., Zdravković, A. S., & Stamenković, J. V. (2014). The effect of the crosslinker content on the swelling properties of intelligent gels. *Advanced Technologies*, *3*(2), 10–15.

Ilić-Stojanović, S. S., Nikolić, L., Nikolić, V., Stanković, M., Stamenković, J., Mladenović-Ranisavljević, I., & Petrović, S. D. (2012). Influence of monomer and crosslinker molar ratio on the swelling behaviour of thermosensitive hydrogels. *Chemical Industry & Chemical Engineering Quarterly*, *18*(1), 1–9. doi:10.2298/CICEQ110711040I

Ilić-Stojanović, S., Nikolić, L., Nikolić, V., Ristić, I., Budinski-Simendić, J., Kapor, A., & Nikolić, G. M. (2014). The structure characterization of thermosensitive poly(*N*-isopropylacrylamide-*co*-2-hydroxypropyl methacrylate) hydrogel. *Polymer International*, *63*(6), 973–981. doi:10.1002/pi.4589

Illum, L. (2015). Intranasal Delivery to the Central Nervous System. In *Blood-Brain Barrier in Drug Discovery: Optimizing Brain Exposure of CNS Drugs and Minimizing Brain Side Effects for Peripheral Drugs.*

Im, J. S., Yun, J., Lim, Y.-M., Kim, H.-I., & Lee, Y.-S. (2010). Fluorination of electrospun hydrogel fibers for a controlled release drug delivery system. *Acta Biomaterialia*, *6*(1), 102–109. doi:10.1016/j.actbio.2009.06.017 PMID:19531386

Immordino, M. L., Dosio, F., & Cattel, L. (2006). Stealth liposomes: Review of the basic science, rationale, and clinical applications, existing and potential. *International Journal of Nanomedicine*, *1*(3), 297. PMID:17717971

Ionescu, L. C., Lee, G. C., Sennett, B. J., Burdick, J. A., & Mauck, R. L. (2010). An anisotropic nanofiber/microsphere composite with controlled release of biomolecules for fibrous tissue engineering. *Biomaterials*, *31*(14), 4113–4120. doi:10.1016/j.biomaterials.2010.01.098 PMID:20149432

Ipsen, J. H., Karlström, G., Mourtisen, O., Wennerström, H., & Zuckermann, M. (1987). Phase equilibria in the phosphatidylcholine-cholesterol system. *Biochimica et Biophysica Acta (BBA)-. Biomembranes*, *905*(1), 162–172. doi:10.1016/0005-2736(87)90020-4

Ishida, T., Harada, M., Wang, X. Y., Ichihara, M., Irimura, K., & Kiwada, H. (2005). Accelerated blood clearance of PEGylated liposomes following preceding liposome injection: Effects of lipid dose and PEG surface-density and chain length of the first-dose liposomes. *Journal of Controlled Release*, *105*(3), 305–317. doi:10.1016/j.jconrel.2005.04.003 PMID:15908032

Ishida, T., & Kiwada, H. (2008). Accelerated blood clearance (ABC) phenomenon upon repeated injection of PEGylated liposomes. *International Journal of Pharmaceutics*, *354*(1), 56–62. doi:10.1016/j.ijpharm.2007.11.005 PMID:18083313

Israelachvili, J. (1994). The science and applications of emulsions- an overview. *Colloids and Surfaces. A, Physicochemical and Engineering Aspects*, *91*, 1–8. doi:10.1016/0927-7757(94)02743-9

Israelachvili, J. N. (2011). *Intermolecular and surface forces* (3rd ed.). Academic Press.

Iwamoto, Y., & Yamakoshi, Y. (2006). A highly water-soluble C60-NVP copolymer: A potential material for photodynamic therapy. *Chemical Communications (Cambridge)*, *46*(46), 4805–4807. doi:10.1039/B614305A PMID:17345735

Jaafar-Maalej, C., Diab, R., Andrieu, V., Elaissari, A., & Fessi, H. (2010). Ethanol injection method for hydrophilic and lipophilic drug-loaded liposome preparation. *Journal of Liposome Research*, *20*(3), 228–243. doi:10.3109/08982100903347923 PMID:19899957

Jacksona, A. W., & Fulton, D. A. (2013). Making polymeric nanoparticles stimuli-responsive with dynamic covalent bonds. *Polymer Chemistry*, *4*(1), 31–45. doi:10.1039/C2PY20727C

Jadhav, S. M., Morey, P., Karpe, M., & Kadam, V. (2012). *Novel vesicular system: An overview*. Academic Press.

Jadhav, M., Nagarsenker, M. S., Gaikwad, R., Samad, A., & Kshirsagar, N. A. (2011). Formulation and evaluation of long circulating liposomal amphotericin B: A scinti-kinetic study using 99mTc in BALB/C mice. *Indian Journal of Pharmaceutical Sciences*, *73*(1), 57. doi:10.4103/0250-474X.89757 PMID:22131622

Jadon, P. S., Gajbhiye, V., Jadon, R. S., Gajbhiye, K. R., & Ganesh, N. (2009). Enhanced oral bioavailability of griseofulvin via niosomes. *AAPS PharmSciTech*, *10*(4), 1186–1192. doi:10.1208/s12249-009-9325-z PMID:19856107

Jafari-Aghdam, Adibkia, Payab, Barzegar-Jalali, Parvizpur, Mohammadi, & Sabzevari. (2014). Methylprednisolone acetate-Eudragit® RS100 electrospuns: Preparation and physicochemical characterization. *Artificial Cells, Nanomedicine, and Biotechnology*, 1-7.

Jafelicci, M. Jr, Davolos, M. R., Santos, F. J., & Andrade, S. J. (1999). Hollow silica particles from microemulsion. *Journal of Non-Crystalline Solids*, *247*(1-3), 98–102. doi:10.1016/S0022-3093(99)00040-X

Jagur-Grodzinski, J. (2010). Polymeric gels and hydrogels for biomedical and pharmaceutical applications. *Polymers for Advanced Technologies*, *21*(1), 27–47.

Jahangiri, A., Davaran, S., Fayyazi, B., Tanhaei, A., Payab, S., & Adibkia, K. (2014). Application of electrospraying as a one-step method for the fabrication of triamcinolone acetonide-PLGA nanofibers and nanobeads. *Colloids and Surfaces. B, Biointerfaces*, *123*, 219–224. doi:10.1016/j.colsurfb.2014.09.019 PMID:25260224

Jain, N. K. (1997). *Controlled and novel drug delivery*. CBS Publishers & Distributors.

Jain, S., Chaudhari, & Swarnakar. (2011). Preparation and characterization of niosomal gel for iontophoresis mediated transdermal delivery of isosorbide dinitrate. *Drug Delivery and Translational Research, 1*(4), 309-321.

Jain, A. S., Goel, P. N., Shah, S. M., Dhawan, V. V., Nikam, Y., Gude, R. P., & Nagarsenker, M. S. (2014). Tamoxifen guided liposomes for targeting encapsulated anticancer agent to estrogen receptor positive breast cancer cells: In vitro and in vivo evaluation. *Biomedicine and Pharmacotherapy, 68*(4), 429–438. doi:10.1016/j.biopha.2014.03.004 PMID:24721327

Jain, C. P., Vyas, S. P., & Dixit, V. K. (2006). Niosomal system for delivery of rifampicin to lymphatics. *International Journal of Pharmaceutics, 68*, 57–58.

Jain, C., & Vyas, S. (1995). Preparation and characterization of niosomes containing rifampicin for lung targeting. *Journal of Microencapsulation, 12*(4), 401–407. doi:10.3109/02652049509087252 PMID:8583314

Jain, C., Vyas, S., & Dixit, V. (2006). Niosomal system for delivery of rifampicin to lymphatics. *Indian Journal of Pharmaceutical Sciences, 68*(5), 575–583. doi:10.4103/0250-474X.29622

Jain, N. (2002). *Targeted and Controlled Drug Delivery*. New Delhi: CBS Publishers and Distributors.

Jain, N. K. (2001). *Advances in controlled and novel drug delivery*. New Delhi: CBS Publishers and Distributers.

Jain, N. K. (2003). Advances. In *Controlled and Novel Drug Delivery* (p. 276). New Delhi, India: CBS Publishers.

Jain, R., Standley, S. M., & Fréchet, J. M. J. (2007). Synthesis and degradation of pH-sensitive linear poly(amidoamine) s. *Macromolecules, 40*(3), 452–457. doi:10.1021/ma062319v

Jain, S., Singh, P., Mishra, V., & Vyas, S. P. (2005). Mannosylated niosomes as adjuvant-carrier system for oral genetic immunization against hepatitis B. *Immunology Letters, 101*(1), 41–49. doi:10.1016/j.imlet.2005.04.002 PMID:15869802

Jalon, G. E., Ygartua, P., & Santoyo, S. (2001). Topical application of acyclovir-loaded microparticles: Quantification of the drug in porcine skin layers. *Journal of Controlled Release, 75*(1-2), 191–197. doi:10.1016/S0168-3659(01)00395-9 PMID:11451509

James, N., Coker, R., Tomlinson, D., Harris, J., Gompels, M., Pinching, A., & Stewart, J. (1994). Liposomal doxorubicin (Doxil): An effective new treatment for Kaposi's sarcoma in AIDS. *Clinical Oncology, 6*(5), 294–296. doi:10.1016/S0936-6555(05)80269-9 PMID:7530036

Jani, P., Halbert, G. W., Langridge, J., & Florence, A. T. (1989). The uptake and translocation of latex nanospheres and microspheres after oral administration to rats. *The Journal of Pharmacy and Pharmacology, 41*(12), 809–812. doi:10.1111/j.2042-7158.1989.tb06377.x PMID:2576440

Jansen, J. F. G. A., Meijer, E. W., & de Brabander-van den Berg, E. M. M. (1995). The Dendritic Box: Shape-Selective Liberation of Encapsulated Guests. *Journal of the American Chemical Society, 117*(15), 4417–4418. doi:10.1021/ja00120a032

Jayaraman, S. C., Ramachandran, C., & Weiner, N. (1996). Topical delivery of erythromycin from various formulations: An in vivo hairless mouse study. *Journal of Pharmaceutical Sciences, 85*(10), 1082–1084. doi:10.1021/js960040u PMID:8897275

Jefferies, W. A., Brandon, M. R., Hunt, S. V., Williams, A. F., Gatter, K. C., & Mason, D. Y. (1984). Transferrin receptor on endothelium of brain capillaries. *Nature, 312*(5990), 162–163. doi:10.1038/312162a0 PMID:6095085

Jennings, L. E., & Long, N. J. (2009). 'Two is better than one'—probes for dual-modality molecular imaging. *Chemical Communications*, (24): 3511–3524. doi:10.1039/b821903f PMID:19521594

Jenquin, M. R., & McGinity, J. W. (1994). Characterization of acrylic resin matrix films and mechanisms of drug-polymer interactions. *International Journal of Pharmaceutics*, *101*(1-2), 23–34. doi:10.1016/0378-5173(94)90072-8

Jia, G., Wang, H., Yan, L., Wang, X., Pei, R., Yan, T., & Guo, X. et al. (2005). Cytotoxicity of carbon nanomaterials: Single-wall nanotube, multi-wall nanotube, and fullerene. *Environmental Science & Technology*, *39*(5), 1378–1383. doi:10.1021/es048729l PMID:15787380

Jiang, H. T., Wu, S. L., Karger, B. L., & Hancock, W. S. (2009). Mass spectrometric analysis of innovator, counterfeit, and follow-on recombinant human growth hormone. *Biotechnology Progress*, *25*(1), 207–218. doi:10.1002/btpr.72 PMID:19224592

Jiang, H., Hu, Y., Li, Y., Zhao, P., Zhu, K., & Chen, W. (2005). A facile technique to prepare biodegradable coaxial electrospun nanofibers for controlled release of bioactive agents. *Journal of Controlled Release*, *108*(2), 237–243. doi:10.1016/j.jconrel.2005.08.006 PMID:16153737

Jiang, H., Hu, Y., Zhao, P., Li, Y., & Zhu, K. (2006). Modulation of protein release from biodegradable core–shell structured fibers prepared by coaxial electrospinning. *Journal of Biomedical Materials Research. Part B, Applied Biomaterials*, *79*(1), 50–57. doi:10.1002/jbm.b.30510 PMID:16544305

Jiang, X. Z., Liu, S. Y., & Narain, R. (2009). Degradable thermoresponsive core cross-linked micelles: Fabrication, surface functionalization, and biorecognition. *Langmuir*, *25*(23), 13344–13350. doi:10.1021/la9034276 PMID:19928937

Jiang, Y.-N., Mo, H.-Y., & Yu, D.-G. (2012). Electrospun drug-loaded core–sheath PVP/zein nanofibers for biphasic drug release. *International Journal of Pharmaceutics*, *438*(1), 232–239. doi:10.1016/j.ijpharm.2012.08.053 PMID:22981688

Jin, G. W., Ji, X. Y., & Choi, J. S. (2009). Preparation of naproxen-loaded poly(ethylene oxide-b-methacrylic acid) micelle and its pH-dependent drug release behavior. *Bulletin of the Korean Chemical Society*, *30*(4), 931–934. doi:10.5012/bkcs.2009.30.4.931

Jin, H., Heller, D. A., & Strano, M. S. (2008). Single-Particle Tracking of Endocytosis and Exocytosis of Single-Walled Carbon Nanotubes in NIH-3T3 Cells. *Nano Letters*, *8*(6), 1577–1585. doi:10.1021/nl072969s PMID:18491944

Jin, H.-J., Chen, J., Karageorgiou, V., Altman, G. H., & Kaplan, D. L. (2004). Human bone marrow stromal cell responses on electrospun silk fibroin mats. *Biomaterials*, *25*(6), 1039–1047. doi:10.1016/S0142-9612(03)00609-4 PMID:14615169

Jin, S., Gu, J., Shi, Y., Shao, K., Yu, X., & Yue, G. (2013). Preparation and electrical sensitive behavior of poly(*N*-vinylpyrrolidone-co-acrylic acid) hydrogel with flexible chain nature. *European Polymer Journal*, *49*(7), 1871–1880. doi:10.1016/j.eurpolymj.2013.04.022

Jin, Y., Ren, X., Wang, W., Ke, L., Ning, E., Du, L., & Bradshaw, J. (2011). A 5-fluorouracil-loaded pH-responsive dendrimer nanocarrier for tumor targeting. *International Journal of Pharmaceutics*, *420*(2), 378–384. doi:10.1016/j.ijpharm.2011.08.053 PMID:21925254

Jin, Y., Tong, L., Ai, P., Li, M., & Hou, X. (2006). Self-assembled drug delivery systems: Properties and in vitro/in vivo behavior of acyclovir self-assembled nanoparticles (SAN). *International Journal of Pharmaceutics*, *309*(1), 199–207. doi:10.1016/j.ijpharm.2005.11.025 PMID:16377106

Jin, Y., Wen, J., Garg, S., Liu, D., Zhou, Y., Teng, L., & Zhang, W. (2013). Development of a novel niosomal system for oral delivery of Ginkgo biloba extract. *International Journal of Nanomedicine*, *8*, 421. doi:10.2147/IJN.S37984 PMID:23378764

Johnson, P. E. (2008). Implications of biosimilars for the future. *American Journal of Health-System Pharmacy*, *65*(Supplement 6). PMID:18591711

Jones, M. C., & Leroux, J. C. (1999). Polymeric micelles - a new generation of colloidal drug carriers. *European Journal of Pharmaceutics and Biopharmaceutics*, *48*(2), 101–111. doi:10.1016/S0939-6411(99)00039-9 PMID:10469928

Jones, R. G., Wilks, E. S., Metanomski, W. V., Kahovec, J., Hess, M., Stepto, R., & Kitayama, T. (2009). *Compendium of Polymer Terminology and Nomenclature: IUPAC Recommendations 2008* (p. 443). Cambridge, UK: Royal Society of Chemistry. doi:10.1039/9781847559425

Jordan-Lloyd, D. (1926). Article. In J. Alexander (Ed.), Colloid Chemistry (Vol. 1, pp. 767–782). New York, NY: The Chemical Catalogue Company.

Juliano, R.L. (1980). Controlled delivery of drugs: an overview and prospectus. *Drug Delivery Systems: Characteristics and Biomedical Application,* 310.

Juntanon, K., Niamlang, S., Rujiravanit, R., & Sirivat, A. (2008). Electrically controlled release of sulfosalicylic acid from crosslinked poly(vinyl alcohol) hydrogel. *International Journal of Pharmaceutics*, *356*(1), 1–11. doi:10.1016/j.ijpharm.2007.12.023 PMID:18242901

Junyaprasert, V., Teeranachaideekul, V., & Supaperm, T. (2008). Effect of charged and non-ionic membrane additives on physicochemical properties and stability of niosomes. *AAPS PharmSciTech*, *9*(3), 851–859. doi:10.1208/s12249-008-9121-1 PMID:18636334

Kaasgaard, T., & Drummond, C. J. (2006). Ordered 2-D and 3-D nanostructured amphiphile self-assembly materials stable in excess solvent. *Physical Chemistry Chemical Physics*, *8*(43), 4957–4975. doi:10.1039/b609510k PMID:17091149

Kabiri, K., Hesarian, S., Jamshidi, A., Zohuriaan-Mehr, M. J., Boohendi, H., Poorheravi, M. R., & Ahmad-Khanbeigi, F. et al. (2011). Minimization of residual monomer content of superabsorbent hydrogels *via* alteration of initiating system. *Journal of Applied Polymer Science*, *120*(5), 2716–2723. doi:10.1002/app.33431

Kageyama, Y., Tanigake, N., Kurokome, Y., Iwaki, S., Takeda, S., Suzuki, K., & Sugawara, T. (2013). Macroscopic motion of supramolecular assemblies actuated by photoisomerization of azobenzene derivatives. *Chemical Communications*, *49*(82), 9386–9388. doi:10.1039/c3cc43488e PMID:23793067

Kakinoki, S., Yasuda, C., Kaetsu, I., Uchida, K., Yukutake, K., Nakayama, M., & Ohyanagi, H. et al. (2003). Preparation of poly-lactic acid microspheres containing the angiogenesis inhibitor TNP-470 with medium-chain triglyceride and the in vitro evaluation of release profiles. *European Journal of Pharmaceutics and Biopharmaceutics*, *55*(2), 155–160. doi:10.1016/S0939-6411(02)00156-X PMID:12637091

Kalshetti, P. P., Rajendra, V. B., Dixit, D. N., & Parekh, P. P. (2012). Hydrogels as a drug delivery system and applications: A review. *International Journal of Pharmacy and Pharmaceutical Sciences*, *4*(1), 1–7.

Kamaly, N., Xiao, Z., Valencia, P. M., Radovic-Moreno, A. F., & Farokhzad, O. C. (2012). Targeted polymeric therapeutic nanoparticles: Design, development and clinical translation. *Chemical Society Reviews*, *41*(7), 2971–3010. doi:10.1039/c2cs15344k PMID:22388185

Kamboj, S., Saini, V., & Bala, S. (2014). Formulation and characterization of drug loaded nonionic surfactant vesicles (niosomes) for oral bioavailability enhancement. *The Scientific World Journal*. PMID:24672401

Kaminskas, L. M., Boyd, B. J., Karellas, P., Krippner, G. Y., Lessene, R., Kelly, B., & Porter, C. J. (2008). The impact of molecular weight and PEG chain length on the systemic pharmacokinetics of PEGylated poly l-lysine dendrimers. *Molecular Pharmaceutics*, *5*(3), 449–463. doi:10.1021/mp7001208 PMID:18393438

Kaminskas, L. M., Kelly, B. D., McLeod, V. M., Sberna, G., Owen, D. J., Boyd, B. J., & Porter, C. J. (2011). Characterisation and tumour targeting of PEGylated polylysine dendrimers bearing doxorubicin via a pH labile linker. *Journal of Controlled Release*, *152*(2), 241–248. doi:10.1016/j.jconrel.2011.02.005 PMID:21315119

Kaminskas, L. M., McLeod, V. M., Kelly, B. D., Sberna, G., Boyd, B. J., Williamson, M., & Porter, C. J. et al. (2012). A comparison of changes to doxorubicin pharmacokinetics, antitumor activity, and toxicity mediated by PEGylated dendrimer and PEGylated liposome drug delivery systems. *Nanomedicine; Nanotechnology, Biology, and Medicine*, *8*(1), 103–111. doi:10.1016/j.nano.2011.05.013 PMID:21704192

Kam, N. W. S., Jessop, T. C., Wender, P. A., & Dai, H. (2004). Nanotube Molecular Transporters: Internalization of Carbon Nanotube–Protein Conjugates into Mammalian Cells. *Journal of the American Chemical Society*, *126*(22), 6850–6851. doi:10.1021/ja0486059 PMID:15174838

Kam, N. W. S., Liu, Z., & Dai, H. (2006). Carbon Nanotubes as Intracellular Transporters for Proteins and DNA: An Investigation of the Uptake Mechanism and Pathway. *Angewandte Chemie International Edition*, *45*(4), 577–581. doi:10.1002/anie.200503389 PMID:16345107

Kaneda, Y. (2000). Virosomes: Evolution of the liposome as a targeted drug delivery system. *Advanced Drug Delivery Reviews*, *43*(2), 197–205. doi:10.1016/S0169-409X(00)00069-7 PMID:10967226

Kang, H. N. (2009). *WHO Guideline on Evaluation of Similar Biotherapeutic Products: The Next Steps*. Presented at the EGA 7th Symposium on Biosimilar Medicines.

Kang, S. I., & Bae, Y. H. (2001). pH-induced volume-phase transition of hydrogels containing sulfonamide side group by reversible crystal formation. *Macromolecules*, *34*(23), 8173–8178. doi:10.1021/ma0021949

Karlsson, H. L., Cronholm, P., Gustafsson, J., & Moller, L. (2008). Copper oxide nanoparticles are highly toxic: A comparison between metal oxide nanoparticles and carbon nanotubes. *Chemical Research in Toxicology*, *21*(9), 1726–1732. doi:10.1021/tx800064j PMID:18710264

Kashyap, N., Kumar, N., & Kumar, M. N. V. R. (2005). Hydrogels for pharmaceutical and biomedical applications. *Critical Reviews™ in Therapeutic Drug Carrier Systems*, *22*(2), 107-150.

Kathmann, E. E., White, L. A., & McCormick, C. L. (1997). Water-Soluble Polymers. 73. Electrolyte-and pH-responsive zwitterionic copolymers of 4-[(2-acrylamido-2-methylpropyl)-dimethylammonio]butanoate with 3-[(2-acrylamido-2-methyl-propyl)dimethylammonio] propanesulfonate. *Macromolecules*, *30*(18), 5297–5304. doi:10.1021/ma961214x

Kato, K., Walde, P., Koine, N., Ichikawa, S., Ishikawa, T., Nagahama, R., & Omokawa, M. et al. (2008). Temperature-sensitive nonionic vesicles prepared from Span 80 (sorbitan monooleate). *Langmuir*, *24*(19), 10762–10770. doi:10.1021/la801581f PMID:18720959

Katono, H., Maruyama, A., Sanui, K., Ogata, N., Okano, T., & Sakurai, Y. (1991). Thermo-responsive swelling and drug release switching of interpenetrating polymer networks composed of poly(acrylamide-co-butyl methacrylate) and poly(acrylic acid). *Journal of Controlled Release*, *16*(1), 215–227. doi:10.1016/0168-3659(91)90045-F

Katzenschlager, R., Ugurluoglu, A., Minar, E., & Hirschl, M. (2003). Liposomal heparin-spraygel in comparison with subcutaneous low molecular weight heparin in patients with superficial venous thrombosis. A randomized, controlled, open multicentre study. *Journal für Kardiologie*, *10*, 375–378.

Katzenschlager, R., Ugurluoglu, A., Sipos, G., Bihari, I., Anyova, E. B., Hirschl, M., & Cencora, A. et al. (2007). Efficacy and tolerability of liposomal heparin spraygel as an add-on treatment in the management of superficial venous thrombosis. *Angiology*, *58*(1SSuppl 1), S27–S35. doi:10.1177/0003319706297741 PMID:17478880

Kaur, & Kanwar, M. (2002). Ocular Preparations: The Formulation Approach. *Drug Development and Industrial Pharmacy, 28*(5), 473–493.

Kaur, I. P., Aggarwal, D., Singh, H., & Kakkar, S. (2010). Improved ocular absorption kinetics of timolol maleate loaded into a bioadhesive niosomal delivery system. *Graefes Archive for Clinical and Experimental Ophthalmology, 248*(10), 1467–1472. doi:10.1007/s00417-010-1383-0 PMID:20437246

Kavitha, D., Sowjanya, J., & Shankar, P. (2012). Pharmacosomes: An Emerging Vesicular System. *International Journal of Pharmaceutical Sciences Review and Research, 5*(3), 168–171.

Kawaguchi, T., Walker, K. L., Wilkins, C. L., & Moore, J. S. (1995). Double Exponential Dendrimer Growth. *Journal of the American Chemical Society, 117*(8), 2159–2165. doi:10.1021/ja00113a005

Kawakami, S., Higuchi, Y., & Hashida, M. (2008). Nonviral approaches for targeted delivery of plasmid DNA and oligonucleotide. *Journal of Pharmaceutical Sciences, 97*(2), 726–745. doi:10.1002/jps.21024 PMID:17823947

Kawamoto, H. (2002). The history of liquid crystal display.*Proceedings of the IEEE*, 460-499.

Kayyali, R., Marriott, C., & Wiseman, H. (1994). Tamoxifen decreases drug efflux from liposomes: Relevance to its ability to reverse multidrug resistance in cancer cells? *FEBS Letters, 344*(2), 221–224. doi:10.1016/0014-5793(94)00378-5 PMID:8187888

Kelner, A., & Schacht, E. H. (2005). Tailor-made polymers for local drug delivery: Release of macromolecular model drugs from biodegradable hydrogels based on poly (ethylene oxide). *Journal of Controlled Release, 101*(1), 13–20. doi:10.1016/j.jconrel.2004.09.010 PMID:15588890

Kenawy, E.-R., Bowlin, G. L., Mansfield, K., Layman, J., Simpson, D. G., Sanders, E. H., & Wnek, G. E. (2002). Release of tetracycline hydrochloride from electrospun poly (ethylene-co-vinylacetate), poly (lactic acid), and a blend. *Journal of Controlled Release, 81*(1), 57–64. doi:10.1016/S0168-3659(02)00041-X PMID:11992678

Kenawy, E.-R., Layman, J. M., Watkins, J. R., Bowlin, G. L., Matthews, J. A., Simpson, D. G., & Wnek, G. E. (2003). Electrospinning of poly (ethylene-co-vinyl alcohol) fibers. *Biomaterials, 24*(6), 907–913. doi:10.1016/S0142-9612(02)00422-2 PMID:12504511

Kersten, G. F., & Crommelin, D. J. (1995). Liposomes and ISCOMS as vaccine formulations. *Biochimica et Biophysica Acta (BBA) -. Reviews on Biomembranes, 1241*(2), 117–138.

Khaksa, G., Souza, R. D., Lewis, S., & Udupa, N. (2000). Pharmacokinetic study of niosome encapsulated insulin. *Indian Journal of Experimental Biology, 38*(9), 901–905. PMID:12561948

Khan, O. F., Zaia, E. W., Jhunjhunwala, S., Xue, W., Cai, W., Yun, D. S., & Anderson, D. G. et al. (2015). Dendrimer-inspired nanomaterials for the in vivo delivery of siRNA to lung vasculature. *Nano Letters, 15*(5), 3008–3016. doi:10.1021/nl5048972 PMID:25789998

Khan, O. F., Zaia, E. W., Yin, H., Bogorad, R. L., Pelet, J. M., Webber, M. J., & Anderson, D. G. et al. (2014). Ionizable Amphiphilic Dendrimer-Based Nanomaterials with Alkyl-Chain-Substituted Amines for Tunable siRNA Delivery to the Liver Endothelium In Vivo. *Angewandte Chemie, 126*(52), 14625–14629. doi:10.1002/ange.201408221 PMID:25354018

Ki, C. S., Kim, J. W., Hyun, J. H., Lee, K. H., Hattori, M., Rah, D. K., & Park, Y. H. (2007). Electrospun three-dimensional silk fibroin nanofibrous scaffold. *Journal of Applied Polymer Science, 106*(6), 3922–3928. doi:10.1002/app.26914

Kidney Disease Improving Global Outcomes (KDIGO) AnemiaWork Group. (2012). KDIGO clinical practice guideline for anemia in chronic kidney disease. *Kidney International. Supplement, 2*, 279–335.

Kikuchi, H., Yokota, M., Hisakado, Y., Yang, H., & Kajiyama, T. (2002). Polymer-stabilized liquid crystal blue phases. *Nature Materials*, *1*(1), 64–68. doi:10.1038/nmat712 PMID:12618852

Killops, K. L., Campos, L. M., & Hawker, C. J. (2008). Robust, Efficient, and Orthogonal Synthesis of Dendrimers via Thiol-ene "Click" Chemistry. *Journal of the American Chemical Society*, *130*(15), 5062–5064. doi:10.1021/ja8006325 PMID:18355008

Kim, G. H. (2008). Electrospun PCL nanofibers with anisotropic mechanical properties as a biomedical scaffold. *Biomedical Materials (Bristol, England)*, *3*(2), 025010. doi:10.1088/1748-6041/3/2/025010 PMID:18458365

Kim, J. O., Sahay, G., Kabanov, A. V., & Bronich, T. K. (2010). Polymeric micelles with ionic cores containing biodegradable cross-links for delivery of chemotherapeutic agents. *Biomacromolecules*, *11*(4), 919–926. doi:10.1021/bm9013364 PMID:20307096

Kim, J. Y., Kim, S., Pinal, R., & Park, K. (2011). Hydrotropic polymer micelles as versatile vehicles for delivery of poorly water-soluble drugs. *Journal of Controlled Release*, *152*(1), 13–20. doi:10.1016/j.jconrel.2011.02.014 PMID:21352878

Kim, K.-H., Jeong, L., Park, H.-N., Shin, S.-Y., Park, W.-H., Lee, S.-C., & Lee, Y.-M. et al. (2005). Biological efficacy of silk fibroin nanofiber membranes for guided bone regeneration. *Journal of Biotechnology*, *120*(3), 327–339. doi:10.1016/j.jbiotec.2005.06.033 PMID:16150508

Kim, K., Luu, Y. K., Chang, C., Fang, D., Hsiao, B. S., Chu, B., & Hadjiargyrou, M. (2004). Incorporation and controlled release of a hydrophilic antibiotic using poly (lactide-co-glycolide)-based electrospun nanofibrous scaffolds. *Journal of Controlled Release*, *98*(1), 47–56. doi:10.1016/j.jconrel.2004.04.009 PMID:15245888

Kim, S., & Martin, G. M. (1981). A method for the preparation of liposomes, a pack for use therein and a composition for use in preparing a liposomal material. *Biochimica et Biophysica Acta*, *646*, 4.

Kim, T. Y., Kim, D. W., Chung, J. Y., Shin, S. G., Kim, S. C., Heo, D. S., & Bang, Y. J. et al. (2004). Phase I and pharmacokinetic study of Genexol-PM, a cremophor-free, polymeric micelle-formulated paclitaxel, in patients with advanced malignancies. *Clinical Cancer Research*, *10*(11), 3708–3716. doi:10.1158/1078-0432.CCR-03-0655 PMID:15173077

Kimura, M., Kato, M., Muto, T., Hanabusa, K., & Shirai, H. (2000). Temperature-sensitive dendritic hosts: Synthesis, characterization, and control of catalytic activity. *Macromolecules*, *33*(4), 1117–1119. doi:10.1021/ma9914671

Kirsch, N., Alexander, C., Lübke, M., Whitcombe, M., & Vulfson, E. (2000). Enhancement of selectivity of imprinted polymers via post-imprinting modification of recognition sites. *Polymer*, *41*(15), 5583–5590. doi:10.1016/S0032-3861(99)00782-X

Kiwada, H., Niimura, H., Fujisaki, Y., Yamada, S., & Kato, Y. (1985). Application of synthetic alkyl glycoside vesicles as drug carriers. I. Preparation and physical properties. *Chemical & Pharmaceutical Bulletin*, *33*(2), 753–759. doi:10.1248/cpb.33.753 PMID:4017121

Kiwada, H., Niimura, H., & Kato, Y. (1985). Tissue distribution and pharmacokinetic evaluation of the targeting efficiency of synthetic alkyl glycoside vesicles. *Chemical & Pharmaceutical Bulletin*, *33*(6), 2475–2482. doi:10.1248/cpb.33.2475 PMID:4064206

Kleinert, H., & Maki, K. (1981). Lattice Textures in Cholesteric Liquid Crystals. *Fortschritte der Physik*, *29*(5), 219–259. doi:10.1002/prop.19810290503

Knight, L. (1986). *Thrombus-localizing radiopharmaceuticals. In Radiopharmaceuticals: Progress and clinical perspectives* (pp. 23–40). Boca Raton, FL: CRC Press.

Koetting, M. C., Peters, J. T., Steichen, S. D., & Peppas, N. A. (2015). Stimulus-responsive hydrogels: Theory, modern advances, and applications. *Materials Science and Engineering R Reports*, *93*, 1–49. doi:10.1016/j.mser.2015.04.001 PMID:27134415

Koh, Y. J., Kim, H. K., Kim, S. W., & Yeo, G. D. (2012). *U.S. Patent Application 14/363,022*. Washington, DC: U.S. Patent and Trademark Office.

Kombath, R., Minumula, S., Sockalingam, A., Subadhra, S., Parre, S., Reddy, T. & David, B. (2012). Critical issues related to transfersomes – Novel vesicular system. *Acta Sci Pol Tech Aliment*, 67-82.

Kono, K., Liu, M., & Fréchet, J. M. (1999). Design of dendritic macromolecules containing folate or methotrexate residues. *Bioconjugate Chemistry*, *10*(6), 1115–1121. doi:10.1021/bc990082k PMID:10563782

Koo, A. N., Lee, H. J., Kim, S. E., Chang, J., Park, C. Y., Kim, C. H., & Lee, S. C. et al. (2008). Disulfide-cross-linked PEG–poly(amino acid)s copolymer micelles for glutathione-mediated intracellular drug delivery. *Chemical Communications*, *48*(48), 6570–6572. doi:10.1039/b815918a PMID:19057782

Koo, O. M., Rubinstein, I., & Onyuksel, H. (2005). Role of nanotechnology in targeted drug delivery and imaging: A concise review. *Nanomedicine; Nanotechnology, Biology, and Medicine*, *1*(3), 193–212. doi:10.1016/j.nano.2005.06.004 PMID:17292079

Kopeček, J., Kopečková, P., Minko, T., & Lu, Z. R. (2000). HPMA copolymer–anticancer drug conjugates: Design, activity, and mechanism of action. *European Journal of Pharmaceutics and Biopharmaceutics*, *50*(1), 61–81. doi:10.1016/S0939-6411(00)00075-8 PMID:10840193

Korenbrot, J. I. (1977). Structural and spectroscopic characteristics of BR in air-water interface films. *Annual Review of Physiology*, *39*, 17.

Koren, E., Apte, A., Jani, A., & Torchilin, V. P. (2012). Multifunctional PEGylated 2C5-immunoliposomes containing pH-sensitive bonds and TAT peptide for enhanced tumor cell internalization and cytotoxicity. *Journal of Controlled Release*, *160*(2), 264–273. doi:10.1016/j.jconrel.2011.12.002 PMID:22182771

Korostynska, O., Arshak, K., Gill, E., & Arshak, A. (2007). Review on State-of-the-art in Polymer Based pH Sensors. *Sensors (Basel, Switzerland)*, *7*(12), 3027–3042. doi:10.3390/s7123027

Kossena, G. A., Charman, W. N., Boyd, B. J., & Porter, C. J. (2004). A novel cubic phase of medium chain lipid origin for the delivery of poorly water soluble drugs. *Journal of Controlled Release*, *99*(2), 217–229. doi:10.1016/j.jconrel.2004.06.013 PMID:15380632

Kostiainen, M. A., Smith, D. K., & Ikkala, O. (2007). Optically Triggered Release of DNA from Multivalent Dendrons by Degrading and Charge-Switching Multivalency. *Angewandte Chemie*, *46*(40), 7600–7604. doi:10.1002/anie.200701200 PMID:17729224

Kostić, M., Krunić, N., Nikolić, L., Nikolić, V., & Najman, S., Kostić, … Petković, D. (2011). Influence of residual monomer reduction on acrylic denture base resins quality. *Hem. Ind.*, *65*(2), 171–177. doi:10.2298/HEMIND101103008K

Kostić, M., Krunić, N., Nikolić, L., Nikolić, V., Najman, S., & Kocić, J. (2009). Residual monomer content determination in some acrylic denture base materials and possibilities of its reduction. *Vojnosanitetski Pregled. Military-Medical and Pharmaceutical Review*, *66*(3), 223–227. doi:10.2298/VSP0903223K PMID:19341229

Kostko, A. F., Cipriano, B. H., Pinchuk, O. A., Ziserman, L., Anisimov, M. A., Danino, D., & Raghavan, S. R. (2005). Salt effects on the phases behavior,structure and rheology of chromonic liquid crystals. *The Journal of Physical Chemistry B*, *109*(41), 19126–19133. doi:10.1021/jp052575u PMID:16853466

Kottari, N., Chabre, Y. M., Shiao, T. C., Rej, R., & Roy, R. (2014). Efficient and accelerated growth of multifunctional dendrimers using orthogonal thiol–ene and SN 2 reactions. *Chemical Communications*, *50*(16), 1983–1985. doi:10.1039/c3cc46633g PMID:24416763

Kotta, S., Khan, A. W., Pramod, K., Ansari, S. H., Sharma, R. K., & Ali, J. (2012). Exploring oral nanoemulsions for bioavailability enhancement of poorly water-soluble drugs. *Expert Opinion on Drug Delivery*, *9*(5), 585–598. doi:10.1517/17425247.2012.668523 PMID:22512597

Koynova, R., Tenchov, B., & Rapp, G. (1997). Low amounts of PEG-lipid induce cubic phase in phosphatidyl ethanolamide dispersions. *Biochimica et Biophysica Acta*, *1326*(2), 167–170. doi:10.1016/S0005-2736(97)00067-9 PMID:9218547

Kraineva, J., Nicolini, C., Thiyagarajan, P., Kondrashkina, E., & Winter, R. (2006). Incorporation of α-chymotrypsin into the 3D channels of bicontinuous cubic lipid mesophases. *Biochimica et Biophysica Acta*, *1764*(3), 424–433. doi:10.1016/j.bbapap.2005.11.004 PMID:16330264

Kremer, J. M., Eskai, M. W., Pathmamanoharan, G., & Wiersema, P. H. (1977). Renal biopsy specimens from patients with rheumatoid arthritis. *Biochemistry*, *16*, 3932. doi:10.1021/bi00636a033 PMID:901761

Kreuter, J. (1994). *Colloidal drug delivery systems* (Vol. 66). CRC Press.

Kreuter, J., & Haenzel, I. (1978). Mode of action of immunological adjuvants: Some physicochemical factors influencing the effectivity of polyacrylic adjuvants. *Infection and Immunity*, *19*, 667–675. PMID:631894

Kreuter, J., Muller, V., & Munz, K. (1989). Quantitative and microautoradiographic study on mouse intestinal distribution of polycyanoacrylate nanoparticles. *International Journal of Pharmaceutics*, *55*(1), 39–45. doi:10.1016/0378-5173(89)90274-3

Kreuter, J., & Speiser, P. P. (1976). In vitro studies of poly(methyl methacrylate) adjuvants. *Journal of Pharmaceutical Sciences*, *65*(11), 1624–1627. doi:10.1002/jps.2600651115 PMID:993993

Krušić, M. K., Ilić, M., & Filipović, J. (2009). Swelling behaviour and paracetamol release from poly(*N*-isopropylacrylamide-itaconic acid) hydrogels. *Polymer Bulletin*, *63*(2), 197–211. doi:10.1007/s00289-009-0086-3

Kucuk, I., & Edirisinghe, M. (2014). Microfluidic preparation of polymer nanospheres. *Journal of Nanoparticle Research*, *16*(12), 2626–2638. doi:10.1007/s11051-014-2626-5 PMID:25484617

Kukowska-Latallo, J. F., Candido, K. A., Cao, Z., Nigavekar, S. S., Majoros, I. J., Thomas, T. P., & Baker, J. R. et al. (2005). Nanoparticle Targeting of Anticancer Drug Improves Therapeutic Response in Animal Model of Human Epithelial Cancer. *Cancer Research*, *65*(12), 5317–5324. doi:10.1158/0008-5472.CAN-04-3921 PMID:15958579

Kulichikhin, V. G., Malkin, A. Y., & Papkov, S. P. (1984). Rheological properties of liquid crystalline polymer systems Review. *Polymer Science USSR*, *26*(3), 499–524. doi:10.1016/0032-3950(84)90384-8

Kulkarni, C. V. (2011). Nanostructural studies on monoelaidin-water systems at low temperatures. *Langmuir*, *27*(19), 11790–11800. doi:10.1021/la201235h PMID:21846133

Kulkarni, S. D., Bakliwal, S. R., Rane, B. R., Pawar, S. P., & Gujarathi, N. A. (2012). Evaluation of Liquisolid Compacts Using Response Surface Methodology. *International Journal of Drug Delivery.*, *4*, 427–433.

Kumar, K. P. S., Bhowmik, D., & Deb, L. (2012). Recent Trends in Liposomes Used As Novel Drug Delivery System. *The Pharma Innovation Journal, 1*, 29-38. Available from The Pharma Innovation Journal Web site: http://www.thepharmajournal.com

Kumar, R. (2008). Enzymatic Hydrolysis of Cellulosic Biomass Solids Prepared by Leading Pretreatments and Identification. Handbook of Particulate Drug Delivery, 2.

Kumar, A., Pathak, K., & Bali, V. (2012). Ultra-adaptable nanovesicular systems: A carrier for systemic delivery of therapeutic agents. *Drug Discovery Today*, *17*(21/22), 1233–1241. doi:10.1016/j.drudis.2012.06.013 PMID:22766375

Kumar, A., Srivastava, A., Galaev, I. Y., & Mattiasson, B. (2007). Smart polymers: Physical forms and bioengineering applications. *Progress in Polymer Science*, *32*(10), 1205–1237. doi:10.1016/j.progpolymsci.2007.05.003

Kumar, D. P., & Arnab, D. (2012). Pharmacosomes: A potential vesicular drug delivery system. *International Research Journal of Pharmacy*, *3*(3), 102–105.

Kumari, A., Yadav, S. K., & Yadav, S. C. (2010). Biodegradable polymeric nanoparticles based drug delivery systems. *Colloids and Surfaces. B, Biointerfaces*, *75*(1), 1–18. doi:10.1016/j.colsurfb.2009.09.001 PMID:19782542

Kumar, M. N. V. R. (2000). Nano and microparticles as controlled drug delivery devices. *Journal of Pharmacy & Pharmaceutical Sciences*, *3*(2), 234–258. PMID:10994037

Kumar, R. (2011). Vesicular System-Carrier for Drug Delivery. *Pelagia Research Library Der Pharmacia Sinica*, *2*(4), 192–202.

Kurtoglu, Y. E., Navath, R. S., Wang, B., Kannan, S., Romero, R., & Kannan, R. M. (2009). Poly (amidoamine) dendrimer–drug conjugates with disulfide linkages for intracellular drug delivery. *Biomaterials*, *30*(11), 2112–2121. doi:10.1016/j.biomaterials.2008.12.054 PMID:19171376

Kushwaha, S. K., Rastogl, A., Rai, A., & Singh, S. (2012). Novel drug delivery system for anticancer drug: A review. *International Journal of Pharm Tech Research*, *4*(2), 542–553.

Kwok, C. S., Mourad, P. D., Crum, L. A., & Ratner, B. D. (2001). Self-assembled molecular structures as ultrasonically-responsive barrier membranes for pulsatile drug delivery. *Journal of Biomedical Materials Research*, *57*(2), 151–164. doi:10.1002/1097-4636(200111)57:2<151::AID-JBM1154>3.0.CO;2-5 PMID:11526905

Kyyrönen, K., Hume, L., Benedetti, L., Urtti, A., Topp, E., & Stella, V. (1992). Methylprednisolone esters of hyaluronic acid in ophthalmic drug delivery: In vitro and in vivo release studies. *International Journal of Pharmaceutics*, *80*(1), 161–169. doi:10.1016/0378-5173(92)90274-6

Labhasetwar, V., Song, C., & Levy, R. J. (1997). Nanoparticle drug delivery system for restenosis. *Advanced Drug Delivery Reviews*, *24*(1), 63–85. doi:10.1016/S0169-409X(96)00483-8

Lachman, L., Lieberman, H. A., & Kanig, J. L. (1986). *The theory and practice of industrial pharmacy*. Academic Press.

Laemmli, U. K. (1970). Cleavage of structural proteins during assembly of head of bacteriophage T4. *Nature*, *227*(5259), 680–685. doi:10.1038/227680a0 PMID:5432063

Laffargue, P., Fialdes, P., Frayssinet, P., Rtaimate, M., Hildebrand, H. F., & Marchandise, X. (2000). Adsorption and release of insulin-like growth factor-I on porous tricalcium phosphate Implant. *Journal of Biomedical Materials Research*, *49*(3), 415–421. doi:10.1002/(SICI)1097-4636(20000305)49:3<415::AID-JBM15>3.0.CO;2-Z PMID:10602075

Lambert, G., Fattal, E., Pinto-Alphandary, H., Gulik, A., & Couvreur, P. (1998). Polyisobutylcyanoacrylate nanocapsules containing an aqueous core as a novel colloidal carrier for the delivery of oligonucleotides. *Biochimie*, *80*, 969–976. doi:10.1016/S0300-9084(99)80002-9 PMID:9924975

Lammers, T., Kiessling, F., Hennink, W. E., & Storm, G. (2012). Drug targeting to tumors: Principles, pitfalls and (pre-) clinical progress. *Journal of Controlled Release*, *161*(2), 175–187. doi:10.1016/j.jconrel.2011.09.063 PMID:21945285

Lancelot, A., Sierra, T., & Serrano, J. L. (2014). Nanostructured liquid crystalline particles for drug delivery. *Expert Opinion on Drug Delivery*, *11*(4), 1–18. doi:10.1517/17425247.2014.884556 PMID:24490701

Langer, R. (1983). Implantable controlled release systems. *Pharmacology & Therapeutics*, *21*(1), 35–51. doi:10.1016/0163-7258(83)90066-9 PMID:6353438

Langer, R. (1998). Drug delivery and targeting. *Nature*, *392*, 5–10. PMID:9579855

Langer, R., & Peppas, N. (1983). Chemical and physical structure of polymers as carriers for controlled release of bioactive agents: A review. *Journal of Macromolecular Science-Reviews in Macromolecular Chemistry and Physics*, *23*(1), 61–126. doi:10.1080/07366578308079439

Lan, M. Y., Hsu, Y. B., Hsu, C. H., Ho, C. Y., Lin, J. C., & Lee, S. W. (2013). Induction of apoptosis by high-dose gold nanoparticles in nasopharyngeal carcinoma cells. *Auris, Nasus, Larynx*, *40*(6), 563–568. doi:10.1016/j.anl.2013.04.011 PMID:23722198

Lanthier, M., Behrman, R., & Nardinelli, C. (2008). Economic issues with follow-on protein products. *Nature Reviews. Drug Discovery*, *7*(9), 733–737. doi:10.1038/nrd2636 PMID:18654570

Laouini, A., Jaafar-Maalej, C., Limayem-Blouza, I., Sfar, S., Charcosset, C., & Fessi, H. (2012). Preparation, characterization and applications of liposomes: state of the art. *Journal of Colloid Science and Biotechnology*, *1*(2), 147-168.

Laouini, A., Jaafar-Maalej, C., Limayem-Blouza, I., Sfar, S., Charcosset, C., & Fessi, H. (2012). Preparation, Characterization and Applications of Liposomes: State of the Art. *Journal of Colloid Science and Biotechnology*, *1*(2), 147–168. doi:10.1166/jcsb.2012.1020

Lapinski, M. M., Castro-Forero, A., Greiner, A. J., Ofoli, R. Y., & Blanchard, G. J. (2007). Comparison of liposomes formed by sonication and extrusion: Rotational and translational diffusion of an embedded chromophore. *Langmuir*, *23*(23), 11677–11683. doi:10.1021/la7020963 PMID:17939695

Lara, M. G., Bentley, M. V., & Collett, J. H. (2005). *In vitro* drug release mechanism and drug loading studies of cubic phase gels. *International Journal of Pharmaceutics*, *293*(1-2), 241–250. doi:10.1016/j.ijpharm.2005.01.008 PMID:15778062

Larsson, K. (1989). Cubic lipid-water phases: Structures and biomembrane aspects. *Journal of Physical Chemistry*, *93*(21), 7304–7314. doi:10.1021/j100358a010

Larsson, K. (2000). Aqueous dispersions of cubic lipid-water phases. *Current Opinion in Colloid & Interface Science*, *5*(1-2), 64–69. doi:10.1016/S1359-0294(00)00040-6

Larsson, K. (2009). Lyotropic liquid crystals and their dispersions relevant in foods. *Current Opinion in Colloid & Interface Science*, *14*(1), 16–20. doi:10.1016/j.cocis.2008.01.006

Lasic, D. D. (1988). The mechanism of vesicle formation. *The Biochemical Journal*, *256*(1), 1–11. doi:10.1042/bj2560001 PMID:3066342

Lasic, D. D. (1998). Novel applications of liposomes. *Trends in Biotechnology*, *16*(7), 307–321. doi:10.1016/S0167-7799(98)01220-7 PMID:9675915

Lasic, D. D., & Barenholz, Y. (1996). *Handbook of nonmedical applications of liposomes: Theory and basic sciences* (Vol. 1). CRC Press.

Lasic, D. D., & Martin, F. J. (1995). *Stealth liposomes* (Vol. 20). CRC press.

Lattin, J., Belnap, D., & Pitt, W. (2012). Formation of Liposomes as a drug delivery vehicle. *Colloids and Surfaces. B, Biointerfaces*, *89*, 93–100. doi:10.1016/j.colsurfb.2011.08.030 PMID:21962853

Lavelle, F., Bissery, M. C., Andre, S., Roquet, F., & Riou, J. F. (1996). Preclinical evaluation of CPT-11 and its active metabolite SN-38. *Seminars in Oncology*, *23*(1), 11–20. PMID:8633248

Laverman, P., Boerman, O. C., Oyen, W. J., Corstens, F. H., & Storm, G. (2001). In vivo applications of PEG liposomes: unexpected observations. *Critical Reviews™ in Therapeutic Drug Carrier Systems, 18*(6).

Laverman, P., Carstens, M. G., Boerman, O. C., Dams, E. T. M., Oyen, W. J., van Rooijen, N., & Storm, G. et al. (2001). Factors affecting the accelerated blood clearance of polyethylene glycol-liposomes upon repeated injection. *The Journal of Pharmacology and Experimental Therapeutics*, *298*(2), 607–612. PMID:11454922

Lawrence, M. J. (1994). Surfactant systems: Their use in drug delivery. *Chemical Society Reviews*, *23*(6), 417–424. doi:10.1039/cs9942300417 PMID:7867669

Lawrie, A., Brisken, A., Francis, S., Cumberland, D., Crossman, D., & Newman, C. (2000). Microbubble-enhanced ultrasound for vascular gene delivery. *Gene Therapy*, *7*(23), 2023–2027. doi:10.1038/sj.gt.3301339 PMID:11175314

LeBourlais, C. A., Chevanne, F., Turlin, B., Acar, L., Zia, H., Sado, P. A., & Leverge, R. et al. (1997). Effect of cyclosporine a formulations on bovine corneal absorption: Ex-vivo study. *Journal of Microencapsulation*, *14*(4), 457–467. doi:10.3109/02652049709033830 PMID:9229345

Lechuga-Ballesteros, D., Abdul-Fattah, A., Stevenson, C. L., & Bennett, D. (2003). Properties and stability of a liquid crystal form of cyclosporine-the first reported naturally occurring peptide that exists as a thermotropic liquid crystal. *Journal of Pharmaceutical Sciences*, *92*(9), 1821–1831. doi:10.1002/jps.10444 PMID:12950000

Lee, C. C., Gillies, E. R., Fox, M. E., Guillaudeu, S. J., Fréchet, J. M., Dy, E. E., & Szoka, F. C. (2006). A single dose of doxorubicin-functionalized bow-tie dendrimer cures mice bearing C-26 colon carcinomas. *Proceedings of the National Academy of Sciences of the United States of America*, *103*(45), 16649–16654. doi:10.1073/pnas.0607705103 PMID:17075050

Lee, C. C., MacKay, J. A., Fréchet, J. M. J., & Szoka, F. C. (2005). Designing dendrimers for biological applications. *Nature Biotechnology*, *23*(12), 1517–1526. doi:10.1038/nbt1171 PMID:16333296

Lee, H. J., Park, Y. H., & Koh, W.-G. (2013). Fabrication of nanofiber microarchitectures localized within hydrogel microparticles and their application to protein delivery and cell encapsulation. *Advanced Functional Materials*, *23*(5), 591–597. doi:10.1002/adfm.201201501

Lee, H. S. (1984). Cloning and expression of human erythropoietin in *Escherichia coli. Proceedings of the National Academy of Sciences of the United States of America*, *81*(9), 2708–2712. doi:10.1073/pnas.81.9.2708 PMID:6371819

Lee, J., & Kellaway, I. W. (2000). *In vitro* peptide release from liquid crystalline buccal delivery systems. *International Journal of Pharmaceutics*, *195*(1-2), 29–33. doi:10.1016/S0378-5173(99)00356-7 PMID:10675679

Lee, K. K., Cussler, E. L., Marchetti, M., & McHugh, M. A. (1990). Pressure-dependent phase transitions in hydrogels. *Chemical Engineering Science*, *45*(3), 766–767. doi:10.1016/0009-2509(90)87019-O

Lee, K. S., Chung, H. C., Im, S. A., Park, Y. H., Kim, C. S., Kim, S. B., & Ro, J. et al. (2008). Multicenter phase II trial of Genexol-PM, a Cremophor-free, polymeric micelle formulation of paclitaxel, in patients withmetastatic breast cancer. *Breast Cancer Research and Treatment*, *108*(2), 241–250. doi:10.1007/s10549-007-9591-y PMID:17476588

Lee, V. H., & Yamamoto, A. (1989). Penetration and enzymatic barriers to peptide and protein absorption. *Advanced Drug Delivery Reviews*, *4*(2), 171–207. doi:10.1016/0169-409X(89)90018-5

Lee, W. Y., Nguyen, T. H., Hanley, T., & Boyd, B. J. (2009). Nanostructure of liquid crystalline matrix determines *in vitro* sustained release and in vivo oral absorption kinetics for hydrophilic model drugs. *International Journal of Pharmaceutics*, *365*(1-2), 190–199. doi:10.1016/j.ijpharm.2008.08.022 PMID:18790030

Lehmann, O. (1889). ÜberfliessendeKrystalle. *Zeitschrift für Physikalische Chemie*, *4*, 462–472.

Leslie, S. B., Puvvada, S., Ratna, B. R., & Rudolph, A. S. (1996). Encapsulation of hemoglobin in a bicontinuous cubic phase lipid. *Biochimica et Biophysica Acta*, *1285*(2), 246–254. doi:10.1016/S0005-2736(96)00169-1 PMID:8972709

Lewis, D. J. M., Huo, Z., Barnett, S., Kromann, I., Giemza, R., Galiza, E., Woodrow, M., Thierry-Carstensen, B., Andersen, P., Novicki, D., Del Giudice, G., Rappuoli, R. (2009). Transient Facial Nerve Paralysis (Bell's Palsy) following Intranasal Delivery of a Genetically Detoxified Mutant of Escherichia coli Heat Labile Toxin. *PLoS One*, *4*(9), e6999. doi:10.1371/journal.pone.0006999

Lian, T., Bui, T., & Ho, R. J. (1999). Formulation of HIV-envelope protein with lipid vesicles expressing ganglioside GM1 associated to cholera toxin B enhances mucosal immune responses. *Vaccine*, *18*(7), 604–611. doi:10.1016/S0264-410X(99)00315-1 PMID:10547418

Lian, T., & Ho, R. J. (2001). Trends and developments in liposome drug delivery systems. *Journal of Pharmaceutical Sciences*, *90*(6), 667–680. doi:10.1002/jps.1023 PMID:11357170

Libster, D., Aserin, A., Wachtel, E., Shoham, G., & Garti, N. (2007). An HII liquid crystal-based delivery system for cyclosporin A: Physical characterization. *Journal of Colloid and Interface Science*, *308*(2), 514–524. doi:10.1016/j.jcis.2006.12.084 PMID:17276444

Lichtenberg, D., & Barenholz, Y. (1988). Liposomes: Preparation, characterization, and preservation. *Methods of Biochemical Analysis*, *33*, 337–462. doi:10.1002/9780470110546.ch7 PMID:3282152

Lieberman, H. A., Rieger, M. M., & Banker, G. S. (1998). *Pharmaceutical Dosage Forms: Disperse Systems*. London: Informa Healthcare.

Lieb, L. M., Flynn, G., & Weiner, N. (1994). Follicular (pilosebaceous unit) deposition and pharmacological behavior of cimetidine as a function of formulation. *Pharmaceutical Research*, *11*(10), 1419–1423. doi:10.1023/A:1018939805601 PMID:7855045

Li, G. L., Danhof, M., & Bouwstra, J. A. (2001). Effect of elastic liquid-state vesicle on apomorphine iontophoresis transport through human skin in vitro. *Pharmaceutical Research*, *18*(11), 1627–1630. doi:10.1023/A:1013098902260 PMID:11758773

Li, H., & Qian, Z. M. (2002). Transferrin/transferrin receptor-mediated drug delivery. *Medicinal Research Reviews*, *22*(3), 225–250. doi:10.1002/med.10008 PMID:11933019

Li, J., Wang, X., Zhang, T., Wang, C., Huang, Y., Luo, X., & Deng, Y. (2015). A review on phospholipids and their main applications in drug delivery systems. *Asian Journal of Pharmaceutical Sciences*, *10*(2), 81–98. doi:10.1016/j.ajps.2014.09.004

Li, L., Bellan, L. M., Craighead, H. G., & Frey, M. W. (2006). Formation and properties of nylon-6 and nylon-6/montmorillonite composite nanofibers. *Polymer*, *47*(17), 6208–6217. doi:10.1016/j.polymer.2006.06.049

Lima-Tenório, M. K., Tenório-Neto, E. T., Guilherme, M. R., Garcia, F. P., Nakamura, C. V., Pineda, E. A., & Rubira, A. F. (2015). Water transport properties through starch-based hydrogel nanocomposites responding to both pH and a remote magnetic field. *Chemical Engineering Journal*, *259*, 620–629. doi:10.1016/j.cej.2014.08.045

Lim, C. T., Tan, E. P. S., & Ng, S. Y. (2008). Effects of crystalline morphology on the tensile properties of electrospun polymer nanofibers. *Applied Physics Letters*, *92*(14), 141908. doi:10.1063/1.2857478

Lim, F., & Sun, A. M. (1980). Microencapsulated islets as bioartificial endocrine pancreas. *Science*, *210*(4472), 908–910. doi:10.1126/science.6776628 PMID:6776628

Lim, J., Guo, Y., Rostollan, C. L., Stanfield, J., Hsieh, J.-T., Sun, X., & Simanek, E. E. (2008). The role of the size and number of polyethylene glycol chains in the biodistribution and tumor localization of triazine dendrimers. *Molecular Pharmaceutics*, *5*(4), 540–547. doi:10.1021/mp8000292 PMID:18672950

Li, N., Li, N., Yi, Q., Luo, K., Guo, C., Pan, D., & Gu, Z. (2014). Amphiphilic peptide dendritic copolymer-doxorubicin nanoscale conjugate self-assembled to enzyme-responsive anti-cancer agent. *Biomaterials*, *35*(35), 9529–9545. doi:10.1016/j.biomaterials.2014.07.059 PMID:25145854

Lindell, K., Engblom, J., Jonstromer, M., Carlsson, A., & Engstrom, S. (1998). Influence of a charged phospholipid on the release pattern of timolol maleate from cubic liquid crystalline phases. *Progress in Colloid & Polymer Science*, *108*, 111–118.

Lin, J., Tang, Q., Hu, D., Sun, X., Li, Q., & Wu, J. (2009). Electric field sensitivity of conducting hydrogels with interpenetrating polymer network structure. *Colloids and Surfaces. A, Physicochemical and Engineering Aspects*, *346*(1), 177–183. doi:10.1016/j.colsurfa.2009.06.011

Linovitz, R. J., & Peppers, T. A. (2002). Use of an advanced formulation of beta-tricalcium phosphate as a bone extender in inter body lumbar fusion. *Orthopedics*, *25*, S585–S589. PMID:12038846

Lin, S. Y., Ho, C. J., & Li, M. J. (2001). Precision and reproducibility of temperature response of a thermo-responsive membrane embedded by binary liquid crystals for drug delivery. *J. Contrl. Rel*, *73*(2-3), 293–301. doi:10.1016/S0168-3659(01)00300-5 PMID:11516506

Lin, Y., Chen, Q., & Luo, H. (2007). Preparation and characterization of N-(2-carboxybenzyl) chitosan as a potential pH-sensitive hydrogel for drug delivery. *Carbohydrate Research*, *342*(1), 87–95. doi:10.1016/j.carres.2006.11.002 PMID:17125756

Li, Q. M., Zhu, L. J., Liu, R. G., Huang, D., Jin, X., Che, N., & Huang, Y. et al. (2012). Biological stimuli responsive drug carriers based on keratin for triggerable drug delivery. *Journal of Materials Chemistry*, *22*(37), 19964–19973. doi:10.1039/c2jm34136k

Li, Q., Li, Z., Zeng, W., Ge, S., Lu, H., Wu, C., & Xu, Y. et al. (2014). Proniosome-derived niosomes for tacrolimus topical ocular delivery: In vitro cornea permeation, ocular irritation, and in vivo anti-allograft rejection. *European Journal of Pharmaceutical Sciences*, *62*, 115–123. doi:10.1016/j.ejps.2014.05.020 PMID:24905830

Li, S.-D., & Huang, L. (2008). Pharmacokinetics and biodistribution of nanoparticles. *Molecular Pharmaceutics*, *5*(4), 496–504. doi:10.1021/mp800049w PMID:18611037

Liu, J. Y., Pang, Y., Huang, W., Huang, X. H., Meng, L. L., Zhu, X. Y., & Yan, D. Y. et al. (2011). Bioreducible micelles self-assembled from amphiphilic hyperbranched multiarm copolymer for glutathione-mediated intracellular drug delivery. *Biomacromolecules*, *12*(5), 1567–1577. doi:10.1021/bm200275j PMID:21456627

Liu, J. Y., Pang, Y., Huang, W., Huang, X. H., Meng, L. L., Zhu, X. Y., & Yan, D. Y. et al. (2011). Redox-responsive polyphosphate nanosized assemblies: A smart drug delivery platform for cancer therapy. *Biomacromolecules*, *12*(6), 2407–2415. doi:10.1021/bm2005164 PMID:21557536

Liu, J., Andya, J. D., & Shire, S. J. (2006). A critical review of analytical ultracentrifugation and field flow fractionation methods for measuring protein aggregation. *The AAPS Journal*, *8*(3), E580–E589. doi:10.1208/aapsj080367 PMID:17025276

Liu, J., Gong, T., Fu, H., Wang, C., Wang, X., Chen, Q., & Zhang, Z. et al. (2008). Solid lipid nanoparticles for pulmonary delivery of insulin. *International Journal of Pharmaceutics*, *356*(1), 333–344. doi:10.1016/j.ijpharm.2008.01.008 PMID:18281169

Liu, K. C., & Yeo, Y. (2013). Zwitterionic Chitosan–Polyamidoamine Dendrimer Complex Nanoparticles as a pH-Sensitive Drug Carrier. *Molecular Pharmaceutics*, *10*(5), 1695–1704. doi:10.1021/mp300522p PMID:23510114

Liu, T. Y., Hu, S. H., Liu, K. H., Liu, D. M., & Chen, S. Y. (2006). Preparation and characterization of smart magnetic hydrogels and its use for drug release. *Journal of Magnetism and Magnetic Materials*, *304*(1), e397–e399. doi:10.1016/j.jmmm.2006.01.203

Liu, T., & Guo, R. (2007). Structure and transformation of the niosome prepared from PEG 6000/Tween 80/Span 80/H2O lamellar liquid crystal. *Colloids and Surfaces. A, Physicochemical and Engineering Aspects*, *295*(1), 130–134. doi:10.1016/j.colsurfa.2006.08.041

Liu, T., Guo, R., Hua, W., & Qiu, J. (2007). Structure behaviors of hemoglobin in PEG 6000/Tween 80/Span 80/H2O niosome system. *Colloids and Surfaces. A, Physicochemical and Engineering Aspects*, *293*(1), 255–261. doi:10.1016/j.colsurfa.2006.07.053

Liu, X., He, B., Xu, Z., Yin, M., Yang, W., Zhang, H., & Shen, J. et al. (2015). A functionalized fluorescent dendrimer as a pesticide nanocarrier: Application in pest control. *Nanoscale*, *7*(2), 445–449. doi:10.1039/C4NR05733C PMID:25429649

Liu, X., Xu, B., Xia, Q. S., Zhao, T. D., & Tang, T. P. (2005). A method of showing thermal effect of iron oxide nanoparticles in alternating magnetic field. *Ai Zheng*, *24*(9), 1148–1150. PMID:16159444

Liu, Y. S., Wen, C. F., & Yang, Y. M. (2012). Development of ethosome-like catanionic vesicles for dermal drug delivery. *Journal of the Taiwan Institute of Chemical Engineers*, *43*(6), 830–838. doi:10.1016/j.jtice.2012.06.008

Liu, Y. Y., Shao, Y. H., & Lü, J. (2006). Preparation, properties and controlled release behaviors of pH-induced thermosensitive amphiphilic gels. *Biomaterials*, *27*(21), 4016–4024. doi:10.1016/j.biomaterials.2006.02.042 PMID:16563494

Liu, Y., Niu, T., Zhang, L., & Yang, J. (2010). Review on nano-drugs. *Natural Science*, *2*(01), 41–48. doi:10.4236/ns.2010.21006

Liu, Y., Servant, A., Guy, O. J., Al-Jamal, K. T., Williams, P. R., Hawkins, K. M., & Kostarelos, K. (2011). An electric-field responsive microsystem for controllable miniaturised drug delivery applications. *Procedia Engineering*, *25*, 984–987. doi:10.1016/j.proeng.2011.12.242

Liu, Z., Tabakman, S., Welsher, K., & Dai, H. (2009). Carbon nanotubes in biology and medicine: *In vitro* and *in vivo* detection, imaging and drug delivery. *Nano Res.*, *2*(2), 85–120. doi:10.1007/s12274-009-9009-8 PMID:20174481

Li, W.-J., Danielson, K. G., Alexander, P. G., & Tuan, R. S. (2003). Biological response of chondrocytes cultured in three-dimensional nanofibrous poly (ϵ-caprolactone) scaffolds. *Journal of Biomedical Materials Research. Part A*, *67*(4), 1105–1114. doi:10.1002/jbm.a.10101 PMID:14624495

Li, W.-J., Tuli, R., Okafor, C., Derfoul, A., Danielson, K. G., Hall, D. J., & Tuan, R. S. (2005). A three-dimensional nanofibrous scaffold for cartilage tissue engineering using human mesenchymal stem cells. *Biomaterials*, *26*(6), 599–609. doi:10.1016/j.biomaterials.2004.03.005 PMID:15282138

Li, Y. L., Zhu, L., Liu, Z. Z., Chemg, R., Meng, F. H., Cui, J. H., & Zhong, Z. Y. et al. (2009). Reversibly Stabilized Multifunctional Dextran Nanoparticles Efficiently Deliver Doxorubicin into the Nuclei of Cancer Cells. *Angewandte Chemie*, *48*(52), 9914–9918. doi:10.1002/anie.200904260 PMID:19937876

Li, Y., Budamaguta, M. S., Luo, J., Xiao, W., Voss, J. C., & Lam, K. S. (2012). Probing of the assembly structure and dynamics within nanoparticls during interaction with bold proteins. *ACS Nano*, *6*(11), 9486–9495. doi:10.1021/nn302317j

Li, Y., He, H., Jia, X., Lu, W.-L., Lou, J., & Wei, Y. (2012). A dual-targeting nanocarrier based on poly(amidoamine) dendrimers conjugated with transferrin and tamoxifen for treating brain gliomas. *Biomaterials*, *33*(15), 3899–3908. doi:10.1016/j.biomaterials.2012.02.004 PMID:22364698

Li, Z., Su, K., Cheng, B., & Deng, Y. (2010). Organically modified MCM-type material preparation and its usage in controlled amoxicillin delivery. *Journal of Colloid and Interface Science*, *342*(2), 607–613. doi:10.1016/j.jcis.2009.10.073 PMID:19948346

Lo, C. T., Jahn, A., Locascio, L. E., & Vreeland, W. N. (2010). Controlled self-assembly of monodisperse niosomes by microfluidic hydrodynamic focusing. *Langmuir*, *26*(11), 8559–8566. doi:10.1021/la904616s PMID:20146467

Locatelli, F., & Roger, S. (2006). Comparative testing and pharmacovigilance of biosimilars. *Nephrology, Dialysis, Transplantation*, *21*(Suppl 5), v13–v16. doi:10.1093/ndt/gfl475 PMID:16959789

Loh, X. J., Lee, T.-C., & Ito, Y. (2012). Hydrogels for Biomedical Applications. In Polymeric and Self Assembled Hydrogels: From Fundamental Understanding to Applications (No. 8, pp. 167-209). Cambridge, UK: The Royal Society of Chemistry.

Lohcharoenkal, W., Wang, L., Chen, Y. C., & Rojanasakul, Y. (2014). Protein nanoparticles as drug delivery carriers for cancer therapy.BioMed Research International.

Loh, X. J., Peh, P., Liao, S., Sng, C., & Li, J. (2010). Controlled drug release from biodegradable thermoresponsive physical hydrogel nanofibers. *Journal of Controlled Release*, *143*(2), 175–182. doi:10.1016/j.jconrel.2009.12.030 PMID:20064568

Loosli, H. R., Kessler, H., Oschkinat, H., Weber, H. P., Petcher, T., & Wider, A. (1985). The conformation of cyclosporin A in the crystal and in solution. *Helvetica Chimica Acta*, *68*, 682–703. doi:10.1002/hlca.19850680319

Lopes, L. B., Ferreira, D. A., De Paula, D., Garcia, M. T. J., Thomazini, J. A., Fantini, M. C. A., & Bentley, M. V. L. B. (2006). Reverse hexagonal phase nano dispersion of monoolein and oleic acid for topical delivery of peptides:in vitro andin vivo skin penetration of cyclosporin A. *Pharmaceutical Research*, *23*(6), 1332–1342. doi:10.1007/s11095-006-0143-7 PMID:16715364

Lopes, L. B., Lopes, J. L. C., Oliveira, D. C. R., Thomazini, J. A., Garcia, M. T. J., Fantini, M. C. A., & Bentley, M. V. L. B. et al. (2006). Liquid crystalline phases of mono olein and water for topical delivery of cyclosporin A: Characterization and study of *in vitro* and *in vivo* delivery. *European Journal of Pharmaceutics and Biopharmaceutics*, *63*(2), 146–155. doi:10.1016/j.ejpb.2006.02.003 PMID:16621488

Lopes, L. B., Speretta, F. F. F., & Bentley, M. V. L. B. (2007). Enhancement of skin penetration of vitamin K using monoolein-based liquid crystalline systems. *European Journal of Pharmaceutical Sciences*, *32*(3), 209–215. doi:10.1016/j.ejps.2007.07.006 PMID:17900879

Losa, C., Marchal-Heussler, L., Orallo, F., Vila Jato, J. L., & Alonso, M. J. (1993). Design of new formulations for topical ocular administration: Polymeric nanocapsules containing metipranolol. *Pharmaceutical Research*, *10*(1), 80–87. doi:10.1023/A:1018977130559 PMID:8094245

Los, M., Roodhart, J. M., & Voest, E. E. (2007). Target practice: Lessons from phase III trials with bevacizumAb and vatalanib in the treatment of advanced colorectal cancer. *The Oncologist*, *12*(4), 443–450. doi:10.1634/theoncologist.12-4-443 PMID:17470687

Lovelyn, C., & Attama, A. A. (2011). Current state of nanoemulsions in drug delivery. *Journal of Biomaterials and Nanobiotechnology*, *2*(05), 626–639. doi:10.4236/jbnb.2011.225075

Lowell, P. A., & El-Aasser, M. S. (1997). *Emulsion Polymerization and Emulsion Polymers* (p. 801). New York: Wiley.

Lowe, P. J., & Temple, C. S. (1994). Calcitonin and Insulin in Isobutylcyanoacrylate nanocapsules: Protection against proteases and effect on intestinal absorption in rats. *The Journal of Pharmacy and Pharmacology*, *46*(7), 547–552. doi:10.1111/j.2042-7158.1994.tb03854.x PMID:7996380

Lu, B., Zhang, J., & Yang, H. (2003). Nonphospholipid vesicles of carboplatin for lung targeting. *Drug Delivery*, *10*(2), 87–94. doi:10.1080/713840364 PMID:12746054

Lu, H. D., Zhao, H. Q., Wang, K., & Lu-Lu, L. (2011). Novel hyaluronic acid–chitosan nanoparticles as non-viral gene delivery vectors targeting osteoarthritis. *International Journal of Pharmaceutics*, *420*(2), 358–365. doi:10.1016/j.ijpharm.2011.08.046 PMID:21911044

Lu, J., Huang, Y., Zhao, W., Chen, Y., Li, J., Gao, X., & Li, S. et al. (2013). Design and characterization of PEG-derivatized vitamin E as a nanomicellar formulation for delivery of paclitaxel. *Molecular Pharmaceutics*, *10*(8), 2880–2890. doi:10.1021/mp300729y PMID:23768151

Lu, J., Huang, Y., Zhao, W., Marquez, R. T., Meng, X., Li, J., & Li, S. et al. (2013). PEGderivatized embelin as a nanomicellar carrier for delivery of paclitaxel to breast and prostate cancers. *Biomaterials*, *34*(5), 1591–1600. doi:10.1016/j.biomaterials.2012.10.073 PMID:23182923

Lu, J., Zhao, W., Liu, H., Marquez, R., Huang, Y., Zhang, Y., & Li, S. et al. (2014). …Li, S. (2014). An improved d-alpha-tocopherol-based nanocarrier for targeted delivery of doxorubicin with reversal of multidrug resistance. *Journal of Controlled Release*, *196*, 272–286. doi:10.1016/j.jconrel.2014.10.016 PMID:25456831

Lukyanov, A. N., & Torchilin, V. P. (2004). Micelles from lipid derivatives of water-soluble polymers as delivery systems for poorly soluble drugs. *Advanced Drug Delivery Reviews*, *56*(9), 1273–1289. doi:10.1016/j.addr.2003.12.004 PMID:15109769

Luo, G., Yu, X., Jin, C., Yang, F., Fu, D., Long, J., & Lu, W. et al. (2010). LyP-1-conjugated nanoparticles for targeting drug delivery to lymphatic metastatic tumors. *International Journal of Pharmaceutics*, *385*(1-2), 150–156. doi:10.1016/j.ijpharm.2009.10.014 PMID:19825404

Luo, M., Shen, Q., & Chen, J. (2011). Transdermal delivery of paeonol using cubic gel and microemulsion gel. *International Journal of Nanomedicine*, *6*, 1603–1610. PMID:21904450

Luo, Y., Ling, Y., Guo, W., Pang, J., Liu, W., Fang, Y., & Gao, X. et al. (2010). Docetaxel loaded oleic acid-coated hydroxyapatite nanoparticles enhance the docetaxel-induced apoptosis through activation of caspase-2 in androgenindependent prostate cancer cells. *Journal of Controlled Release*, *147*(2), 278–288. doi:10.1016/j.jconrel.2010.07.108 PMID:20655966

Lu, W., Zhan, C., & Hou, H. (2014). *Targeted Liposomes and Micelles as Carriers for Cancer Therapy. In Nano-Oncologicals* (pp. 95–122). Springer.

Lu, Y., & Low, P. S. (2012). Folate-mediated delivery of macromolecular anticancer therapeutic agents. *Advanced Drug Delivery Reviews*, *64*, 342–352. doi:10.1016/j.addr.2012.09.020 PMID:12204598

Madduri, S., Papaloizos, M., & Gander, B. (2010). Trophically and topographically functionalized silk fibroin nerve conduits for guided peripheral nerve regeneration. *Biomaterials*, *31*(8), 2323–2334. doi:10.1016/j.biomaterials.2009.11.073 PMID:20004018

Maeda, H., Bharate, G., & Daruwalla, J. (2009). Polymeric drugs for efficient tumor-targeted drug delivery based on EPR-effect. *European Journal of Pharmaceutics and Biopharmaceutics*, *71*(3), 409–419. doi:10.1016/j.ejpb.2008.11.010 PMID:19070661

Maeda, H., Sawa, T., & Konno, T. (2001). Mechanism of tumor-targeted delivery of macromolecular drugs, including the EPR effect in solid tumor and clinical overview of the prototype polymeric drug SMANCS. *Journal of Controlled Release*, *74*(1), 47–61. doi:10.1016/S0168-3659(01)00309-1 PMID:11489482

Maeda, H., Wu, J., Sawa, T., Matsumura, Y., & Hori, K. (2000). Tumor vascular permeability and the EPR effect in macromolecular therapeutics: A review. *Journal of Controlled Release*, *65*(1-2), 271–284. doi:10.1016/S0168-3659(99)00248-5 PMID:10699287

Magee, W. E., Goff, C. W., Schoknecht, J., Smith, M. D., & Cherian, K. (1974). The interaction of cationic liposomes containing entrapped horseradish peroxidase with cells in culture. *The Journal of Cell Biology*, *63*(2), 492–504. doi:10.1083/jcb.63.2.492 PMID:4138544

Maghraby, E. I., Williams, M., & Barry, B. W. (1998). Optimization of deformable vesicles for epidermal delivery of oestradiol. *The Journal of Pharmacy and Pharmacology*, *50*(S9), 146. doi:10.1111/j.2042-7158.1998.tb02346.x

Mahmoudi, M., Simchi, A., Imani, M., Shokrgozar, M. A., Milani, A. S., Häfeli, U. O., & Stroeve, P. (2010). A new approach for the in vitro identification of the cytotoxicity of superparamagnetic iron oxide nanoparticles. *Colloids and Surfaces. B, Biointerfaces*, *75*(1), 300–309. doi:10.1016/j.colsurfb.2009.08.044 PMID:19781921

Mainardes, R. M., & Silva, L. P. (2004). Drug delivery systems: Past, present, and future. *Current Drug Targets*, *5*(5), 449–455. doi:10.2174/1389450043345407 PMID:15216911

Majumdar, S., & Chowdhury, S. (2010). Novel therapeutic application of microbubbles for targeted drug delivery. *International Journal of Pharma and Bio Sciences, 1*(3).

Makai, M., Csanyi, E., Dekany, I., Nemeth, Z., & Eros, I. (2003). Structural properties of non-ionic surfactant/glycerol/paraffin lyotropic crystals. *Colloid & Polymer Science*, *281*, 839–844. doi:10.1007/s00396-002-0851-4

Makai, M., Csányi, E., Németh, Z., Pálinkás, J., & Erős, I. (2003). Structure and drug release of lamellar liquid crystals containing glycerol. *International Journal of Pharmaceutics*, *256*(1-2), 95–107. doi:10.1016/S0378-5173(03)00066-8 PMID:12695015

Malam, Y., Loizidou, M., & Seifalian, A. M. (2009). Liposomes and nanoparticles: Nanosized vehicles for drug delivery in cancer. *Trends in Pharmacological Sciences*, *30*(11), 592–599. doi:10.1016/j.tips.2009.08.004 PMID:19837467

Malhotra, M., & Jain, N. (1994). Niosomes as drug carriers. *Indian Drugs-Bombay*, *31*, 81–81.

Mali, N., Darandale, S., & Vavia, P. (2013). Niosomes as a vesicular carrier for topical administration of minoxidil: formulation and in vitro assessment. *Drug Delivery and Translational Research, 3*(6), 587-592.

Malik, N., Evagorou, E. G., & Duncan, R. (1999). Dendrimer-platinate: A novel approach to cancer chemotherapy. *Anti-Cancer Drugs*, *10*(8), 767–776. doi:10.1097/00001813-199909000-00010 PMID:10573209

Mamaeva, V., Sahlgren, C., & Lindén, M. (2013). Mesoporous silica nanoparticles in medicine- Recent advances. *Advanced Drug Delivery Reviews*, *65*(5), 689–702. doi:10.1016/j.addr.2012.07.018 PMID:22921598

Manconi, M., Sinico, C., Fadda, A., Vila, A., Figueruelo, J., & Molina, F. (2005). Thermodynamical aspects regarding the formation of self-assembly decylpolyglucoside structures. *Colloids and Surfaces. A, Physicochemical and Engineering Aspects*, *270*, 124–128. doi:10.1016/j.colsurfa.2005.05.051

Manconi, M., Sinico, C., Valenti, D., Lai, F., & Fadda, A. (2006). Niosomes as carriers for tretinoin III. A study into the in vitro cutaneous delivery of vesicle-incorporated tretinoin. *International Journal of Pharmaceutics*, *311*(1-2), 11–19. doi:10.1016/j.ijpharm.2005.11.045 PMID:16439071

Manconi, M., Sinico, C., Valenti, D., Loy, G., & Fadda, A. (2002). Niosomes as carriers for tretinoin. I. Preparation and properties. *International Journal of Pharmaceutics*, *234*(1-2), 237–248. doi:10.1016/S0378-5173(01)00971-1 PMID:11839454

Manconi, M., Valenti, D., Sinico, C., Lai, F., Loy, G., & Fadda, A. (2003). Niosomes as carriers for tretinoin. II. Influence of vesicular incorporation on tretinoin photostability. *International Journal of Pharmaceutics*, *260*(2), 261–272. doi:10.1016/S0378-5173(03)00268-0 PMID:12842345

Manconi, M., Vila, A., Sinico, C., Figueruelo, J., Molina, F., & Fadda, A. (2006). Theoretical and experimental evaluation of decypolyglucoside vesicles as potential drug delivery systems. *Journal of Drug Delivery Science and Technology*, *16*(2), 141–146. doi:10.1016/S1773-2247(06)50021-8

Mann, B. K., Gobin, A. S., Tsai, A. T., Schmedlen, R. H., & West, J. L. (2001). Smooth muscle cell growth in photopolymerized hydrogels with cell adhesive and proteolytically degradable domains: Synthetic ECM analogs for tissue engineering. *Biomaterials*, *22*(22), 3045–3051. doi:10.1016/S0142-9612(01)00051-5 PMID:11575479

Manosroi, A., Ruksiriwanich, W., Manosroi, W., Abe, M., & Manosroi, J. (2012). In Vivo Hair Growth Promotion Activity of Gel Containing Niosomes Loaded with the Oryza sativa Bran Fraction (OSF3). Advanced Science Letters, 16(1),222-228.

Manosroi, A., Chutoprapat, R., Abe, M., & Manosroi, J. (2008). Characteristics of niosomes prepared by supercritical carbon dioxide (scCO2) fluid. *International Journal of Pharmaceutics*, *352*(1-2), 248–255. doi:10.1016/j.ijpharm.2007.10.013 PMID:18036754

Manosroi, A., Chutoprapat, R., Abe, M., Manosroi, W., & Manosroi, J. (2012). Transdermal absorption enhancement of rice bran bioactive compounds entrapped in niosomes. *AAPS PharmSciTech*, *13*(1), 323–335. doi:10.1208/s12249-012-9751-1 PMID:22258804

Manosroi, A., Jantrawut, P., & Manosroi, J. (2008). Anti-inflammatory activity of gel containing novel elastic niosomes entrapped with diclofenac diethylammonium. *International Journal of Pharmaceutics*, *360*(1-2), 156–163. doi:10.1016/j.ijpharm.2008.04.033 PMID:18539416

Manosroi, A., Khanrin, P., Werner, R., Götz, F., Manosroi, W., & Manosroi, J. (2010). Entrapment enhancement of peptide drugs in niosomes. *Journal of Microencapsulation*, *27*(3), 272–280. doi:10.3109/02652040903131293 PMID:20113169

Mantripragada, S. (2002). A lipid based depot (DepoFoam® technology) for sustained release drug delivery. *Progress in Lipid Research*, *41*(5), 392–406. doi:10.1016/S0163-7827(02)00004-8 PMID:12121719

Marchal-Heussler, L., Fessi, H., Devissaguet, J. P., Hoffman, M., & Maincent, P. (1992). Colloidal drug delivery systems for the eye. A comparison of the efficacy of three different polymers: Polyisobutylcyanoacrylate, poly (lactic-co-glycolic Acid, poly-epsilon caprolactone. *S.T.P. Pharma*, *2*, 98–104.

Marchal-Heussler, L., Sirbat, D., Hoffman, M., & Maincent, P. (1993). Poly(epsilon-caprolactone) nanocapsules in carteolol ophthalmic delivery. *Pharmaceutical Research*, *10*(3), 386–390. doi:10.1023/A:1018936205485 PMID:8464811

Marcolis, L. B. (1984). Cell interaction with model membranes probing, modification and simulation of cell surface functions. *Biochimica et Biophysica Acta (BBA)-. Reviews on Biomembranes*, *779*(2), 161–189.

Marianeci, C., Marzio, L., Rinaldi, F., Celia, F., Paolino, D., Alhaique, F., & Carafa, M. et al. (2014). Niosomes from 80s to present: The state of the art. *Advances in Colloid and Interface Science*, *205*, 187–206. doi:10.1016/j.cis.2013.11.018 PMID:24369107

Mark, H. F. (2013). *Encyclopedia of polymer science and technology, concise*. John Wiley & Sons.

Markman, J. L., Rekechenetskiy, A., Holler, E., & Ljubimova, J. Y. (2013). Nanomedicine therapeutic approaches to overcome cancer drug resistance. *Advanced Drug Delivery Reviews*, *65*(13-14), 1866–1879. doi:10.1016/j.addr.2013.09.019 PMID:24120656

Marsh, D. (1990). Spin label ESR and 31P-NMR studies of the cubic and inverted hexagonal phases of dimyristoyl phosphatidylcholine/myristic acid (1:2, mol/mol) mixtures. *Biochimica et Biophysica Acta*, *1024*(1), 89–94. doi:10.1016/0005-2736(90)90211-6 PMID:2159807

Martin, A. (2001). *Physical pharmacy* (4th ed.). Lippincott Williams and Wilkins. Printed in India at Gopsons Papers Ltd, Noida.

Martin-Bertelsen, B., Korsholm, K. S., Rose, F., Nordly, P., Franzyk, H., Andersen, P., & Foged, C. (2013). The supra molecular structure is decisive for the immune stimulatory properties of synthetic analogues of a mycobacterial lipid in vitro. *RSC Advances*, *3*(43), 20673–20683. doi:10.1039/C3RA42737D

Martin-James, D., Keary-Cristin, L., Thornton-Todd, A., & Novotnak-Mark, P. (2006). Metallotropic liquid crystals formed by surfactant templating of molten metal halides. *Nature Materials*, *5*(4), 271–275. doi:10.1038/nmat1610 PMID:16547520

Martins, A., Reis, R. L., & Neves, N. M. (2008). Electrospinning: Processing technique for tissue engineering scaffolding. *International Materials Reviews*, *53*(5), 257–274. doi:10.1179/174328008X353547

Martín-Saavedra, F. M., Ruíz-Hernández, E., Boré, A., Arcos, D., Vallet-Regí, M., & Vilaboa, N. (2010). Magneticmesoporous silica spheres for hyperthermia therapy. *Acta Biomaterialia*, *6*(12), 4522–4531. doi:10.1016/j.actbio.2010.06.030 PMID:20601238

Marty, J. J., Oppenheim, R. C., & Speiser, P. (1978). Nanoparticles: A new colloidal drug delivery systems. *Pharmaceutica Acta Helvetiae*, *53*, 17–23. PMID:643885

Masotti, A., Vicennati, P., Alisi, A., Marianecci, C., Rinaldi, F., Carafa, M., & Ortaggi, G. (2010). Novel Tween® 20 derivatives enable the formation of efficient pH-sensitive drug delivery vehicles for human hepatoblastoma. *Bioorganic & Medicinal Chemistry Letters*, *20*(10), 3021–3025. doi:10.1016/j.bmcl.2010.04.010 PMID:20427183

Matsumura, Y. (2011). Preclinical and clinical studies of NK012, an SN-38-incorporating polymeric micelles, which is designed based on EPR effect. *Advanced Drug Delivery Reviews*, *63*(3), 184–192. doi:10.1016/j.addr.2010.05.008 PMID:20561951

Matsumura, Y., Hamaguchi, T., Ura, T., Muro, K., Yamada, Y., Shimada, Y., & Watanabe, N. et al. (2004). Phase I clinical trial and pharmacokinetic evaluation of NK911, a micelle-encapsulated doxorubicin. *British Journal of Cancer*, *91*(10), 1775–1781. doi:10.1038/sj.bjc.6602204 PMID:15477860

Matsumura, Y., & Maeda, H. (1986). A new concept for macromolecular therapeutics in cancer chemotherapy: Mechanism of tumoritropic accumulation of proteins and the antitumor agent smancs. *Cancer Research*, *46*(12 Part 1), 6387–6392. PMID:2946403

Matsumura, Y., & Maeda, H. (1986). A new concept formacromolecular therapeutics in cancer chemotherapy: Mechanism of tumouritropic accumulation of proteins and the antitumour agent smancs. *Cancer Research*, *46*, 6387–6392. PMID:2946403

Matthews, J. A., Boland, E. D., Wnek, G. E., Simpson, D. G., & Bowlin, G. L. (2003). Electrospinning of collagen type II: A feasibility study. *Journal of Bioactive and Compatible Polymers*, *18*(2), 125–134. doi:10.1177/0883911503018002003

Matthews, J. A., Wnek, G. E., Simpson, D. G., & Bowlin, G. L. (2002). Electrospinning of collagen nanofibers. *Biomacromolecules*, *3*(2), 232–238. doi:10.1021/bm015533u PMID:11888306

Matthias, R., Egbert, J., Priscilla, M., Stefan, M., Ulrich, V., & Ilka, R. (2009). Efficacy of epicutaneous diractin® (ketoprofen in transfersome® gel) for the treatment of pain related to eccentric muscle contractions. *Drug Des Devel Ther*, *3*, 143–149. PMID:19920930

Maurya, S., Aggarwal, S., Tilak, V., Dhakar, R., Singh, A., & Maurya, G. (2010). Enhanced transdermal delivery of indinavir sulfate via transfersomes. *IJCP*, *1*(06), 1–7.

Maver, U., Godec, A., Bele, M., Planinšek, O., Gaberšček, M., Srčič, S., & Jamnik, J. (2007). Novel hybrid silica xerogels for stabilization and controlled release of drug. *International Journal of Pharmaceutics*, *330*(1), 164–174. doi:10.1016/j.ijpharm.2006.09.024 PMID:17055199

Mayer, L. D., Hope, M. J., Cullis, P. R., & Janoff, A. S. (1985). Solute distributions and trapping efficiencies observed in freeze-thawed multilamellar vesicles. *Biochimica et Biophysica Acta*, 817–193. PMID:4005257

Mbah, C. C., Builders, P. F., & Attama, A. A. (2014). Nanovesicular carriers as alternative drug delivery systems: Ethosomes in focus. *Expert Opinion on Drug Delivery*, *11*(1), 45–59. doi:10.1517/17425247.2013.860130 PMID:24294974

McGurk, J., Ross, A., & Gilroy, G. (1986). A Novel Method for the In-Situ Preparation of Liposomes Using an Aerosol Delivery System. *The Journal of Pharmacy and Pharmacology*, *38*(S12), 20P–20P. doi:10.1111/j.2042-7158.1986.tb14249.x

Medina, O. P., Zhu, Y., & Kairemo, K. (2004). Targeted liposomal drug delivery in cancer. *Current Pharmaceutical Design*, *10*(24), 2981–2989. doi:10.2174/1381612043383467 PMID:15379663

Medina, S. H., & El-Sayed, M. E. H. (2009). Dendrimers as Carriers for Delivery of Chemotherapeutic Agents. *Chemical Reviews*, *109*(7), 3141–3157. doi:10.1021/cr900174j PMID:19534493

Mehta, S., & Jindal, N. (2013). Formulation of tyloxapol niosomes for encapsulation, stabilization and dissolution of anti-tubercular drugs. *Colloids and Surfaces. B, Biointerfaces*, *101*, 434–441. doi:10.1016/j.colsurfb.2012.07.006 PMID:23010052

Meinel, A. J., Germershaus, O., Luhmann, T., Merkle, H. P., & Meinel, L. (2012). Electrospun matrices for localized drug delivery: Current technologies and selected biomedical applications. *European Journal of Pharmaceutics and Biopharmaceutics*, *81*(1), 1–13. doi:10.1016/j.ejpb.2012.01.016 PMID:22342778

Melanko, J. B., Pearce, M. E., & Salem, A. K. (2009). *Nanotubes, nanorods, nanofibers, and fullerenes for nanoscale drug delivery. In Nanotechnology in Drug Delivery* (pp. 105–127). Springer.

Mellin, L., Borg, N., & Kaellrot, M. J. (2014). *Patent Application JP 2014177460.*

Mellman, I., Fuchs, R., & Helenius, A. (1986). Acidification of the endocytic and exocytic pathways. *Annual Review of Biochemistry*, *55*(1), 663–700. doi:10.1146/annurev.bi.55.070186.003311 PMID:2874766

Mellstedt, H., Niederwieser, D., & Ludwig, H. (2008). The challenge of biosimilars. *Ann Omol.*, *19*, 411–419. PMID:17872902

Memisoğlu, E., Oner, F., Ayhan, A., Basaran, I., & Hincal, A. (1997). In vivo evaluation for rhGM-CSF wound-healing efficacy in topical vehicles. *Pharmaceutical Development and Technology*, *2*(2), 171–180. doi:10.3109/10837459709022622 PMID:9552443

Meng, F. H., Cheng, R., Deng, C., & Zhong, Z. Y. (2012). Intracellular drug release nanosystems. *Materials Today*, *15*(10), 436–442. doi:10.1016/S1369-7021(12)70195-5

Meng, H. A., Liong, M., Xia, T., Li, Z., Ji, Z., Zink, J. I., & Nel, A. E. (2010). Engineered design of mesoporous silica nanoparticles to deliver doxorubicin & P-glycoprotein siRNA to overcome drug resistance in a cancer cell line. *ACS Nano*, *4*(8), 4539–4550. doi:10.1021/nn100690m PMID:20731437

Merrigan, S. R., Schechtman, L. A., Goldman, S. A., Beck, M., Gorth, F. C., Weidl, … Stephan, O. (2004). *U.S. Patent Application 2004/0068093*. Washington, DC: U.S. Patent and Trademark Office.

Mezzenga, R., Meyer, C., Servais, C., Romoscanu, A. I., Sagalowicz, L., & Hayward, R. C. (2005). Shear rheology of lyotropic liquid crystals: A case study. *Langmuir*, *21*(8), 3322–3333. doi:10.1021/la046964b PMID:15807570

Mezzenga, R., Schurtenberger, P., Burbidge, A., & Michel, M. (2005). Understanding foods as soft materials. *Nature Materials*, *4*(10), 729–740. doi:10.1038/nmat1496 PMID:16195765

Michalet, X., Pinaud, F. F., Bentolila, L. A., Tsay, J. M., Doose, S., Li, J. J., & Weiss, S. et al. (2005). Quantum dots for live cells, in vivo imaging, and diagnostics. *Science*, *307*(5709), 538–544. doi:10.1126/science.1104274 PMID:15681376

Michel, C., Aprahamian, M., Defontaine, L., Couvreur, P., & Damge, C. (1991). The effect of site of administration in the gastrointestinal tract on the absorption of insulin from nanocapsules in diabetic rats. *The Journal of Pharmacy and Pharmacology*, *43*(1), 1–5. doi:10.1111/j.2042-7158.1991.tb05437.x PMID:1676051

Mickova, A., Buzgo, M., Benada, O., Rampichova, M., Fisar, Z., Filova, E., & Amler, E. et al. (2012). Core/shell nanofibers with embedded liposomes as a drug delivery system. *Biomacromolecules*, *13*(4), 952–962. doi:10.1021/bm2018118 PMID:22401557

Milić, J., & Petrović, S. D. (2003). The characteristics of novel dosage forms. *Hem. Ind.*, *57*(10), 424–436. doi:10.2298/HEMIND0310424M

Miller, L. L. (1988). Electrochemically controlled release of drug ions from conducting polymers. *Molecular Crystals and Liquid Crystals*, *160*(1), 297–301.

Milsmann, M. H., Schwendener, R. A., & Weder, H.-G. (1978). The preparation of large single bilayer liposomes by a fast and controlled dialysis. *Biochimica et Biophysica Acta (BBA)-. Biomembranes*, *512*(1), 147–155. doi:10.1016/0005-2736(78)90225-0

Milton, N., & Nail, S. L. (1996). The physical state of nafcillin sodium in frozen aqueous solutions and freezedried powders. *Pharmaceutical Development and Technology*, *1*(3), 269–277. doi:10.3109/10837459609022595 PMID:9552309

Min, B.-M., Lee, G., Kim, S. H., Nam, Y. S., Lee, T. S., & Park, W. H. (2004). Electrospinning of silk fibroin nanofibers and its effect on the adhesion and spreading of normal human keratinocytes and fibroblasts in vitro. *Biomaterials*, *25*(7), 1289–1297. doi:10.1016/j.biomaterials.2003.08.045 PMID:14643603

Mintzer, M. A., & Grinstaff, M. W. (2011). Biomedical applications of dendrimers: A tutorial. *Chemical Society Reviews*, *40*(1), 173–190. doi:10.1039/B901839P PMID:20877875

Mishra, B., Patel, B. B., & Tiwari, S. (2010). Colloidal nanocarriers: A review on formulation technology, types and applications toward targeted drug delivery. *Nanomedicine; Nanotechnology, Biology, and Medicine*, *6*(1), 9–24. doi:10.1016/j.nano.2009.04.008 PMID:19447208

Misra, R., Acharya, S., & Sahoo, S. K. (2010). Cancer nanotechnology: Application of nanotechnology in cancer therapy. *Drug Discovery Today*, *15*(19-20), 842–850. doi:10.1016/j.drudis.2010.08.006 PMID:20727417

Mittur, A. (2005). *U.S. Patent Application 11/304,335*. Washington, DC: U.S. Patent and Trademark Office.

Mi, Y., Liu, Y., & Feng, S. S. (2011). Formulation of docetaxel by folic acid conjugated D-α-tocopheryl polyethylene glycol succinate 2000 (Vitamin E TPGS2k) micelles for targeted and synergistic chemotherapy. *Biomaterials*, *32*(16), 4058–4066. doi:10.1016/j.biomaterials.2011.02.022 PMID:21396707

Miyaji, F., Davis, S. A., Charmant, J. P. H., & Mann, S. (1999). Organic crystal templating of hollow silica fibers. *Chemistry of Materials*, *11*(11), 3021–3024. doi:10.1021/cm990449v

Miyata, T., Uragami, T., & Nakamae, K. (2002). Biomolecule-sensitive hydrogels. *Advanced Drug Delivery Reviews*, *54*(1), 79–98. doi:10.1016/S0169-409X(01)00241-1 PMID:11755707

Miyazaki, M., Kaneno, J., Kohama, R., Uehara, M., Kanno, K., Fujii, M., & Maeda, H. et al. (2004). Preparation of functionalized nanostructures on micro channel surface and their use for enzyme micro reactors. *Chemical Engineering Journal*, *101*(1-3), 277–284. doi:10.1016/j.cej.2003.11.010

Miyazaki, S., Yokouchi, C., & Takada, M. (1988). External control of drug release: Controlled release of insulin from a hydrophilic polymer implant by ultrasound irradiation in diabetic rats. *The Journal of Pharmacy and Pharmacology*, *40*(10), 716–717. doi:10.1111/j.2042-7158.1988.tb07001.x PMID:2907539

Moazeni, E., Gilani, K., Sotoudegan, F., Pardakhty, A., Najafabadi, A. R., Ghalandari, R., & Jamalifar, H. et al. (2010). Formulation and in vitro evaluation of ciprofloxacin containing niosomes for pulmonary delivery. *Journal of Microencapsulation*, *10*, 1–10. PMID:20681747

Moerkerke, R., Koningsveld, R., Berghmans, H., Dusek, K., & Solc, K. (1995). Phase transitions in swollen networks. *Macromolecules*, *28*(4), 1103–1107. doi:10.1021/ma00108a043

Moghassemi, S., Parnian, E., Hakamivala, A., Darzianiazizi, M., Vardanjani, M. M., Kashanian, S., & Omidfar, K. et al. (2015). Uptake and transport of insulin across intestinal membrane model using trimethyl chitosan coated insulin niosomes. *Materials Science and Engineering C*, *46*, 333–340. doi:10.1016/j.msec.2014.10.070 PMID:25491995

Moghimi, S. (2005). Nanomedicine: Current status and future prospects. *The FASEB Journal*, *19*(3), 311–330. doi:10.1096/fj.04-2747rev PMID:15746175

Mohammady, S. Z., Pouzot, M., & Mezzenga, R. (2009). Oleoylethanolamide-based lyotropic liquid crystals as vehicles for delivery of amino acids in aqueous environment. *Biophysical Journal*, *96*(4), 1537–1546. doi:10.1016/j.bpj.2008.10.057 PMID:19217870

Mohanraj, V. J., & Chen, Y. (2007). Nanoparticles-a review. *Tropical Journal of Pharmaceutical Research*, *5*(1), 561–573. doi:10.4314/tjpr.v5i1.14634

Mokhtar, M., Sammour, O. A., Hammad, M. A., & Megrab, N. A. (2008). Effect of some formulation parameters on flurbiprofen encapsulation and release rates of niosomes prepared from proniosomes. *International Journal of Pharmaceutics*, *361*(1-2), 104–111. doi:10.1016/j.ijpharm.2008.05.031 PMID:18577437

Molla, M. R., Rangadurai, P., Pavan, G. M., & Thayumanavan, S. (2015). Experimental and theoretical investigations in stimuli responsive dendrimer-based assemblies. *Nanoscale*, *7*(9), 3817–3837. doi:10.1039/C4NR04563G PMID:25260107

Momma, K. (1996). Lipo-PGE 1 treatment of the neonate with critical congenital heart disease and ductus-arteriosus dependent circulation. *Advanced Drug Delivery Reviews*, *20*(2), 177–180. doi:10.1016/0169-409X(95)00121-M

Monteiro, N., Martins, A., Reis, R. L., & Neves, N. M. (2014). Liposomes in tissue engineering and regenerative medicine. *Journal of the Royal Society, Interface*, *11*(101), 1–24. doi:10.1098/rsif.2014.0459 PMID:25401172

Moon, I. J., Kim, H. Y., & Choi, H. J. (2015). Conducting poly(*N*-methylaniline)-coated cross-linked poly(methyl methacrylate) nanoparticle suspension and its steady shear response under electric fields. *Colloids and Surfaces. A, Physicochemical and Engineering Aspects*, *481*, 506–513. doi:10.1016/j.colsurfa.2015.05.051

Mora-Huertas, C. E., Fessi, H., & Elaissari, A. (2010). Polymer-based nanocapsules for drug delivery. *International Journal of Pharmaceutics*, *385*(1-2), 113–142. doi:10.1016/j.ijpharm.2009.10.018 PMID:19825408

Morgan, M. T., Carnahan, M. A., Immoos, C. E., Ribeiro, A. A., Finkelstein, S., Lee, S. J., & Grinstaff, M. W. (2003). Dendritic molecular capsules for hydrophobic compounds. *Journal of the American Chemical Society*, *125*(50), 15485–15489. doi:10.1021/ja0347383 PMID:14664594

Mozafari, M. R. (2005). Liposomes: An overview of manufacturing techniques. *Cellular & Molecular Biology Letters*, *10*, 711–719. PMID:16341279

Muchow, M., Maincent, P., & Müller, R. H. (2008). Lipid nanoparticles with a solid matrix (SLN®, NLC®, LDC®) for oral drug delivery. *Drug Development and Industrial Pharmacy*, *34*(12), 1394–1405. doi:10.1080/03639040802130061 PMID:18665980

Mueller-Goymann, C. C. (2002). Liquid crystals in drug delivery. In J. Swarbrick & J. C. Boylan (Eds.), *Encyclopedia of Pharmaceutical Technology* (pp. 834–853). New York, Basel: Marcel Dekker.

Mueller-Goymann, C. C., & Frank, S. G. (1986). Interaction of lidocaine and lidocaine hydrochloride with liquid crystal structure of topical preparation. *International Journal of Pharmaceutics*, *29*(2-3), 147–159. doi:10.1016/0378-5173(86)90112-2

Mueller-Goymann, C. C., & Hamann, H. J. (1993). Sustained release from reverse micellar solutions by phase transformation into lamellar liquid crystals. *Journal of Controlled Release*, *23*(2), 165–174. doi:10.1016/0168-3659(93)90042-4

Muggia, F., Hainsworth, J., Jeffers, S., Groshen, S., Tan, M., & Greco, F. (1996). *Liposomal doxorubicin (Doxil) is active against refractory ovarian cancer.* Paper presented at the Proc Am Soc Clin Oncol.

Mu, L., Elbayoumi, T. A., & Torchilin, V. P. (2005). Mixed micelles made of poly(ethylene glycol)–phosphatidylethanolamine conjugate and d-α-tocopheryl polyethylene glycol 1000 succinate as pharmaceutical nanocarriers for camptothecin. *International Journal of Pharmaceutics*, *306*(1–2), 142–149. doi:10.1016/j.ijpharm.2005.08.026 PMID:16242875

Mullaicharam, A., & Murthy, R. (2004). Lung accumulation of niosome-entrapped rifampicin following intravenous and intratracheal administration in the rat. *Journal of Drug Delivery Science and Technology*, *14*(2), 99–104. doi:10.1016/S1773-2247(04)50020-5

Mullaicharam, A., & Murthy, R. (2006). Lung accumulation of niosome-entrapped gentamicin sulfate follows intravenous and intratracheal administration in rats. *Journal of Drug Delivery Science and Technology*, *16*(2), 109–113. doi:10.1016/S1773-2247(06)50016-4

Mullen, D. G., McNerny, D. Q., Desai, A., Cheng, X.-, DiMaggio, S. C., Kotlyar, A., & Banaszak Holl, M. M. et al. (2011). Design, Synthesis, and Biological Functionality of a Dendrimer-Based Modular Drug Delivery Platform. *Bioconjugate Chemistry*, *22*(4), 679–689. doi:10.1021/bc100360v PMID:21425790

Muller, F., Salonen, A., & Glatter, O. (2010). Monoglyceride-based cubosomes stabilized by Laponite: Separating the effects of stabilizer, pH and temperature. *Colloids and Surfaces. A, Physicochemical and Engineering Aspects*, *358*(1–3), 50–56. doi:10.1016/j.colsurfa.2010.01.021

Müller-Goymann, C. C. (2004). Physicochemical characterization of colloidal drug delivery systems such as reverse micelles, vesicles, liquid crystals and nanoparticles for topical administration. *European Journal of Pharmaceutics and Biopharmaceutics*, *58*(2), 343–356. doi:10.1016/j.ejpb.2004.03.028 PMID:15296960

Muller-Goymann, C. C., & Hamann, H. J. (1991). Pharmacosomes: Multilamellar vesicles consisting of Pure Drug. *European Journal of Pharmaceutics and Biopharmaceutics*, *37*, 113–117.

Müller, R. H., & Keck, C. M. (2004). Challenges and solutions for the delivery of biotech drugs – a review of drug nanocrystals technology and lipid nanoparticles. *Journal of Biotechnology*, *113*(1-3), 151–170. doi:10.1016/j.jbiotec.2004.06.007 PMID:15380654

Muller, R. H., Mader, K., & Gohla, S. (2000). Solid lipid nanoparticles (SLN) for controlled drug delivery – a review of the state of the art. *European Journal of Pharmaceutics and Biopharmaceutics*, *50*, 161–177. doi:10.1016/S0939-6411(00)00087-4 PMID:10840199

Müller, R. H., Radtke, M., & Wissing, S. A. (2002). Nanostructured lipid matrices for improved microencapsulation of drugs. *International Journal of Pharmaceutics*, *242*(1-2), 121–128. doi:10.1016/S0378-5173(02)00180-1 PMID:12176234

Mura, S., Manconi, M., Sinico, C., Valenti, D., & Fadda, A. M. (2009). Penetration enhancer-containing vesicles (PEVs) as carriers for cutaneous delivery of minoxidil. *International Journal of Pharmaceutics*, *380*(1), 72–79. doi:10.1016/j.ijpharm.2009.06.040 PMID:19589377

Mura, S., Manconi, M., Valenti, D., Sinico, C., Vila, A. O., & Fadda, A. M. (2011). Transcutol containing vesicles for topical delivery of minoxidil. *Journal of Drug Targeting*, *19*(3), 189–196. doi:10.3109/1061186X.2010.483516 PMID:20446805

Mura, S., Nicolas, J., & Couvreur, P. (2013). Stimuli-responsive nanocarriers for drug delivery. *Nature Materials*, *12*(11), 991–1003. doi:10.1038/nmat3776 PMID:24150417

Mura, S., Pirot, F., Manconi, M., Falson, M., & Fadda, A. M. (2007). Liposomes and niosomes as potential carriers for dermal delivery of minoxidil. *Journal of Drug Targeting*, *15*(2), 101–108. doi:10.1080/10611860600991993 PMID:17365280

Murdan, S. (2003). Electro-responsive drug delivery from hydrogels. *Journal of Controlled Release*, *92*(1), 1–17. doi:10.1016/S0168-3659(03)00303-1 PMID:14499181

Murgia, S., Bonacchi, S., Falchi, A. M., Lampis, S., Lippolis, V., Meli, V., & Caltagirone, C. (2013). Drug-loaded fluorescent cubosomes: Versatile nanoparticles for potential the ranostic applications. *Langmuir*, *29*(22), 6673–6679. doi:10.1021/la401047a PMID:23642193

Mutha, S., Patil, S., & Bhosale, A. (2013). Thermoreversible niosomal gel as a potential ophthalmic drug delivery system for Ganciclovir. *Indo American Journal of Pharmaceutical Research*, *3*(11), 1990–9201.

Muzzalupo, R., Nicoletta, F. P., Trombino, S., Cassano, R., Iemma, F., & Picci, N. (2007). A new crown ether as vesicular carrier for 5-fluoruracil: Synthesis, characterization and drug delivery evaluation. *Colloids and Surfaces. B, Biointerfaces*, *58*(2), 197–202. doi:10.1016/j.colsurfb.2007.03.010 PMID:17434295

Muzzalupo, R., Tavano, L., Trombino, S., Cassano, R., Picci, N., & La Mesa, C. (2008). Niosomes from [alpha],[omega]-trioxyethylene-bis (sodium 2-dodecyloxy-propylenesulfonate): Preparation and characterization. *Colloids and Surfaces. B, Biointerfaces*, *64*(2), 200–207. doi:10.1016/j.colsurfb.2008.01.026 PMID:18378125

Myung, D., Waters, D., Wiseman, M., Duhamel, P. E., Noolandi, J., Ta, C. N., & Frank, C. W. (2008). Progress in the development of interpenetrating polymer network hydrogels. *Polymers for Advanced Technologies*, *19*(6), 647–657. doi:10.1002/pat.1134 PMID:19763189

Nademi, M., Mozaffari, A., & Farrokhabadi, A. (2011). A New Self Healing Method in Composite Laminates Using the Hollow Glass Fiber. *Key Engineering Materials*, *471*, 548–551. doi:10.4028/www.scientific.net/KEM.471-472.548

Nagarsenker, M., Amin, L., & Date, A. A. (2008). Potential of cyclodextrin complexation and liposomes in topical delivery of ketorolac: In vitro and in vivo evaluation. *AAPS PharmSciTech*, *9*(4), 1165–1170. doi:10.1208/s12249-008-9157-2 PMID:19016331

Nagarsenker, M., & Londhe, V. (2003). Preparation and evaluation of a liposomal formulation of sodium cromoglicate. *International Journal of Pharmaceutics*, *251*(1), 49–56. doi:10.1016/S0378-5173(02)00583-5 PMID:12527174

Nagle, P., & Gerancher, J. C. (2011). DepoDur® (extended-release epidural morphine): A review of an old drug in a new vehicle. *Techniques in Regional Anesthesia & Pain Management*, *11*(1), 9–18. doi:10.1053/j.trap.2007.02.011

Naik, B., & Nagarsenker, M. (2006). Novel drug delivery systems: Potential in improving topical delivery of antiacne agents. *Skin Pharmacology and Physiology*, *19*(1), 2–16. doi:10.1159/000089138 PMID:16247244

Nakada, Y., Fattal, E., Foulquier, M., & Couvreur, P. (1996). Pharmacokinetics and biodistribution of oligonucleotide adsorbed onto poly(isobutylcyanoacrylate) nanoparticles after intravenous administration in mice. *Pharmaceutical Research*, *13*(1), 38–43. doi:10.1023/A:1016017014573 PMID:8668676

Namgung, R., Singh, K., Yu, M. K., Jon, S., Kim, Y. S., Ahn, Y., & Kim, W. J. et al. (2010). Hybrid superparamagneticiron oxide nanoparticle-branched polyethyleniminemagnetoplexes for gene transfection of vascular endothelial cells. *Biomaterials*, *31*(14), 4204–4213. doi:10.1016/j.biomaterials.2010.01.123 PMID:20170956

Nanda, A., Nanda, S., Dhall, M., & Rao, R. (2005). Transferosomes: A novel ultradeformable vesicular carrier for transdermal drug delivery. *Drug Delivery Technology*, *5*(8), 59–64.

Nasr, M. (2010). In vitro and in vivo evaluation of proniosomes containing celecoxib for oral administration. *AAPS PharmSciTech*, *11*(1), 85–89. doi:10.1208/s12249-009-9364-5 PMID:20058106

Nasr, M., Mansour, S., Mortada, N. D., & Elshamy, A. (2008). Vesicular aceclofenac systems: A comparative study between liposomes and niosomes. *Journal of Microencapsulation*, *25*(7), 499–512. doi:10.1080/02652040802055411 PMID:18608811

Nässander, U., Storm, G., Peeters, P., & Crommelin, D. (1990). Liposomes. *Drugs and the Pharmaceutical Sciences*, *45*, 261 338.

Nasseri, B. (2005). Effect of cholesterol and temperature on the elastic properties of niosomal membranes. *International Journal of Pharmaceutics*, *300*(1-2), 95–101. doi:10.1016/j.ijpharm.2005.05.009 PMID:16006080

Nayak, A. P., Tiyaboonchai, W., Patankar, S., Madhusudhan, B., & Souto, E. B. (2010). Curcuminoids-loaded lipid nanoparticles: Novel approach towards malaria treatment. *Colloids and Surfaces. B, Biointerfaces*, *81*(1), 263–273. doi:10.1016/j.colsurfb.2010.07.020 PMID:20688493

Nazemi, A., Schon, T. B., & Gillies, E. R. (2013). Synthesis and degradation of backbone photodegradable polyester dendrimers. *Organic Letters*, *15*(8), 1830–1833. doi:10.1021/ol4004367 PMID:23545015

Nazli, C., Demirer, G. S., Yar, Y., Acar, H. Y., & Kizilel, S. (2014). Targeted delivery of doxorubicin into tumor cells via MMP-sensitive PEG hydrogel-coated magnetic iron oxide nanoparticles (MIONPs). *Colloids and Surfaces. B, Biointerfaces*, *122*, 674–683. doi:10.1016/j.colsurfb.2014.07.049 PMID:25183059

Negrini, R., & Mezzenga, R. (2011). PH-responsive lyotropic liquid crystals for controlled drug delivery. *Langmuir*, *27*(9), 5296–5303. doi:10.1021/la200591u PMID:21452814

Nesseem, D. I. (2001). Formulation and evaluation of itraconazole via liquid crystal for topical delivery system. *Journal of Pharmaceutical and Biomedical Analysis*, *26*(3), 387–399. doi:10.1016/S0731-7085(01)00414-9 PMID:11489384

Neubert, R. H. H. (2011). Potentials of new nanocarriers for dermal and transdermal drug delivery. *European Journal of Pharmaceutics and Biopharmaceutics*, *77*(1), 1–2. doi:10.1016/j.ejpb.2010.11.003 PMID:21111043

Neumann, R., Ringsdorf, H., Patton, E. V., & O'Brien, D. F. (1987). Preparation and characterization of long chain amino acid and peptide vesicle membranes. *Biochimica et Biophysica Acta (BBA)-. Biomembranes*, *898*(3), 338–348. doi:10.1016/0005-2736(87)90075-7

New, R. R. (1990). *Liposomes: a practical approach*. IRL Press.

Newkome, G. R., Yao, Z., Baker, G. R., & Gupta, V. K. (1985). Micelles. Part 1. Cascade molecules: A new approach to micelles. A [27]-arborol. *The Journal of Organic Chemistry*, *50*(11), 2003–2004. doi:10.1021/jo00211a052

New, R. R. C. (Ed.). (1990). *Liposomes a pratical approach*. Oxford, UK: Oxford University Press.

New, R. R., Philippot, J., & Schuber, F. (1995). *Influence of liposome characteristics on their properties and fate*. New York, NY: CRC Press.

Nguyen, T. H., Hanley, T., Porter, C. J. H., & Boyd, B. J. (2011). Nanostructured liquid crystalline particles provide long duration sustained-release effect for a poorly water soluble drug after oral administration. *Journal of Controlled Release*, *153*(2), 180–186. doi:10.1016/j.jconrel.2011.03.033 PMID:21497623

Nguyen, T. H., Hanley, T., Porter, C. J. H., Larson, I., & Boyd, B. J. (2010). Phytantriol and glyceryl monooleate cubic liquid crystalline phases as sustained-release oral drug delivery systems for poorly water-soluble drugs II. In-vivo evaluation. *The Journal of Pharmacy and Pharmacology*, *62*(7), 856–865. doi:10.1211/jpp.62.07.0006 PMID:20636873

Niamlang, S., Buranut, T., & Niansiri, A. (2011). Electrically controlled Aloe-vera extraction release from polyacrylamide hydrogel. *Energy Procedia*, *9*, 468–473. doi:10.1016/j.egypro.2011.09.053

Nick, C. (2012). The US Biosimilars Act: Challenges Facing RegulatoryApproval. *Pharm Med.*, *26*(3), 145–152. doi:10.1007/BF03262388

Nicolas, J., Mura, S., Brambilla, D., Mackiewicz, N., & Couvreur, P. (2013). Design, functionalization strategies and biomedical applications of targeted biodegradable/biocompatible polymer-based nanocarriers for drug delivery. *Chemical Society Reviews*, *42*(3), 1147–1235. doi:10.1039/C2CS35265F PMID:23238558

Niederwieser, D., & Schmitz, S. (2011). Biosimilar agents in oncology/haematology: From approval to. *European Journal of Haematology*, *86*(4), 277–288. doi:10.1111/j.1600-0609.2010.01566.x PMID:21175852

Niederwieser, H. D., & Ludwig, H. (2007). The challenge of biosimilars. *Annals of Oncology*, *19*(3), 411–419. doi:10.1093/annonc/mdm345 PMID:17872902

Nie, H., & Wang, C.-H. (2007). Fabrication and characterization of PLGA/HAp composite scaffolds for delivery of BMP-2 plasmid DNA. *Journal of Controlled Release*, *120*(1), 111–121. doi:10.1016/j.jconrel.2007.03.018 PMID:17512077

Niemiec, S. M., Ramachandran, C., & Weiner, N. (1995). Influence of nonionic liposomal composition on topical delivery of peptide drugs into pilosebaceous units: An in vivo study using the hamster ear model. *Pharmaceutical Research*, *12*(8), 1184–1188. doi:10.1023/A:1016268027854 PMID:7494832

Nilesh. (2007). *Pharmacosomes*. Retrieved from farmavita.net

Nilsson, C., Barrios-Lopez, B., Kallinen, A., Laurinmäki, P., Butcher, S. J., Raki, M., & Yaghmur, A. (2013). SPECT/CT imaging of radiolabeled cubosomes and hexosomes forpotential theranostic applications. *Biomaterials, 34*(33), 8491–8503. doi:10.1016/j.biomaterials.2013.07.055 PMID:23932247

Ning, M., Guo, Y., Pan, H., Chen, X., & Gu, Z. (2005). Preparation, in vitro and in vivo evaluation of liposomal/niosomal gel delivery systems for clotrimazole. *Drug Development and Industrial Pharmacy, 31*(4-5), 375–383. doi:10.1081/DDC-54315 PMID:16093203

Ning, M., Guo, Y., Pan, H., Yu, H., & Gu, Z. (2005). Niosomes with sorbitan monoester as a carrier for vaginal delivery of insulin: Studies in rats. *Drug Delivery, 12*(6), 399–407. doi:10.1080/10717540590968891 PMID:16253956

Nishiyama, N., Bae, Y., Miyata, K., Fukushima, S., & Kataoka, K. (2005). Smart polymeric micelles for gene and drug delivery. *Drug Discovery Today. Technologies, 2*(1), 21–26. doi:10.1016/j.ddtec.2005.05.007 PMID:24981751

Nizam El-Din, H. M. (2011). Characterization and caffeine release properties of N-isopropylacrylamide/hydroxypropyl methacrylate copolymer hydrogel synthesized by gamma radiation. *Journal of Applied Polymer Science, 119*(1), 577–585. doi:10.1002/app.32675

Noori, A. P. (2012). Preparation, characterization and anti-inflammatory evaluation of indomethacin niosomes in carrageenan inflammation model. *Research in Pharmaceutical Sciences, 7*(5), S381.

Norlen, L., & Al-Amoudi, A. (2004). Stratum corneum keratin structure, function, and formation: The cubic rod-packing and membrane templating model. *The Journal of Investigative Dermatology, 123*(4), 715–732. doi:10.1111/j.0022-202X.2004.23213.x PMID:15373777

Norling, T., Lading, P., Engstrom, S., Larsson, K., Krog, N., & Nissen, S. S. (1992). Formulation of a drug delivery system based on a mixture of monoglycerides and triglycerides for use in the treatment of periodontal disease. *Journal of Clinical Periodontology, 19*(9), 687–692. doi:10.1111/j.1600-051X.1992.tb02529.x PMID:1447387

Nounesis, G., Shi, Y., & Kumars, S. (1995). *X-ray Diffraction and Calorimetric Studies of Nematic – Nematic and Smectic – Sematic phase Transitions.* ACS Meeting, Anaheim, CA.

Nyarko, K. A. (2009). *Regulatory Approach for Subsequent Entry Biologics in Canada, Health Canada.* Presented at the PMDA 3rd International Symposium on Biologics.

O'brien, M., Wigler, N., Inbar, M., Rosso, R., Grischke, E., Santoro, A., & Ackland, S. et al. (2004). Reduced cardiotoxicity and comparable efficacy in a phase III trial of pegylated liposomal doxorubicin HCl (CAELYX™/Doxil®) versus conventional doxorubicin for first-line treatment of metastatic breast cancer. *Annals of Oncology, 15*(3), 440–449. doi:10.1093/annonc/mdh097 PMID:14998846

O'Hagan, D. T., Palin, K., & Davis, S. S. (1989). Poly(butyl2cyanoacrylate) particles as adjuvant for oral immunization. *Vaccine, 7*(3), 213–216. doi:10.1016/0264-410X(89)90231-4 PMID:2781856

Oberdörster, G., Oberdörster, E., & Oberdörster, J. (2005). Nanotoxicology: An emerging discipline evolving from studies of ultrafine particles. *Environmental Health Perspectives, 113*(7), 823–839. doi:10.1289/ehp.7339 PMID:16002369

Ogihara, U., Sasaki, T., Toyama, H., Odak, S. M., & Nishigori, H. (1997). Pharmacosomes: An emerging vesicular system. *Cancer Detection and Prevention, 21*(6), 56–62.

Ohki, Y. (2010). Development of epoxy resin composites with high thermal conductivity. *IEEE Electrical Insulation Magazine, 26*(1), 1–49. doi:10.1109/MEI.2010.5383936

Okahata, Y., Tanamachi, S., Nagai, M., & Kunitake, T. (1981). Synthetic bilayer membranes prepared from dialkyl amphiphiles with nonionic and zwitterionic head groups. *Journal of Colloid and Interface Science*, *82*(2), 401–417. doi:10.1016/0021-9797(81)90382-9

Okamoto, Y., Masum, S. M., Miyazawa, H., & Yamazaki, M. (2008). Low-pH-induced transformation of bilayer membrane into bicontinuous cubic phase in dioleoyl phosphatidyl serine/monoolein membranes. *Langmuir*, *24*(7), 3400–3406. doi:10.1021/la7036795 PMID:18302439

Okuda, T., Kawakami, S., Akimoto, N., Niidome, T., Yamashita, F., & Hashida, M. (2006). PEGylated lysine dendrimers for tumor-selective targeting after intravenous injection in tumor-bearing mice. *Journal of Controlled Release*, *116*(3), 330–336. doi:10.1016/j.jconrel.2006.09.012 PMID:17118476

Okuda, T., Tominaga, K., & Kidoaki, S. (2010). Time-programmed dual release formulation by multilayered drug-loaded nanofiber meshes. *Journal of Controlled Release*, *143*(2), 258–264. doi:10.1016/j.jconrel.2009.12.029 PMID:20074599

Okumura, Y., & Iwata, Y. (2011). Electroformation of Giant Vesicles and Electrode Polarity. *Bulletin of the Chemical Society of Japan*, *84*(10), 1147–1149. doi:10.1246/bcsj.20110097

Omidian, H., Gavrilas, C., Han, W., Li, G., & Rocca, J. G. (2008). *U.S. Patent Application 12/036,680*. Washington, DC: U.S. Patent and Trademark Office.

Omray, L. K. (2013). Liquid crystals as novel vesicular delivery system: A review. *Current Trends in Technology and Science*, *II*(VI), 347–353.

O'Reilly, M. A., & Hynynen, K. (2012). Ultrasound enhanced drug delivery to the brain and central nervous system. *International Journal of Hyperthermia*, *28*(4), 386–396. doi:10.3109/02656736.2012.666709 PMID:22621739

Orle, G. W., Drechsler, M., Koch, M. H. J., Siekmann, B., Westesen, K., & Bunjes, H. (2007). Influence of composition and preparation parameters on the properties of aqueous monoolein dispersions. *International Journal of Pharmaceutics*, *329*(1-2), 150–157. doi:10.1016/j.ijpharm.2006.08.023 PMID:16987623

Owens, D. E. III, & Peppas, N. A. (2006). Opsonization, biodistribution, & pharmacokinetics of polymeric nanoparticles. *International Journal of Pharmaceutics*, *307*(1), 93–102. doi:10.1016/j.ijpharm.2005.10.010 PMID:16303268

Özer, A., Turker, S., Çolak, S., Korkmaz, M., Kiliç, E., & Özalp, M. (2013). The effects of gamma irradiation on diclofenac sodium, liposome and niosome ingredients for rheumatoid arthritis. *Interventional Medicine and Applied Science*, *5*(3), 122–130. doi:10.1556/IMAS.5.2013.3.5 PMID:24265902

Paavola, A., Kilpelaine, I., Yliruusi, J., & Rosenberg, P. (2005). Controlled release of vancomycine from poloxamer 407 gels. *International Journal of Pharmaceutics*, *288*(2), 235–244. doi:10.1016/j.ijpharm.2004.09.028 PMID:15620863

Packhaeuser, C., Schnieders, J., Oster, C., & Kissel, T. (2004). In situ forming parenteral drug delivery systems: An overview. *European Journal of Pharmaceutics and Biopharmaceutics*, *58*(2), 445–455. doi:10.1016/j.ejpb.2004.03.003 PMID:15296966

Pagano, R. E., & Weinstein, J. N. (1978). Interactions of liposomes with mammalian cells. *Annual Review of Biophysics and Bioengineering*, *7*(1), 435–468. doi:10.1146/annurev.bb.07.060178.002251 PMID:352245

Pal, K., Banthia, A. K., & Majumdar, D. K. (2009). Polymeric hydrogels: Characterization and biomedical applications. *Designed Monomers and Polymers*, *12*(3), 197–220. doi:10.1163/156855509X436030

Panchagnula, R. (1997). Transdermal delivery of drugs. *Indian Journal of Pharmacology*, *29*, 140–156.

Pande, S., Kshirsagar, M., & Chandewar, A. (2011). Ion exchange resins pharmaceutical applications and recent advancement. *International Journal of Advances in Pharmaceutical Sciences, 2*(1).

Pansuriya, M., Gupta, A., & Gadhvi, V. (n.d.). Pharmacosomes: A Novel Vesicular System. *GTC.*

Panyam, J., & Labhasetwar, V. (2003). Biodegradable nanoparticles for drug and gene delivery to cells and tissue. *Advanced Drug Delivery Reviews, 55*(3), 329–347. doi:10.1016/S0169-409X(02)00228-4 PMID:12628320

Panyosak, A., Manosroi, J., Rojanasakul, Y., & Manosroi, A. (2009). Safety assessment of azelaic acid and its derivatives entrapped in nanovesicles. *Human and Experimental Toxicology, 28*(6-7), 387–392. doi:10.1177/0960327109105164 PMID:19755450

Paolino, D., Cosco, D., Molinaro, R., Celia, C., & Fresta, M. (2011). Supramolecular devices to improve the treatment of brain diseases. *Drug Discovery Today, 16*(7), 311–324. doi:10.1016/j.drudis.2011.02.006 PMID:21335100

Paolino, D., Cosco, D., Muzzalupo, R., Trapasso, E., Picci, N., & Fresta, M. (2008). Innovative bola-surfactant niosomes as topical delivery systems of 5-fluorouracil for the treatment of skin cancer. *International Journal of Pharmaceutics, 353*(1-2), 233–242. doi:10.1016/j.ijpharm.2007.11.037 PMID:18191509

Paolino, D., Muzzalupo, R., Ricciardi, A., Celia, C., Picci, N., & Fresta, M. (2007). In vitro and in vivo evaluation of Bola-surfactant containing niosomes for transdermal delivery. *Biomedical Microdevices, 9*(4), 421–433. doi:10.1007/s10544-007-9046-6 PMID:17252206

Papahadjopoulos, D., Allen, T., Gabizon, A., Mayhew, E., Matthay, K., Huang, S., & Redemann, C. et al. (1991). Sterically stabilized liposomes: Improvements in pharmacokinetics and antitumor therapeutic efficacy. *Proceedings of the National Academy of Sciences of the United States of America, 88*(24), 11460–11464. doi:10.1073/pnas.88.24.11460 PMID:1763060

Paramonov, S. E., Bachelder, E. M., Beaudette, T. T., Standley, S. M., Lee, C. C., Dashe, J., & Fréchet, J. M. J. (2008). Fully acid-degradable biocompatible polyacetal microparticles for drug delivery. *Bioconjugate Chemistry, 19*(4), 911–919. doi:10.1021/bc7004472 PMID:18373356

Pardakhty, A., & Moazeni, E. (2013). Nano-niosomes in drug, vaccine and gene delivery: A rapid overview. *Nanomedicine Journal, 1*(1), 1–12.

Pardakhty, A., Moazeni, E., Varshosaz, J., Hajhashemi, V., & Najafabadi, A. R. (2011). Pharmacokinetic study of niosome-loaded insulin in diabetic rats. *DARU Journal of Pharmaceutical Sciences, 19*(6), 404. PMID:23008685

Pardakhty, A., Varshosaz, J., & Rouholamini, A. (2007). In vitro study of polyoxyethylene alkyl ether niosomes for delivery of insulin. *International Journal of Pharmaceutics, 328*(2), 130–141. doi:10.1016/j.ijpharm.2006.08.002 PMID:16997517

Park, K., & Mersny, R.J. (2000). Controlled drug delivery: present and future. *Controlled Drug Delivery: Designing Technology for the Future,* 2–13.

Park, H. J., Sohn, J. H., Kim, Y.-J., Park, Y. H., Han, H., Park, K. H., & Lee, J.-H. et al. (2015). Acute exposure to silica nanoparticles aggravate airway inflammation: Different effects according to surface characteristics. *Experimental & Molecular Medicine, 47*(7), e173. doi:10.1038/emm.2015.50 PMID:26183169

Park, J.-Y., & Lee, I.-H. (2011). Controlled release of ketoprofen from electrospun porous polylactic acid (PLA) nanofibers. *Journal of Polymer Research, 18*(6), 1287–1291. doi:10.1007/s10965-010-9531-0

Park, K. (1997). *Controlled Drug Delivery: Challenges and Strategies.* Washington, DC: American Chemical Society.

Park, K. (2007). Nanotechnology: What it can do for drug delivery. *Journal of Controlled Release*, *120*(1-2), 1–3. doi:10.1016/j.jconrel.2007.05.003 PMID:17532520

Park, S. S., Park, J., Ko, J., Chen, L., Meriage, D., Crouse-Zeineddini, J., & Kerwin, B. A. et al. (2009). Biochemical assessment of erythropoietin products from Asia versus Epoetin alfa manufactured by Amgen. *Journal of Pharmaceutical Sciences*, *98*(5), 1688–1699. doi:10.1002/jps.21546 PMID:18781649

Park, T. G. (1999). Temperature modulated protein release from pH/temperature-sensitive hydrogels. *Biomaterials*, *20*(6), 517–521. doi:10.1016/S0142-9612(98)00197-5 PMID:10213354

Parmar, K. R., Shah, S. R., & Sheth, N. R. (2011). Studies in dissolution enhancement of ezetimibe by solid dispersions in combination with a surface adsorbent. *Dissolut Technol*, *8*(3), 55–61. doi:10.14227/DT180311P55

Parthasarathi, G., Udupa, N., Umadevi, P., & Pillai, G. (1994). Niosome encapsulated of vincristine sulfate: Improved anticancer activity with reduced toxicity in mice. *Journal of Drug Targeting*, *2*(2), 173–182. doi:10.3109/10611869409015907 PMID:8069596

Passirani, C., Barratt, G., Devissaguet, J. P., & Labarre, D. (1998). Interactions of nanoparticles bearing heparin or dextran covalently bound to poly(methylmethacrylate) with the complement system. *Life Sciences*, *62*(8), 775–785. doi:10.1016/S0024-3205(97)01175-2 PMID:9489513

Passirani, C., Ferrarini, L., Barratt, G., Devissaguet, J. P., & Labarre, D. (1999). Preparation and characterization of nanoparticles bearing heparin or dextran covalently-linked to poly(methylmethacrylate). *J. Biomater. Sci. Polym*, *10*(1), 47–62. doi:10.1163/156856299X00270 PMID:10091922

Patel, S. (2007). Ethosomes: A promising tool for transdermal delivery of drug. *Pharmainfo. Net, 5*(3), 345-350.

Patel, D., Jani, R., & Patel, C. (2011). Ufasomes: A vesicular drug delivery. *Systematic Reviews in Pharmacy*, *2*(2), 72. doi:10.4103/0975-8453.86290

Patel, J., Bharadia, P., Amin, A., & Patel, M. (2004). Formulation optimisation and evaluation of controlled release mucoadhesive microspheres of glipizide for oral delivery using factorial design. *Drug Delivery*, *4*, 48–53.

Patel, R., & Patel, K. P. (2010). Advances in novel parentral drug delivery systems. *Asian Journal of Pharmaceutics*, *4*(3), 193. doi:10.4103/0973-8398.72117

Patel, R., Singh, S., Singh, S., Sheth, N., & Gendle, R. (2009). Development and characterization of curcumin loaded transfersome for transdermal delivery. *Journal of Pharm Sci Res*, *1*(4), 71–80.

Patel, T., Zhou, J., Piepmeier, J. M., & Saltzman, W. M. (2012). Polymeric nanoparticles for drug delivery to the central nervous system. *Advanced Drug Delivery Reviews*, *64*(7), 701–705. doi:10.1016/j.addr.2011.12.006 PMID:22210134

Patel, V., & Agrawal, Y. K. (2011). Current Status and Advanced Approaches In Ocular Drug Delivery System. *Journal of Global Trends In Pharmaceutical Sciences*, *2*(2), 131–148.

Pathak, C. P., Sawhney, A. S., & Hubbell, J. A. (1992). Rapid photopolymerization of immunoprotective gels in contact with cells and tissue. *Journal of the American Chemical Society*, *114*(21), 8311–8312. doi:10.1021/ja00047a065

Pathak, P. O., Nagarsenker, M. S., Barhate, C. R., Padhye, S. G., Dhawan, V. V., Bhattacharyya, D., & Fahr, A. et al. (2015). Cholesterol anchored arabinogalactan for asialoglycoprotein receptor targeting: Synthesis, characterization, and proof of concept of hepatospecific delivery. *Carbohydrate Research*, *408*, 33–43. doi:10.1016/j.carres.2015.03.003 PMID:25841057

Patil, Y. P., & Jadhav, S. (2014). Novel methoda for liposome preparation. *Chemistry and Physics of Lipids*, *177*, 8–18. doi:10.1016/j.chemphyslip.2013.10.011 PMID:24220497

Patterson, J., Bary, A., & Rades, T. (2002). Physical stability and solubility of the thermotropic mesophases of fenoprofen calcium as pure drug and in a tablet formulation. *International Journal of Pharmacy and Pharmaceutical Sciences*, *247*, 147–157. PMID:12429493

Paul, A., & Cevec, G. (1998). Non-invasive administration of protein antigens epicutaneous with bovin serum albulmine. *Vaccine Research*, *4*, 145–164.

Paul, A., Cevec, G., & Bachhavat, B. K. (1995). Transdermal immunization with large proteins by means of ultradeformable drug carriers. *European Journal of Immunology*, *25*(12), 3551–3524. doi:10.1002/eji.1830251248 PMID:8566048

Pawan, C., & Hemchand, P. (2009). Magnetic microsphere: as targeted drug delivery. *Journal of Pharmacy Research, 2*(5).

Payab, Davaran, Tanhaei, Fayyazi, Jahangiri, Farzaneh, & Adibkia. (2014). Triamcinolone acetonide-Eudragit® RS100 nanofibers and nanobeads: Morphological and physicochemical characterization. *Artificial Cells, Nanomedicine, and Biotechnology*, 1-8.

Peng, C., Qin, J., Zhou, B., Chen, Q., Shen, M., Zhu, M., & Shi, X. et al. (2013). Targeted tumor CT imaging using folic acid-modified PEGylated dendrimer-entrapped gold nanoparticles. *Polymer Chemistry*, *4*(16), 4412–4424. doi:10.1039/c3py00521f

Peng, C., Zheng, L., Chen, Q., Shen, M., Guo, R., Wang, H., & Shi, X. et al. (2012). PEGylated dendrimer-entrapped gold nanoparticles for in vivo blood pool and tumor imaging by computed tomography. *Biomaterials*, *33*(4), 1107–1119. doi:10.1016/j.biomaterials.2011.10.052 PMID:22061490

Peng, F. Y., Qin, Z., Bin, W., Ming, Y., & Mu-Sheng, W. (2012). Process optimization by response surface design and characterization study on geniposidepharmacosomes. *Pharmaceutical Development and Technology*, *17*(1), 94–102. doi:10.3109/10837450.2010.516439 PMID:20919929

Peng, X., Wen, X., Pan, X., Wang, R., Chen, B., & Wu, C. (2010). Design and In Vitro evaluation of capsaicin transdermal controlled release cubic phase gels. *AAPS PharmSciTech*, *11*(3), 1405–1410. doi:10.1208/s12249-010-9481-1 PMID:20839080

Peppas, N. A. (1986). Hydrogels of poly(vinyl alcohol) and its copolymers. In N. A. Peppas (Ed.), *Hydrogels in medicine and pharmacy* (Vol. 2, pp. 1–48). Boca Raton, FL: CRC Press.

Peppas, N. A. (1991). Physiologically responsive hydrogels. *Journal of Bioactive and Compatible Polymers*, *6*(3), 241–246. doi:10.1177/088391159100600303

Peppas, N. A., Bures, P., Leobandung, W., & Ichikawa, H. (2000). Hydrogels in pharmaceutical formulations. *European Journal of Pharmaceutics and Biopharmaceutics*, *50*(1), 27–46. doi:10.1016/S0939-6411(00)00090-4 PMID:10840191

Peppas, N. A., & Khare, A. R. (1993). Preparation, structure and diffusional behavior of hydrogels in controlled release. *Advanced Drug Delivery Reviews*, *11*(1), 1–35. doi:10.1016/0169-409X(93)90025-Y

Peracchia, M. T., Fattal, E., Desmaële, D., Besnard, M., Noël, J. P., Gomis, J. M., & Couvreur, P. et al. (1999). Stealth (R) PEGylated polycyanoacrylate nanoparticles for intravenous administration and splenic targeting. *Journal of Controlled Release*, *60*(1), 121–128. doi:10.1016/S0168-3659(99)00063-2 PMID:10370176

Perini, G., Saettone, M., Carafa, M., Santucci, E., & Alhaique, F. (1996). Niosomes as carriers for ophthalmic drugs: In vitro/in vivo evaluation. *Bollettino Chimico Farmaceutico*, *135*(2), 145. PMID:8791827

Perry, G. (2009). *Biosimilar Medicines: Towards Global Development and Monoclonal Antibodies*. Presented at the 7th EGA Annual Symposium on Biosimilar Medicines, EGA.

Petre, C. E., & Dittmer, D. P. (2007). Liposomal daunorubicin as treatment for Kaposi's sarcoma. *International Journal of Nanomedicine*, *2*(3), 277. PMID:18019828

Petros, R. A., & DeSimone, J. M. (2010). Strategies in the design of nanoparticles for therapeutic applications. *Nature Reviews. Drug Discovery*, *9*(8), 615–627. doi:10.1038/nrd2591 PMID:20616808

Pham, Q. P., Sharma, U., & Mikos, A. G. (2006). Electrospinning of polymeric nanofibers for tissue engineering applications: A review. *Tissue Engineering*, *12*(5), 1197–1211. doi:10.1089/ten.2006.12.1197 PMID:16771634

Pharmaphorum. (2012). *Biosimilars 2012 – what does the current landscape look like?* Author.

Pidgeon, C., Hunt, A. H., & Dittrich, K. (1986). Formation of multilayered vesicles from water/organic-solvent (W/O) emulsions: Theory and practice. *Pharmaceutical Research*, *3*(1), 23–34. doi:10.1023/A:1016316730560 PMID:24271353

Pillay V., Indermun S., Du Toit L. C., Choonara Y. E., & Kumar P. (2014). *WO Patent Application, WO 2014/191979.*

Ping, A., Jin, Y., & Dawei, C. (2005). Preparation and In Vivo Behavior of DidanosinePharmacosomes in Rats. *Chinese Journal of Pharmaceuticals*, *3*, 227–235.

Piplani, P., Kumar, P., Rohilla, A., Singla, S., & Kaur, I. P. (2015). Development and evaluation of an ocular niosomal delivery system for some newly synthesized Beta blockers. *Asian Journal of Biomedical and Pharmaceutical Sciences*, *4*(40), 8–17. doi:10.15272/ajbps.v4i40.634

Planas, M., Gonzalez, P., Rodriguez, S., Sanchez, G. & Cevc, G. (1992). Noninvasive percutaneous induction of topical analgesia by a new type of drug carrier, and prolongation of local pain insensitivity by anesthetic liposomes. *Anesthia Analoge*, 615-621.

Plummer, R., Wilson, R. H., Calvert, H., Boddy, A. V., Griffin, M., Sludden, J., & Nishiya, T. et al. (2011, February15). …Nishiya, T. A Phase I clinical study of cisplatin-incorporated polymeric micelles (NC-6004) in patients with solid tumours. *British Journal of Cancer*, *104*(4), 593–598. doi:10.1038/bjc.2011.6 PMID:21285987

Podual, K., Doyle, F. J., & Peppas, N. A. (2000). Preparation and dynamic response of cationic copolymer hydrogels containing glucose oxidase. *Polymer*, *41*(11), 3975–3983. doi:10.1016/S0032-3861(99)00620-5

Poland, C. A., Duffin, R., Kinloch, I., Maynard, A., Wallace, W. A., Seaton, A., & Donaldson, K. et al. (2008). Carbon nanotubes introduced into the abdominal cavity of mice show asbestos-like pathogenicity in a pilot study. *Nature Nanotechnology*, *3*(7), 423–428. doi:10.1038/nnano.2008.111 PMID:18654567

Polidori, A., Braun, O., Mora, N., & Pucci, B. (1997). Synthesis of polymerizable double-chain glycolipids derived from Tris. Polymerization in aqueous media. Preliminary investigation of their colloidal behavior. *Tetrahedron Letters*, *38*(14), 2475–2478. doi:10.1016/S0040-4039(97)00413-9

Polidori, A., Pucci, B., Riess, J. G., Zarif, L., & Pavia, A. A. (1994). Synthesis of double-chain glycolipids derived from aspartic acid: Preliminary investigation of their colloidal behavior. *Tetrahedron Letters*, *35*(18), 2899–2902. doi:10.1016/S0040-4039(00)76654-8

Poon, Z., Chang, D., Zhao, X., & Hammond, P. T. (2011). Layer-by-layer nanoparticles with a pH-sheddable layer for in vivo targeting of tumor hypoxia. *ACS Nano*, *5*(6), 4284–4292. doi:10.1021/nn200876f PMID:21513353

Popescu, M. T., Tsitsilianis, C., Papadakis, C. M., Adelsberger, J., Balog, S., Busch, P., & Patrickios, C. S. et al. (2012). Stimuli-Responsive Amphiphilic Polyelectrolyte Heptablock Copolymer Physical Hydrogels: An Unusual pH-Response. *Macromolecules*, *45*(8), 3523–3530. doi:10.1021/ma300222d

Popovici, R., Seftel, E., Mihai, G., Popovici, E., & Voicu, V. (2011). Controlled drug delivery system based on ordered mesoporous silica matrices of captopril as angiotensin-converting enzyme inhibitor drug. *Journal of Pharmaceutical Sciences*, *100*(2), 704–714. doi:10.1002/jps.22308 PMID:20740675

Poste, G., Kirsch, R., & Koestler, T. (1983). Liposomes Technology. CRC Press Inc.

Powell, M. F., Fleitman, J., Sanders, L. M., & Si, V. C. (1994). Peptide liquid crystals: Inverse correlation of kinetic formation and thermodynamic stability in aqueous solution. *Pharmaceutical Research*, *11*(9), 1352–1354. doi:10.1023/A:1018963016079 PMID:7816768

Powell, M. F., Sanders, L. M., Rogerson, A., & Si, V. (1991). Parenteral Peptide formulations: Chemical and physical properties of native luteinizing hormone releasing hormone and hydrophobic analogues in aqueous solution. *Pharmaceutical Research*, *8*(10), 1258–1263. doi:10.1023/A:1015847628047 PMID:1839059

Poznansky, M. J., & Juliano, R. L. (1983). Liposome targeting in vivo: Problems and opportunities. *Pharmacological Reviews*, *36*, 277. PMID:6395142

Pozzi, D., Caminiti, R., Marianecci, C., Carafa, M., Santucci, E., De Sanctis, S. C., & Caracciolo, G. (2009). Effect of cholesterol on the formation and hydration behavior of solid-supported niosomal membranes. *Langmuir*, *26*(4), 2268–2273. doi:10.1021/la9026877 PMID:19761205

Prabhu, P., Koland, M., Vijaynarayan, K., Harish, N., Ganesh, D., Charyulu, R., & Satynarayana, D. (2010). Preaparation and evaluation of niosomes of Brimonidine tartrate as ocular drug delivery system. *Journal of Pharmaceutical Research and Health Care*, *2*(4), 293–301.

Prajapati, S. K., Kumar, S., Sahu, V. K., & Prakash, G. (2012). Proniosomal gel of flurbiprofen: Formulation and evaluation. *Journal of Drug Delivery & Therapeutics*, *2*, 105–114.

Prajapati, S. T., Patel, C. G., & Patel, C. N. (2011). Transfersomes: A vesicular carrier system for transdermal drug delivery. *Asian J Biochemical Pharma Res*, *1*(2), 507–524.

Prasanthi,N.L., Manikiran,S.S., Rama Rao, N.(2010) Pharmacosomes: An Alternative Carrier System for Drug Delivery. *The Pharma Review*, 93-96.

Prasanthi, D., & Lakshmi, K. (2013). Iontophoretic transdermal delivery of finasteride in vesicular invasomal carriers. *Pharmaceutical Nanotechnology*, *1*(2), 136–150. doi:10.2174/2211738511301020009

Prasanth, V., Moy, A. C., Mathew, S. T., & Mathapan, R. (2011). Microspheres-An Overview. *International Journal of Research in Pharmaceutical and Biomedical Sciences*, *2*(2), 332–338.

Primo, F. L., Michieleto, L., Rodrigues, M. A., Macaroff, P. P., Morais, P. C., Lacava, Z. G., & Tedesco, A. C. et al. (2007). Magnetic nanoemulsions as drug delivery system for Foscan®: Skin permeation and retention in vitro assays for topical application in photodynamic therapy (PDT) of skin cancer. *Journal of Magnetism and Magnetic Materials*, *311*(1), 354–357. doi:10.1016/j.jmmm.2006.10.1183

Prokopowicz, M. (2010). Synthesis and in vitro characterization of freeze-dried doxorubicin-loaded silica xerogels. *Journal of Sol-Gel Science and Technology*, *53*(3), 525–533. doi:10.1007/s10971-009-2126-8

Puri, A. (2013). Phototriggerable liposomes: Current research and future perspectives. *Pharmaceutics*, *6*(1), 1–25. doi:10.3390/pharmaceutics6010001 PMID:24662363

Qian, S., Li, C., & Zuo, Z. (2012). Pharmacokinetics and disposition of various drug loaded liposomes. *Current Drug Metabolism*, *13*(4), 372–395. doi:10.2174/138920012800166562 PMID:22443534

Qian, X., Peng, X.-H., Ansari, D. O., Yin-Goen, Q., Chen, G. Z., Shin, D. M., & Nie, S. et al. (2008). In vivo tumor targeting and spectroscopic detection with surface-enhanced Raman nanoparticle tags. *Nature Biotechnology*, *26*(1), 83–90. doi:10.1038/nbt1377 PMID:18157119

Qiao, Z., & Shi, X. (2014). Dendrimer-based molecular imaging contrast agents. *Progress in Polymer Science*, *44*, 1–27. doi:10.1016/j.progpolymsci.2014.08.002

Qiu, Y., & Park, K. (2012). Environment-sensitive hydrogels for drug delivery. *Advanced Drug Delivery Reviews*, *64*, 49–60. doi:10.1016/j.addr.2012.09.024 PMID:11744175

Qizhen, L., Pengtao, L., Cheng, L., Xigao, J., Dingyi, H., & Yang, L. (2005). Synthesis and Properties of Lyotropic Liquid Crystalline Copolyamides Containing Phthalazinone Moieties and Ether Linkages. *Polymer*, *46*(16), 6258–6265. doi:10.1016/j.polymer.2005.05.059

Quan, C. Y., Chen, J., Wang, H.-Y., Li, C., Chang, C., Zhang, X.-Z., & Zhuo, R.-X. (2010). Core–shell nanosized assemblies mediated by the cyclodextrindimer with a tumor-triggered targeting property. *ACS Nano*, *4*(7), 4211–4219. doi:10.1021/nn100534q PMID:20521828

Quintanar-Guerrero, D., Ganem-Quintanar, A., Nava-Arzaluz, M. G., & Piñón-Segundo, E. (2009). *Silica xerogels as pharmaceutical drug carriers*. Academic Press.

Quintanar-Guerrero, D., Alle'man, E., Doelker, E., & Fessi, H. (1998a). Preparation and characterization of nanocapsules from preformed polymers by a new process based on emulsification–diffusion technique. *Pharmaceutical Research*, *15*(7), 1056–1062. doi:10.1023/A:1011934328471 PMID:9688060

Quintanar-Guerrero, D., Alle'man, E., Fessi, H., & Doelker, E. (1998b). Preparation techniques and mechanisms of formation of biodegradable nanoparticles from preformed polymers. *Drug Development and Industrial Pharmacy*, *24*(12), 1113–1128. doi:10.3109/03639049809108571 PMID:9876569

Quintanar-Guerrero, D., Alle'man, E., Fessi, H., & Doelker, E. (1999). Pseudolatex preparation using a novel emulsion–diffusion process involving direct displacement of partially water-miscible solvents by distillation. *International Journal of Pharmaceutics*, *188*(2), 155–164. doi:10.1016/S0378-5173(99)00216-1 PMID:10518671

Rades, T., Gerke, A., Schutze, W., & Muller-Goymann, C. C. (1997). Characterization of a commercial liposome spray. *Die Pharmazie*, *52*(1), 44–50. PMID:9035234

Rades, T., & Muller-Goymann, C. C. (1992). Structural investigations on the liquid crystalline phases of fenoprofen. *Pharmacol Biochem Prop Drug Sust*, *2*, 131–134.

Rades, T., & Muller-Goymann, C. C. (1997). Electron and light microscopical investigation of defect structures in mesophases of pharmaceutical substances. *Colloid & Polymer Science*, *275*(12), 1169–1178. doi:10.1007/s003960050198

Radomski, A., Jurasz, P., Alonso-Escolano, D., Drews, M., Morandi, M., Malinski, T., & Radomski, M. W. (2005). Nanoparticle-induced platelet aggregation and vascular thrombosis. *British Journal of Pharmacology*, *146*(6), 882–893. doi:10.1038/sj.bjp.0706386 PMID:16158070

Raghupathi, K. R., Guo, J., Munkhbat, O., Rangadurai, P., & Thayumanavan, S. (2014). Supramolecular Disassembly of Facially Amphiphilic Dendrimer Assemblies in Response to Physical, Chemical, and Biological Stimuli. *Accounts of Chemical Research*, *47*(7), 2200–2211. doi:10.1021/ar500143u PMID:24937682

Rahimpour, Y., & Hamishehkar, H. (2012). Niosomes as Carrier in Dermal Drug Delivery, Recent Advances in Novel Drug Carrier Systems. Current Pharmaceutical Design, 21(20), 2883-2891.

Rai, M., Yadav, A., & Gade, A. (2009). Silver nanoparticles as a new generation of antimicrobials. *Biotechnology Advances*, *27*(1), 76–83. doi:10.1016/j.biotechadv.2008.09.002 PMID:18854209

Raja, N., Pillai, G., Udupa, N., & Chandrashekar, G. (1994). Anti-inflammatory activity of niosome encapsulated diclofenac sodium in arthritic rats. *Indian Journal of Pharmacology*, *26*(1), 46.

Rajput, M., Sharma, R., Kumar, S., Jamil, F., Sissodia, N., & Sharma, S. (2012). Pulsatile drug delivery system: A review. *International Journal of Research in Pharmaceutical and Biomedical Sciences*, *3*(1), 118–124.

Ramireddy, , R., Raghupathi, K., Torres, D. A., & Thayumanavan, S. (2012). Stimuli sensitive amphiphilic dendrimers. *New Journal of Chemistry*, *36*(2), 340–349. doi:10.1039/c2nj20879b PMID:24039387

Ramsammy, L. S., & Brockerhoff, H. (1982). Lysophosphatidylcholine-cholesterol complex. *The Journal of Biological Chemistry*, *257*(7), 3570–3574. PMID:7061497

Ramteke, K., Jadhav, V., & Dhole, S. (2012). Microspheres: As carriers used for novel drug delivery system. *IOSR Journal of Pharmacy*, *2*(4), 44–48. doi:10.9790/3013-24204448

Rand, R. P., & Parsegian, V. A. (1989). Hydration forces between phospholipid bilayers. *Biochimica et Biophysica Acta*, *988*(3), 351–377. doi:10.1016/0304-4157(89)90010-5

Rapoport, N., Pitt, W. G., Sun, H., & Nelson, J. L. (2003). Drug delivery in polymeric micelles: From in vitro to in vivo. *Journal of Controlled Release*, *91*(1), 85–95. doi:10.1016/S0168-3659(03)00218-9 PMID:12932640

Rasve, G., Borade, G., Deshmukh, S., & Tagalpallewar, A. (2011). Pulsatile drug delivery system: current scenario. *International Journal of Pharma and Bio Science, 2*(3).

Ratner, B. D., & Hoffman, A. S. (1976). Synthetic hydrogels for biomedical applications. In J. D. Andrade (Ed.), *Hydrogels for medical and related applications* (Vol. 31, pp. 1–36). Washington, DC: American Chemical Society. doi:10.1021/bk-1976-0031.ch001

Ravouru, N., Kondreddy, P., Korakanchi, D., & M, H. (2013). Formulation and evaluation of niosomal nasal drug delivery system of folic acid for brain targeting. *Current Drug Discovery Technologies*, *10*(4), 270–282. doi:10.2174/15701638113109990031 PMID:23863098

Razin, S. (1972). Physiology of michoplasm: Advance in microbiology. *Biochimica et Biophysica Acta*, *265*, 241. doi:10.1016/0304-4157(72)90004-4 PMID:4555471

Reddy, D. N., & Udupa, N. (1993). Formulation and evaluation of oral and transdermal preparations of flurbiprofen and piroxicam incorporated with different carriers. *Drug Development and Industrial Pharmacy*, *19*(7), 843–852. doi:10.3109/03639049309062986

Rego, J. A., Harvey, J. A. A., MacKinnon, A. L., & Gatdula, E. (2010). Asymmetric synthesis of a highly soluble 'trimeric' analogue of the chiral nematic liquid crystal twist agent Merck S1011. *Liquid Crystals.*, *37*(1), 37–43. doi:10.1080/02678290903359291

Reichert, J. M. (2010). Metrics for antibody therapeutics development. *mAbs*, *2*, 695–700.

Reinitzer, F. (1888). BeiträgezurKenntniss des Cholesterins. *MonatsheftefürChemie (Wien)*, *9*(1), 421–441.

Ren, T. B., Feng, Y., Zhang, Z. H., Lia, L., & Li, Y. Y. (2011). Shell-sheddable micelles based on star-shaped poly(3-caprolactone)-SS-poly(ethylglycol) copolymer for intracellular drug release. *Soft Matter*, *7*(6), 2329–2331. doi:10.1039/c1sm05020f

Ren, T. B., Xia, W. J., Dong, H. Q., & Li, Y. Y. (2011). Sheddable micelles based on disulfide-linked hybrid PEG–poly-peptide copolymer for intracellular drug delivery. *Polymer*, *52*(16), 3580–3586. doi:10.1016/j.polymer.2011.06.013

Riaz, M. (1996). Liposomes preparation methods. *Pakistan Journal of Pharmaceutical Sciences*, *19*, 65–77. PMID:16414777

Richard, B., Merryman, T., Newton, P., Ott, L., Haan, D., Brubaker, A., . . . One, E. (2011). *Safety Evaluation of a Novel Pharmaceutical Excipient (DEPC) in EXPAREL™, an Extended-Release Liposomal Formulation of Bupivacaine*. The 38th Annual Meeting & Exposition of the Controlled Release Society, National Harbor, MD. Retrieved from Pacira Pharmaceuticals Inc. Web site: http://investor.pacira.com/phoenix.zhtml?c=220759&p=irol-newsArticle&ID=1591609

Rijcken, C. J., Snel, C. J., Schiffelers, R. M., van Nostrum, C. F., & Hennink, W. E. (2007). Hydrolysable core-crosslinked thermosensitive polymeric micelles: Synthesis, characterization and in vivo studies. *Biomaterials*, *28*(36), 5581–5593. doi:10.1016/j.biomaterials.2007.08.047 PMID:17915312

Ritika, S.L., & Aggarwal G.H. (2012). Formulation Tactics for the Delivery of Poorly Soluble Drugs. *International Journal of Physical Therapy and Rehabilitation,* 915-919.

Rizwan, S. B., Hanley, T., Boyd, B. J., Rades, T., & Hook, S. (2009). Liquid crystalline systems of phytantriol and glyceryl mono oleate containing a hydrophilic protein: Characterisation, swelling and release kinetics. *Journal of Pharmaceutical Sciences*, *98*(11), 4191–4204. doi:10.1002/jps.21724 PMID:19340889

Roger, E., Lagarce, F., Garcion, E., & Benoit, J. P. (2010). Biopharmaceutical parameters to consider in orderto alter the fate of nanocarriers after oral delivery. *Nanomedicine, 5,* 287–306.

Roger, S. D. (2006). Biosimilars: How similar or dissimilar are they? *Nephrology (Carlton, Vic.)*, *11*(4), 341–346. doi:10.1111/j.1440-1797.2006.00594.x PMID:16889575

Roger, S. D. (2010). Biosimilars: Current status and future directions. *Expert Opinion on Biological Therapy*, *10*(7), 1011–1018. doi:10.1517/14712591003796553 PMID:20384525

Roger, S. D., & Goldsmith, D. (2008). Biosimilars: It's not as simple as cost alone. *Journal of Clinical Pharmacy and Therapeutics*, *33*(5), 459–464. doi:10.1111/j.1365-2710.2008.00942.x PMID:18834359

Rogerson, A., Cummings, J., & Florence, A. T. (1987). Adriamycin-loaded niosomes: Drug entrapment, stability and release. *Journal of Microencapsulation*, *4*(4), 321–328. doi:10.3109/02652048709021824 PMID:3504513

Rosenblatt, J., Devereux, B., & Wallace, D. G. (1994). Injectable collagen as a pH-sensitive hydrogel. *Biomaterials*, *15*(12), 985–995. doi:10.1016/0142-9612(94)90079-5 PMID:7841296

Roshkova, A. (2009). Quantitative analysis of monoclonal antibodies by cationexchange chromatofocusing. *Journal of Chromatography. A*, *1216*(32), 5989–5994. doi:10.1016/j.chroma.2009.06.045 PMID:19560777

Rosier, R. N., Gunter, T. E., Tucker, D. A., & Gunter, K. K. (1979). A rapid method for separating small vesicles from suspension. *Analytical Biochemistry*, *120*, 113. PMID:474964

Rösler, A., Vandermeulen, G. W. M., & Klok, H.-A. (2012). Advanced drug delivery devices via self-assembly of amphiphilic block copolymers. *Advanced Drug Delivery Reviews, 64,* 270-279.

Ruel-Gariepy, E., & Leroux, J.-C. (2004). In situ-forming hydrogels—review of temperature-sensitive systems. *European Journal of Pharmaceutics and Biopharmaceutics*, *58*(2), 409–426. doi:10.1016/j.ejpb.2004.03.019 PMID:15296964

Russell, J., Carden, J., & Herron, H. (1988). Dosimetry calculations for yttrium-90 used in the treatment of liver cancer. *Endocurietherapy/Hyperthermia Oncology, 4*(171-1), 86.

Ryu, E. K., Ross, R. J., Matsushita, T., MacCoss, M., Hong, C. I., & West, C. R. (1982). Phospholipid-nucleoside conjugates. 3. Syntheses and preliminary biological evaluation of 1-. beta.-D-arabinofuranosylcytosine 5'-monophosphate-L-1, 2-dipalmitin and selected 1-. beta.-D-arabinofuranosylcytosine 5'-diphosphate-L-1, 2-diacylglycerols. *Journal of Medicinal Chemistry*, *25*(11), 1322–1329. doi:10.1021/jm00353a010 PMID:7143370

Ryu, J. H., Roy, R., Ventura, J., & Thayumanavan, S. (2010). Redox-sensitive disassembly of amphiphilic copolymer based micelles. *Langmuir*, *26*(10), 7086–7092. doi:10.1021/la904437u PMID:20073533

Saad, M., Garbuzenko, O. B., Ber, E., Chandna, P., Khandare, J. J., Pozharov, V. P., & Minko, T. (2008). Receptor targeted polymers, dendrimers, liposomes: Which nanocarrier is the most efficient for tumor-specific treatment and imaging? *Journal of Controlled Release*, *130*(2), 107–114. doi:10.1016/j.jconrel.2008.05.024 PMID:18582982

Sachan, R., Parashar, T., Singh, V., Singh, G., Tyagi, S., Patel, C., & Gupta, A. (2013). Drug carrier transfersomes: A novel tool for transdermal drug delivery system. *IJRDPLS*, *2*(2), 309–316.

Sackmann, E. (1995). Physical basis of self-organization and function of membranes: physics of vesicles. Handbook of Biological Physics, 1, 213-304.

Sadhale, Y., & Shah, J. C. (1998). Glyceryl monooleate cubic phase gel as chemical stability enhancer of cefazolin and cefuroxime. *Pharmaceutical Development and Technology*, *3*(4), 549–556. doi:10.3109/10837459809028637 PMID:9834958

Sadhale, Y., & Shah, J. C. (1999a). Biological activity of insulin in GMO gels and the effect of agitation. *International Journal of Pharmaceutics*, *191*(1), 65–74. doi:10.1016/S0378-5173(99)00287-2 PMID:10556741

Sadhale, Y., & Shah, J. C. (1999b). Stabilization of insulin against agitation-induced aggregation by the GMO cubic phase gel. *International Journal of Pharmaceutics*, *191*(1), 51–64. doi:10.1016/S0378-5173(99)00288-4 PMID:10556740

Sagalowicz, L., Leser, M. E., Watzke, H. J., & Michel, M. (2006). Monoglyceride self-assembly structures as delivery vehicles. *Trends in Food Science & Technology*, *17*(5), 204–214. doi:10.1016/j.tifs.2005.12.012

Sagalowicz, L., Mezzenga, R., & Leser, M. E. (2006). Investigating reversed liquid crystalline mesophases. *Current Opinion in Colloid & Interface Science*, *11*(4), 224–229. doi:10.1016/j.cocis.2006.07.002

Sahin, N. O. (2007). Niosomes as nanocarrier systems. *Nanomaterials and Nanosystems for Biomedical Applications*, 67-81.

Saito, G., Swanson, J. A., & Lee, K. D. (2003). Drug delivery strategy utilizing conjugation via reversible disulfide links: Role and site of cellular reducing activities. *Advanced Drug Delivery Reviews*, *55*(2), 199–215. doi:10.1016/S0169-409X(02)00179-5 PMID:12564977

Sakai, S., Yamada, Y., Yamaguchi, T., & Kawakami, K. (2006). Prospective use of electrospun ultra-fine silicate fibers for bone tissue engineering. *Biotechnology Journal*, *1*(9), 958–962. doi:10.1002/biot.200600054 PMID:16941440

Salama, A. H., & Aburahma, M. H. (2015). Ufasomes nano-vesicles-based lyophilized platforms for intranasal delivery of cinnarizine: Preparation, optimization, ex-vivo histopathological safety assessment and mucosal confocal imaging. *Pharmaceutical Development and Technology*, 1–10. doi:10.3109/10837450.2015.1048553 PMID:25996631

Sallam, A. S., Khalil, E., Ibrahim, H., & Freij, I. (2002). Formulation of an oral dosage form utilizing the properties of cubic liquid crystalline phases of glyceryl monooleate. *European Journal of Pharmaceutics and Biopharmaceutics*, *53*(3), 343–352. doi:10.1016/S0939-6411(02)00016-4 PMID:11976023

Samad, A., Sultana, Y., & Aqil, M. (2007). Liposomal Drug Delivery Systems: An Update Review. *Current Drug Delivery*, *4*(4), 297–305. doi:10.2174/156720107782151269 PMID:17979650

Samra, B., Galaev, I., & Mattiasson, B. (2003). *U.S. Patent No. 6,538,089.* Washington, DC: U.S. Patent and Trademark Office.

Sandoz. (2009). *Sandoz Canada receives approval for recombinant human-growth hormone Omnitrope, the first Subsequent Entry Biologic in Canada*. Sandoz.

Sankar, V., Babu, E., Siram, K., Penmetsa, S. D., Kabila, B., Srinavas, C. R., & Rai, R. (2013). Formulation and Clinical Evaluation of Triamcinolone Acetonide Niosomes: Effect of Iontophoresis on the Permeation Across Skin. *Pharmaceutical Nanotechnology*, *1*(4), 282–289. doi:10.2174/22117385113016660008

Sant, V. P., & Nagarsenker, M. S. (2011). Synthesis of Monomethoxypolyethyleneglycol—Cholesteryl Ester and Effect of its Incorporation in Liposomes. *AAPS PharmSciTech*, *12*(4), 1056–1063. doi:10.1208/s12249-011-9674-2 PMID:21853369

Sant, V. P., Nagarsenker, M. S., Rao, S. A., & Gude, R. P. (2003). Sterically stabilized etoposide liposomes: Evaluation of antimetastatic activity and its potentiation by combination with sterically stabilized pentoxifylline liposomes in mice. *Cancer Biotherapy & Radiopharmaceuticals*, *18*(5), 811–817. doi:10.1089/108497803770418355 PMID:14629829

Sant, V., Nagarsenker, M., Rao, S., & Gude, R. (2000). Enhancement of Anti-metastatic Activity of Pentoxifylline by Encapsulation in Conventional Liposomes and Sterically Stabilized Liposomes in Murine Experimental B16F10 Melanoma Model. *The Journal of Pharmacy and Pharmacology*, *52*(12), 1461–1466. doi:10.1211/0022357001777667 PMID:11197073

Saraf, S., Gupta, D., Kaur, C. D., & Saraf, S. (2011). Sphingosomes a novel approach to vesicular drug delivery. *Int J Cur Sci Res.*, *1*(2), 63–68.

Saraf, S., Jeswani, G., Deep Kaur, C., & Saraf, S. (2011). Development of novel herbal cosmetic cream with curcuma longa extract loaded transfersomes for anti-wrinkle effect. *African J Pharm Pharmacol*, *5*(8), 1054–1062.

Saraogia, G. K., Gupta, P., Gupta, U. D., Jain, N. K., & Agrawala, G. P. (2010). Gelatin nanocarriers as potential vectors for effective management of tuberculosis. *International Journal of Pharmaceutics*, *385*(1-2), 143–149. doi:10.1016/j.ijpharm.2009.10.004 PMID:19819315

Sassi, A. P., Shaw, A. J., Han, S. M., Blanch, H. W., & Prausnitz, J. M. (1996). Partitioning of proteins and small biomolecules in temperature-and pH-sensitive hydrogels. *Polymer*, *37*(11), 2151–2164. doi:10.1016/0032-3861(96)85860-5

Saul, J. M., Annapragada, A., Natarajan, J. V., & Bellamkonda, R. V. (2003). Controlled targeting of liposomal doxorubicin via the folate receptor in vitro. *Journal of Controlled Release*, *92*(1), 49–67. doi:10.1016/S0168-3659(03)00295-5 PMID:14499185

Sawahata, K., Hara, M., Yasunaga, H., & Osada, Y. (1990). Electrically controlled drug delivery system using polyelectrolyte gels. *Journal of Controlled Release*, *14*(3), 253–262. doi:10.1016/0168-3659(90)90165-P

Sawant, R. R., & Torchilin, V. P. (2012). Challenges in development of targeted liposomal therapeutics. *The AAPS Journal*, *14*(2), 303–315. doi:10.1208/s12248-012-9330-0 PMID:22415612

Schafer, F. Q., & Buettner, G. R. (2001). Redox environment of the cell as viewed through the redox state of the glutathione disulfide/glutathione couple. *Free Radical Biology & Medicine*, *30*(11), 1191–1212. doi:10.1016/S0891-5849(01)00480-4 PMID:11368918

Schatzlein, A., & Cevc, G. (1995). *Skin penetration by phospholipids vesicles, transfersomes as visualized by means of the confocal scanning laser microscopy, in characterization, metabolism, and novel biological applications*. Champaign, IL: AOCS Press.

Schatzlein, A., & Cevc, G. (1998). Non-uniform cellular packing of the stratum corneum and permeability barrier function of intact skin: A high-resolution confocal laser scanning microscopy study using highly deformable vesicles (Transfersomes). *The British Journal of Dermatology*, *138*(4), 583–598. doi:10.1046/j.1365-2133.1998.02166.x PMID:9640361

Scheffel, U., Rhodes, B. A., Natarajan, T. K., & Wagner, H. N. (1972). Albumin microspheres for the study of the reticulo-endothelial system. *Journal of Nuclear Medicine*, *13*, 498–503. PMID:5033902

Scheffler, P., Gross, J., Markwirth, T., Maier, J., & Schieffer, H. (1996). Progress in the prostaglandin E1-therapy of the intermittent claudication by means of bolus injections of LIPO-prostaglandin E1 (LIPO-PGE1). *European Journal of Clinical Pharmacology*, *51*(3-4), 235–239. doi:10.1007/s002280050190 PMID:9010691

Schellekens, H. (2003). Relationship between biopharmaceutical immunogenicity of epoetin alfa and pure red cell aplasia. *Current Medical Research and Opinion*, *19*(5), 433–434. doi:10.1185/030079903125002072 PMID:13678481

Schellekens, H. (2005). Follow-on biologics: Challenges of the next generation. *Nephrology, Dialysis, Transplantation*, *20*(4), 31–36. PMID:15827057

Schellekens, H. (2009). Biosimilar therapeutics- what do we need to consider? *NDT Plus*, *2*(Supplement 1), 27–36. doi:10.1093/ndtplus/sfn177 PMID:19461855

Schellekens, H., Lisman, J., & Bols, T. (2008). Biosimilars in clinical practice – the challenges for hospital pharmacists. *EJHPP Practice.*, *14*, 32–33.

Schenk, P., Ausborn, M., Bendas, F., Nuhn, P., Arndt, D., & Meyer, H. W. (1989). The preparation and characterization of lipid vesicles containing esters of sucrose and fatty acids. *Journal of Microencapsulation*, *6*(1), 95–103. doi:10.3109/02652048909019906 PMID:2715918

Scherer, F., Anton, M., Schillinger, U., Henke, J., Bergemann, C., Kruger, A., & Plank, C. et al. (2002). Magnetofection: Enhancing and targeting gene delivery by magnetic force *in vitro* and *in vivo*. *Gene Therapy*, *9*(2), 102–109. doi:10.1038/sj.gt.3301624 PMID:11857068

Schieran, H., Rudolph, S., Fiukelstein, M., Coleman, P., & Weisman, G. (1978). Comparison of large unilamellar vesicles prepared by a petroleum ether vaporization method with multilamellar vesicles: ESR, diffusion and entrapment analyses. *Biochimica et Biophysica Acta*, *646*, 4.

Schiffelers, R., Storm, G., & Bakker-Woudenberg, I. (2001). Liposome-encapsulated aminoglycosides in pre-clinical and clinical studies. *The Journal of Antimicrobial Chemotherapy*, *48*(3), 333–344. doi:10.1093/jac/48.3.333 PMID:11532996

Schiffman, J. D., & Schauer, C. L. (2008). A review: Electrospinning of biopolymer nanofibers and their applications. *The Polish Review*, *48*(2), 317–352. doi:10.1080/15583720802022182

Schmid, G. (2011). *Nanoparticles: from theory to application*. John Wiley & Sons.

Schneider, Y., Abarca, J., Pirak, A. E., Baurain, R., Ceulemans, F., Campeneere, D. D., ... Trouet, A. (1984). Drug targeting in human cancer chemotherapy. In Receptor-Mediated Targeting of Drugs. Springer. doi:10.1007/978-1-4684-4862-7_1

Schwab, G., Duroux, I., Chavany, C., Helene, C., & Saison-Behmoaras, E. (1994). An approach for new anticancer drugs: Oncogene-targeted antisense DNA. *Annals of Oncology*, *5*(suppl 4), 55–58. doi:10.1093/annonc/5.suppl_4.S55 PMID:8060898

Seema, M., & Jadhav, P.M. (n.d.). Novel Vesicular System: An Overview. *Journal of Pharmaceutical Sciences*, 193-202.

Seideman, T. (1990). The liquid-crystalline blue phases. *Reports on Progress in Physics*, *53*(6), 659–705. doi:10.1088/0034-4885/53/6/001

Seijo, B., Fattal, E., Roblot-Treupel, L., & Couvreur, P. (1990). Design of nanoparticles of less than 50nm in diameter. Preparation, characterization and drug loading. *International Journal of Pharmaceutics*, *62*(1), 1–7. doi:10.1016/0378-5173(90)90024-X

Selvamuthukumar, S., Anandam, S., Krishnamoorthy, K., & Rajappan, M. (2012). Nanosponges: A novel class of drug delivery system-Review. *Journal of Pharmacy & Pharmaceutical Sciences*, *15*(1), 103–111. doi:10.18433/J3K308 PMID:22365092

Semalty, A., Semalty, M., Rawat, B. S., Singh, D., & Rawat, M. (2009). *Pharmacosomes: the lipid-based new drug delivery system.* Academic Press.

Semple, S. C., Akinc, A., Chen, J., Sandhu, A. P., Mui, B. L., Cho, C. K., & Yaworski, E. et al. (2010). Rational design of cationic lipids for siRNA delivery. *Nature Biotechnology*, *28*(2), 172–176. doi:10.1038/nbt.1602 PMID:20081866

Sennato, S., Bordi, F., Cametti, C., Marianecci, C., Carafa, M., & Cametti, M. (2008). Hybrid niosome complexation in the presence of oppositely charged polyions. *The Journal of Physical Chemistry B*, *112*(12), 3720–3727. doi:10.1021/jp0775449 PMID:18307334

Sessa, G., & Weissmann, G. (1968). Phospholipid spherules (liposomes) as a model for biological membranes. *Journal of Lipid Research*, *9*(3), 310–318. PMID:5646182

Seyler, I., Appel, M., Devissaguet, J. P., Legrand, P., & Barratt, G. (1999). Macrophage activation by a lipophilic derivative of muramyldipeptide. *Journal of Nanoparticle Research*, *1*(1), 91–97. doi:10.1023/A:1010016128378

Sezaki, H., & Hashida, M. (1985). Macromolecules as drug delivery systems *Directed*[Springer.]. *Drug Delivery*, 189–208.

Sezgin-Bayindir, Z., Antep, M. N., & Yuksel, N. (2015). Development and Characterization of Mixed Niosomes for Oral Delivery Using Candesartan Cilexetil as a Model Poorly Water-Soluble Drug. *AAPS PharmSciTech*, *16*(1), 108–117. doi:10.1208/s12249-014-0213-9 PMID:25204859

Shafer-Peltier, K. E., Haynes, C. L., Glucksberg, M. R., & Van Duyne, R. P. (2003). Toward a glucose biosensor based on surface-enhanced Raman scattering. *Journal of the American Chemical Society*, *125*(2), 588–593. doi:10.1021/ja028255v PMID:12517176

Shafiq, S., Shakeel, F., Talegaonkar, S., Ahmad, F. J., Khar, R. K., & Ali, M. (2007). Development and bioavailability assessment of ramipril nanoemulsion formulation. *European Journal of Pharmaceutics and Biopharmaceutics*, *66*(2), 227–243. doi:10.1016/j.ejpb.2006.10.014 PMID:17127045

Shahiwala, A., & Misra, A. (2002). Studies in topical application of niosomally entrapped nimesulide. *Journal of Pharmacy and Pharmaceutical Sciences*, *5*(3), 220–225.

Shah, J. C., Sadhale, Y., & Chilukuri, D. M. (2001). Cubic phase gels as drug delivery systems. *Advanced Drug Delivery Reviews*, *47*(2-3), 229–250. doi:10.1016/S0169-409X(01)00108-9 PMID:11311994

Shah, M. H., & Paradkar, A. (2005). Cubic liquid crystalline glyceryl monooleate matrices for oral delivery of enzyme. *International Journal of Pharmaceutics*, *294*(1-2), 161–171. doi:10.1016/j.ijpharm.2005.01.019 PMID:15814241

Shah, M. H., & Paradkar, A. (2007). Effect of HLB of additives on the properties and drug release from the glyceryl monooleate matrices. *European Journal of Pharmaceutics and Biopharmaceutics*, *67*(1), 166–174. doi:10.1016/j.ejpb.2007.01.001 PMID:17353118

Shah, S. M., Ashtikar, M., Jain, A. S., Makhija, D. T., Nikam, Y., Gude, R. P., & Fahr, A. et al. (2015). LeciPlex, invasomes, and liposomes: A skin penetration study. *International Journal of Pharmaceutics*, *490*(1-2), 391–403. doi:10.1016/j.ijpharm.2015.05.042 PMID:26002568

Shah, S. M., Goel, P. N., Jain, A. S., Pathak, P. O., Padhye, S. G., Govindarajan, S., & Gopal, V. et al. (2014). Liposomes for targeting hepatocellular carcinoma: Use of conjugated arabinogalactan as targeting ligand. *International Journal of Pharmaceutics*, *477*(1), 128–139. doi:10.1016/j.ijpharm.2014.10.014 PMID:25311181

Shah, S. M., Pathak, P. O., Jain, A. S., Barhate, C. R., & Nagarsenker, M. S. (2013). Synthesis, characterization, and in vitro evaluation of palmitoylated arabinogalactan with potential for liver targeting. *Carbohydrate Research*, *367*, 41–47. doi:10.1016/j.carres.2012.11.025 PMID:23298829

Shamsi Meymandi, S., Amiri, R., Aflatunian, M., & Pardakhty, A. (2014). Comparison of the efficacy of niosomal minoxidil with conventional minoxidil in the treatment of androgenetic alopecia: A randomized, controlled, double-blind clinical trial. *Dermatology and Cosmetic*, *5*(2), 53–60.

Shao, S., Li, L., Yang, G., Li, J., Luo, C., Gong, T., & Zhou, S. (2011). Controlled green tea polyphenols release from electrospun PCL/MWCNTs composite nanofibers. *International Journal of Pharmaceutics*, *421*(2), 310–320. doi:10.1016/j.ijpharm.2011.09.033 PMID:21983092

Shao, Y., & Zerda, T. W. (1998). Phase Transitions of Liquid Crystal PAA in Confined Geometries. *The Journal of Physical Chemistry B*, *102*(18), 3387–3394. doi:10.1021/jp9734437

Shapria, A., Livney, Y. D., Broxterman, H. J., & Assaraf, Y. G. (2011). Nanomedicine for targeted cancer therapy: towards the overcoming of drug resistance. *Drug Resistance Updates: Reviews and Commentaries in Antimicrobial and Anticancer Chemotherapy, 14*(3), 150-163.

Sharma, R., & Pathak, K. (2010). Nanosponges: emerging drug delivery system. *Pharma Stud*, 33-35.

Sharma, A., & Sharma, U. S. (1997). Liposomes in drug delivery: Progress and limitations. *International Journal of Pharmaceutics*, *154*(2), 123–140. doi:10.1016/S0378-5173(97)00135-X

Sharma, P., Tyrell, D. A., & Ryman, B. T. (1977). Use of ordination and other multivariate descriptive methods to study. *Biochemical Society Transactions*, *5*, 1146. doi:10.1042/bst0051146 PMID:913809

Sheena, I., Singh, U., Aithal, K., & Udupa, N. (1997). Pilocarpine β-cyclodextrin Complexation and Niosomal Entrapment. *Pharmacy and Pharmacology Communications*, *3*(8), 383–386.

Shen, S. C., Ng, W. K., Shi, Z., Chia, L., Neoh, K. G., & Tan, R. B. H. (2011). Mesoporous silica nanoparticle-functionalized poly (methylmethacrylate)-based bone cement for effective antibiotics delivery. *Journal of Materials Science. Materials in Medicine*, *22*(10), 2283–2292. doi:10.1007/s10856-011-4397-1 PMID:21786132

Sheo, D., Shweta, A., Ram, C., Ghanshyam, M., Girish, K., & Sunil, K. (2010). Transfersomes- a novel vesicular carrier for enhanced transdermal delivery of stavudine: Development, characterization and performance evaluation. *Journal of Scientific Speculations and Res*, *1*(1), 30–36.

Shi, B., Fang, C., & Pei, Y. (2006). Stealth PEG-PHDCA niosomes: Effects of chain length of PEG and particle size on niosomes surface properties, in vitro drug release, phagocytic uptake, in vivo pharmacokinetics and antitumor activity. *Journal of Pharmaceutical Sciences*, *95*(9), 1873–1887. doi:10.1002/jps.20491 PMID:16795003

Shields, K. J., Beckman, M. J., Bowlin, G. L., & Wayne, J. S. (2004). Mechanical properties and cellular proliferation of electrospun collagen type II. *Tissue Engineering*, *10*(9-10), 1510–1517. doi:10.1089/ten.2004.10.1510 PMID:15588410

Shi, J., Votruba, A. R., Farokhzad, O. C., & Langer, R. (2010). Nanotechnology in Drug Delivery and Tissue Engineering: From Discovery to Applications. *Nano Letters*, *10*(9), 3223–3230. doi:10.1021/nl102184c PMID:20726522

Shi, M. Q., Zhang, M. Z., Rong, B., Wetzel, K., & Friedrich, K. (2004). Sliding wear behavior of epoxy containing nano-Al_2O_3 particles with different pretreatments. *Wear*, *256*(11-12), 1072–1081. doi:10.1016/S0043-1648(03)00533-7

Shinto, Y., Uchida, A., Korkusuz, F., Araki, N., & Ono, K. (1992). Calcium hydroxyapatite ceramic used as a delivery system for antibiotics. *The Journal of Bone and Joint Surgery. British Volume*, *74*, 600–604. PMID:1320622

Shin, Y., Chang, J. H., Liu, J., Williford, R., Shin, Y. K., & Exarhos, G. J. (2001). Hybrid nanogels for sustainable positive thermosensitive drug release. *Journal of Controlled Release*, *73*(1), 1–6. doi:10.1016/S0168-3659(01)00247-4 PMID:11337054

Shirwaikar, A., Kumar, S., Jacob, S., Rashi, W., & Ravi, K. (2006). Recent developments in floating drug delivery systems for gastric retention of drugs, an overview. *INDIAN DRUGS-BOMBAY*, *43*(9), 697.

Shi, X., Wang, S. H., Swanson, S. D., Ge, S., Cao, Z., Van Antwerp, M. E., & Baker, J. R. et al. (2008). Dendrimer-Functionalized Shell-crosslinked Iron Oxide Nanoparticles for In-Vivo Magnetic Resonance Imaging of Tumors. *Advanced Materials*, *20*(9), 1671–1678.

Shortencarier, M. J., Dayton, P., Bloch, S. H., Schumann, P., Matsunaga, T. O., & Ferrara, K. W. (2004). A method for radiation-force localized drug delivery using gas-filled lipospheres. *Ultrasonics, Ferroelectrics, and Frequency Control. IEEE Transactions on*, *51*(7), 822–831.

Shukla, R., Thomas, T. P., Peters, J. L., Desai, A. M., Kukowska-Latallo, J., Patri, A. K., & Baker, J. R. et al. (2006). HER2 specific tumor targeting with dendrimer conjugated anti-HER2 mAb. *Bioconjugate Chemistry*, *17*(5), 1109–1115. doi:10.1021/bc050348p PMID:16984117

Shukla, R., Thomas, T. P., Peters, J., Kotlyar, A., Myc, A., & Baker, J. R. Jr. (2005). Tumor angiogenic vasculature targeting with PAMAM dendrimer–RGD conjugates. *Chemical Communications*, (46): 5739–5741. doi:10.1039/b507350b PMID:16307130

Sill, T. J., & von Recum, H. A. (2008). Electrospinning: Applications in drug delivery and tissue engineering. *Biomaterials*, *29*(13), 1989–2006. doi:10.1016/j.biomaterials.2008.01.011 PMID:18281090

Silva, J., Fernandes, A. R., & Baptista, P. V. (2014). Application of nanotechnology in drug delivery. *Application of Nanotechnology in Drug Delivery*.

Silva, G. A., Czeisler, C., Niece, K. L., Beniash, E., Harrington, D. A., Kessler, J. A., & Stupp, S. I. (2004). Selective differentiation of neural progenitor cells by high-epitope density nanofibers. *Science*, *303*(5662), 1352–1355. doi:10.1126/science.1093783 PMID:14739465

Singh, M., Kumar, M., Manikandan, S., Chandrasekaran, N., & Mukherjee, A. (2014). Drug delivery system for controlled cancer therapy using physico-chemically stabilized bioconjugated gold nanoparticles synthesized from marine macroalgae, *PadinaGymnospora. J. Nanomed Nanotechol.*, *5*, 9.

Singh, D., Singh, R., Singh, P., & Gupta, R. S. (2009). Effect of embelin on lipid peroxidation and free radical scavenging activity against liver damage in rats. *Basic & Clinical Pharmacology & Toxicology*, *105*(4), 243–248. doi:10.1111/j.1742-7843.2009.00429.x PMID:19496777

Singh, P., Gonzalez, M. J., & Manchester, M. (2006). Viruses & their uses in nanotechnology. *Drug Development Research*, *6*(1), 23–41. doi:10.1002/ddr.20064

Singh, P., Gupta, U., Asthana, A., & Jain, N. K. (2008). Folate and Folate–PEG–PAMAM Dendrimers: Synthesis, Characterization, and Targeted Anticancer Drug Delivery Potential in Tumor Bearing Mice. *Bioconjugate Chemistry*, *19*(11), 2239–2252. doi:10.1021/bc800125u PMID:18950215

Sirisha, V. N. L., BhavaniHarika, I., Sruthi, B., Namrata, M., Kirankumar, P., Kiran Kumar Rao, Y., … UmaMaheshwaraRao, O. (2012). Liposomes – the potential drug carriers. *IOSR Journal of Pharmacy, 2*, 26-38.

Six, K., Berghmans, H., Leuner, C., Dressman, J., Van Werde, K., Mullens, J., & Van den Mooter, G. et al. (2003). Characterization of solid dispersions of itraconazole and hydroxyl propyl methyl cellulose prepared by melts extrusion, part II. *Pharmaceutical Research*, *20*(7), 1047–1054. doi:10.1023/A:1024414423779 PMID:12880291

Six, K., Verreck, G., Peeters, J., Augustijns, P., Kinget, R., & Van den Mooter, G. (2001). Investigation of thermal properties of glassy itraconazole: Identification of a monotropic mesophase. *Thermochimica Acta*, *376*(2), 175–181. doi:10.1016/S0040-6031(01)00563-9

Sjolund, M., Lindblom, G., Rilfors, L., & Arvidson, G. (1987). Hydrophobic molecules in lecithin-water systems. I. Formation of reversed hexagonal phases at high and low water contents. *Biophysical Journal*, *52*(2), 145–153. doi:10.1016/S0006-3495(87)83202-2 PMID:2822159

Slomkowski, S., Alemán, J. V., Gilbert, R. G., Hess, M., Horie, K., Jones, R. G., & Stepto, R. F. (2011). Terminology of polymers and polymerization processes in dispersed systems (IUPAC Recommendations 2011). *Pure and Applied Chemistry*, *83*(12), 2229–2259. doi:10.1351/PAC-REC-10-06-03

Slowing, I. I., Trewyn, B. G., Giri, S., & Lin, V. Y. (2007). Mesoporous silica nanoparticles for drug delivery and biosensing applications. *Advanced Functional Materials*, *17*(8), 1225–1236. doi:10.1002/adfm.200601191

Sluckin, T. J., Dunmur, D. A., & Stegemeyer, H. (2004). *Crystals That Flow – classic papers from the history of liquid crystals*. London: Taylor & Francis.

Sojka, R. E., Bjorneberg, D. L., Entry, J. A., Lentz, R. D., & Orts, W. J. (2007). Polyacrylamide in agriculture and environmental land management. *Advances in Agronomy*, *92*, 75–162. doi:10.1016/S0065-2113(04)92002-0

Solanki, A. B., Parikh, J. R., & Parikh, R. H. (2007). Formulation and optimization of piroxicam proniosomes by 3-factor, 3-level Box-Behnken design. *AAPS PharmSciTech*, *8*(4), 43–49. doi:10.1208/pt0804086 PMID:18181547

Solanki, A., Parikh, J., & Parikh, R. (2010). Preparation, characterization, optimization, and stability studies of aceclofenac proniosomes. *Iranian Journal of Pharmaceutical Research*, 237–246.

Soma, C. E., Dubernet, C., Barratt, G., Nemati, F., Appel, M., Benita, S., & Couvreur, P. (1999). Ability of doxorubicin-loaded nanoparticles to overcome multidrug resistance of tumor cells after their capture by macrophages. *Pharmaceutical Research*, *16*(11), 1710–1716. doi:10.1023/A:1018902031370 PMID:10571276

Song, M., Raphaelli, K., Jones, M. L., Aliabadi-Zadeh, K., Leung, K. M., Crowley, D., & Chin, D. Y. (2011). Clonal selection of high producing, stably transfected HEK293 cell lines utilizing modified, high-throughput FACS screening. *Journal of Chemical Technology and Biotechnology (Oxford, Oxfordshire)*, *86*(7), 935–941. doi:10.1002/jctb.2618

Song, W., Yu, X., Markel, D. C., Shi, T., & Ren, W. (2013). Coaxial PCL/PVA electrospun nanofibers: Osseointegration enhancer and controlled drug release device. *Biofabrication*, *5*(3), 035006. doi:10.1088/1758-5082/5/3/035006 PMID:23799653

Son, Y. J., Kim, W. J., & Yoo, H. S. (2014). Therapeutic applications of electrospun nanofibers for drug delivery systems. *Archives of Pharmacal Research*, *37*(1), 69–78. doi:10.1007/s12272-013-0284-2 PMID:24234913

Son, Y. J., & Yoo, H. S. (2012). Dexamethasone-incorporated nanofibrous meshes for antiproliferation of smooth muscle cells: Thermally induced drug-loading strategy. *Journal of Biomedical Materials Research. Part A*, *100*(10), 2678–2685. doi:10.1002/jbm.a.34197 PMID:22619069

Sourkohi, B. K., Cunningham, A., Zhang, Q., & Oh, J. K. (2011). Biodegradable block copolymer micelles with thiol-responsive sheddable coronas. *Biomacromolecules*, *12*(10), 3819–3825. doi:10.1021/bm2011032 PMID:21879701

Souto, E. B., & Muller, R. H. (2010). Lipid nanoparticles: Effect on bioavailability and pharmacokinetic changes. *Handbook of Experimental Pharmacology*, *197*, 115–141. doi:10.1007/978-3-642-00477-3_4 PMID:20217528

Spasojević, J., Radosavljević, A., Krstić, J., Jovanović, D., Spasojević, V., Kalagasidis-Krušić, M., & Kačarević-Popović, Z. (2015). Dual responsive antibacterial Ag-poly(*N*-isopropylacrylamide/itaconic acid) hydrogel nanocomposites synthesized by gamma irradiation. *European Polymer Journal*, *69*, 168–185. doi:10.1016/j.eurpolymj.2015.06.008

Speir, J.A., Munshi, S., Wang, G.J., Baker, T.S., & Johnson, J.E. (1995). Structures of the native &swollen forms of cowpea chlorotic mottle virus determined by X-ray crystallography & cryoelectron microscopy. *Structure, 3*, 63–78.

Sperling, L. H., & Mishra, V. (1996). The current status of interpenetrating polymer networks. *Polymers for Advanced Technologies*, *7*(4), 197–208. doi:10.1002/(SICI)1099-1581(199604)7:4<197::AID-PAT514>3.0.CO;2-4

Spicer, P. T. (2005). Progress in liquid crystalline dispersions: Cubosomes. *Current Opinion in Colloid & Interface Science*, *10*(5-6), 274–279. doi:10.1016/j.cocis.2005.09.004

Spicer, P. T., Hayden, K. L., Lynch, M. L., Ofori-Boateng, A., & Burns, J. L. (2001). Novel process for producing cubic liquid crystalline nanoparticles (cubosomes). *Langmuir*, *17*(19), 5748–5756. doi:10.1021/la010161w

Srikanth, M., Sunil, S., Rao, N., Uhumwangho, M., & Murthy, K. R. (2010). Ion-exchange resins as controlled drug delivery carriers. *Journal of Scientific Research*, *2*(3), 597. doi:10.3329/jsr.v2i3.4991

Srinivas, S., Kumar, Y. A., Hemanth, A., & Anitha, M. (2010). Preparation and evaluation of niosomes containing aceclofenac. *Digest Journal of Nanomaterials and Biostructures*, *5*(1), 249–254.

Stainmesse, S. (1990). *Etude gale'nique D'un Nouveau Proce'de´ D'obtention De Vecteurs Colloı¨daux Submicroniques a` Partir D'une Prote'ine Ou D'un Polyme`re Synthe'tique*. (Thesis). Universite´ De Paris Sud.

Stankus, J. J., Guan, J., & Wagner, W. R. (2004). Fabrication of biodegradable elastomeric scaffolds with sub-micron morphologies. *Journal of Biomedical Materials Research. Part A*, *70*(4), 603–614. doi:10.1002/jbm.a.30122 PMID:15307165

Stella, B., Arpicco, S., & Peracchia, M. T. (2000). Characterization of Folic Acid-Nanoparticles Conjugates for Tumoral Targeting. *Proceedings of the 27th International Symposium on Controlled Release of Bioactive Materials of the Controlled Release Society, Inc.*

Stephenson, G. A., & Diseroad, B. A. (2000). Structural relationship and desolvation behavior of cromolyn, cefazolin and fenoprofen sodium hydrates. *International Journal of Pharmaceutics*, *198*(2), 167–177. doi:10.1016/S0378-5173(00)00331-8 PMID:10767566

Stevenson, C. L., Bennett, D. B., & Ballesteros, D. L. (2005). Pharmaceutical liquid crystals: The relevance of partially ordered systems. *Journal of Pharmaceutical Sciences*, *94*(9), 1861–1879. doi:10.1002/jps.20435 PMID:16052511

Storm, G., & Crommelin, D. (1998). Liposomes: Quo vadis? *Pharmaceutical Science & Technology Today*, *1*(1), 19–31. doi:10.1016/S1461-5347(98)00007-8

Such, G. K., Yan, Y., Johnston, A. P. R., Gunawan, S. T., & Caruso, F. (2015). Interfacing Materials Science and Biology for Drug Carrier Design. *Advanced Materials*, *27*(14), 2278–2297. doi:10.1002/adma.201405084 PMID:25728711

Sun, H. L., Guo, B. N., Cheng, R., Meng, F. H., Liu, H. Y., & Zhong, Z. Y. (2009). Biodegradable micelles with sheddable poly(ethylene glycol) shells for triggered intracellular release of doxorubicin. *Biomaterials*, *30*(31), 6358–6366. doi:10.1016/j.biomaterials.2009.07.051 PMID:19666191

Sun, H. L., Guo, B. N., Cheng, R., Meng, F. H., Liu, H. Y., & Zhong, Z. Y. (2010). Shellsheddable micelles based on dextran-SS-poly(ε-caprolactone) diblock copolymer for efficient intracellular release of doxorubicin. *Biomacromolecules*, *11*(4), 848–854. doi:10.1021/bm1001069 PMID:20205476

Sun, I. C., Eun, D. K., Na, J. H., Lee, S., Kim, I. J., Youn, I. C., & Choi, K. et al. (2009). Heparin-Coated Gold Nanoparticles for Liver-Specific CT Imaging. *Chemistry (Weinheim an der Bergstrasse, Germany)*, *15*(48), 13341–13347. doi:10.1002/chem.200902344 PMID:19902441

Sunoqrot, S., Bugno, J., Lantvit, D., Burdette, J. E., & Hong, S. (2014). Prolonged blood circulation and enhanced tumor accumulation of folate-targeted dendrimer-polymer hybrid nanoparticles. *Journal of Controlled Release*, *191*(0), 115–122. doi:10.1016/j.jconrel.2014.05.006 PMID:24837188

Sun, Y., Yan, X. L., Yuan, T. M., Liang, J., Fan, Y. J., Gu, Z. W., & Zhang, X. D. (2010). Disassemblable micelles based on reduction-degradable amphiphilic graft copolymers for intracellular delivery of doxorubicin. *Biomaterials*, *31*(27), 7124–7131. doi:10.1016/j.biomaterials.2010.06.011 PMID:20580429

Sun, Z., Zussman, E., Yarin, A. L., Wendorff, J. H., & Greiner, A. (2003). Compound core-shell polymer nanofibers by co-electrospinning. *Advanced Materials*, *15*(22), 1929–1932. doi:10.1002/adma.200305136

Suri, S. S., Fenniri, H., & Singh, B. (2007). Nanotechnology-based drug delivery systems. *Journal of Occupational Medicine and Toxicology (London, England)*, *2*(1), 16. doi:10.1186/1745-6673-2-16 PMID:18053152

Suryanarayanan, R., Venkatesh, S., Hodgin, L. P., & Hanson, P. (1992). Hanson. Determination of the physical state of salicylic acid in hydrogel formulations by x-ray diffractometry. *International Journal of Pharmaceutics*, *78*(1-3), 77–83. doi:10.1016/0378-5173(92)90357-8

Suwakul, W., Ongpipattanakul, B., & Vardhanabhuti, N. (2006). Preparation and characterization of propylthiouracil niosomes. *Journal of Liposome Research*, *16*(14), 391–401. doi:10.1080/08982100600992542 PMID:17162580

Suzuki, A., & Tanaka, T. (1990). Phase transition in polymer gels induced by visible light. *Nature, 346*(6282), 345-347.

Swarbrick, J., & Boylan, J. C. (1993). *Encyclopedia of Pharmaceutical Technology: Volume 9-Liposomes as Pharmaceutical Dosage Forms to Microencapsulation.* CRC Press.

Swarnakar, N. K., Jain, V., Dubey, V., Mishra, D., & Jain, N. K. (2007). Enhanced oromucosal delivery of progesterone via hexosomes. *Pharmaceutical Research*, *24*(12), 2223–2230. doi:10.1007/s11095-007-9409-y PMID:17828445

Sznitowska, M., Gajewska, M., Janicki, S., Radwanska, A., & Lukowski, G. (2001). Bioavailability of diazepam from aqueous-organic solution, submicron emulsion and solid lipid nanoparticles after rectal administration in rabbits. *European Journal of Pharmaceutics and Biopharmaceutics*, *52*(2), 159–163. doi:10.1016/S0939-6411(01)00157-6 PMID:11522481

Szoka, F. Jr, & Papahadjopoulos, D. (1980). Comparative properties and methods of preparation of lipid vesicles (liposomes). *Annual Review of Biophysics and Bioengineering*, *9*(1), 467–508. doi:10.1146/annurev.bb.09.060180.002343 PMID:6994593

Szoka, F., & Papahadjopoulos, D. (1978). Procedure for preparation of liposomes with large internal aqueous space and high capture by reverse-phase evaporation. *Proceedings of the National Academy of Sciences of the United States of America*, *75*(9), 4194–4198. doi:10.1073/pnas.75.9.4194 PMID:279908

Tabbakhian, M., Daneshamouz, S., Tavakoli, N., & Jaafari, M. R. (2005). Influence of liposomes and niosomes on the in vitro permeation and skin retention of finasteride. *Indian Journal of Pharmaceutical Sciences*, *1*(3), 119–130.

Tabbakhian, M., Tavakoli, N., Jaafari, M. R., & Daneshamouz, S. (2006). Enhancement of follicular delivery of finasteride by liposomes and niosomes 1. In vitro permeation and in vivo deposition studies using hamster flank and ear models. *International Journal of Pharmaceutics*, *323*(1-2), 1–10. doi:10.1016/j.ijpharm.2006.05.041 PMID:16837150

Taepaiboon, P., Rungsardthong, U., & Supaphol, P. (2006). Drug-loaded electrospun mats of poly (vinyl alcohol) fibres and their release characteristics of four model drugs. *Nanotechnology*, *17*(9), 2317–2329. doi:10.1088/0957-4484/17/9/041

Taepaiboon, P., Rungsardthong, U., & Supaphol, P. (2007). Vitamin-loaded electrospun cellulose acetate nanofiber mats as transdermal and dermal therapeutic agents of vitamin A acid and vitamin E. *European Journal of Pharmaceutics and Biopharmaceutics*, *67*(2), 387–397. doi:10.1016/j.ejpb.2007.03.018 PMID:17498935

Tafreshi, S.-H., & Mirdamadi, S. (2015). Survey Study of Lipid Effect on Nisin Nanoliposome Formation and Application in Pasteurized Milk as a Food Model. *Applied Food Biotechnology*, *3*(2), 7–14.

Tai, H. S., & Lee, J. Y. (1990). Phase transition behaviors and selective optical properties of a binary cholesteric liquid crystals system: Mixtures of cholesteryloleyl carbonate and cholesteryl nonanoate. *Journal of Applied Physics*, *67*(2), 1001–1006. doi:10.1063/1.345807

Takahashi, H., Hatta, I., & Quinn, P. J. (1996). Cubic phases in hydrated 1:1 and 1:2 dipalmitoyl phosphatidyl choline- dipalmitoyl glycerol mixtures. *Biophysical Journal*, *70*(3), 1407–1411. doi:10.1016/S0006-3495(96)79699-6 PMID:8785296

Takeuchi, T., & Haginaka, J. (1999). Separation and sensing based on molecular recognition using molecularly imprinted polymers. *Journal of Chromatography. B, Biomedical Sciences and Applications*, *728*(1), 1–20. doi:10.1016/S0378-4347(99)00057-2 PMID:10379652

Talanov, V. S., Regino, C. A., Kobayashi, H., Bernardo, M., Choyke, P. L., & Brechbiel, M. W. (2006). Dendrimer-based nanoprobe for dual modality magnetic resonance and fluorescence imaging. *Nano Letters*, *6*(7), 1459–1463. doi:10.1021/nl060765q PMID:16834429

Talsma, H., Van Steenbergen, M. J., Borchert, J. C., & Crommelin, D. J. (1994). A novel technique for the one-step preparation of liposomes and nonionic surfactant vesicles without the use of organic solvents. Liposome formation in a continuous gas stream: The 'Bubble'method. *Journal of Pharmaceutical Sciences*, *83*(3), 276–280. doi:10.1002/jps.2600830303 PMID:8207668

Tamizharasi, S., Dubey, A., Rathi, V., & Rathi, J. (2009). Development and characterization of niosomal drug delivery of gliclazide. *Journal of Young Pharmacists*, *1*(3), 205. doi:10.4103/0975-1483.57065

Tanaka, T., & Fillmore, D. J. (1979). Kinetics of swelling of gels. *The Journal of Chemical Physics*, *70*(3), 1214–1218. doi:10.1063/1.437602

Tang, L. Y., Wang, Y. C., Li, Y., Du, J. Z., & Wang, J. (2009). Shell-detachable micelles based on disulfide-linked block copolymer as potential carrier for intracellular drug delivery. *Bioconjugate Chemistry*, *20*(6), 1095–2009. doi:10.1021/bc900144m PMID:19438224

Tang, R., Ji, W., Panus, D., Palumbo, R. N., & Wang, C. (2011). Block copolymer micelles with acid-labile ortho ester side-chains: Synthesis, characterization, and enhanced drug delivery to human glioma cells. *Journal of Controlled Release, 151*(1), 18–27. doi:10.1016/j.jconrel.2010.12.005 PMID:21194551

Tang, T. Y. D., Brooks, N. J., Jeworrek, C., Ces, O., Terrill, N. J., Winter, R., & Seddon, J. M. (2012). Hydrostatic pressure effects on the lamellar to gyroid cubic phase transition of monolinolein at limited hydration. *Langmuir, 28*(36), 13018–13024. doi:10.1021/la3025843 PMID:22894718

Tan, M. M., Corley, C. A., & Stevenson, C. L. (1998). Effect of gelation on the chemical stability and conformation of leuprolide. *Pharmaceutical Research, 15*(9), 1442–1448. doi:10.1023/A:1011914007940 PMID:9755898

Taratula, O., Schumann, C., Duong, T., Taylor, K. L., & Taratula, O. (2015). Dendrimer-encapsulated naphthalocyanine as a single agent-based theranostic nanoplatform for near-infrared fluorescence imaging and combinatorial anticancer phototherapy. *Nanoscale, 7*(9), 3888–3902. doi:10.1039/C4NR06050D PMID:25422147

Tarekegn, A., Joseph, Palani, Zacharia, & Ayenew. (2010). Niosomes in targeted drug delivery some recent advances. *Int j pharm sci res, 29*(1), 9.

Tavano, L., Muzzalupo, R., Cassano, R., Trombino, S., Ferrarelli, T., & Picci, N. (2010). New sucrose cocoate based vesicles: Preparation, characterization and skin permeation studies. *Colloids and Surfaces. B, Biointerfaces, 75*(1), 319–322. doi:10.1016/j.colsurfb.2009.09.003 PMID:19782543

Tenchov, B., Koynova, R., & Rapp, G. (1998). Accelerated formation of cubic phases in phosphatidyl ethanolamine dispersions. *Biophysical Journal, 75*(2), 853–866. doi:10.1016/S0006-3495(98)77574-5 PMID:9675186

Tenchov, B., Rappolt, M., Koynova, R., & Rapp, G. (1996). New phases induced by sucrose in saturated phosphatidyl ethanolamines: An expanded lamellar gel phase and a cubic phase. *Biochimica et Biophysica Acta, 1285*(1), 109–122. doi:10.1016/S0005-2736(96)00156-3 PMID:8948481

Thandavamoorthy, S., Gopinath, N., & Ramkumar, S. S. (2006). Self-assembled honeycomb polyurethane nanofibers. *Journal of Applied Polymer Science, 101*(5), 3121–3124. doi:10.1002/app.24333

Thassu, D., Deleers, M., & Pathak, Y. V. (2007). *Nanoparticulate drug delivery systems* (Vol. 166). CRC Press. doi:10.1201/9781420008449

The Chemical Industry and its Development. (1950). *Nature, 165*, 413-415.

Theeuwes, F., Hussain, A., & Higuchi, T. (1974). Quantitative analytical method for determination of drugs dispersed in polymers using differential scanning calorimetry. *Journal of Pharmaceutical Sciences, 63*(3), 427–429. doi:10.1002/jps.2600630325 PMID:4820377

Thewalt, J. L., & Bloom, M. (1992). Phosphatidylcholine: Cholesterol phase diagrams. *Biophysical Journal, 63*(4), 1176–1181. doi:10.1016/S0006-3495(92)81681-8 PMID:19431848

Thiagarajan, P. (2011). Nanoemulsions for drug delivery through different routes. *Research in Biotechnology, 2*(3).

Tomalia, D. A., Baker, H., Dewald, J., Hall, M., Kallos, G., Martin, S., & Smith, P. et al. (1985). A New Class of Polymers: Starburst-Dendritic Macromolecules. *Polymer Journal, 17*(1), 117–132. doi:10.1295/polymj.17.117

Tomlinson, R., Klee, M., Garrett, S., Heller, J., Duncan, R., & Brocchini, S. (2002). Pendent chain functionalized polyacetals that display pH-dependent degradation: A platform for the development of novel polymer therapeutics. *Macromolecules, 35*(2), 473–480. doi:10.1021/ma0108867

Tono,. Y., Kojima, C., Haba, Y., Takahashi, T., Harada, A., Yagi, S., & Kono, K. (2006). Thermosensitive properties of poly (amidoamine) dendrimers with peripheral phenylalanine residues. *Langmuir*, *22*(11), 4920–4922. doi:10.1021/la060066t PMID:16700575

Torchilin, V. (2008). *Multifunctional Pharmaceutical Nanocarriers*. Springer Science + Business Media, LLC.

Torchilin, V. (2005). Recent advances with liposomes as pharmaceutical carriers. *Nature Reviews. Drug Discovery*, *4*(2), 145–160. doi:10.1038/nrd1632 PMID:15688077

Torchilin, V. (2011). Tumor delivery of macromolecular drugs based on the EPR effect. *Advanced Drug Delivery Reviews*, *63*(3), 131–135. doi:10.1016/j.addr.2010.03.011 PMID:20304019

Torchilin, V. (2012). *Liposomes in drug delivery. In Fundamentals and Applications of Controlled Release Drug Delivery* (pp. 289–328). Springer. doi:10.1007/978-1-4614-0881-9_11

Torchilin, V. P. (2010). Passive and active drug targeting: Drug delivery to tumors as an example. *Drug Delivery*, 3–53. PMID:20217525

Torchilin, V. P. (2014). Multifunctional, stimuli-sensitive nanoparticulate systems for drug delivery. *Nature Reviews. Drug Discovery*, *13*(11), 813–827. doi:10.1038/nrd4333 PMID:25287120

Torchilin, V. P., & Trubetskoy, V. S. (1995). Which polymers can make nanoparticulate drug carriers long-circulating. *Advanced Drug Delivery Reviews*, *16*(2-3), 141–155. doi:10.1016/0169-409X(95)00022-Y

Touitou, E., Dayan, N., Bergelson, L., Godin, B., & Eliaz, M. (2000). Ethosomes – novel vesicular carriers for enhanced delivery: Characterization and skin penetration properties. *Journal of Controlled Release*, *65*(3), 403–418. doi:10.1016/S0168-3659(99)00222-9 PMID:10699298

Trotta, M., Peira, E., Carlotti, M., & Gallarate, M. (2004). Deformable liposomes for dermal administration of methotrexate. *International Journal of Pharmaceutics*, *270*(1-2), 119–125. doi:10.1016/j.ijpharm.2003.10.006 PMID:14726128

Trubetskoy, V. S., & Torchilin, V. P. (1995). Use of polyoxyethylene-lipid conjugates as long-circulating carriers for delivery of therapeutic and diagnostic agents. *Advanced Drug Delivery Reviews*, *16*(2–3), 311–320. doi:10.1016/0169-409X(95)00032-3

Tsai, C., Jamison, J., & Miller, T. (2007). New liquid crystal technology hope for treatment of cancer and other diseases. Kent State University.

Tsang, L., & Kracov, D. (2008). Biosimilars, developments in the EU and US. In *PLC Life Sciences Handbook* (pp. 17-21). Academic Press.

Tsutsui, J. M., Xie, F., & Porter, R. T. (2004). The use of microbubbles to target drug delivery. *Cardiovascular Ultrasound*, *2*(1), 23. doi:10.1186/1476-7120-2-23 PMID:15546496

Türker, S., Erdoğan, S., Ozer, A., Ergün, E., Tuncel, M., Bilgili, H., & Deveci, S. (2005). Scintigraphic imaging of radiolabelled drug delivery systems in rabbits with arthritis. *International Journal of Pharmaceutics*, *296*(1-2), 34–43. doi:10.1016/j.ijpharm.2005.02.017 PMID:15885453

Tyagi, L. K., Kumar, S., Maurya, S. S., & Kori, M. L. (2013). Ethosomes: Novel Vesicular Carrier for enhanced transdermaldrug delivery system. *Bulletin of Pharmaceutical Research*, *3*(1), 6–13.

U.S. Food and Drug Administration (USFDA). (2012). Guidance for Industry: Quality considerations in demonstration biosimilarity to a reference protein product. Washington, DC: U.S. Food and Drug Administration.

U.S. Food and Drug Administration. (2015). *Guidance for Industry. Scientific Considerations in Demonstrating Biosimilarity to a Reference Product. Draft Guidance*. U.S. Food and Drug Administration. Retrieved from http://www.fda.gov/downloads/DrugsGuidanceComplianceRegulatoryInformation/Guidances/UCM291128.pdf

Ubbink, J., Burbidge, A., & Mezzenga, R. (2008). Food structure and functionality: A soft matter perspective. *Soft Matter*, *4*(8), 1569–1581. doi:10.1039/b802183j

Uchegbu, I. (1998). The biodistribution of novel 200-nm palmitoyl muramic acid vesicles. *International Journal of Pharmaceutics*, *162*(1), 19–27. doi:10.1016/S0378-5173(97)00408-0

Uchegbu, I. F., & Vyas, S. P. (1998). Non-ionic surfactant based vesicles (niosomes) in drug delivery. *International Journal of Pharmaceutics*, *172*(1-2), 33–70. doi:10.1016/S0378-5173(98)00169-0

Uchegbu, I., Double, J., Kelland, L., Turton, J., & Florence, A. (1996). The activity of doxorubicin niosomes against an ovarian cancer cell line and three in vivo mouse tumour models. *Journal of Drug Targeting*, *3*(5), 399–409. doi:10.3109/10611869608996831 PMID:8866659

Uchegbu, I., Double, J., Turton, J., & Florence, A. (1995). Distribution, metabolism and tumoricidal activity of doxorubicin administered in sorbitan monostearate (Span 60) niosomes in the mouse. *Pharmaceutical Research*, *12*(7), 1019–1024. doi:10.1023/A:1016210515134 PMID:7494796

Üner, M., & Yener, G. (2007). Importance of solid lipid nanoparticles (SLN) in various administration routes and future perspectives. *International Journal of Nanomedicine*, *2*, 289–300. PMID:18019829

Vadas, E., Toma, P., & Zografi, G. (1991). Solid state phase transitions initiated by water vapor sorption of crystalline L-660-711, a leukotriene D4 receptor antagonist. *Pharmaceutical Research*, *8*(2), 148–155. doi:10.1023/A:1015871415925 PMID:2023861

Vakkalanka, S. K., Brazel, C. S., & Peppas, N. A. (1997). Temperature-and pH-sensitive terpolymers for modulated delivery of streptokinase. *Journal of Biomaterials Science. Polymer Edition*, *8*(2), 119–129. doi:10.1163/156856296X00192 PMID:8957708

van den Bergh, B. A., Wertz, P. W., Junginger, H. E., & Bouwstra, J. A. (2001). Elasticity of vesicles assessed by electron spin resonance, electron microscopy and extrusion measurements. *International Journal of Pharmaceutics*, *217*(1-2), 13–24. doi:10.1016/S0378-5173(01)00576-2 PMID:11292538

van der Linden, H. J., Herber, S., Olthuis, W., & Bergveld, P. (2003). Stimulus-sensitive hydrogels and their applications in chemical (micro) analysis. *Analyst (London)*, *128*(4), 325–331. doi:10.1039/b210140h PMID:12741636

van Hal, D. A., Bouwstra, J. A., van Rensen, A., Jeremiasse, E., de Vringer, T., & Junginger, H. E. (1996). Preparation and characterization of nonionic surfactant vesicles. *Journal of Colloid and Interface Science*, *178*(1), 263–273. doi:10.1006/jcis.1996.0114 PMID:10479441

van Hoogevest, P., & Wendel, A. (2014). The use of natural and synthetic phospholipids as pharmaceutical excipients. *European Journal of Lipid Science and Technology*, *116*(9), 1088–1107. doi:10.1002/ejlt.201400219 PMID:25400504

Van Vlerken, L. E., Vyas, T. K., & Amiji, M. M. (2007). Poly(ethylene glycol)-modified nanocarriers for tumor-targeted and intracellular delivery. *Pharmaceutical Research*, *24*(8), 1405–1414. doi:10.1007/s11095-007-9284-6 PMID:17393074

Varga, Z., Filipcsei, G., & Zrínyi, M. (2006). Magnetic field sensitive functional elastomers with tuneable elastic modulus. *Polymer*, *47*(1), 227–233. doi:10.1016/j.polymer.2005.10.139

Varshosaz, J., Taymouri, Pardakhty, Asadi-Shekaari, & Babaee (2014). *Niosomes of Ascorbic Acid and α-Tocopherol in the Cerebral Ischemia-Reperfusion Model in Male Rats*. BioMed Research International.

Varshosaz, J., Pardakhty, A., Hajhashemi, V.-I., & Najafabadi, A. R. (2003). Development and physical characterization of sorbitan monoester niosomes for insulin oral delivery. *Drug Delivery*, *10*(4), 251–262. doi:10.1080/drd_10_4_251 PMID:14612341

Vasita, R., & Katti, D. S. (2006). Nanofibers and their applications in tissue engineering. *International Journal of Nanomedicine*, *1*(1), 15–30. doi:10.2147/nano.2006.1.1.15 PMID:17722259

Vauthier, C., & Couvreur, P. (2000). Development of polysaccharide nanoparticles as novel drug carrier systems. In C. Trantolo & S. Inyang (Eds.), *Handbook of Pharmaceutical Controlled Release Technology; Wise* (pp. 413–429). New York: Marcel Dekker, Inc.

Vemuri, S., & Rhodes, C. (1995). Preparation and characterization of liposomes as therapeutic delivery systems: A review. *Pharmaceutica Acta Helvetiae*, *70*(2), 95–111. doi:10.1016/0031-6865(95)00010-7 PMID:7651973

Venkatesan, P., Manavalan, R., & Valliappan, K. (2009). Microencapsulation: A vital technique in novel drug delivery system. *J Pharm Sci Res*, *1*(4), 26–35.

Venugopal, J., Zhang, Y. Z., & Ramakrishna, S. (2005). Fabrication of modified and functionalized polycaprolactone nanofibre scaffolds for vascular tissue engineering. *Nanotechnology*, *16*(10), 2138–2142. doi:10.1088/0957-4484/16/10/028 PMID:20817986

Verreck, G., Chun, I., Rosenblatt, J., Peeters, J., Van Dijck, A., Mensch, J., & Brewster, M. E. et al. (2003). Incorporation of drugs in an amorphous state into electrospun nanofibers composed of a water-insoluble, nonbiodegradable polymer. *Journal of Controlled Release*, *92*(3), 349–360. doi:10.1016/S0168-3659(03)00342-0 PMID:14568415

Vögtle, F., Buhleier, E., & Wehner, W. (1978). Cascade and Nonskid-Chain-Like Syntheses of Molecular Cavity Topologies. *Synthesis*, *2*, 155–158.

Volkering, F. (1995). Influence of Nonionic Surfactants on Bioavailability and Biodegradation of Polycyclic Aromatic Hydrocarbons. *Applied and Environmental Microbiology*, *61*(5), 1699–1705. PMID:16535016

Vo, T. N., Kasper, F. K., & Mikos, A. G. (2012). Strategies for controlled delivery of growth factors and cells for bone regeneration. *Advanced Drug Delivery Reviews*, *64*(12), 1292–1309. doi:10.1016/j.addr.2012.01.016 PMID:22342771

Wadsten-Hindrichsen, P., Bender, J., Unga, J., & Engstrom, S. (2007). Aqueous self-assembly of phytantriol in ternary systems: Effect of monoolein, distearoyl phosphatidyl glycerol and three watermiscible solvents. *Journal of Colloid and Interface Science*, *315*(2), 701–713. doi:10.1016/j.jcis.2007.07.011 PMID:17655855

Wagner, A., & Vorauer-Uhl, K. (2011). Liposome Technology for Industrial Purposes. *Journal of Drug Delivery*. 10.1155/2011/591325

Wagner, E. (1994). Panthenol and phytantriol in cosmetics. *Parfumerie Und Kosmetik*, *75*(4), 260–267.

Wagner, M. E., & Rizvi, S. S. (2015). Novel method of niosome generation using supercritical carbon dioxide part I: Process mechanics. *Journal of Liposome Research*, (0): 1–13. doi:10.3109/08982104.2015.1088868 PMID:25945392

Walsh, G. (2010). Biopharmaceutical Benchmarks. *Nature Biotechnology*, *28*(9), 917–924. doi:10.1038/nbt0910-917 PMID:20829826

Walve, J., Bakliwal, S., Rane, B., & Pawar, S. (2011). Transfersomes: A surrogated carrier for transdermal drug delivery system. *IJABPT*, *2*(1), 204–213.

Wang, A. Z., Yuet, K., Zhang, L., Gu, F. X., Huynh-Le, M., Radovic-Moreno, A. F., & Farokhzad, O. C. et al. (2010). Chemo Rad nanoparticles: A novel multifunctional nanoparticle platform for targeted delivery of concurrent chemo radiation. *Nanomedicine (London)*, *5*(3), 361–368. doi:10.2217/nnm.10.6 PMID:20394530

Wang, G., & Uludag, H. (2008). Recent developments in nanoparticle-based drug delivery and targeting systems with emphasis on protein-based nanoparticles. *Expert Opinion on Drug Delivery*, *5*(5), 499–515. doi:10.1517/17425247.5.5.499 PMID:18491978

Wang, H., Zheng, L., Peng, C., Guo, R., Shen, M., Shi, X., & Zhang, G. (2011). Computed tomography imaging of cancer cells using acetylated dendrimer-entrapped gold nanoparticles. *Biomaterials*, *32*(11), 2979–2988. doi:10.1016/j.biomaterials.2011.01.001 PMID:21277019

Wang, J., Sun, J., Chen, Q., Gao, Y., Li, L., Li, H., & He, Z. (2012). Star-shape copolymer of lysine linked di-tocopherol polyethylene glycol 2000 succinate for doxorubicin delivery with reversal of multidrug resistance. *Biomaterials*, *28*(28), 6877–6888. doi:10.1016/j.biomaterials.2012.06.019 PMID:22770799

Wang, K., Liu, Y., Yi, W. J., Li, C., Li, Y. Y., Zhuo, R. X., & Zhang, X. Z. (2013). Novel shell-cross-linked micelles with detachable PEG corona for glutathione-mediated intracellular drug delivery. *Soft Matter*, *9*(3), 692–699. doi:10.1039/C2SM27028E

Wang, L., Li, X., Zhang, G., Dong, J., & Eastoe, J. (2007). Oil-in-water nanoemulsions for pesticide formulations. *Journal of Colloid and Interface Science*, *314*(1), 230–235. doi:10.1016/j.jcis.2007.04.079 PMID:17612555

Wang, N. X., & Recum, H. A. (2011). Affinity-Based Drug Delivery. *Macromolecular Bioscience*, *11*(3), 321–332. doi:10.1002/mabi.201000206 PMID:21108454

Wang, X., Cai, X., Hu, J., Shao, N., Wang, F., Zhang, Q., & Cheng, Y. et al. (2013). Glutathione-triggered "off–on" release of anticancer drugs from dendrimer-encapsulated gold nanoparticles. *Journal of the American Chemical Society*, *135*(26), 9805–9810. doi:10.1021/ja402903h PMID:23789713

Wang, X., Gu, X., Yuan, C., Chen, S., Zhang, P., Zhang, T., & Chen, G. et al. (2004). Evaluation of biocompatibility of polypyrrole *in vitro* and *in vivo*. *Journal of Biomedical Materials Research. Part A*, *68*(3), 411–422. doi:10.1002/jbm.a.20065 PMID:14762920

Wang, Y. C., Li, Y., Sun, T. M., Xiong, M. H., Wu, J. J., Yang, Y. Y., & Wang, J. (2010). Core–shell-corona micelle stabilized by reversible cross-link for intracellular drug delivery. *Macromolecular Rapid Communications*, *31*(13), 1201–1206. doi:10.1002/marc.200900863 PMID:21590876

Wang, Y., Qiao, W., & Yin, T. (2010). A novel controlled release drug delivery system for multiple drugs based on electrospun nanofibers containing nanoparticles. *Journal of Pharmaceutical Sciences*, *99*(12), 4805–4811. doi:10.1002/jps.22189 PMID:20821381

Wang, Y., Tu, S., Pinchuk, A. N., & Xiong, M. P. (2013). Active drug encapsulation and release kinetics from hydrogel-in-liposome nanoparticles. *Journal of Colloid and Interface Science*, *406*, 247–255. doi:10.1016/j.jcis.2013.05.081 PMID:23809875

Wang, Y., Zhang, Y., Wang, B., Cao, Y., Yu, Q., & Yin, T. (2013). Fabrication of core–shell micro/nanoparticles for programmable dual drug release by emulsion electrospraying. *Journal of Nanoparticle Research*, *15*(6), 1–12. doi:10.1007/s11051-013-1726-y

Wang, Z., Zhou, B., Liu, D., & Fan, X. (2010). Thermosensitive Poly (N-isopropylacrylamide)-g-Polyamidoamine Dendrimer Derivatives: Preparation and the Drug Release Behaviors. *Macromolecular Symposia*, *297*(1), 158–166. doi:10.1002/masy.200900055

Waranuch, N., Ramachandran, C., & Weiner, N. D. (1998). Controlled topical delivery of cyclosporin-A from nonionic liposomal formulations: Mechanistic aspects. *Journal of Liposome Research*, *8*(2), 225–238. doi:10.3109/08982109809035528

Watnasirichaikul, S., Rades, R., Tucker, I. G., & Davies, N. M. (2000). Manipulating the Release of Insulin from Nanocapsules Prepared by Interfacial Polymerization of Microemulsions. *Proceedings of the 27th International Symposium on Controlled Release of Bioactive Materials of the Controlled Release Society, Inc.*

Wearner, R. R., Myers, M. C., & Taylor, D. A. (1988). Electron probe analysis of human skin: Determination of the water concentration profile. *The Journal of Investigative Dermatology*, *90*(2), 218–224. doi:10.1111/1523-1747.ep12462252 PMID:3339263

Weber, C., Coester, C., Kreuter, J., & Langer, K. (2000). Dessolvation process and surface characterization of protein nanoparticles. *International Journal of Pharmaceutics*, *194*(1), 94–102. doi:10.1016/S0378-5173(99)00370-1

Wei, H., Cheng, S.-X., Zhang, X.-Z., & Zhuo, R.-X. (2009). Thermo-sensitive polymeric micelles based on poly (N-isopropylacrylamide) as drug carriers. *Progress in Polymer Science*, *34*(9), 893–910. doi:10.1016/j.progpolymsci.2009.05.002

Wei, L., Hu, N., & Zhang, Y. (2010). Synthesis of polymer—mesoporous silica nanocomposites. *Materials (Basel)*, *3*(7), 4066–4079. doi:10.3390/ma3074066

Wei, L., Lu, J., Xu, H., Patel, A., Chen, Z., & Chen, G. (2015, May). Silver nanoparticles: Synthesis, properties, & therapeutic applications. *Drug Discovery Today*, *20*(5), 595–601. doi:10.1016/j.drudis.2014.11.014 PMID:25543008

Weissig, V. (2010). *Liposomes: Methods and protocols* (Vol. 2). Humana Press USA.

Weiss, W. F. IV, Young, T. M., & Roberts, C. J. (2009). Princples, approaches, and challenges for predicting protein aggregation rates and shelf life. *Journal of Pharmaceutical Sciences*, *98*(4), 1247–1277. doi:10.1002/jps.21521 PMID:18683878

Weisz, B., Giehl, K., Gana-Weisz, M., Egozi, Y., Ben-Baruch, G., Marciano, D., & Kloog, Y. et al. (1999). A new functional Ras antagonist inhibits human pancreatic tumor growth in nude mice. *Oncogene*, *18*(16), 2579–2588. doi:10.1038/sj.onc.1202602 PMID:10353601

Wei, T., Chen, C., Liu, J., Liu, C., Posocco, P., Liu, X., & Fermeglia, M. et al. (2015). Anticancer drug nanomicelles formed by self-assembling amphiphilic dendrimer to combat cancer drug resistance. *Proceedings of the National Academy of Sciences of the United States of America*, *112*(10), 2978–2983. doi:10.1073/pnas.1418494112 PMID:25713374

Wen, H. Y., Dong, H. Q., Xie, W. J., Li, Y. Y., Wang, K., Pauletti, G. M., & Shi, D. L. (2011). Rapidly disassembling nanomicelles with disulfide-linked PEG shells for glutathione-mediated intracellular drug delivery. *Chemical Communications*, *47*(12), 3550–3562. doi:10.1039/c0cc04983b PMID:21327187

Wen, S., Li, K., Cai, H., Chen, Q., Shen, M., Huang, Y., & Zhang, G. et al. (2013). Multifunctional dendrimer-entrapped gold nanoparticles for dual mode CT/MR imaging applications. *Biomaterials*, *34*(5), 1570–1580. doi:10.1016/j.biomaterials.2012.11.010 PMID:23199745

Wen, Y., Zhang, Z., & Li, J. (2014). Highly Efficient Multifunctional Supramolecular Gene Carrier System Self-Assembled from Redox-Sensitive and Zwitterionic Polymer Blocks. *Advanced Functional Materials*, *24*(25), 3874–3884. doi:10.1002/adfm.201303687

White, P. F., Ardeleanu, M., Schooley, G., & Burch, R. M. (2009). *Pharmacokinetics of DepoBupivacaine Following Infiltration in Patients Undergoing Two Types of Surgery and in Normal Volunteers*. The International Anesthesia Research Society Annual Meeting, San Diego, CA. Retrieved from: http://www.google.rs/url?sa=t&rct=j&q=&esrc=s&frm=1&source=web&cd=1&ved=0CBwQFjAA&url=http%3A%2F%2Fphx.corporate-ir.net%2FExternal.File%3Fitem%3D-UGFyZW50SUQ9NDI4NTE2fENoaWxkSUQ9NDQ1NDk1fFR5cGU9MQ%3D%3D%26t%3D1&ei=DDOHVfTGBoSrUePzmbAN&usg=AFQjCNH6FX5VmgkfXPINYvRCdmKCUx0B-g&sig2=QB1d8uciRRRy5RpYJLHqEQ

Wilczewska, A. Z., Niemirowicz, K., Markiewicz, K. H., & Car, H. (2012). Nanoparticles as drug delivery systems. *Pharmacological Reports*, *64*(5), 1020–1037. doi:10.1016/S1734-1140(12)70901-5 PMID:23238461

Williams, K. J., Werth, V. P., & Wolff, J. A. (1984). Intravenously administered lecithin liposomes: A synthetic antiatherogenic lipid particle. *Perspectives in Biology and Medicine*, *27*(3), 417–431. doi:10.1353/pbm.1984.0031 PMID:6374607

Winsor, P. A. (1968). Binary and multicomponent solution of amphiphilic compounds solubilization and the formation structure and theoretical significance of liquid crystalline solutions. *Chemical Reviews*, *68*(1), 1–40. doi:10.1021/cr60251a001

Wissing, S., Kayser, O., & Müller, R. (2004). Solid lipid nanoparticles for parenteral drug delivery. *Advanced Drug Delivery Reviews*, *56*(9), 1257–1272. doi:10.1016/j.addr.2003.12.002 PMID:15109768

Wohlfart, S., Gelperina, S., & Kreuter, J. (2012). Transport of drugs across the blood–brain barrier by nanoparticles. *Journal of Controlled Release*, *161*(2), 264–273. doi:10.1016/j.jconrel.2011.08.017 PMID:21872624

Wooley, K. L., Hawker, C. J., & Fréchet, J. M. (1994). A "Branched-Monomer Approach" for the Rapid Synthesis of Dendimers. *Angewandte Chemie*, *33*(1), 82–85. doi:10.1002/anie.199400821

World Health Organisation (WHO). (2009). *Expert Committee on Biological standardization. Guidelines on evaluation of similar biotherapeutic products (SBPs)*. Retrieved from http://www.who.int/biologicals/areas/biological_therapeutics/BIOTHERAPEUTICS_FOR_WEB_22APRIL2010.pdf

Wulff, G. (1995). Molecular imprinting in cross-linked materials with the aid of molecular templates—a way towards artificial antibodies. *Angewandte Chemie International Edition in English*, *34*(17), 1812–1832. doi:10.1002/anie.199518121

Wu, P., Chen, X., Hu, N., Tam, U. C., Blixt, O., Zettl, A., & Bertozzi, C. R. (2008). Biocompatible Carbon Nanotubes Generated by Functionalization with Glycodendrimers. *Angewandte Chemie International Edition in English*, *47*(27), 5022–5025. doi:10.1002/anie.200705363 PMID:18509843

Wu, W., Driessen, W., & Jiang, X. (2014). Oligo (ethylene glycol)-based thermosensitive dendrimers and their tumor accumulation and penetration. *Journal of the American Chemical Society*, *136*(8), 3145–3155. doi:10.1021/ja411457r PMID:24506735

Wyatt, D., & Dorschel, D. (1992). A cubic-phase delivery system composed of glyceryl monooleate and water for sustained release of water-soluble drugs. *Pharmaceutical Technology*, *16*(10), 116–130.

Xiao, K., Luo, J., Fowler, W. L., Li, Y., Lee, J. S., Xing, L., & Lam, K. S. et al. (2009). A self-assembling nanoparticle for paclitaxel delivery in ovarian cancer. *Biomaterials*, *30*(30), 6006–6016. doi:10.1016/j.biomaterials.2009.07.015 PMID:19660809

Xiao, K., Luo, J., Li, Y., Lee, J. S., Fung, G., & Lam, K. S. (2011). PEG-oligocholic acid telodendrimer micelles for the targeted delivery of doxorubicin to B-cell lymphoma. *Journal of Controlled Release*, *155*(2), 272–281. doi:10.1016/j.jconrel.2011.07.018 PMID:21787818

Xiao, X. C., Chu, L. Y., Chen, W. M., Wang, S., & Li, Y. (2003). Positively thermo-sensitive monodisperse core–shell microspheres. *Advanced Functional Materials*, *13*(11), 847–852. doi:10.1002/adfm.200304513

Xia, T. A., Kovochich, M., Liong, M., Meng, H., Kabehie, S., George, S., & Nel, A. E. et al. (2009). Polyethyleneimine coating enhances the cellular uptake of mesoporous silica nanoparticles and allows safe delivery of siRNA and DNA constructs. *ACS Nano*, *3*(10), 3273–3286. doi:10.1021/nn900918w PMID:19739605

Xie, J., & Wang, C.-H. (2006). Electrospun micro-and nanofibers for sustained delivery of paclitaxel to treat C6 glioma in vitro. *Pharmaceutical Research*, *23*(8), 1817–1826. doi:10.1007/s11095-006-9036-z PMID:16841195

Xue, J., He, M., Liu, H., Niu, Y., Crawford, A., Coates, P. D., & Zhang, L. et al. (2014). Drug loaded homogeneous electrospun PCL/gelatin hybrid nanofiber structures for anti-infective tissue regeneration membranes. *Biomaterials*, *35*(34), 9395–9405. doi:10.1016/j.biomaterials.2014.07.060 PMID:25134855

Xu, X., Chen, X., Xu, X., Lu, T., Wang, X., Yang, L., & Jing, X. (2006). BCNU-loaded PEG–PLLA ultrafine fibers and their in vitro antitumor activity against Glioma C6 cells. *Journal of Controlled Release*, *114*(3), 307–316. doi:10.1016/j.jconrel.2006.05.031 PMID:16891029

Xu, X., Jian, Y., Li, Y., Zhang, X., Tu, Z., & Gu, Z. (2014). Bio-Inspired Supramolecular Hybrid Dendrimers Self-Assembled from Low-Generation Peptide Dendrons for Highly Efficient Gene Delivery and Biological Tracking. *ACS Nano*, *8*(9), 9255–9264. doi:10.1021/nn503118f PMID:25184443

Xu, Y. M., Meng, F. H., Cheng, R., & Zhong, Z. Y. (2009). Reduction-sensitive reversibly crosslinked biodegradable micelles for triggered release of doxorubicin. *Macromolecular Bioscience*, *9*(12), 1254–1261. doi:10.1002/mabi.200900233 PMID:19904724

Xu, Z., He, B., Shen, J., Yang, W., & Yin, M. (2013). Fluorescent water-soluble perylenediimide-cored cationic dendrimers: Synthesis, optical properties, and cell uptake. *Chemical Communications*, *49*(35), 3646–3648. doi:10.1039/c3cc40330k PMID:23529155

Yaghmur, A., Campo, L., & De, . (2005). Emulsified microemulsions and oil-containing liquid crystalline phases. *Langmuir*, *21*(2), 569–577. doi:10.1021/la0482711 PMID:15641825

Yaghmur, A., Campo, L., & De, . (2006). Control of the internal structure of MLO-based isasomes by the addition of diglycerol monooleate and soybean Phosphatidyl choline. *Langmuir*, *22*(24), 9919–9927. doi:10.1021/la061303v PMID:17106981

Yaghmur, A., & Glatter, O. (2009). Characterization and potential applications of nanostructured aqueous dispersions. *Advances in Colloid and Interface Science*, *147-148*, 333–342. doi:10.1016/j.cis.2008.07.007 PMID:18804754

Yaghmur, A., Kriechbaum, M., Amenitsch, H., Steinhart, M., Laggner, P., & Rappolt, M. (2010). Effects of pressure and temperature on the self-assembled fully hydrated nanostructures of monoolein-oil systems. *Langmuir*, *26*(2), 1177–1185. doi:10.1021/la9023019 PMID:19681634

Yaghmur, A., Laggner, P., Sartori, B., & Rappolt, M. (2008). Calcium triggered *Lα -H2*phase transition monitored by combined rapid mixing and time-resolved synchrotron SAXS. PLo*S ONE, 3*(*4*), e2072. doi:10.1371/journal.pone.0002072 PMID:18446202

Yaghmur, A., Larsen, W., Schmitt, M., Ostergaard, J., Larsen, C., Jensen, H., & Rappolt, M. (2011). In situ characterization of lipidic bupivacaine-loaded formulations. So*ft Matter,* 7(*18*), 8291–8295. doi:10.1039/c1sm05854a

Yaghmur, A., Rappolt, M., Ostergaard, J., Larsen, C., & Larsen, S. W. (2012). Characterization of bupivacaine-loaded formulations based on liquid crystalline phases and microemulsions: The effect of lipid composition. *Langmuir, 28*(5), 2881–2889. doi:10.1021/la203577v PMID:22247936

Yaghmur, A., Sartori, B., & Rappolt, M. (2011). The role of calcium in membrane condensation and spontaneous curvature variations in model lipidic systems. *Physical Chemistry Chemical Physics*, *13*(8), 3115–3125. doi:10.1039/C0CP01036G PMID:21049109

Yamada, K., Yamashita, J., Todo, H., Miyamoto, K., Hashimoto, S., Tokudome, Y., & Sugibayashi, K. (2011). Preparation and evaluation of liquid-crystal formulations with skin-permeation enhancing abilities for entrapped drug. *Journal of Oleo Science*, *60*(1), 31–40. doi:10.5650/jos.60.31 PMID:21178315

Yamamoto, J., Nishiyama, I., Inoue, M., & Yokoyama, H. (2005). Optical isotropy and iridescence in a smectic blue phase. *Nature Materials*, *437*(7058), 525–528. doi:10.1038/nature04034 PMID:16177785

Yamauchi, H., Yano, T., Kato, T., Tanaka, I., Nakabayashi, S., Higashi, K., & Yamada, H. et al. (1995). Effects of sialic acid derivative on long circulation time and tumor concentration of liposomes. *International Journal of Pharmaceutics*, *113*(2), 141–148. doi:10.1016/0378-5173(94)00188-B

Yang, Chang, Yang, & Lin. (2010). Pharmacokinetics and physiologically-based pharmacokinetic modeling of nanoparticles. *Journal of Nanoscience and Nanotechnology, 10*(12), 8482-8490.

Yang, H., Deng, A., Zhang, J., Wang, J., & Lu, B. (2013). Preparation, characterization and anticancer therapeutic efficacy of cisplatin-loaded niosomes. *Journal of Microencapsulation*, *30*(3), 237–244. doi:10.3109/02652048.2012.717116 PMID:23272761

Yang, J., Luo, Y., Xu, Y., Li, J., Zhang, Z., Wang, H., & Zhang, G. et al. (2015). Conjugation of Iron Oxide Nanoparticles with RGD-Modified Dendrimers for Targeted Tumor MR Imaging. *ACS Applied Materials & Interfaces*, *7*(9), 5420–5428. doi:10.1021/am508983n PMID:25695661

Yang, Q., Yang, Y., Li, L., Sun, W., Zhu, X., & Huang, Y. (2015). Polymeric Nanomedicine for Tumor-Targeted Combination Therapy to Elicit Synergistic Genotoxicity against Prostate Cancer. *ACS Applied Materials & Interfaces*, *7*(12), 6661–6673. doi:10.1021/am509204u PMID:25775367

Yang, Y., Li, X., Qi, M., Zhou, S., & Weng, J. (2008). Release pattern and structural integrity of lysozyme encapsulated in core–sheath structured poly (DL-lactide) ultrafine fibers prepared by emulsion electrospinning. *European Journal of Pharmaceutics and Biopharmaceutics*, *69*(1), 106–116. doi:10.1016/j.ejpb.2007.10.016 PMID:18078743

Yang, Z., Tan, Y., Chen, M., Dian, L., Shan, Z., Peng, X., & Wu, C. (2013). Development of amphotericin B-loaded cubosomes through the Sol Emuls technology for enhancing the oral bioavailability. *AAPS PharmSciTech*, *13*(4), 1483–1491. doi:10.1208/s12249-012-9876-2 PMID:23090113

Yariv, D., Efrat, R., Libster, D., Aserin, A., & Garti, N. (2010). In vitro permeation of diclofenac salts from lyotropic liquid crystalline systems. *Colloids and Surfaces. B, Biointerfaces*, *78*(2), 185–192. doi:10.1016/j.colsurfb.2010.02.029 PMID:20363601

Yarmolenko, P. S., Zhao, Y., Landon, C., Spasojevic, I., Yuan, F., Needham, D., & Dewhirst, M. W. et al. (2010). Comparative effects of thermosensitive doxorubicin-containing liposomes and hyperthermia in human and murine tumours. *International Journal of Hyperthermia*, *26*(5), 485–498. doi:10.3109/02656731003789284 PMID:20597627

Ye, Q., Asherman, J., Stevenson, M., Brownson, E., & Katre, N. V. (2000). DepoFoam® technology: A vehicle for controlled delivery of protein and peptide drugs. *Journal of Controlled Release*, *64*(1-3), 155–166. doi:10.1016/S0168-3659(99)00146-7 PMID:10640654

Yesilyurt, V., Ramireddy, R., Azagarsamy, M. A., & Thayumanavan, S. (2012). Accessing Lipophilic Ligands in Dendrimer-Based Amphiphilic Supramolecular Assemblies for Protein-Induced Disassembly. *Chemistry (Weinheim an der Bergstrasse, Germany)*, *18*(1), 223–229. doi:10.1002/chem.201102727 PMID:22127994

Yesilyurt, V., Ramireddy, R., & Thayumanavan, S. (2011). Photoregulated Release of Noncovalent Guests from Dendritic Amphiphilic Nanocontainers. *Angewandte Chemie*, *123*(13), 3094–3098. doi:10.1002/ange.201006193 PMID:21404394

Yildirimera, L., Thanhb, N. T. K., Loizidoua, M., & Seifaliana, A. M. (2011). Toxicology and clinical potential of nanoparticles. *Nano Today*, *6*(6), 585–607. doi:10.1016/j.nantod.2011.10.001 PMID:23293661

Yoo, H. S., Kim, T. G., & Park, T. G. (2009). Surface-functionalized electrospun nanofibers for tissue engineering and drug delivery. *Advanced Drug Delivery Reviews*, *61*(12), 1033–1042. doi:10.1016/j.addr.2009.07.007 PMID:19643152

Yoshida, H., Lehr, C.-M., Kok, W., Junginger, H., Verhoef, J., & Bouwstra, J. (1992). Niosomes for oral delivery of peptide drugs. *Journal of Controlled Release*, *21*(1), 145–153. doi:10.1016/0168-3659(92)90016-K

Yoshimoto, H., Shin, Y. M., Terai, H., & Vacanti, J. P. (2003). A biodegradable nanofiber scaffold by electrospinning and its potential for bone tissue engineering. *Biomaterials*, *24*(12), 2077–2082. doi:10.1016/S0142-9612(02)00635-X PMID:12628828

Yoshioka, T., Sternberg, B., & Florence, A. (1994). Preparation and properties of vesicles (niosomes)of sorbitan monoesters (Span 20, 40, 60, and 80) and a sorbitan triester (Span 85). *International Journal of Pharmaceutics*, *105*(1), 1–6. doi:10.1016/0378-5173(94)90228-3

Yuan, H., Luo, K., Lai, Y., Pu, Y., He, B., Wang, G., & Gu, Z. et al. (2010). A novel poly (L-glutamic acid) dendrimer based drug delivery system with both pH-sensitive and targeting functions. *Molecular Pharmaceutics*, *7*(4), 953–962. doi:10.1021/mp1000923 PMID:20481567

Yuan, X. B., Yuan, Y., Jiang, W., Liu, J., Tian, E., Shun, H., & Sheng, J. et al. (2008). Preparation of rapamycin-loaded chitosan/PLA nanoparticles for immunosuppression in corneal transplantation. *International Journal of Pharmaceutics*, *349*(1-2), 241–248. doi:10.1016/j.ijpharm.2007.07.045 PMID:17919859

Yuan, Z. F., Huang, J. Y., Liu, J., Cheng, S. X., Zhuo, R. X., & Li, F. (2011). PEG-detachable and acid-labile cross-linked micelles based on orthoester linked graft copolymer for paclitaxel release. *Nanotechnology*, *22*(33), 335601. doi:10.1088/0957-4484/22/33/335601 PMID:21788685

Yu, C. C. (2013). Non-metallic nanomaterials in cancer theranostics: A review of silica- and carbon-based drug delivery systems. *Science and Technology of Advanced Materials*, *14*(4), 044407. doi:10.1088/1468-6996/14/4/044407

Yu, D. G., Wang, X., Li, X. Y., Chian, W., Li, Y., & Liao, Y. Z. (2013). Electrospun biphasic drug release polyvinylpyrrolidone/ethyl cellulose core/sheath nanofibers. *Acta Biomaterialia*, *9*(3), 5665–5672. doi:10.1016/j.actbio.2012.10.021 PMID:23099302

Yu, D.-G., Li, X.-Y., Wang, X., Chian, W., Liao, Y.-Z., & Li, Y. (2013). Zero-order drug release cellulose acetate nanofibers prepared using coaxial electrospinning. *Cellulose (London, England)*, *20*(1), 379–389. doi:10.1007/s10570-012-9824-z

Yu, H., Jia, Y., Yao, C., & Lu, Y. (2014). PCL/PEG core/sheath fibers with controlled drug release rate fabricated on the basis of a novel combined technique. *International Journal of Pharmaceutics*, *469*(1), 17–22. doi:10.1016/j.ijpharm.2014.04.045 PMID:24751343

Yulin, C., Ping, M., & Shuangying, G. (2014). Cubic and Hexagonal Liquid Crystals as Drug Delivery Systems. *BioMed Research International*, *2014*, 815981. PMID:24995330

Yu-Nam, Y., & Lead, R. (2008). Manufactured nanoparticles: An overview of their chemistry, interactions and potential environmental implications. *The Science of the Total Environment*, *400*(1-3), 396–414. doi:10.1016/j.scitotenv.2008.06.042 PMID:18715626

Zambaux, M. F., Bonneauz, F., Gref, R., Maincent, P., Dellacherie, E., Alonso, M. J., & Vigneron, C. et al. (1998). Influence of experimental parameters on the characteristics of poly(lactic acid) nanoparticles prepared by a double emulsion method. *Journal of Controlled Release*, *50*(1-3), 31–40. doi:10.1016/S0168-3659(97)00106-5 PMID:9685870

Zarif, L. (2002). Elongated supramolecular assemblies in drug delivery. *Journal of Controlled Release*, *81*(1), 7–23. doi:10.1016/S0168-3659(02)00010-X PMID:11992674

Zarif, L., Gulik-Krzywicki, T., Riess, J. G., Pucci, B., Guedj, C., & Pavia, A. A. (1994). Alkyl and perfluoroalkyl glycolipid-based supramolecular assemblies. *Colloids and Surfaces. A, Physicochemical and Engineering Aspects*, *84*(1), 107–112. doi:10.1016/0927-7757(93)02680-D

Zeng, F., & Zimmerman, S. C. (1996). Rapid synthesis of dendrimers by an orthogonal coupling strategy. *Journal of the American Chemical Society*, *118*(22), 5326–5327. doi:10.1021/ja960317s

Zeng, J., Aigner, A., Czubayko, F., Kissel, T., Wendorff, J. H., & Greiner, A. (2005). Poly (vinyl alcohol) nanofibers by electrospinning as a protein delivery system and the retardation of enzyme release by additional polymer coatings. *Biomacromolecules*, *6*(3), 1484–1488. doi:10.1021/bm0492576 PMID:15877368

Zenotech Builds Pipeline of 'Generic' Monoclonals. (2007). *Scrip*, (3237), 10.

Zhanga, H., Xiaolin, L. A., Jing, D., Xu, H., & Daid, X. (2013). Delivery of ursolic acid in polymeric nanoparticles effectively promotesthe apoptosis of gastric cancer cells through enhanced inhibition of cyclooxygenase 2. *International Journal of Pharmaceutics*, *441*(1-2), 261–268. doi:10.1016/j.ijpharm.2012.11.034 PMID:23194884

Zhang, C., Pan, D., Luo, K., She, W., Guo, C., Yang, Y., & Gu, Z. (2014). Peptide Dendrimer-Doxorubicin Conjugate-Based Nanoparticles as an Enzyme-Responsive Drug Delivery System for Cancer Therapy. *Advanced Healthcare Materials*, *3*(8), 1299–1308. doi:10.1002/adhm.201300601 PMID:24706635

Zhang, J. Y., Jiang, X. Z., Zhang, Y. F., Li, Y. T., & Liu, S. Y. (2007). Facile fabrication of reversible core cross-linked micelles possessing thermosensitive swellability. *Macromolecules*, *40*(25), 9125–9132. doi:10.1021/ma071564r

Zhang, L., Gu, F. X., Chan, J. M., Wang, A. Z., Langer, R. S., & Farokhzad, O. C. (2008). Nanoparticles in medicine: Therapeutic applications and developments. *Clinical Pharmacology and Therapeutics*, *83*(5), 761–769. doi:10.1038/sj.clpt.6100400 PMID:17957183

Zhang, L., Liu, W. G., Lin, L., Chen, D. Y., & Stenzel, M. H. (2008, November10). (208). Degradable disulfide core-cross-linked micelles as a drug delivery system prepared from vinyl functionalized nucleosides via the RAFT process. *Biomacromolecules*, *9*(11), 3321–3331. doi:10.1021/bm800867n PMID:18842025

Zhang, X., Huang, Y., Zhao, W., Liu, H., Marquez, R., Lu, J., & Li, S. et al. (2014). Targeted delivery of anticancer agents via a dual function nanocarrier with an interfacial drug-interactive motif. *Biomacromolecules*, *10*(15), 4326–4335. doi:10.1021/bm501339j PMID:25325795

Zhang, X., Li, Y., Hu, Z., & Littler, C. L. (1995). Bending of *N*-isopropylacrylamide gel under the influence of infrared light. *The Journal of Chemical Physics*, *102*(1), 551–555. doi:10.1063/1.469434

Zhang, X., Lu, J., Huang, Y., Zhao, W., Li, J., Gao, X., & Li, S. et al. (2013). PEGfarnesylthiosalicylate conjugate as a nanomicellar carrier for delivery of paclitaxel. *Bioconjugate Chemistry*, *24*(3), 464–472. doi:10.1021/bc300608h PMID:23425093

Zhang, X., Wu, D., & Chu, C. C. (2004). Synthesis and characterization of partially biodegradable, temperature and pH sensitive Dex–MA/PNIPAAm hydrogels. *Biomaterials*, *25*(19), 4719–4730. doi:10.1016/j.biomaterials.2003.11.040 PMID:15120518

Zhang, Y., Huang, Y., Zhao, W., Lu, J., Zhang, P., Zhang, X., & Li, S. et al. (2014). Design and evaluation of a PEGylated lipopeptide equipped with drug-interactive motifs as an improved drug carrier. *The AAPS Journal*, *16*(1), 114–124. doi:10.1208/s12248-013-9536-9 PMID:24281690

Zhang, Y., Huang, Y., Zhao, W., Lu, J., Zhang, P., Zhang, X., & Li, S. et al. (2014). Fmoc-conjugated PEG-vitamin E micelles for tumor-targeted delivery of paclitaxel: Enhanced drug−carrier interaction and loading capacity. *The AAPS Journal*, *16*(6), 1282–1291. doi:10.1208/s12248-014-9651-2 PMID:25193267

Zhang, Y., Huang, Z.-M., Xu, X., Lim, C. T., & Ramakrishna, S. (2004). Preparation of core-shell structured PCL-r-gelatin bi-component nanofibers by coaxial electrospinning. *Chemistry of Materials*, *16*(18), 3406–3409. doi:10.1021/cm049580f

Zhang, Y., Sun, Y., Xu, X., Zhang, X., Zhu, H., Huang, L., & Shen, Y.-M. et al. (2010). Synthesis, Biodistribution, and Microsingle Photon Emission Computed Tomography (SPECT) Imaging Study of Technetium-99m Labeled PEGylated Dendrimer Poly (amidoamine)(PAMAM)-Folic Acid Conjugates. *Journal of Medicinal Chemistry*, *53*(8), 3262–3272. doi:10.1021/jm901910j PMID:20350006

Zhang, Z., Tan, S., & Feng, S. S. (2012). Vitamin E TPGS as a molecular biomaterial for drug delivery. *Biomaterials*, *33*(19), 4889–4906. doi:10.1016/j.biomaterials.2012.03.046 PMID:22498300

Zhao, L., Liu, J., Zhang, L., Gao, Y., Zhang, Z., & Luan, Y. (2013). Self-assembly properties, aggregation behavior and prospective application for sustained drug delivery of a drug-participating catanionic system. *International Journal of Pharmaceutics*, *452*(1-2), 108–115. doi:10.1016/j.ijpharm.2013.04.072 PMID:23644346

Zhao, Y., Fan, X., Liu, D., & Wang, Z. (2011). PEGylated thermo-sensitive poly(amidoamine) dendritic drug delivery systems. *International Journal of Pharmaceutics*, *409*(1–2), 229–236. doi:10.1016/j.ijpharm.2011.02.005 PMID:21316434

Zhen, X., Wang, X., Xie, C., Wu, W., & Jiang, X. (2013). Cellular uptake,antitumor response and tumor penetration of cisplatin-loaded milk protein nanoparticles. *Biomaterials*, *34*(4), 1372–1382. doi:10.1016/j.biomaterials.2012.10.061 PMID:23158934

Zhong, M., Feng, Y., Liao, H., Hu, X., Wan, S., Zhu, B., & Zhang, J. et al. (2014). Azithromycin cationic non-lecithoid nano/microparticles improve bioavailability and targeting efficiency. *Pharmaceutical Research*, *31*(10), 2857–2867. doi:10.1007/s11095-014-1382-7 PMID:25208873

Zhong, X., Wang, Y. X., & Wang, S. C. (1996). Pressure dependence of the volume phase-transition of temperature-sensitive gels. *Chemical Engineering Science*, *51*(12), 3235–3239. doi:10.1016/0009-2509(95)00344-4

Zhou, F., Xing, D., Ou, Z., Wu, B., Resasco, D. E., & Chen, W. R. (2009). Cancer photothermal therapy in the near-infra red region by using single-walled carbon nanotubes. *Journal of Biomedical Optics*, *14*(2), 021009. doi:10.1117/1.3078803 PMID:19405722

Zhou, L. J., Liang, D., He, X., Li, J., Tan, H., Li, J., & Gu, Q. et al. (2012). The degradation and biocompatibility of pH-sensitive biodegradable polyurethanes for intracellular multifunctional antitumor drug delivery. *Biomaterials*, *33*(9), 2734–2745. doi:10.1016/j.biomaterials.2011.11.009 PMID:22236829

Zhou, T., Chen, P., Niu, L., Jin, J., Liang, D., Li, Z., & Liu, D. et al. (2012). pH-Responsive Size-Tunable Self-Assembled DNA Dendrimers. *Angewandte Chemie*, *124*(45), 11433–11436. doi:10.1002/ange.201205862 PMID:23037637

Zhu, H., Xu, J., Varlashkin, P., Long, S., & Kidd, C. (2001). Dehydration, hydration behavior and structural analysis of fenoprofen calcium. *Journal of Pharmaceutical Sciences*, *90*(7), 845–859. doi:10.1002/jps.1038 PMID:11458334

Zhu, S., Qian, L., Hong, M., Zhang, L., Pei, Y., & Jiang, Y. (2011). RGD-Modified PEG-PAMAM-DOX Conjugate: In Vitro and In Vivo Targeting to Both Tumor Neovascular Endothelial Cells and Tumor Cells. *Advanced Materials*, *23*(12), H84–H89. doi:10.1002/adma.201003944 PMID:21360776

Zidan, A. S., & Habib, M. J. (2014). Maximized Mucoadhesion and Skin Permeation of Anti-AIDS-Loaded Niosomal Gels. *Journal of Pharmaceutical Sciences*, *103*(3), 952–964. doi:10.1002/jps.23867 PMID:24464823

Zidan, A. S., Rahman, Z., & Khan, M. A. (2011). Product and process understanding of a novel pediatric anti-HIV tenofovir niosomes with a high-pressure homogenizer. *European Journal of Pharmaceutical Sciences*, *44*(1), 93–102. doi:10.1016/j.ejps.2011.06.012 PMID:21726640

Zimmermann, T. S., Lee, A. C., Akinc, A., Bramlage, B., Bumcrot, D., Fedoruk, M. N., & John, M. et al. (2006). RNAi-mediated gene silencing in non-human primates. *Nature*, *441*(7089), 111–114. doi:10.1038/nature04688 PMID:16565705

Zong, X., Kim, K., Fang, D., Ran, S., Hsiao, B. S., & Chu, B. (2002). Structure and process relationship of electrospun bioabsorbable nanofiber membranes. *Polymer*, *43*(16), 4403–4412. doi:10.1016/S0032-3861(02)00275-6

Zrinyi, M., Barsi, L., & Büki, A. (1996). Deformation of ferrogels induced by non uniform magnetic fields. *The Journal of Chemical Physics*, *104*(21), 8750–8756. doi:10.1063/1.471564

Zrinyi, M., Barsi, L., & Büki, A. (1997). Ferrogel: A new magneto-controlled elastic medium. *Polymer Gels and Networks*, *5*(5), 415–427. doi:10.1016/S0966-7822(97)00010-5

About the Contributors

Raj K. Keservani has more than 7 years of academic (Teaching) experience in various institutes of India imparting Pharmaceutical education. Mr. Keservani did his graduation (B. Pharmacy) from Department of Pharmacy, Kumaun University, Nainital (U.A.), India in 2005. Afterwards he qualified GATE in same year conducted by IIT Mumbai. He received Master of Pharmacy (M. Pharmacy) from School of Pharmaceutical Sciences, Rajiv Gandhi Proudyogiki Vishwavidyalaya, Bhopal (M.P.), India in 2008 with specialization in Pharmaceutics. Further, he has published 25 peer reviewed papers in the field of Pharmaceutical Sciences in national and international reputed journals, 10 book chapters, 2 co-authored books. He is also active as a reviewer in several scientific international journals. His research interest encompasses Nutraceutical and Functional Foods, Novel Drug Delivery Systems (NDDS), Transdermal Drug Delivery/ Drug Delivery, Health Science/Life Science, Biology/Cancer Biology/Neurobiology.

Anil K. Sharma has more than 6 years of academic experience in Pharmaceutical sciences. He did his graduation (B. Pharmacy) from University of Rajasthan, Jaipur, India in 2005. Afterwards he qualified GATE in same year conducted by IIT Mumbai. He received Master of Pharmacy (M. Pharmacy) from School of Pharmaceutical Sciences, Rajiv Gandhi Proudyogiki Vishwavidyalaya, Bhopal (M.P.), India in 2007 with specialization in Pharmaceutics. Further, he has published 25 peer reviewed papers in the field of Pharmaceutical Sciences in national and international reputed journals, 10 book chapters. His research interest encompasses Nutraceutical and Functional Foods, Novel Drug Delivery Systems (NDDS), Drug Delivery, Nanotechnology, Health Science/Life Science, Biology/Cancer Biology/Neurobiology. Currently he is working as lecture at Delhi Institute of Pharmaceutical Sciences & Research, University of Delhi, India.

Rajesh K. Kesharwani has more than 7 years of research and 2 years of teaching experience in various institutes of India imparting bioinformatics and biotechnology education. Dr. Kesharwani did his graduation (B.Sc. Biology) from Ewing Christian College, Allahabad, an autonomous college of University of Allahabad and post-graduation (M.Sc. Biochemistry) from Singh University, Rewa, Madhya Pradesh, India. He has qualified GATE 2005 and 2006, received Ministry of Human Resource Development, India fellowship to complete M.Tech-IT (specialization in Bioinformatics) degree from Indian Institute of Information Technology, Allahabad, India in 2008. He has completed doctorate (Ph.D.) from Indian Institute of Information Technology, Allahabad in 2014 and received Ministry of Human Resource Development, India fellowship and Senior Research Fellowship from Indian Council of Medical Research, India. Dr. Kesharwani is recipient of Swarna Jayanti Puruskar by The National Academy of Sciences, India for best paper presentation. He has authored 29+ peer-reviewed articles, 5 book chapters and, one book as co-editor together with more than 10 book chapters has been accepted for publication with international publishers. He has been members of many scientific communities and reviewer of many international journals. His research fields of interest are Medical Informatics, Protein Structure and Function Prediction, Computer Aided Drug Designing, Structural Biology, Drug Delivery, Cancer Biology and Next Generation Sequence Analysis.

* * *

Khosro Adibkia is currently Associate Professor of Pharmaceutics at Tabriz University of Medical Sciences. Dr. Khosro Adibkia received his Ph.D. from Tabriz University of Medical Sciences. He was a research fellow in Pharmaceutical nanobiotechnology in the Gent University (Belgium). He has authored over 90 publications in various areas of nanotechnology and pharmaceutics. He is editor of several scientific journals. Dr. Khosro Adibkia has received several honors and awards in his career of well-being.

Solmaz Maleki Dizaj has PhD in pharmaceutical nanotechnology from Tabriz University of Medical Sciences. She has more than 30 publications in the field of physical chemistry and pharmaceutical nanotechnology. She had received several awards in her field of action.

Ljiljana Djekic received her B. Sc, M. Sc., and Ph.D. in Pharmaceutical technology from the University of Belgrade – Faculty of pharmacy. She is currently Assistant Professor at Department of Pharmaceutical Technology and Cosmetology, University of Belgrade – Faculty of Pharmacy, Belgrade, Serbia. She is the author of more than 70 publications including scientific monographs, edited book chapters, scientific papers, abstracts and conference proceedings. She is the author or coauthor of several textbooks in the field of Pharmaceutical Technology, Preformulation and Formulation of Drugs. She is a member of the Pharmaceutical Association of Serbia. She reviewed a numerous scientific articles in leading international journals relevant for pharmaceutical science. Her research interests are focused on development and characterization of colloidal carriers of drugs and cosmetic active substance, including surfactant self-assembly based nanocarriers.

Anuj Garg has earned his B.Pharm, M.Pharm and Ph.D degree from Indian Institute of Technology, (Banaras Hindu University), Varanasi. He is recipient of Gold medal and GP Nair IDMA Award. Presently, he is serving as faculty in Department of Pharmaceutics at National Institute of Pharmaceutical Education and Research, Raebareli. His research area is mainly focused on lipid based nanoparticles for drug delivery.

Nayan Ashok Gujarathi is presently working as head at department of Pharmaceutics, P.S.G.V.P. Mandal's, College of Pharmacy, Shahada. He published number of research and review articles in national and international journals (IJP published by Elseiver and DDIP published by Informa Healthcare). An invited as speaker at national level seminars and conferences. He completed his basic education from Shahada, Dist.Nandurbar, (M.S) India. Onwards he completed graduation in pharmacy from P.S.G.V.P.Mandal;s, College of Pharmacy, Shahada affiliated to North MaharashtraUniversity, Jalgaon in 2004. For post graduation in pharmacy he migrated to RGPV, Mandhya Pradesh and completed his doctorate in 2013 from Jodhpur National University, Jodhpur, India.

Snežana S. Ilić-Stojanović works at the Faculty of Technology, University of Niš, Republic of Serbia. She received her PhD in the field of intelligent hydrogels synthesis and their pharmaceutical application as drug carriers. Also, she has thirteen years experience in pharmaceutical industry "Zdravlje Actavis" as a patent engineer for intellectual property protection, especially for patent and trademark protection.

Song Li is a Professor at Department of Pharmaceutical Sciences and a member of the Center for Pharmacogenetics, University of Pittsburgh School of Pharmacy. He received his M.D. and Ph.D. from the Fourth Military Medical University, Xi'an, China, and pursued his postdoctoral training with Dr. Leaf Huang. He became a faculty at the University of Pittsburgh School of Pharmacy in 2000. Dr. Li has broad knowledge in medicine, biology, and drug and gene delivery and is the author or co-author of over 100 peer-reviewed articles and 27 review articles or book chapters. Dr. Li is an Associate Editor for Journal of Gene Medicine and also serves on the editorial boards of several other journals. He frequently serves on the review panels of NIH, DOD and other funding agencies. Research in Dr. Li's lab has been continuously supported by grants from various funding agencies including NIH, DOD, and American Heart Association (AHA).

Megha S. Marwah has completed her B.Pharm from Institute of Chemical Technology, Mumbai and M.Pharm in Pharmaceutics from Bombay College of Pharmacy, Mumbai. She is currently pursuing Ph.D in Pharmaceutics under the guidance of Dr. (Mrs.) Mangal S. Nagarsenker. She has received the prestigious J.R.D Tata Scholarship for academic excellence (2009-10, 2010-11). She has presented six research papers at conferences of national and international calibre and won accolades for the same. She is one of the inventors in a patent filed with the Indian patent office on bioavailability improvement of poorly soluble drugs. Her key research interests include design, formulation, optimisation and characterization of polymeric nanosystems, targeted liposomes, lipid nanosystems and solid oral dosage forms.

Nidhi Mishra is an Assistant Professor in Department of Applied Sciences in IIIT-Allahabad. Prior to this she was Assistant Professor in Chemistry at BITS Pilani The author has obtained PH.D. from University of Delhi.

Mangal S. Nagarsenker completed her B.Pharm from Institute of Chemical Technology, Mumbai University, Mumbai with University Gold Medal in 1978. She received her Ph.D in Pharmaceutical Sciences from Mumbai University in 1989. She has been a recipient of several awards, few of which include Prof. (Mrs.) M. R. Baichwal Visiting fellow in Pharmaceutical Sciences and Technology in UICT (2005-2006), Amrut Mody Research Fund, Distinguished Researcher National Award (2012), Association of Pharmaceutical Teachers of India (APTI) Dr. (Mrs.) Manjushree Pal Best Researcher National Award (2013). Besides, she has reviewed several articles in different national and international journals, is a member of the editorial board of Indian Journal of Pharmaceutical Sciences and has authored around 100 research articles (national and international), 6 review articles, 3 book chapters and 2 books. She has more than 100 research papers presented at various national and international conferences to her credit. In addition, she has been granted two Indian patents and three trademarks. Also, she has delivered numerous lectures as an invited speaker at various conferences, both national and international. She has 34 years of research experience and mentored more than 40 M.Pharm and 30 Ph.D students. Her key areas of research interest entail design, formulation, optimisation and characterization of nanosystems like targeted liposomes, lipid based nanosystems, polymeric nanosystems, cyclodextrin based drug delivery, controlled release systems for oral, parenteral, topical, pulmonary and ophthalmic routes and gene delivery. Her research group is the first to design and report the utility of nanosystems like Gelupearl and Leciplex. She is currently Professor and Head, Dept. of Pharmaceutics, Bombay College of Pharmacy, Mumbai and is a Member of several esteemed scientific organisations like Society for Pharmaceutical Dissolution Sciences, Indian Pharmaceutical Association, Controlled Release Society and Association of Pharmaceutical Teachers of India.

Ljubiša B. Nikolić was born in 1963 in Leskovac, Serbia. He graduated from the Faculty of Technology in Leskovac in 1990 and in 2003 he defended his doctoral dissertation and qualified for the title of Doctor of Technical Sciences. Since 1991 he has worked at the Faculty of Technology in Leskovac, University of Niš. Ljubiša Nikolić is engaged in scientific research work in the field of organic chemical technology and polymer engineering.

Vesna D. Nikolić studied Organic Chemical Technology on the Faculty of Technology in Leskovac at University of Nis. Full Professor on the Faculty of Technology in Leskovac. Fields of Research: Organic Chemistry, Synthesis Pharmaceutical Compounds.

Abbas Pardakhty is a professor of Pharmaceutics which has been graduated from Isfahan University of Medical Sciences, Iran, in 2002. His main field of research is lipid vesicular drug delivery systems, especially niosomes in drug, vaccine and gene delivery. He is also the Vice Chancellor of Research and Technology in Kerman University of Medical Sciences from 2013 and also the Director of Kerman Innovation Center from 2015.

Slobodan D. Petrović, full professor at the Faculty of Technology and Metallurgy, University of Belgrade, was born in 1950 in Belgrade. He earned his B.Sc (1974), M.Sc (1976) and PhD (1984). Fields of interests: Organic Chemistry and Chemistry of Natural Products, especially compounds with amide bond and pharmaceutically active organic compounds.

Bhushan Rajendra Rane is presently working as head at department of Pharmaceutics, Shri D.D.Vispute College of Pharmacy and Research Center, Panvel, New Mumbai. He has more than 9 years of experience in academics and research. He published number of research and review articles in national and international journals (DDIP published by Informa Healthcare and IJP published by Elseiver). An invited as speaker at national level seminars and conferences. He is life time member of different associations such as APTI, IGPA and MSPC. He completed his basic education from Nijampur, Tal. Sakri, Dist. Dhule, (M.S) India. Onwards he completed graduation in pharmacy from R.C.Patel, College of Pharmacy, Shirpur affiliated to North MaharashtraUniversity, Jalgaon in 2005. For post graduation in pharmacy he migrated to Annamalai University, Tamilnadu and completed his doctorate in 2013 from Jodhpur National University, Jodhpur, India.

Vijay Kumar Singh is working as Asst. Professor at Institute of Pharmacy, Bundelkhand University, Jhansi, UP, India. He has published reviews and research articles in various reputed national and international journals of repute. He is presently a member of the editorial board of two international journals (IJPSR and IJRDPL).

Jingjing Sun received her PhD Degree majoring in Polymer Chemistry and Physics from Shanghai Institute of Organic Chemistry, Chinese Academy of Science in 2015. Now She is studying as a postdoctoral associate under the supervision of Dr. Song Li at University of Pittsburgh. Her research interests include the design and synthesis of multi-functional polymers for anti-cancer drug delivery.

Sandeep Waghulde is working as Asst. Professor at KGRDCP & RI, Karjat, University of Mumbai.

Shadi Yaqoubi is a PhD student of Pharmaceutics in Tabriz University of Medical Sciences.

Tingbin Zhang received his BS degree from HeFei University of Technology in 2012. Currently, he is a PhD candidate in the Department of School of Chemical Engineering and Technology, Tianjin University, co-supervised by Associate Professor Jinfeng Xing and Professor Xing-jie Liang from the National Center for Nanoscience and Technology (NCNST). His research is mainly on the development of novel small molecules for drug/gene delivery.

Index

A

B

C

D

E

F

G

H

T

U

V

www.ingramcontent.com/pod-product-compliance
Lightning Source LLC
LaVergne TN
LVHW060349300926
849162LV00006B/1231